D1218203

RECONSTRUCTION OF LIFE FROM THE SKELETON

RECONSTRUCTION OF LIFE FROM THE SKELETON

Editors

Mehmet Yaşar İşcan
Department of Anthropology
Florida Atlantic University
Boca Raton, Florida

Kenneth A. R. Kennedy
Ecology and Systematics
Division of Biological Sciences
Cornell University
Ithaca, New York

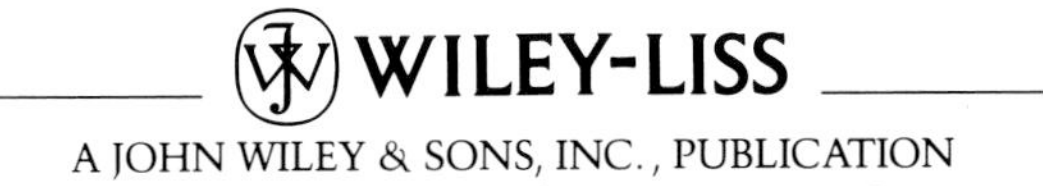

A JOHN WILEY & SONS, INC., PUBLICATION
New York • Chichester • Brisbane • Toronto • Singapore

Address All Inquiries to the Publisher
Wiley-Liss, Inc., 605 Third Avenue, New York, NY 10158-0012

Printed in the United States of America.

Library of Congress Cataloging-in-Publication Data

Reconstruction of life from the skeleton / [edited by] M. Yaşar İşcan,
Kenneth A. R. Kennedy
p. cm.
Includes bibliographies and indexes.
ISBN 0-471-56229-7
1. Paleopathology. I. İşcan, M. Yaşar. II. Kennedy, Kenneth A. R.
[DNLM: 1. Paleopathology. QZ 11.5 R311]
R134.8.R43 1989
616.07—dc20
DNLM/DLC
for Library of Congress 89-12533
CIP

The text of this book is printed on acid-free paper.

Book design and front cover illustration by
Jeff A. Menges

10 9 8 7 6 5 4

Dedicated to
Muzaffer Süleyman Şenyürek, Ph.D. (1915–1961)
for his pioneering work in Paleodemography

Contents

Contributors

Arthur C. Aufderheide (M.D., University of Minnesota, 1946) is currently professor of pathology at the University of Minnesota–Duluth School of Medicine, Duluth. Specializing in pathology, his numerous publications include "Lead in bone. II: Skeletal lead contact as an indicator of lifetime lead ingestion and the social correlates in an archaeological population" (with Neiman FD, Wittmers LE, and Rapp G), *Am. J. Phys. Anthropol.,* 1981; "Lead in bone. III: Prediction of social correlates from skeletal lead content in four colonial American populations (Catoctin Furnace, College Landing, Governor's Land and Irene Mound)" (with Angel JL et al.), *Am. J. Phys. Anthropol.,* 1985; "Lead contact and poisoning in Barbados slaves: Historical, chemical and biological evidence" (with Handler JS, Corruccini RS, et al.), *Social Science History,* 1986; and "Comparison of two in vitro methods of bone lead analysis and the implications for in vivo measurements" (with Somervaille LJ, Chettle DR, Scott MC, et al.) *Phys. Med. Biol.,* 1986. Dr. Aufderheide is a member of the American Society of Clinical Pathologists, the American Association of Physical Anthropologists, and the New York Academy of Sciences.

Mehmet Yaşar İşcan (Ph.D., Cornell University, 1976) is currently professor and chairman of the Department of Anthropology, Florida Atlantic University in Boca Raton and a board certified diplomate of the American Board of Forensic Anthropology. Specializing in human osteology and forensic anthropology, he has published numerous books and articles including *The Human Skeleton in Forensic Medicine* (with Krogman WM), C.C. Thomas, 1986; *Age Markers in the Human Skeleton* (editor), C.C. Thomas, 1989; "The rise of forensic anthropology," *Yrbk. Phys. Anthropol.,* 1988; and "An odontometric profile of a prehistoric southeastern Florida population," *Am. J. Phys. Anthropol.,* 1989. Dr. İşcan was the recipient of the Aleš Hrdlička Fellowship (1968) and has been awarded grants from Florida Atlantic University and the Smithsonian Institution. He is the founder and past president of the Dental Anthropological Association and is a member of the American Anthropological Association, the American Association of Physical Anthropologists, and a fellow of the American Academy of Forensic Sciences.

Francis E. Johnston (Ph.D., University of Pennsylvania, 1962) is currently professor and chairman of the Department of Anthropology, University of Pennsylvania, Philadelphia. Specializing in biological anthropology, his many publications include *Nutritional Anthropology* (editor), Alan R. Liss, 1987; *Human Physical Growth and Maturation* (editor), Plenum, 1980; *Biosocial Interrelationships in Population Adaptation* (editor), Mouton, 1974; and *Social and Biological Predictors of Nutritional Status, Physical Growth and Neurological Development* (editor), Academic Press, 1980. Dr. Johnston is a past president of the American Association of Physical Anthropologists, two-term editor of the *American Journal of Physical Anthropology,* and is currently editor of the *American Journal of Human Biology.* He is a member of the

American Association of Physical Anthropologists, the Human Biology Council, and the American Institute of Nutrition.

William F. Keegan (Ph.D., University of California, Los Angeles, 1985) was a Visiting Scholar in North American Prehistory at Southern Illinois University and is currently an assistant curator of anthropology at the Florida Museum of Natural History, Gainesville. Specializing in archaeology and prehistoric Carribean Islanders, his publications include "The optimal foraging analysis of horticulture production," *Am. Anthropol.*, 1986; "The ecology of Lucayan Arawak fishing practices" (with Diamond JM), *Am. Antiquity,* 1986; *Emergent Horticultural Economies of the Eastern Woodlands* (editor), Southern Illinois University Center for Archaeological Investigations, 1987; and "Stable carbon—and nitrogen—isotope ratios of bone collagen used to study coral-reef and terrestrial components of prehistoric Bahamian diet" (with DeNiro MJ), *Am. Antiquity,* 1988. He is a member of the Society for American Archaeology, the American Anthropological Association, and the Florida Anthropological Society.

Marc Allen Kelley (Ph.D., Case Western Reserve University, 1980) is presently associate professor of anthropology at the University of Rhode Island, Kingston. Specializing in paleopathology and forensic anthropology, his publications include *Atlas of Human Paleopathology* (with Zimmerman MR), Praeger, 1982; "The evolution of mycobacterial disease in human populations: A reevaluation" (with Clark GA, Grange JM, and Hill MC), *Current Anthropol.*, 1987; and Rib lesions and chronic pulmonary tuberculosis (with Micozzi MS), *Am. J. Phys. Anthropol.*, 1984. Dr. Kelley received an NSF award for Research Experiences for Undergraduates, a 1987 training program, Biosocial Adaptation: Assessment of Paleonutritional Techniques, and led a group of students in studies of paleonutrition and paleopathology in northern Chile. He is a member of the American Association of Physical Anthropologists and the Paleopathology Association, and he is on the Executive Board of the Dental Anthropological Association.

Kenneth A. R. Kennedy (Ph.D., University of California, Berkeley, 1962) is currently professor in the Section of Ecology and Systematics at Cornell University, Ithaca, New York. Specializing in human palaeontology, palaeodemography, forensic anthropology, biological anthropology history, and human anatomy, he has conducted extensive field research in India, Pakistan, and Sri Lanka. His publications include "Upper Pleistocene fossil hominids from Sri Lanka" (with Deraniyagala SU, Reortgen WJ, Chiment J, and Disotell T), *Am. J. Phys. Anthropol.*, 1987; *Mesolithic Human Remains from the Gangetic Plain: Sarai Nahar Rai* (with Lovell NC and Burrow CB), Cornell University South Asia Program, Occasional Papers and Theses, 1986; "Principal-components analysis of prehistoric south Asian crania" (with Chiment J and Disotell T), *Am. J. Phys. Anthropol.*, 1984; and "Morphological variation in ulnar supinator crests and fossae as identifying markers of occupational stress," *J. Forensic Sci.*, 1983. Dr. Kennedy was the recipient of the T. Dale Stewart Award in Forensic Anthropology (1987) and was a guest at the White House State Dinner for the President of Sri Lanka (1984). His research has been supported by N.S.F., the American Institute for Indian Studies, and the Howard Foundation. He was chairman of the Biological Anthropology Unit of the American Anthropological Association, and is a fellow of the Royal Anthropological Institute, the American Academy of Forensic Sciences, and a member of the American Association of Physical Anthropologists.

Susan R. Loth (B.A., New York University) is a 1989 M.A. candidate in the Department of Anthropology at Florida Atlantic University, Boca Raton. She currently serves as editor of the *Dental Anthropology Newsletter*. Specializing in human skeletal biology, her numerous publications include "Age estimation from the rib by phase analysis: White males" (with İşcan MY and Wright RK), *J. Forensic Sci.*, 1984; "Metamorphosis at the sternal rib end: A new method to estimate age at death in White males" (with İşcan MY and Wright RK), *Am. J. Phys. Anthropol.*, 1984; "Age estimation from the rib by phase analysis: White females" (with İşcan MY and Wright RK), *J. Forensic Sci.*, 1985; and "Racial variation at the sternal extremity of the rib and its effect on age determination" (with İşcan MY and Wright RK), *J. Forensic Sci.*, 1987. Ms. Loth was awarded the Lambda Alpha National Scholarship Award and Certificate of Distinguished Achievement, a Grant-in-Aid of Research from Sigma Xi, a Short Term Visitor's Grant from the Smithsonian Institution, and has been inducted into The Honor Society of Phi Kappa Phi. She is a member of the American Association of Physical Anthropologists, the Dental Anthropological Association, and the Florida Academy of Sciences.

John R. Lukacs (Ph.D., Cornell University, 1977) is now professor of anthropology at the University of Oregon, Eugene. Specializing in dental anthropology, human evolution, and South Asia, he has done extensive fieldwork studying the dental morphology and pathology of prehistoric Pakistan in collaboration with the French Archaeological Mission and the University of California. Among his publications are *People of South Asia* (editor), Plenum, 1984; "Dental disease in prehistoric Baluchistan" (with Retief DH and Jarrige JF), National Geographic Research, 1985; *Excavations at Inamgaon. Vol II: Physical Anthropology of Human Skeletal Remains. Part 1: An Osteobiographic Analysis*, Deccan College Press, 1986; and "Dental morphology and odontometrics of early agriculturalists from Neolithic Mehrgarh, Pakistan," in DE Russell et al. (eds): *Teeth Revisited*, Editions Du Museum, 1988. Dr. Lukacs has been awarded grants from the National Geographic Society and is a member of the American Association of Physical Anthropologists, the Human Biology Council, and Sigma Xi.

Charles F. Merbs (Ph.D., University of Wisconsin, Madison, 1969) is presently professor of anthropology at Arizona State University, Tempe. Specializing in physical anthropology and medical genetics, he organized and chaired the first Conference on Health and Disease in the Prehistoric Southwest. His publications include *Health and Disease in the Prehistoric Southwest* (editor), Arizona State University Anthropological Research Papers, 1985; *Patterns of Activity-Induced Pathology in a Canadian Inuit Population*, National Museum of Man Mercury Series, 1983; and "Atlanto-occipital fusion and spondylolisthesis in an Anasazi skeleton from Bright Angel Ruin, Grand Canyon National Park, Arizona" (with Euler RC), *Am. J. Phys. Anthropol.*, 1985. Dr. Merbs was the recipient of the ASU Dean's Quality Teaching Award (Liberal Arts) in 1984. He is a member of the American Association of Physical Anthropologists, the Arctic Institute of North America, and a Fellow of the Canadian Association for Physical Anthropology.

Lucile E. St. Hoyme (D. Phil., Oxford University, 1963) is currently curator emeritus of Anthropology at the Smithsonian Institution, Washington, D.C. Her publications include "On the origins of New World paleopathology," *Am. J. Phys. Anthropol.*, 1969; "Significance of canine wear in pongid evolution" (with Koritzer RT), *Am. J. Phys. Anthropol.*, 1971; "Ecology of dental disease" (with Koritzer RT), *Am. J. Phys. Anthropol.*, 1976; and "Sex determination in the posterior pelvis," *Collegium Antropologicum*, 1984. Dr. St. Hoyme is a member of the American Association of Physical Anthropologists.

Frank P. Saul (Ph.D., Harvard University, 1972) is now associate professor of anatomy and assistant dean for Research at the Medical College of Ohio, Toledo. Specializing in biomedical anthropology, he is also a diplomate of the American Board of Forensic Anthropology. His publications include *The Human Skeletal Remains From Altar de Sacrificios, Guatemala: An Osteobiographic Analysis*, Peabody Museum of Harvard Press, 1972; *Paleobiologia en la Zona Maya—Investigaciones Recientes en el Area Maya—XVII Mesa Redonda* (with Saul JM), Sociedad Mexicana de Antropologia, 1984; "La osteopatologia de los Mayas de las tierras bajas del sur" (with Saul JM), in L Austin and C Viesca Trevino (eds): *Mexico Antigua,* 1984; and *Life History as Recorded in Maya Skeletons From Cozumel, Mexico* (with Saul JM), National Geographic Society Press, 1985. Dr. Saul has been the recipient of National Geographic Society Research and NSF Grants, and is a member of the Paleopathology Association, American Association of Physical Anthropologists, and the American Academy of Forensic Sciences.

Julie Mather Saul (B.A., Pennsylvania State University, 1963) is currently a research associate in anatomy at the Medical College of Ohio, Toledo. Specializing in chemistry and zoology, she has published *Paleobiologia en la Zona Maya—Investigaciones Recientes en el Area Maya—XVII Mesa Redonda* (with Saul FP), Sociedad Mexicana de Antropologia, 1984; "La osteopatologia de los mayas de las tierras bajas del sur" (with Saul FP), in L Austin and C Viesca Trevino (eds): *Mexico Antigua,* 1984; and *Life History as Recorded in Maya Skeletons From Cozumel, Mexico* (with Saul FP), National Geographic Society Press, 1985. With her husband Frank, Ms. Saul has received National Geographic Society Research and NSF Grants and is a member of the Paleopathology Association, the American Anthropological Association, and the American Association of Physical Anthropologists.

Shelley R. Saunders (Ph.D., University of Toronto, 1977) is currently associate professor of Anthropology at McMaster University, Hamilton, Ontario, Canada. Specializing in physical anthropology and skeletal biology, she is chairman of the Ontario Council of Professional Osteologists. Her publications include "Growth remodeling of the human femur," *Canad. Rev. Phys. Anthropol.,* 1987; "Dimensional and discrete dental trait asymmetry relationships," *Am. J. Phys. Anthropol.,* 1986; "Surface and cross-sectional comparisons of bone growth remodeling," *Growth,* 1985; and "The inheritance of acquired characteristics: A concept that will not die" in LR Godfrey (ed): *What Darwin Began,* Allyn & Bacon, 1985. Dr. Saunders is the secretary/treasurer of the Canadian Association for Physical Anthropology and is also a member of the American Association of Physical Anthropologists and the Human Biology Council.

Sam D. Stout (Ph.D., Washington University, St. Louis, 1975) is currently professor of Anthropology at the University of Missouri, Columbia. Specializing in skeletal biology, bone histomorphometry, and forensic anthropology, he was a member of the scientific team commissioned by the government of Peru to authenticate the remains of Francisco Pizarro. His publications include "Histological structure and its preservation in ancient bone," *Current Anthropol.,* 1978; "The effects of long-term immobilization on the histomorphology of human cortical bone," *Calcif. Tissue Int.,* 1982; "Use of histology in ancient bone research" (with Simmons DJ), *Yrbk. Phys. Anthropol.,* 1979; and "Histomorphometric determination of formation rates of archaeological bone" (with Teitelbaum SL), *Calcif. Tissue Res.,* 1976. Dr. Stout is a member of the American Association of Physical Anthropologists, the American Academy of Forensic Sciences, and the American Association for the Advancement of Science.

Patricia Lea Stuart-Macadam (Ph.D., University of Cambridge) is now assistant professor of anthropology at the University of Toronto, Canada. Specializing in skeletal biology, she is the physical anthropologist affiliated with the ongoing excavation of a medieval site in Moroduice, Macedonia. Her publications include "Porotic hyperostosis: Representative of a childhood condition," *Am. J. Phys. Anthropol.,* 1985; "Porotic hyperostosis: New evidence to support the anemia theory," *Am. J. Phys. Anthropol.,* 1987; "A radiographic study of porotic hyperostosis," *Am. J. Phys. Anthropol.,* 1987; and "Preparation and further study of the Singa skull from Sudan" (with Stinger CB and Cornish L), *Bull. Br. Mus. Nat. Hist. (Geol.),* 1985. Dr. Stuart-Macadam was the recipient of a Smithsonian Short Term visitor Award, the Commonwealth Scholarship, and the Emslie

Hoeniman Anthropological Research Award. She is a member of the Canadian Association for Physical Anthropology, the Human Biology Council, and the Paleopathology Association.

Spencer Jay Turkel (Ph.D., Cornell University, 1982) is presently associate professor of anthropology at the New York Institute of Technology, Old Westbury. Specializing in physical and forensic anthropology and functional anatomy, he has published "The stabilizing mechanisms preventing anterior dislocation of the glenohumeral joint," *J. Bone Joint Surg.*, 1981. Dr. Turkel is treasurer of the New York Society of Forensic Sciences and is also a member of the American Anthropological Association and the New York Academy of Sciences.

Louise O. Zimmer (B.A., Smith College) is currently a Ph.D. candidate in the Department of Anthropology at the University of Pennsylvania, Philadelphia. She is specializing in nutritional anthropology.

Preface

The purpose of this book, *Reconstruction of Life From the Skeleton,* is to present the state of the art of elucidating biological characteristics from skeletal remains. The book features a critical review of the scientific literature and an assessment of methodological advances and problems. The topics addressed include growth and aging, racial variation, sexual dimorphism, markers of occupational stress and related trauma, dental biology, nutrition and diet, disease, and osteogenetics.

The idea for this volume originated with a symposium of the same name organized by M. Y. İşcan and P. Miller-Shaivitz at the 1986 annual meeting of the American Anthropological Association in Philadelphia, PA. When Alan R. Liss, Inc., agreed to publish the book, İşcan and Kennedy rounded out their treatment of the subject by enlisting the expertise of some of the most respected members of the profession. It goes without saying that the book would not have materialized without the diligence and enthusiasm of these contributors.

The authors are grateful to Susan R. Loth for her editorial assistance and her organization of the "Contributors" section. We also appreciate the patience of Mr. Glen Campbell of Alan R. Liss, Inc. Finally, the authors wish to thank production editor Martin Berkenwald for his helpfulness and conscientious attention to every detail.

Mehmet Yaşar İşcan
Kenneth A. R. Kennedy

Reconstruction of Life From the Skeleton
© 1989 Alan R. Liss, Inc., pages 1–10

Chapter 1

Reconstruction of Life From the Skeleton: An Introduction

Mehmet Yaşar İşcan and Kenneth A. R. Kennedy
Department of Anthropology, Florida Atlantic University, Boca Raton, Florida 33431-0991 (M.Y.İ.); Ecology and Systematics, Division of Biological Sciences, Cornell University, Ithaca, New York 14853-2701 (K.A.R.K.)

> Is the seashell's shape determined exclusively by its inner biological structure? We happen to know otherwise. The configuration of the outer form that confines the inner structure—in this case, the animal—actually results from an interaction between the inner nucleus and its external environment. . . . A form cannot evolve exclusively from unilateral action of something inside or outside! An entity always exists in its environment, living entities in a biological and ecological environment. . . . Whether the entity is biological or inanimate, it owes its integrity to the interplay of offensive and defensive forces of action and reaction. (Bredendieck, 1981:385)

Efforts to explain how natural entities assume their characteristic qualities of size and shape, their mass and morphology, rest upon distinguishing those properties intrinsic to the entity from modifications imposed by extrinsic forces. This dynamic of *innate* vs. *acquired, inside* vs. *outside, natural* vs. *artificial* finds its intellectual roots in the platonic conception of an interface of idealized forms and their perceptual manifestations. This dualistic approach to nature is recognized in the above quotation. It was not written by a biologist, as the subject of the seashell's shape might suggest, but by an industrial designer of building interiors, furniture, toys, and appliances. Hin Bredendieck holds a Bauhaus Diploma and taught at the New Bauhaus in Chicago, which was founded in 1937 by Moholy-Nagy with the advice of the German architect Walter Gropius. He makes his statement in the context of refuting the claim of the French architect Le Corbusier (1959) that design must develop primarily from the inside outwards, as a seashell is not simply a facade of a beautiful natural entity but assumes its shape from internal forces. Within the *gestalt* that combines art, science, technology, and the anatomy of the human body, which are the components of the Bauhaus movement, emerges the classic debate over *outside-in* and *inside-out*. This theoretical orientation to industrial design and architecture finds a parallel in biology, where the search to make sense of the anatomical morphology of living things is the heart of evolutionary theory.

At the close of the nineteenth century, the anatomist Julius Wolff (1892) described responses of bone to mechanical forces. He observed that every change in the form and the function of a bone, or of its function alone, is followed by certain definite changes in its internal architecture and secondary alterations in its external conformation. Remodeling takes place in resistance to stress. Because bone form reflects function, it follows that changes in function result in structural modifications. Wolff's law is applicable to those specific tissues of bone, cartilage, enamel, and dentine that have unique properties of composition, development, and function, as well as to macroscopic bone that is a skeletal component. Mechanical adaptations of bones are interpreted by anatomists using the model of an interface of form and function, of morphology and activity patterns.

Vertebrate species share many of the same form–function relationships, but adaptations to varied ecological settings have contributed to their exploitation of different lifeways and the evolution of distinctive form–function responses. Vestiges of earlier adaptations may be preserved in bone and tooth morphology, and variables of this kind form the bases of phylogenetic reconstructions and assessments of degrees of biological affinities between species by paleontologists. The bones and teeth of the fossil record preserve the morphological inheritance of extinct organisms upon which outside forces have exerted their influence and left diagnostic markers of patterns of ontogenetic development, trauma, disease, and indicators of individual life histories. Scientific interpretation of form and function in the osteological systems of extinct organisms demands a broad knowledge of comparative anatomy as well as a keen sensitivity to nongenetic forces affecting the phenotype.

Intrinsic properties of the skeleton include the organic cellular components and inorganic constituents of calcium, phosphate, carbonate, and citrate, plus lesser quantities of water, sodium, magnesium, potassium, fluorine, and chlorine. These minerals provide the relatively rigid structures that support muscles and tendons, nerves, integument, vascular structures, and soft tissues. In addition to its function as a frame to support the body and protect organs, bone contains in its hollow cavities the marrow that produces most of the cells of the blood. Bone stores minerals and repairs itself when injury occurs. It grows as a living tissue by a process of destruction and buildup and provides for movement and locomotion by means of levers and struts operated by muscles. Allied to bone's developmental properties is the process of aging and the manifestation of the secondary sexual characteristics that distinguish the male and female skeleton.

Extrinsic forces affecting bone correspond to Bredendieck's offensive and defensive forces of action and reaction, as exemplified by changes wrought by trauma, disease, nutritional history of the individual, habitat, occupation, and myriad environmental factors that shape the individual from conception to death. The form–function approach to human skeletal biology is presented in many modern anatomy textbooks (Shipman et al., 1985) and studies of bone physiology (McLean and Urist, 1968) and bone mechanics (Currey, 1984). Bone growth (Hall, 1978; Watts, 1986) and skeletal evolution (Hanken and Hall, 1983) are other aspects of the study of the human osteological system that use the form–function concept. Not the least of these studies are the growing contributions of research and writings by forensic anthropologists and paleodemographers.

The challenge of reconstructing the life of human beings from their skeletal remains is the domain of those anthropologists who apply their knowledge of skeletal biology to medical-legal problems and to paleodemographic questions that contribute to archaeological investigations of extinct populations. The field and laboratory methods practiced by the biological anthropologist in the course of describing and analyzing mortuary data of ancient populations from cemeteries are brought to bear upon questions of personal identification in police investigations and in the laboratory of the medical examiner (Ubelaker, 1978). The forensic anthropologist is familiar with the appearance and variables of dried bone through training in archaeology and skeletal biology, a realm of expertise seldom mastered by medical pathologists and other clinically trained health care specialists who come into contact more frequently with wet tissues and articulated bones of the cadaver in the settings of hospitals and morgues.

In the protocol of a forensic investigation, the anthropologist seeks answers to a standard set of questions (İşcan, 1988). In cases of identification of individuals, one must know if the remains are human or belong to animals. How many individuals are represented in the collection of bones if these are identified as human? What is the sex of the individual? What is the individual's age at time of death? How tall was the individual in life, as determined by stature reconstruction from measurements of long bone lengths? Can weight and body form variables be determined? What is the race, or ancestry, of the individual? Can nutritional and health history be reconstructed from the osteological evidence? Are markers of occupational stress and other individual features wrought by habitual activities, trauma, or other lifetime events present? Finally, is it possible to make a positive identification of the skeletal subject with a missing or otherwise unidentified person?

These essentials of forensic anthropology are described by T. Dale Stewart (1979) in one of the few textbooks written on the subject, for the literature is diffuse and contained primarily in scientific journals. The second and revised edition of *The Human Skeleton in Forensic Medicine* by Krogman and İşcan was published in 1986. Collections of case histories and research reports that document advances in the field have been published recently in edited volumes (Rathbun and Buikstra, 1984; Reichs, 1986). The most recent review of the entire field to date appears in the 1988 edition of the *Yearbook of Physical Anthropology* (İşcan, 1988).

Seventeen authors have contributed the originally written articles that make up this book. After the introductory chapter, the first few chapters address basic skeletal variation with growth, age, sex, and race.

In Chapter 2, Frank Johnston and Louise Zimmer describe the types of growth studies carried out by auxologists and indicate how the results can be used to understand and make inferences about the growth patterns of prehistoric populations. They also compare and contrast skeletal growth studies with those carried out on the living. Their paper makes it clear that one of the main problems confronting skeletal biologists when trying to study prehistoric material is the nature and availability of the remains. Most of the time these bones are very fragile or badly damaged, if present at all. The most serious situation is the overall lack of archaeological fetal and infant skeletons which, in turn, makes it extremely difficult to assess variations in rates of growth and thus may lead to erroneous interpretations. This underrepresentation of the young may, in part, be explained by variation in cultural norms whereby, for example, a new infant might not be buried in a cemetery with the rest of the population.

Johnston and Zimmer examine those specific studies that provide a relationship between growth rate and conditions such as protein-calorie malnutrition and episodes of arrested development. As expected, the authors point out that these conditions may register a wide range of discrepancy between the chronological (or calendar) age and skeletal age. These problems are difficult to solve and, in most cases, they are population specific. The primary dilemma facing nearly all osteologists is the identification and control of factors affecting growth rate that cause variation both between and within individuals.

The subject of age estimation is continued in Chapter 3 by Yaşar İşcan and Susan Loth, who shift from the ordered, sequential changes characteristic of youth to the much more subtle, unpredictable metamorphoses of the adult. Classified by method of observation, the authors systematically present, analyze, and evaluate existing age determination techniques from their origins in the latter part of the nineteenth century to the present. They begin with methods based on directly observable gross morphological changes ranging from T. Wingate Todd's first formal methodological works on the pubic symphysis and cranial sutures in the 1920s to the authors' rib techniques of the 1980s (e.g., Todd, 1920; Todd and Lyon, 1924; McKern and Stewart, 1957; İşcan et al., 1984). This is followed by a presentation of the radiographic approach. Although roentgenographic technology has been available since the last century, this is the method of choice only when the soft tissues cannot be removed or the bones cannot be sacrificed for histomorphometric analysis. Schranz's work (1959) from the 1930s onward provided the basis for x-ray assessment for aging the adult skeleton. The more recent studies of the 1970s and 1980s have offered improvements, but even the strongest proponents warn of technical difficulties.

The third section is an overview of the use of bone and tooth histology. (Histomorphometric analysis is further elaborated in Chapter 4.) In their review of the field of adult age estimation, İşcan and Loth reiterate the problems inherent in estimating age from a single isolated region of a skeleton. Although a number of researchers as early as Graves (1922) and Todd (1939) have criticized this tendency, there has not been a study that assesses age-related variation between different bones in the same individual using different techniques. Finally, the authors stress that there are racially and sexually—possibly even temporally—linked differences in the aging process. Therefore, they recommend that one must first analyze these factors separately when standards are being developed or the applicability of a given technique to another race or sex group must be questioned.

Examination of bone at the cellular level can provide evidence of the effects of the environment, diet, genetics, aging, and musculoskeletal disease and trauma on bone remodeling. We see its first application in biological anthropology by Kerley (1965) in assessing age from the cross section of long bones. In Chapter 4, Sam Stout discusses the development and advancement of thin sectioning and age determination techniques used on undecalcified tissue. The method basically assumes that bone is a dynamic tissue that first goes through the changes of modeling (growth and development) in youth and remodeling (old bone cells being replaced by new ones) in the adult. The most common application is to estimate age at death either in a cross section (Kerley, 1965; Ahlqvist and Damsten, 1969) or core segment (Thompson, 1981) of a long bone. The most recent addition has been the author's introduction of histomorphometric standards from the rib. Stout points out that each of these techniques varies in terms of the effectiveness of the parameters selected, and he claims that the revised version of Kerley's original technique provides the greatest accuracy (Kerley and Ubelaker, 1978). He also notes the effects of such conditions as osteoporosis, polio, dietary factors, and disuse as in quadriplegia.

Aging is an important characteristic that can be determined from the bones, but it is only one component of an individual's biography. The chapter by Lucile St. Hoyme and Yaşar İşcan presents the skeletal variation arising from sex and race differences. These authors outline the current theories—taxonomic, hormonal, environment, ecological, and behavioral—formulated to explain racial origin and variation and discuss the sociopolitical problems arising from race differences in the United States. St. Hoyme and İşcan use all pertinent literature to illustrate the variation in body dimensions and proportions in the living. A detailed discussion of the differences in the skull, pelvic girdle, and extremities is offered, along with current explanations for variations among populations. They point out problems and discrepancies that can arise from the use of skeletal collections as data bases. These sources are usually composed of individuals of lower socioeconomic status and less admixture than represented in modern populations. Unfortunately, there are no large, well-documented skeletal collections representing post-1950 populations. In these discussions, the reader is reminded that our scientific knowledge of race and sex differences is far from complete and is compromised by cultural factors.

The chapter continues with discriminant function comparisons. Although the authors do not list the formulas, they compare the accuracy of estimations each bone or bone fragment can provide. These studies indicate that the skull is the most useful region for the determination of race, and the pelvis is best for sexing. This type of analysis not only has obvious forensic applications, but is also of value in the study of human morphological variation. These osteometric data can be used to gauge genetic distances between populations.

St. Hoyme and İşcan state that to determine sex or race, one must use all available anatomical sites, and each trait must be weighted based on its relative contribution to the discrimination process. Finally, they stress the need for an energetic program of skeletal collection that would contain as detailed documentation as possible for everything from age to steroid consumption.

Another way of addressing population or genetic characteristics is through the observation of nonmetric traits in the skeleton (Berry and Berry, 1967; Ossenberg, 1969; Saunders, 1978). In Chapter 6, Shelley Saunders considers these morphological markers in terms of their presence or absence, but cautions that this is an oversimplification because there is considerable variation in the expression of a trait. In her detailed introduction, the author gives a brief history of research and attempts to clarify some sticky terminological complications. Much of the confusion results from the classification of some traits as discontinuous, that is, presumably controlled by the rules of simple Mendelian genetics. However, as the author points out, this view is not unanimous. A number of sources disagree with this assumption because it has been noted that some of these traits are actually polygenic in origin and thus show continuity in their range of expressions.

An important application of nonmetric trait analysis is based on our knowledge of the extent to which these traits can be used to separate one population from another. In this area, Berry and Berry's (1967) approach is considered to be the pioneering one. Saunders states that their observations and the studies that followed made the assumption that these traits can be considered familial tendencies, because of either genetic or environmental factors. This is particularly helpful in establishing kinship patterns in cemetery populations. Modern efforts on this subject have been toward the calculation of heritability and population distance.

As in all studies that compare one population with another, there are several problems. Saunders indicates that certain issues arise from unsettled methodological considerations leading to premature conclusions. She suggests that further progress is dependent upon answering the questions as to how to deal with symmetry vs. asymmetry, sex and age differences, the effects of the expression of one trait on the expression of another, and the very basic problem of interobserver error. Each of these areas has been intensely investigated, yet the results have been generally discouraging.

In Chapter 7, Spencer Turkel turns to another type of skeletal variation that includes osseus malformations or defects encountered with varying frequencies in archaeological populations (Steinbock, 1976; Ortner and Putschar, 1981). As in nonmetric trait analysis, the study of congenital anomalies also suffers from the lack of precise definitions of what constitutes an abnormality. The approach that the World Health Organization takes in defining the terminological problem is simply that they are not only malformations but also functional and biochemical entities. The variation in congenital abnormalities ranges in a continuum between "normal" and "extremely abnormal," thus creating problems in definition and introducing statistical snags as well. After describing them, Turkel presents examples of congenital problems that can be assessed anthropometrically, such as achondroplastic dwarfism (short limbs) and Morquio's disease (short trunk).

Another aspect of this area of research is the etiology and pathogenesis of a particular disorder. Turkel is critical of those studies that isolate one trait without relevance to other malformations, physiological conditions, or secondary factors later in life that can lead to the same abnormalities, such as rickets and the anemias. He supplements his medical and epidemiological considerations of congenital abnormalities with anthropological studies, especially those pertaining to skeletal remains of different geographic and local populations. He notes that certain malformations are more frequent in some populations than in others, which suggests racial (genetic) and possibly even cultural linkage. For example, polydactyly is more common in blacks of Africa and North America, whereas the highest frequency of several types of cleft palate is seen in Malaysia and Hong Kong. Some of the anthropological studies of skeletal populations are particularly significant because they show the effects of inbreeding (e.g., Ferembach, 1963, and Bennett, 1973, on spina bifida).

Turkel concludes his chapter by discussing the cultural implications that can be derived from these studies. He cites examples such as the differential burial of malformed individuals, the possible role of dwarfs in mythology, and indications of class differences in ancient Egyptian burials.

Obviously, differential morphological characteristics of the skeletal system can also be related to occupational stress and physical activity (Merbs, 1983; Krogman and İşcan, 1986). In the next chapter, Kenneth A.R. Kennedy assembles a critical synthesis of this topic. He begins with a rich historical background, reaching back to Agricola of the sixteenth century and continuing with the studies of Ramazzini in 1705 on the disease of tradesman and Lane's observations of the working classes and their skeletons in the latter part of the nineteenth century. Kennedy then incorporates the contributions of more recent anatomists and biological anthropologists to illustrate how they laid the foundation of contemporary thinking on the subject of skeletal markers of occupational stress.

After his historical summary, Kennedy attempts to establish the relationships between occupational stress and industrialization and between medical and orthopedic problems. He states that anthropological concerns with occupational stress originated independently from those of the medical community. The former arose from studies of human paleontology, skeletal biology, and, most recently, forensic anthropology. However, all approaches have the common aim of reconstructing group and individual lifeways.

Kennedy offers a rationale for bone response to stress by citing Wolff's Law of Transformation, which states that bone responds to mechanical forces, whereby remodeling takes place in well-vascularized subchondral areas in order to resist stress. After describing the processes leading to the development of these markers, Kennedy classifies them into several types, including dental attrition, enthesopathic lesions caused by muscular hypertrophy, sex and racial variation, etc., and adds an extensive table listing skeletal structures that are assumed to vary by occupation. The author indicates that a number of skeletal modifications may result from a single pattern of behavior, such as squatting or running over rough terrain. However, he cautions that there is little documented data about markers of occupational stress and most conclusions have been drawn from anecdotal material that seldom finds its way to published literature.

In Chapter 9, Charles Merbs examines the importance of trauma in the reconstruction of the behavior of ancient populations. In spite of its importance, the subject matter has not been adequately investigated and clarified until now. Merbs presents a number of classifications of trauma types (following Steinbock, 1976; Ortner and Putschar, 1981; and Knowles, 1983) that include, for example, fractures, dental trauma, weapon wounds, dislocation, scalping, surgery, perimortem cuts and fractures, and related lesions like anthropathy. To clarify confusing terminology, terms are defined and tabulated. Diagnosis of each trauma is described and illustrated with relevant figures along with rates and physiological processes of healing. The author also provides numerous examples to demonstrate the significance of trauma analysis in studying individuals and populations from the Pleistocene to the present time. Merbs's earlier study, published in 1983, is an excellent example of reconstructing behavior of an ancient population of the Arctic region.

The author concludes with a discussion of how trauma analysis can provide greater understanding of two important issues: the health status of ancient individuals and non-Western medical practices ranging from simple bone setting to amputation.

Anthropologists deem the interplay between culture and infectious disease a measure of adaptation. When the interplay does not maximize the gain in terms of population size and minimize energy expenditure, it is held that the population lacks an adaptive cultural repertoire (Alland, 1970). One health problem especially devastating for earlier peoples was infectious disease. In Chapter 10, Marc Kelley describes the difficulties associated with the differential diagnosis of various lesions and problems inherent in dealing with ancient skeletons. The author also outlines the evolutionary implications of these lesions and how the types of infectious diseases have changed as humans modified their subsistence strategy from hunting and gathering (which has been associated with parasitic infestation and nonspecific infections like staphylococcus) to a settled way of life (where increased population density led to the domination and spread of pathogens like those causing smallpox and cholera). Kelley writes that the evolutionary host–parasite relationship, as proposed by epidemiologists, appears to be supported by skeletal paleopathological studies.

Kelley discusses the synergistic interactions between culture, environment, and disease with examples from native North Americans, specifically, the case of a seventeenth century burial ground in Rhode Island. He illustrates this ecological model with malaria and hemolytic anemias and the associated cultural responses. The author states that the study of infectious disease is complex and requires proper methodology for accurate interpretation of the lifeways of ancient peoples.

Another difficulty that skeletal biologists face is the interpretation of nutritional problems associated with archaeological populations. Patricia Stuart-Macadam's chapter on this subject focuses on scurvy, rickets, and iron deficiency anemia. She systematically surveys these three conditions in terms of pathophysiology, clinical manifestations, history, and archaeological evidence. It becomes clear that anemia has attracted considerable attention because its marks on the skeleton are numerous and may be caused by a multitude of factors. This contrasts with the relatively minor interest anthropologists have shown in the effects of scurvy and rickets on skeletal remains. The author concludes her chapter by stressing that these three diseases result from improper or incomplete nutrition rather than from overall malnutrition. She notes that children under two years of age are most often affected. Stuart-Macadam reminds us that these conditions are of relatively recent origin and very likely find their origins in the settled way of life that began in the Neolithic. Rickets and scurvy are associated with the intensified urbanization of medieval times in the Western world.

In addition to gross and radiologic assessment of nutrition in the context of its association with disease, a new trend in forensic anthropology and paleodemography is the reconstruction of diet from trace element and stable isotope analyses. In essence these studies seek to establish subsistence practices and general dietary conditions. In Chapter 12, William Keegan is concerned with stable isotope analysis from bone collagen. After a brief introduction on how both stable and unstable isotopic analysis became a significant research method in anthropology, there follows a detailed description of the chemistry of the stable isotope method.

Analysis of the pathways whereby carbon enters food chains through plants shows that aquatic vegetation differs from terrestrial varieties. While, theoretically, carbon (and to a lesser extent nitrogen) isotopes should be able to produce a record of plants consumed, there are numerous problems that skeletal biologists must face. Some of these include the pitfalls inherent in small sample size, alterations in bone chemistry from collagen to apatite, and diagenesis. In the laboratory, special care must be taken in sample preparation, and Keegan provides detailed instructions. The author cautions that stable isotopic analysis should be complemented by other techniques to reconstruct diet. This method is more effective in allowing anthropologists to distinguish between food groups in order to reveal the subsistence activity of a past population rather than distinguish between individuals.

Chemical analysis has become an important aspect of human skeletal analysis; Arthur Aufderheide has already demonstrated this in his studies of lead levels in the human skeleton. In Chapter 13, he presents a comprehensive treatise on the use of chemical techniques to provide a better picture of the health and nutrition of historic and prehistoric people. The trace element analysis portion of his chapter is the most comprehensive and includes discussions of how strontium, zinc, and lead can be used to analyze health, diet, and social status as well as define subsistence activity. There is also an important consideration of the instrumentation necessary for light and mass spectrometry and neutron activation analysis to obtain dietary profiles.

Aufderheide continues with a discussion of other techniques, including paleoserology and amino acid racemization. The determination of the ABO system antigens from bone has long been of interest to anthropologists (Candela, 1936; Thieme and Otten, 1957; Heglar, 1972; Lengyel, 1984). He mentions primary methods like agglutination-inhibition, immunodiffusion, and antibody induction, and illustrates their effectiveness in population genetics and paternity studies that have been attempted using mummy tissues. However, the results and reliability of these techniques are often less than satisfactory when used on bone (Thieme and Otten, 1957; Heglar, 1972).

Analysis of the dental pathology of a skeletal population has provided a wealth of insights into health, nutrition, subsistence, and social organization. Yet, in Chapter 14, John Lukacs makes it clear that there are still many problematic areas that curtail the potential reconstructive and comparative value of this assessment. Foremost of these are the inadequate consideration of dental health in standard osteological sources and lack of standards for the analysis of data. Lukacs clarifies some of these issues and offers a method of investigation. He states that the progress of this specialty requires an understanding of how dental disease is classified, how a lesion is described and recorded, and how interobserver error can be minimized. He describes the conditions of caries, enamel hypoplasia, calculus, antemortem tooth loss, abscesses, and alveolar resorption. With methodological standardization, a particular community can be analyzed properly. Furthermore, standardization will allow valid comparisons to be made between populations. The chapter also includes examples from his analyses of several dental series from Pakistan and India.

The concluding chapter represents the latest installment of Frank Saul's (1972, 1976) continuing quest to reveal the world of the ancient Mayans using an approach he terms "osteobiography." Osteobiography involves all of the techniques available to the skeletal biologist. In Chapter 15, Frank and Julie Saul use this synthesis to try to answer questions about the Mayans. They attempt to elucidate their demographic profile and the genetic, cultural, and environmental variables; the interconnections of these concepts are represented with a flow chart. Like Edynak (1976), Saul and Saul use a total integrative ecologic approach. Their chapter starts with the question "Who was there?" The answer is sought in the paleodemographic composition of the population, including age, sex, and parity.

They then turn to the question of the origin of the Mayan people and use genetic distance studies as one way of answering this question. Questions on the interpretation of skeletal morphological characteristics follow. Some of these morphological features result from the practice of cranial deformation, dental mutilation and attrition, and occupational stress; others may be pathological in origin. The chapter concludes that the osteobiographic approach to the analysis of ancient individuals and populations is now being put to the test on modern forensic cases.

As the chapters in this book illustrate, the attempt to reconstruct the lives of extinct and extant people from their skeletons has long been a challenging goal for physical anthropologists (e.g., Hooton, 1930; Krogman, 1935, 1938; Hoyme [now St. Hoyme] and Bass, 1962; Angel, 1971). To this distinguished list, we must also include Muzaffer Şenyürek, a Harvard graduate (class of 1939) and student of Hooton, Coon, and Romer (Sayılı, 1962). Before his untimely death at 46, he conducted extensive field work and research on material in his native Turkey and also in Africa and the Middle East. Şenyürek's broad range of research extended to patterns of dental anomalies (1949a) and attrition (1949b), cranial anomalies (1946, 1951a), and trephination (1958). His prolific publications in the area of dental growth and development were highlighted by his studies of the fossil Shanidar infant (1957a,b, 1959) and ancient Anatolians (1955, 1956a,b). Şenyürek can be credited with crafting many of the basic tools we now use to reconstruct life from the skeleton.

Today the search for methods to answer the many questions that remain has accelerated. Edynak (now y'Edynak) (1976) attributes the increasing interest in life-style reconstruction from skeletal remains to the decline in typological thinking. The pioneering works of Şenyürek (1947, 1951b, 1957c) and Angel (1969) on paleodemography and Hooton (1930) and Angel (1966) on paleopathology signaled this theoretical shift in physical anthropology. Excellent publications have proliferated in these areas, including those by Brothwell and Sandison (1967), Acsádi and Nemeskéri (1970), Steinbock (1976), Morse (1978), Ortner and Putschar (1981), and Živanović (1982). This move has been followed by a further expansion beyond biological concerns to the elucidation of the biocultural history of various populations and geographic regions. For example, Edynak (1976) interrelates paleopathological variables with age and sex and finds correlates in the ethnographic data. It is also notable that her study treats not only the population as a whole, but establishes the place and the importance of the individual within the group. This approach is also illustrated by the works of Angel (1971), Pfeiffer (1977), Kennedy (1981), Lipták (1983), Bennike (1985), Lukacs (1986), and Powell (1988).

The purpose of the present volume is to offer to our colleagues in archaeology, paleodemography, paleopathology, and human anatomy—

as well as to specialists in the legal and medical fields—a clear profile of current research activities in skeletal anthropology, thereby documenting the progress achieved within this century. This book shows what has already been accomplished and, more importantly, points the way for research to continue in the twenty-first century.

REFERENCES

Acsádi G, and Nemeskéri J (1970) History of Human Life Span and Mortality. Budapest: Akadémiai Kiadó.

Ahlqvist J, and Damsten O (1969) A modification of Kerley's method for the microscopic determination of age in human bone. J Forensic Sci 14:205–212.

Alland A (1970) Adaptation in Cultural Evolution: An Approach to Medical Anthropology. New York: Columbia University Press.

Angel JL (1966) Porotic hyperostosis, anemias, malarias, and marshes in the prehistoric eastern Mediterranean. Science 153(3737):760–763.

Angel JL (1969) The bases of paleodemography. Am J Phys Anthropol 30:427–437.

Angel JL (1971) The People of Lerna: Analysis of a Prehistoric Aegean Population. Washington, DC: Smithsonian Institution Press.

Bennett KA (1973) Lumbo-sacral malformations and spina bifida occulta in a group of proto-historic Modoc Indians. Am J Phys Anthropol 36:435–440.

Bennike P (1985) Palaeopathology of Danish Skeletons: A Comparative Study of Demography, Disease and Injury. Copenhagen: Akademisk Forlag.

Berry RJ, and Berry AC (1967) Epigenetic variation in the human cranium. J Anat 101:361–379.

Bredendieck H (1981) The determination of form. Impact of Science on Society 31(4):381–388.

Brothwell D, and Sandison AT (eds) (1967) Diseases in Antiquity: A Survey of the Diseases, Injuries, and Surgery of Early Populations. Springfield, IL: Charles C Thomas.

Candela PB (1936) Blood group reactions in ancient human skeletons. Am J Phys Anthropol 21:429–432.

Currey JD (1984) The Mechanical Adaptations of Bones. Princeton: Princeton University Press.

Edynak GJ (1976) Life-styles from skeletal material: A medieval Yugoslav example. In E Giles and JS Friedlaender (eds): The Measures of Man: Methodologies in Biological Anthropology. Cambridge, MA: Peabody Museum Press, pp 408–432.

Ferembach D (1963) Frequency of spina bifida occulta in prehistoric human skeletons. Nature 199:100–101.

Graves WW (1922) Observations on age changes in the scapula. Am J Phys Anthropol 5:21–33.

Hall BK (1978) Developmental and Cellular Skeletal Biology. New York: Academic Press.

Hanken J, and Hall BK (1983) Evolution of the skeleton. Nat History 4:28–39.

Heglar R (1972) Paleoserology technique applied to skeletal identification. J Forensic Sci 17:358–363.

Hooton EA (1930) The Indians of Pecos Pueblo: A Study of Their Skeletal Remains. New Haven: Yale University Press.

Hoyme LE, and Bass WM (1962) Human skeletal remains from the Tollifero (Ha6) and Clarksville (Mc14) sites, John H. Kerr Reservoir Basin, Virginia. Bureau Am Ethnol Bull 182:329–400.

İşcan MY (1988) Rise of forensic anthropology. Yrbk Phys Anthropol 31:203–230.

İşcan MY, Loth SR, and Wright RK (1984) Estimation from the rib by phase analysis: White males. J Forensic Sci 29: 1094–1104.

Kennedy B (1981) Marriage Patterns in an Archaic Population: A Study of Skeletal Remains from Port au Choix, Newfoundland. Mercury Series, Archaeological Survey of Canada, No. 104. Ottawa: National Museums of Canada.

Kerley ER (1965) The microscopic determination of age in human bone. Am J Phys Anthropol 23:149–163.

Kerley ER, and Ubelaker DH (1978) Revisions in the microscopic method of estimating age at death in human cortical bone. Am J Phys Anthropol 49:545–546.

Knowles AK (1983) Acute traumatic lesion. In GD Hart (ed): Disease in Ancient Man. Toronto: Clarke Irwin, pp 61–83.

Krogman WM (1935) Life histories recorded in the skeleton. Am Anthropol 37:92–103.

Krogman WM (1938) The skeleton talks. Sci Am 159:61–64.

Krogman WM, and İşcan MY (1986) The Human Skeleton in Forensic Medicine. Springfield, IL: Charles C Thomas.

Le Corbusier (Charles Edouard Jeanneret) (1959) Time Magazine 30(November):81.

Lengyel I (1984) ABO typing of human skeletal remains in Hungary. Am J Phys Anthropol 63:283–290.

Lipták P (1983) Avars and Ancient Hungarians. Budapest: Akadémiai Kiadó.

Lukacs JR (1986) Excavations at Inamgaon, Vol. 2: The Physical Anthropology of Human Skeletal Remains, Part 1: An Osteobiographic Analysis. Pune: Deccan College Press.

McKern TW, and Stewart TD (1957) Skeletal age changes in young American males, analyzed from the standpoint of identification. Headquarters QM Research and Development Command, Technical Report EP-45, Natick, MA.

McLean FC, and Urist MR (1968) Bone: An Introduction to the Physiology of Skeletal Tissue. Chicago: University of Chicago Press.

Merbs CF (1983) Patterns of activity-induced pathology in a Canadian population. Mercury Series, Archaeological Survey of Canada, No. 119. Ottawa: National Museums of Canada.

Morse D (1978) Ancient Disease in the Midwest. Reports of Investigations, No. 15. Springfield: Illinois State Museum.

Ortner DJ, and Putschar WGJ (1981) Identification of Pathological Conditions in Human Skeletal Remains. Smithsonian Contributions to Anthropology, No. 28. Washington, DC: Smithsonian Institution Press.

Ossenberg NS (1969) Discontinuous morphological variation in the human cranium. Doctoral dissertation, University of Toronto.

Pfeiffer S (1977) The Skeletal Biology of Archaic Populations of the Great Lakes Region. Mercury Series, Archaeological Survey of Canada, No. 64. Ottawa: National Museums of Canada.

Powell ML (1988) Status and Health in Prehistory: A Case Study of the Moundville Chiefdom. Washington, DC: Smithsonian Institution Press.

Rathbun TA, and Buikstra JE (eds) (1984) Human Identification: Case Studies in Forensic Anthropology. Springfield, IL: Charles C. Thomas.

Reichs KJ (ed) (1986) Forensic Osteology: Advances in the Identification of Human Remains. Springfield, IL: Charles C Thomas.

Saul F (1976) Osteobiography: Life history recorded in bone. In E Giles and JS Friedlaender (eds): The Measures of Man: Methodologies in Biological Anthropology. Cambridge, MA: Peabody Museum Press, pp 372–382.

Saul FP (1972) The Human Skeletal Remains from Altar de Sacrificios, Guatemala: An Osteobiographic Analysis. Paper of the Peabody Museum, Harvard 63:2:1–123. Cambridge, MA: Peabody Museum of Harvard Press.

Saunders SR (1978) The Development and Distribution of Discontinuous Morphological Variation of the Human Infracranial Skeleton. Mercury Series, Archaeological Survey of Canada, No. 81. Ottawa: National Museums of Canada.

Sayılı A (1962) Ordinaryüs Profesör Dr. Muzaffer Süleyman (1915–1961). Belleten 24:181–201.

Schranz D (1959) Age determination from the internal structure of the humerus. Am J Phys Anthropol 17:273–278.

Şenyürek MS (1946) The multiplicity of foramina mentalia in human mandible from the Copper Age of Anatolia. Nature 157:792.

Şenyürek MS (1947) A note on the duration of life of the ancient inhabitants of Anatolia. Am J Phys Anthropol 5: 55–66.

Şenyürek MS (1949a) The occurrence of taurodontism in the ancient inhabitants of Anatolia. Belleten 13:215–227.

Şenyürek MS (1949b) The attrition of molars in the ancient inhabitants of Anatolia. Belleten 13:229–244.

Şenyürek MS (1951a) Two cases of premature suture closure among the ancient inhabitants of Anatolia. Belleten 15:247–262.

Şenyürek MS (1951b) The longevity of the Chalcolithic and Copper Age inhabitants of Anatolia. Belleten 15:447–468.

Şenyürek MS (1955) A review of the order of eruption of the permanent teeth in fossil hominids. Belleten 19:407–444.

Şenyürek MS (1956a) Order of eruption of the permanent teeth in the Chalcolithic and Copper Age inhabitants of Anatolia. Belleten 20:1–28.

Şenyürek MS (1956b) The time of eruption of the third molars in the Chalcolithic and Copper Age inhabitants of Anatolia. Belleten 20:201–212.

Şenyürek MS (1957a) The skeletons of the fossil infant found in the Shanidar Cave, northern Iraq. Anatolia 2: 49–55.

Şenyürek MS (1957b) A further note on the Paleolithic Shanidar infant. Anatolia 2:111–121.

Şenyürek MS (1957c) The duration of life of the Chalcolithic and Copper Age populations of Anatolia. Anatolia 2: 95–110.

Şenyürek MS (1958) A case of trepanation among the inhabitants of the Assyrian trading colony at Kültepe. Anatolia 3:49–52.

Şenyürek MS (1959) A study of deciduous teeth of the fossil Shanidar infant: A comparative study of the milk teeth of fossil man. Ankara Üniv. Dil ve Tarih-Cografya Fak. Yayinlari 24:693–698.

Shipman P, Walker A, and Bichell D (1985) The Human Skeleton. Cambridge, MA: Harvard University Press.

Steinbock RT (1976) Paleopathological Diagnosis and Interpretation. Springfield, IL: Charles C Thomas.

Stewart TD (1979) Essentials of Forensic Anthropology: Especially as Developed in the United States. Springfield, IL: Charles C Thomas.

Thieme FP, and Otten CM (1957) The unreliability of blood typing aged bone. Am J Phys Anthropol 15:387–398.

Thompson DD (1981) Microscopic determination of age at death in an autopsy series. J Forensic Sci 26:470–475.

Todd TW (1920) Age changes in the pubic bone: I. The male white pubis. Am J Phys Anthropol 3:285–334.

Todd TW (1939) Skeleton, locomotor system, and teeth. In EV Cowdry (ed): Problems of Ageing. Baltimore: Williams and Wilkins, pp 278–338.

Todd TW, and Lyon DW Jr (1924) Endocranial suture closure, its progress and age relationship: Part I. Adult males of white stock. Am J Phys Anthropol 7:325–384.

Ubelaker DH (1978) Human Skeletal Remains: Excavation, Analysis, Interpretation. Washington, DC: Taraxacum.

Watts ES (1986) Skeletal development. In WR Dukelow and J Erwin (eds): Comparative Primate Biology, Vol. 3: Reproduction and Development. New York: Alan R. Liss, pp 415–439.

Wolff J (1892) Das Gesetz der Transformation der Knocken. Berlin: A. Hirschwald.

Živanović S (1982) Ancient Diseases: The Elements of Paleopathology. New York: Pica Press.

Reconstruction of Life From the Skeleton

Chapter 2

Assessment of Growth and Age in the Immature Skeleton

Francis E. Johnston and Louise O. Zimmer
Department of Anthropology, University of Pennsylvania, Philadelphia, Pennsylvania 19104-6398

INTRODUCTION

The study of growth and development has been, for several decades, a basic concern of physical anthropologists. Studies of growth changes in samples of both human and nonhuman primates may be classified into four categories:

1. Studies of the growth process itself, which seek largely to describe the changes that occur with age. Such studies may use relatively simple techniques (Ostyn et al., 1980) or complex mathematical models (Bock, 1980).

2. Studies that interpret evolutionary change in the context of growth (Jungers, 1984; Watts, 1985). This approach is based on the understanding that altering the rate of growth and maturation is an efficient strategy for effecting morphological change.

3. Studies that seek to understand the interaction of hereditary and environmental factors in regulating the course of development (Frisancho, 1975; Townsend et al., 1982). Many researchers employing this approach see growth as an adaptive mechanism, responding to the pressures of the environment.

4. Studies that use the adequacy of the growth of the children of a community as an index of overall community health. Poor growth is seen to be an indicator of unfavorable conditions in the community (Johnston, 1981; Tanner, 1986).

For those physical anthropologists who study the skeletal biology of earlier human populations, growth studies are also important, though they were begun much more recently. The analysis of variability in the subadult skeleton, focusing originally on epiphyseal formation and epiphyseo-diaphyseal union, dates back only to the 1920s (e.g., Pryor, 1923; Krogman and İşcan, 1986). Studies of growth itself only begin to appear in the literature in the 1960s (Johnston, 1962; Mahler, 1968; Armelagos et al., 1972). Despite such a short history, there is essential agreement among workers that interpretation of variation in skeletal populations requires data on the patterns of development in children and youth like that needed for an understanding of variability in living populations.

This chapter will consider the study of growth and development in human skeletal populations. It will deal with methodological issues as well as summarize the existing studies that have analyzed the skeletal remains of children and youth from prehistoric time periods. We will focus on the information that may be obtained from such studies in the reconstruction of the lifeways of peoples whose remains are being analyzed.

ISSUES OF METHODOLOGY AND DESIGN

Methodological issues are basic to any scientific endeavor because, without a rigorous research design and reliable techniques, no study can be acceptable. In studying the growth of children from a skeletal sample there are some specific problems that need to be addressed. These problems affect not only the design of the research but also interpretation and generalization from the results. Even though they have been discussed by other authors (Mahler, 1968; Johnston, 1969; Armelagos et al., 1972), the issues involved are important enough to warrant their discussion here.

The skeletal remains of subadults, especially infants and younger children, are likely to be underrepresented in a given sample. Immature bones are small and fragile and more likely to become lost either through decay or taphonomic processes. Furthermore, the burial practices of various societies differ, especially with regard to the very young; often, infants who die in the perinatal period may not be buried. As a result, it is particularly difficult to attain a sample size sufficiently large for adequate analysis; the younger the age, the greater the likelihood of underrepresentation.

As will be discussed below, the age at death of immature skeletons is usually estimated by determining the maturation stages of the various bones. As a result, the investigator obtains a "skeletal" (or "bone") age (SA) rather than a true chronological age (CA). A bone age represents an equivalent level of skeletal development (e.g., epiphyseal union) attained by children of a given (and known) CA in some standard, reference population. (This is analogous to our use of a mental age to indicate a level of intellectual function.)

Two sources of error are introduced by using skeletal development as an indicator of CA. The first reflects the fact that individual children of the same CA will vary in their levels of skeletal maturation, resulting in a margin of error in the assignment of age at death (for example, ±2.0 years). The second source of error occurs because environmental and/or genetic factors can affect the rate of skeletal maturation in the population under study. We know, for example, that chronic malnutrition can delay maturation by two to three years (Himes, 1978). This means that, in a well-nourished society, a given level of skeletal maturation may be associated with a CA of 5.0 years, whereas in a population where there is malnutrition, children may not attain the same level until 7.0 years.

The truth is we do not know the CAs of the children of a sample with certainty. We estimate their SAs and interpret them as the CAs that would have been attained if they had been maturing at the same rate as the children of the reference population. The results must be interpreted with caution.

Another problem associated with growth studies of skeletal populations involves the measurement of bone lengths. Given that body length can only be measured on rare occasions, if at all, data on growth are usually obtained as long bone lengths. Prior to the union of the epiphyses with their diaphyses, only the diaphyseal length is measured. This is done because epiphyses, being very small, are frequently not recovered by the excavators; even if they were, there would be no reliable estimate of the thickness of the epiphyseal cartilage between the diaphysis and epiphysis. However, as epiphyses begin to fuse to diaphyses (typically in the mid-teens), the lengths measured include the associated epiphyses. Hence, there can be no continuous curve representing long bone growth from infancy through the second decade of life.

Finally, any conclusions drawn from growth data obtained from skeletal samples must be drawn carefully. Growth curves of such samples do not necessarily represent the growth of the healthy members of the population. The skeletons of all immature subjects represent individuals who died prematurely, many because of diseases (including malnutrition) that might have affected their growth as well as longevity. In short, skeletal samples cannot be compared to normal healthy groups in a straightforward way.

CONTRIBUTIONS OF GROWTH STUDIES TO THE RECONSTRUCTION OF LIFEWAYS OF SKELETAL POPULATIONS

Despite the above problems, the study of the growth patterns of skeletal populations can provide important and essential data in the reconstruction of the lifeways of populations from the past. Growth processes are the pathways by which variation among adults arises. Therefore, the first step to understanding morphological differences among individuals or populations is to understand the differences in the growth patterns that gave rise to the variants being studied.

In some instances, the patterns of growth variation observed seem to reflect genetic mechanisms (see, e.g., Eveleth and Tanner, 1976, for a worldwide survey of population variation among the living). For example, y'Edynak (1976) reported a study of 109 prehistoric Eskimo and Aleut skeletons from Kodiak Island. She found the characteristically short legs, relative to the trunk, of Eskimos and Aleuts; furthermore, this pattern is shown to have arisen through a reduced rate of long bone growth. Y'Edynak's results agree with studies of the growth of living Eskimo and Aleut children (e.g., Jamison, 1976; Johnston et al., 1982) and suggests possible genetic continuity between prehistoric and contemporary groups from this geographical area.

Even more important in the reconstruction of lifeways from the skeleton is the observation that growth patterns reflect the severity of environmental stressors experienced by a population. These stressors include nutritional factors and disease, as well as their interactions. In discussing the skeleton, Huss-Ashmore (1981) notes that "nutritional stress produces characteristic patterns of disturbance in bone . . . [and that] . . . an analysis of such patterns . . . should indicate the degree and (to some extent) the kind of nutritional deficiency encountered."

Other authors have made similar observations. Hughes (1968) summarized a broad range of data on the dead and the living in his discussion of the plasticity of the skeleton. He notes that biologic differences between peoples are not "merely anthropometric or genetic." Rather they result from differences in response to the demands and opportunities that compose their ecosystems. In a comprehensive review of the effects of protein-energy malnutrition (PEM) on bone growth and development in the living, Himes (1978) notes that the major effect of PEM is in slowing the rate and hence the amount of growth. This slowing of the growth process occurs in general throughout the skeleton; centers of ossification appear and epiphyses fuse, though at a slower tempo than is found in well-nourished groups. The reduction in the amount of growth and slowing of the tempo of development are straightforward functions of the severity and the chronicity of the malnutrition.

In skeletal populations, individuals with deviations from the normal course of development may often have died at younger ages. Clark et al. (1986) have reported on their analyses of the relationship between vertebral growth and life span in 90 skeletons from the Dickson Mound, a prehistoric site (950–1300 A.D.) in Illinois. They found that reduced growth of the vertebrae was associated with a shortened life span. This is important evidence in support of a point made earlier in this paper, namely, deviations from normal growth provide an indication of impaired health and reduced life expectancy. Put another way, growth mirrors the conditions in which the group lived.

Although this chapter is devoted to the skeleton, it is important to note that defects of the dental enamel may also reflect responses during childhood to environmental, primarily nutritional, stress (Rudney, 1983). El-Najjar et al. (1978) suggest that, while the etiology seems to be nonspecific, nutritional factors are likely to be involved. Goodman and coworkers (1980) have analyzed the frequency of enamel hypoplasia in the skeletons of 111 adults from three cultural levels of the Dickson Mound; these hypoplasias provide a "memory" of growth disruption during childhood resulting from environmental stresses, with the distance of the hypoplasia from the cemento-enamel junction providing an estimate of the age of occurrence. The authors found differences over time in the frequency of hypoplasias that they attributed to poorer nutritional status associated with an increased reliance on maize agriculture. The repetitive nature of the hypoplasias in individual teeth was interpreted as indicative of periodic nutritional stress, probably resulting from a cycle of food shortages.

In a more recent analysis of Dickson Mound skeletons, Blakey and Armelagos (1985) examined enamel defects in the skeletons of children. They were able to demonstrate a greater prevalence of defects during the prenatal period than after birth, which suggested that the stresses experienced by this population affected dental development during the fetal period to such an extent that an increased rate of death could be observed.

The analysis of growth and development of skeletal samples thus provides important information beyond the children whose skeletons are measured. Findings from analyses of growth may be extrapolated to the entire population being studied. Growth status is an excellent mirror of the conditions under which a group lived and of their success at adapting to those conditions.

SKELETAL MINERALIZATION AND GROWTH

Bone provides the basic reservoir for the storage of calcium in the body. Calcium provides the rigidity for the musculoskeletal system and, when released into the bloodstream, plays an essential role in the transmission of nerve impulses. Several endogenous and exogenous mechanisms; operating in a complex manner, regulate the deposition and release of calcium from bone. However, the dietary intake of calcium is an important factor, and reductions in bone mineralization are seen in malnourished living children (Garn et al., 1964; Himes, 1978).

A number of techniques have been used to evaluate the degree of mineralization of the skeleton. For example, one of the earliest approaches estimated bone density visually from x-rays. However, this method is subject to serious errors and reliable estimates of bone density cannot be obtained.

More common has been the measurement of the thickness of the layer of compact bone as visualized on a radiograph of a long bone, such as the second metacarpal or the tibia. Using standard techniques, the thickness of the cortices may be measured accurately on x-rays of either the living or deceased (Johnston, 1969) and related to the ability of specific bones to support body weight (Ruff and Hayes, 1983). Hummert (1983), for example, measured the compact bone thicknesses of the tibiae of 174 children from a prehistoric site in Sudanese Nubia. He found a decreased amount of compact bone, brought about not by a reduction in the deposition of bone on the periosteal surface, but by an increased resorption of bone from the endosteal surface. These observations were consistent with those made on x-rays of skeletons of living children suffering from PEM and led Hummert to conclude that his sample was stressed nutritionally. In a more recent study of this site, Van Gerven et al. (1985) analyzed cortical measurements of the tibia; they also calculated the moments of inertia. The authors noted a reduction in the percentage of the total cross-sectional area made up of compact bone. However, they also found that the biomechanical quality of the bone was not compromised by this reduction, leading them to conclude that if nutritional stress had been responsible, it had not resulted in a weakness of the bone.

PROBLEM OF ASSIGNING AGE AT DEATH

As noted above, the assignment of age at death is a major problem in the study of physical growth in skeletal samples. The issue is, of course, one of concern for all ages, but it is particularly acute for research dealing with children. Because of the many complex and often rapid changes that occur as part of development, age categories must be made narrower than among adults, preferably only one year in width (though this is often not possible in skeletal studies). Fortunately, the skeleton and teeth undergo many changes during the growing years, making it possible to be far more specific in estimating age in that time span than among adults.

Dental indicators can provide useful estimates of age, especially in younger children. Dental emergence (eruption) is frequently used, and, where available, radiographs can reveal the amount of calcification that has occurred in the enamel and the root (Demirjian, 1980) (see Fig. 1). The Miles method (Miles, 1963) is also useful for older children and youth, because dental wear has begun to occur.

For the skeleton itself, age estimates are usually based on the fusion of the centers of ossification of a particular bone, for example of those bones that fuse to make up the innominate, or the union of secondary epiphyseal centers of ossification to primary centers (Fig. 2).

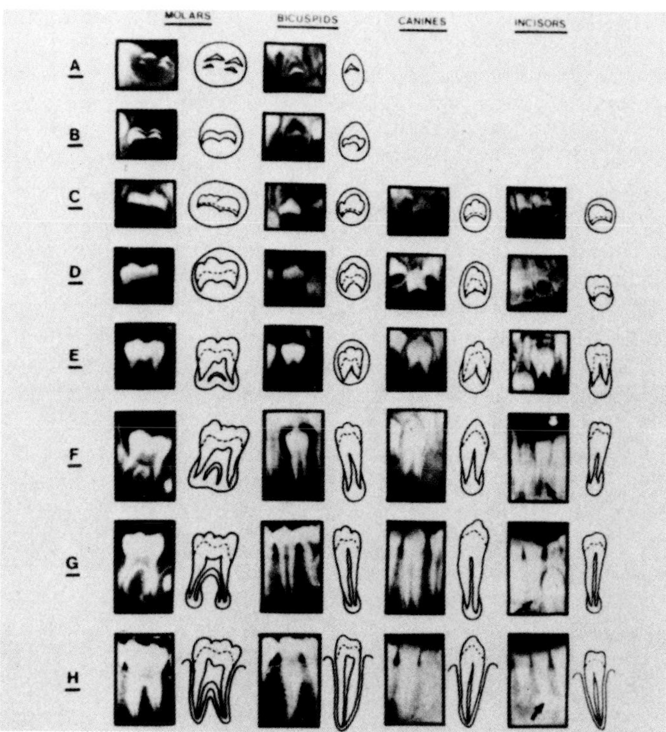

Fig. 1. Developmental stages of the permanent dentition (reproduced from Demirjian, 1980, with permission of Plenum Publishing Corp).

Many, but not all, bones of the skeleton undergo this process of fusion, which provides, in conjunction with the teeth, an adequate number of indicators of age for a skeleton, assuming that enough bones have been recovered.

Epiphyseal union is primarily a phenomenon of the teenage years; the most precise estimates of age are therefore possible during this period. A number of tables are available that give the ages at which epiphyseo-diaphyseal fusion of various centers occurs (Table 1). The issues involved, along with many of the earlier tables, have been presented and discussed in depth by Krogman and İşcan (1986). The sequence in which the various epiphyses fuse has not been shown to differ significantly among the major ethnic groups, so one table is about as useful as another, providing that it has been based on a large sample of well-nourished individuals. Such tables are drawn from children of known age and, almost without exception, were published before 1960. New data occasionally appear; for example, Webb and Suchey (1985) give ages at which the epiphyses at the anterior iliac crest and the medial aspect of the clavicle unite with their diaphyseal surfaces. These indicators are useful after approximately 12 years of age.

Fewer bony indicators of age are available to the researcher working with skeletons of infants and young children. As a consequence, dental features are most often used in working with these ages. However, some skeletal indicators have been proposed. For example, Becker (1986) has reported on the union of the left and right halves of the mandible in the midline as an aid to researchers working with skeletons from the first year of life. Fusion occurs at the mandibular symphysis between 6 and 9 months of age and therefore is useful for identifying the young infant.

The tympanic plate of the temporal bone develops from the formation of the tympanic ring through a series of stages, culminating with its

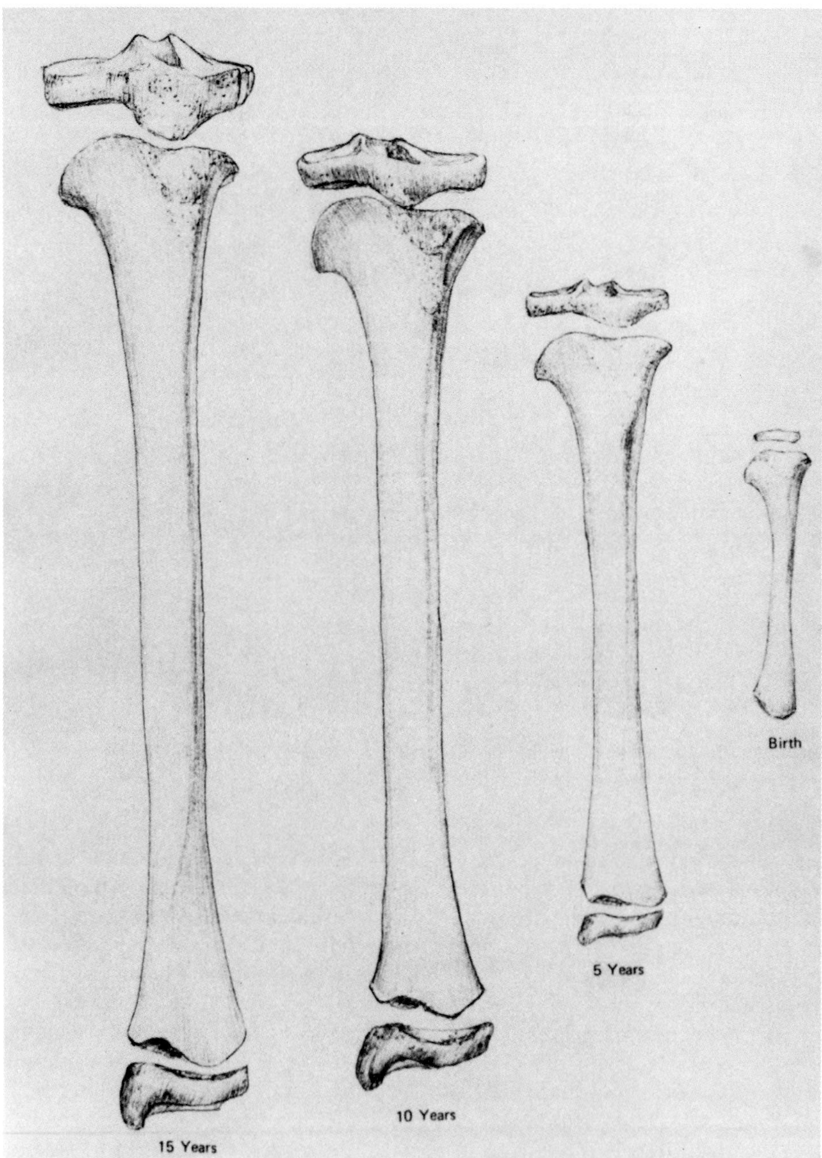

Fig. 2. Anterior view of the tibia at various ages showing development of proximal and distal epiphyses (reproduced from Bass WM, 1971, with permission of Missouri Archeological Society).

fusion to the temporal bone. Because this process occurs over a short period of time and because it spans birth, it is especially useful in attempting to differentiate fetuses from neonates. Curran and Weaver (1982) developed a set of three stages using likelihood tests to determine its reliability as an indicator of age. Although the results were not perfect, they did permit age grouping into one of three stages: 1) fetal, 2) fetal/neonatal, and 3) neonatal.

Perhaps the most vexing problem in studying the growth of children from skeletal samples is in the utilization and interpretation of the assigned ages at death. As noted earlier,

TABLE 1. Postnatal Ages, in Years, of Union of Centers of Ossification in U.S. Youth

Center	Age range
Scapula	
Acromion	18.0–19.0
Vertebral margin	20.0–21.0
Inferior angle	20.0–21.0
Clavicle	
Sternal end	25.0–28.0
Acromial end	19.0–20.0
Humerus	
Head	19.5–20.5
Distal	14.0–15.0
Medial epicondyle	15.0–16.0
Radius	
Proximal	14.5–15.5
Distal	18.0–19.0
Ulna	
Proximal	14.5–15.5
Distal	18.0–19.0
Hand	
Metacarpals	15.5–16.5
Phalanges I	15.0–16.0
Phalanges II	15.0–16.0
Phalanges III	14.5–15.5
Pelvis	
Primary elements	13.0–15.0
Iliac crest	18.0–19.0
Ischial tuberosity	19.0–20.0
Femur	
Head	17.0–18.0
Greater trochanter	17.0–18.0
Lesser trochanter	17.0–18.0
Distal	17.5–18.5
Tibia	
Proximal	17.5–18.5
Distal	15.5–16.5
Fibula	
Proximal	17.5–18.5
Distal	15.5–16.5
Calcaneus	14.5–15.5
Foot	
Metatarsals	15.0–16.0
Phalanges I	14.5–15.5
Phalanges II	14.0–15.0
Phalanges III	14.0–15.0

Modified from Krogman and İşcan (1986, Table 3.5, p 65).

these are not true CAs, but are SAs. Skeletal ages are CA equivalents, representing the age at which, e.g., the union of a particular epiphysis occurs in a well-nourished, contemporary population (Roche, 1980). As such, they are subject to two kinds of errors.

The first error is a random one, representing individual variability in the attainment of a given stage of skeletal development. Random error reduces the precision with which one can analyze the data. For example, in their study of the usefulness of the tympanic plate in differentiating between fetal and newborn skeletons, Curran and Weaver (1982) found that individuals judged as stage 1 were almost certain to be fetuses, and those in stage 3, neonates. However, the variation among individuals was great enough that those in stage 2 could not be placed with confidence into either a fetal or a neonatal category.

The same uncertainty occurs at later ages. Studies of the living have shown that normal children of a given SA will vary over a three-year range (i.e., ±1.5 years) in chronological age. As a consequence, any CA category based on skeletal age will include children outside of that category. For example, the 7-year-old age group will include children ranging at least from 6.5 through 8.5 years; a significant proportion of the variability in a measure of growth will thus be due to the rather heterogeneous and uncontrollable variation in true CA. The statistical power to detect differences between samples or groups within samples will be reduced considerably.

The second error is a systematic one, reflecting the effect of environmental stress on the tempo of growth. The children of the reference data are assumed to be healthy. If the children of the skeletal sample are subject to malnutrition and infectious disease, they will move more slowly through the stages of bone maturation. The result is that a skeleton judged to be, say, 8 years old, will most likely be older by one to three years. The greater the stress, the greater the delay, and the more that the true CA will be underestimated. Himes (1978) notes that the bone ages of children from upper and lower socioeconomic strata in India may differ by three years in children of the same CA.

A further complication arises from the fact that the delay in bone maturation is not constant across ages. The longer children are exposed to a harsh environment, the greater the lag in SA. In children from a poor environment, therefore, the difference between CA and age assigned from the skeleton will be greater in older than in younger children.

In the final analysis, the ages assigned to the skeletons being studied should not be termed chronological at all, but rather skeletal, for that is what they are. This is especially significant if the populations under study have been subjected to environmental stress.

STUDIES OF THE GROWTH OF CHILDREN FROM SKELETAL SAMPLES

The earliest studies of the growth of children from skeletal samples date back only to the late 1950s, as investigators began to realize the significance of growth in human biological studies. The first published study did not deal with long bones, but rather with age changes in the skull and face of a sample of native Americans from Indian Knoll, a site in Kentucky dating to the Archaic period (Sarnas, 1957). Sarnas utilized radiographs of the skulls, which allowed him to visualize the internal bony architecture and to compare the results to similar x-rays of Swedes, Africans, and native Australians.

By and large, studies of native American samples reveal little overall difference from group to group, especially when compared to measurements of the long bones of living North American children. The prehistoric samples all lag behind the living ones, indicative of the poorer environments of the former. Merchant and Ubelaker (1977) analyzed the growth of a sample of protohistoric Arikara Indians from South Dakota, comparing their results to other samples. The other samples included two studies of children from Indian Knoll. The first study was published by Johnston (1962) and the second by Sundick (1978). Despite the fact that Johnston and Sundick studied many of the same skeletons, Merchant and Ubelaker noted that the Indian Knoll results differed more from each other than either did from the Arikara data.

Merchant and Ubelaker attributed this difference to the methods used to assign age. Johnston utilized dental and osseous criteria, whereas Sundick relied exclusively on dental staging. When allowances were made for these methodological differences, the Arikara and the two Indian Knoll studies showed very similar growth curves.

Jantz and Owsley have also analyzed the growth of the Arikara in a series of papers (Jantz and Owsley, 1984a,b; Owsley and Jantz, 1985). Their samples were drawn from three populations ranging in time from 1550 to 1862 A.D. and differing in environmental quality. The most recent population experienced the harshest environment. The change from earlier times resulted from depopulation, disease, sociocultural deterioration, and severe food shortages. With only a few exceptions, differences in growth patterns among the three samples were consistent with the environmental differences. The exceptions led Jantz and Owsley to suggest tentatively that various bones may respond differently to environmental stress.

Owsley and Jantz (1985) have also focused more specifically on the perinatal component of their sample (i.e., late fetal/early neonatal). In the most recent time period, with increasing morbidity and a decreasing subsistence base, they found smaller bone lengths than in earlier periods. The authors concluded that the poorer environment affected fetal growth through the maternal organism, and also postnatal growth, because of increased disease and poorer nutritional intake.

A similar analysis was conducted by Mensforth (1985), who compared two sites located in Ohio. The first, Bt-5, was from an Archaic (hunter-gatherer) time period and the second, Libben, Late Woodland (settled farming). He found that the differences in growth of the tibia between the two samples appeared during the years of early childhood, when the growth of Libben children lagged. This was attributed to ecological differences related to food availability, disease, and population density accompanying the beginnings of sedentary communities.

Hummert and Van Gerven (1983) studied the growth of 180 children from Sudanese Nubia, spanning a time range from 550 to 1450 A.D. In their analyses, in contrast to those reported above, the authors analyzed differences in growth in order to ascertain differences in environmental quality between their sample and another from Lower Nubia. They also utilized other data, e.g., age at death and the presence or absence of specific indicators of bone pathology. The growth data were consistent with the other observations and led the authors to conclude that the environments of the two Nubian groups differed significantly.

An overview of the above studies reveals three themes emerging from the research. The first theme is that growth differences between groups, especially during childhood, are primarily the result of environmental factors. Genetic mechanisms may play a role if the groups being compared are not closely related biologically to each other. However, the primacy of the environment in the genesis of between-group differences in childhood growth is consistent with studies on living children from lesser-developed countries.

The second theme is that environmental variation becomes a key factor in the differentiation of populations from one other. The differences in growth that are observed are interpreted as resulting from environmental factors. In research following this model, growth patterns are interpreted as adaptations to environmental stress rather than as indicators of genetic differences between populations.

The third theme uses growth patterns as indicators of the environment. Developmental retardation indicates a poor environment and allows the investigator to assess environmental quality in the absence of other data. In this approach growth becomes an evaluative tool for the entire population.

USE OF GROWTH DATA IN SKELETAL ANALYSES

Researchers who analyze the skeletal material recovered from archaeological investigations are usually interested in using the information gathered from that analysis to help in reconstructing the lifeways of the people who lived at the site. Such a reconstruction is a basic step in realizing the objectives of the research being undertaken. For example, we may want to know how well a population was adapted to the rigors of their environment. An evaluation of the growth patterns, obtained from a study of the bones of the children and adolescents, will provide valuable data to help answer the question.

The transition from a hunting and gathering subsistence pattern to a farming one was accompanied by a wide range of other changes. Whereas hunter-gatherers move over a wide geographical area, farmers are sedentary, living in villages and towns. Matters of sanitation and hygiene, of disease transmission, and of crowding become problems to which the society must adapt. This situation was made more acute by the radical change in food sources, from a diet containing a significant amount of animal products to one emphasizing vegetable materials. Protein consumption went down and carbohydrate intake increased. This isn't necessarily bad; however, the shift represented yet another stress to which a population had to adapt.

It is now known that the development of agriculture was not a "marvelous invention" that provided more leisure time for a society. Rather, agriculture was a change in subsistence that accompanied increases in the size of the human population. Taken in conjunction with the changes mentioned above, it is clear that this was a period of intense adjustment, one requiring major adaptive responses. Some societies adapted better and more quickly than others. The growth studies described above, carried out in eastern North America, have shown a negative impact on the populations living during those times. Growth data have been essential in leading researchers to such a conclusion.

The skeletal studies by Jantz and Owsley on the growth of Arikara children have also documented stresses that increased with time, due at least in part to the increasing pressure of white Americans moving westward. The social disruption is well documented in the historical literature; the biological effects on the children are seen through an analysis of skeletal growth.

At the beginning of this chapter, four types of growth study were listed as characteristic of research in biological anthropology. Of the four, the first three are generally not appropriate for samples of skeletons from prehistoric time periods. Documentation of age and sex is not reliable enough to allow analyses of the growth process itself and is better left for investigators who work with living children. Nor is there the vast time perspective necessary for studies of human and primate evolution. And, as with the first type of study, the individuals in a skeletal sample cannot be characterized with the precision needed for genetic studies.

However, the fourth type of study, which uses growth data as an evaluative tool, is highly relevant for skeletal analysis. In fact, given what we know about the effects of a harsh environment on the growth of disadvantaged children from the Third World, no data are potentially more useful than measurements of the children of skeletal samples. Unfortunately, this fact has not been realized for much more than a decade. However, given the interest of anthropology in adaptation to the environment, and especially the success of adaptations to an increasing complexity of culture, studies of growth are even more valuable than before. It is important that those who conduct such research be aware of its potential value; however, it is equally important that the limitations be recognized. A successful balance of the potential and the limitations will result in the addition of a valuable source of data to the information analyzed by those interested in prehistoric lifeways.

CONCLUSIONS

It is clear that the study of growth is becoming an increasingly important part of the reconstruction of the lifeways of skeletal populations. As research design and analytic methods become more incisive and more sophisticated, the questions being asked extend beyond mere description into areas of hypothesis testing and ecological investigation. The sensitivity of the growth process to the environment provides the biological anthropologist, as well as the archaeologist, with an excellent tool for assessing the relationship between a population and its environment. The increasing sensitivity of the excavator to the preservation of the skeletons of the very young will ensure an even greater data base for the application of this tool.

ACKNOWLEDGMENTS

The assistance of Virginia Lathbury is gratefully acknowledged.

REFERENCES

Armelagos GJ, Mielke JH, Owen KH, Van Gerven DP, Dewey JR, and Mahler PE (1972) Bone growth and development in prehistoric populations from Sudanese Nubia. J Hum Evol 1:89–119.

Bass WM (1971) Human Osteology. Columbia: Missouri Archeological Society.

Becker MJ (1986) Mandibular symphysis (medial suture) closure in modern *Homo sapiens:* Preliminary evidence from archaeological populations. Am J Phys Anthropol 69:499–501.

Blakey ML, and Armelagos GJ (1985) Deciduous enamel defects in prehistoric Americans from Dickson Mounds: Prenatal and postnatal stress. Am J Phys Anthropol 66: 371–380.

Bock DB (1980) Statistical problems of fitting individual growth curves. In FE Johnston, AF Roche, and C Susanne (eds): Human Physical Growth and Maturation: Methodologies and Factors. New York: Plenum Press, pp 265–290.

Clark GA, Hall NR, Armelagos GJ, Borkan GA, Panjabi MM, and Wetzel FT (1986) Poor growth prior to early childhood: Decreased health and life-span in the adult. Am J Phys Anthropol 70:145–160.

Curran BK, and Weaver DS (1982) The use of the coefficient of agreement and the likelihood ratio test to examine the development of the tympanic plate using a known-age sample of fetal and infant skeletons. Am J Phys Anthropol 58:343–346.

Demirjian A (1980) Dental development: A measure of physical maturation. In FE Johnston, AF Roche, and C Susanne (eds): Human Physical Growth and Maturation: Methodologies and Factors. New York: Plenum Press, pp 83–100.

El-Najjar MY, DeSanti MV, and Ozebek L (1978) Prevalence and possible etiology of dental enamel hypoplasia. Am J Phys Anthropol 48:185–192.

Eveleth PH, and Tanner JM (1976) Worldwide Variation in Human Growth. New York: Cambridge University Press.

Frisancho AR (1975) Functional adaptation to high altitude hypoxia. Science 187:313–319.

Garn SM, Rohmann CG, Behar M, Viteri F, and Guzman MA (1964) Compact bone deficiency in protein-calorie malnutrition. Science 145:1444–1445.

Goodman AH, Armelagos GJ, and Rose JC (1980) Enamel hypoplasias as indicators of stress in three prehistoric populations from Illinois. Hum Biol 52:515–528.

Himes JH (1978) Bone growth and development in protein-calorie malnutrition. World Rev Nutr Diet 28:143–187.

Hughes DR (1968) Skeletal plasticity and its relevance in the study of earlier populations. In DR Brothwell (ed): The Skeletal Biology of Earlier Human Populations. New York: Pergamon Press, pp 31–56.

Hummert JR (1983) Cortical bone growth and dietary stress among subadults from Nubia's Batn el Hajar. Am J Phys Anthropol 62:167–176.

Hummert JR, and Van Gerven DP (1983) Skeletal growth in a medieval population from Sudanese Nubia. Am J Phys Anthropol 60:471–478.

Huss-Ashmore R (1981) Bone growth and remodeling as a measure of nutritional stress. In DL Martin and MP Bumsted (eds): Biocultural Adaptation, Comprehensive Approaches to Skeletal Analysis. Research Report 20:84–95. Amherst: University of Massachusetts Department of Anthropology.

Jamison PL (1976) Growth of Eskimo children in northwestern Alaska. In RJ Shepherd and S Itoh (eds): Circumpolar Health. Toronto: University of Toronto Press, pp 223–229.

Jantz RL, and Owsley DW (1984a) Temporal changes in limb proportionality among skeletal samples of Arikara Indians. Ann Hum Biol 11:157–164.

Jantz RL, and Owsley DW (1984b) Long bone growth variation among Arikara skeletal populations. Am J Phys Anthropol 63:13–20.

Johnston FE (1962) Growth of the long bones of infants and children at Indian Knoll. Am J Phys Anthropol 20:249–254.

Johnston FE (1969) Approaches to the study of developmental variability in human skeletal populations. Am J Phys Anthropol 31:335–341.

Johnston FE (1981) Anthropometry and nutritional status. In Assessing Changing Food Consumption Patterns: Committee on Food Consumption Patterns. Washington, DC: National Academy Press, pp 252–264.

Johnston FE, Laughlin WS, Harper AB, and Ensroth AE (1982) Physical growth of St. Lawrence Island Eskimos:

Body size, proportion, and composition. Am J Phys Anthropol 58:397–401.

Jungers WL (1984) Aspects of size and scaling in primate biology with special reference to the locomotor skeleton. Yrbk Phys Anthropol 27:73–98.

Krogman WM, and İşcan MY (1986) The Human Skeleton in Forensic Medicine. Springfield, IL: Charles C Thomas.

Mahler PE (1968) Growth of the long bones in a prehistoric population from Sudanese Nubia. PhD dissertation, University of Utah, Salt Lake City.

Mensforth RP (1985) Relative tibia long bone growth in the Libben and Bt-5 prehistoric skeletal populations. Am J Phys Anthropol 68:247–262.

Merchant VL, and Ubelaker DH (1977) Skeletal growth of the protohistoric Arikara. Am J Phys Anthropol 46:61–72.

Miles AEW (1963) The dentition in the assessment of individual age in skeletal material. In DR Brothwell (ed): Dental Anthropology. New York: Macmillan, pp 191–209.

Ostyn M, Simons J, Beunen G, Renson R, and Van Gerven D (1980) Somatic and Motor Development of Belgian Secondary Schoolboys. Norms and Standards. Leuven: Leuven University Press.

Owsley DW, and Jantz RL (1985) Long bone lengths and gestational age distributions of post-contact period Arikara Indian perinatal infant skeletons. Am J Phys Anthropol 68:321–328.

Pryor JW (1923) Differences in the time of development of centres of ossification in the male and female skeleton. Anat Rec 25:257–273.

Roche AF (1980) The measurement of skeletal maturation. In FE Johnston, AF Roche, and C Susanne (eds): Human Growth and Maturation: Methodologies and Factors. New York: Plenum Press, pp 61–82.

Rudney JD (1983) Dental indicators of growth disturbance in a series of ancient Lower Nubian populations: Changes over time. Am J Phys Anthropol 60:463–470.

Ruff CB, and Hayes WC (1983) Cross-sectional geometry of Pecos Pueblo femora and tibiae—A biomechanical investigation. I. Method and general patterns of variation. Am J Phys Anthropol 60:359–382.

Sarnas KV (1957) Growth changes in skulls of ancient man in North America. Acta Odontol Scand 15:213–271.

Sundick RI (1978) Human skeletal growth and age determination. Homo 29:228–249.

Tanner JM (1986) Growth as a mirror of the condition of society: Secular trends and class distinctions. In A Demirjian and M Dubuc (eds): Human Growth, A Multidisciplinary Review. London: Taylor & Francis, pp 3–34.

Townsend JW, Klein RE, Irwin MH, Owens W, Yarbrough C, and Engle PL (1982) Nutrition and preschool mental development. In DA Wagner and HW Stevenson (eds): Cultural Perspectives on Child Development. San Francisco: W.H. Freeman, pp 124–145.

Van Gerven DP, Hummert JR, and Burr DB (1985) Cortical bone maintenance and geometry of the tibia in prehistoric children from Nubia's Batn el Hajar. Am J Phys Anthropol 66:275–280.

Watts ES (ed) (1985) Nonhuman Primate Models for Human Growth and Development. New York: Alan R. Liss.

Webb PAO, and Suchey JM (1985) Epiphyseal union of the anterior iliac crest and medial clavicle in a modern multiracial sample of American males and females. Am J Phys Anthropol 68:457–466.

y'Edynak G (1976) Long bone growth in western Eskimo and Aleut skeletons. Am J Phys Anthropol 45:569–574.

Reconstruction of Life From the Skeleton
© 1989 Alan R. Liss, Inc., pages 23–40

Chapter 3

Osteological Manifestations of Age in the Adult

Mehmet Yaşar İşcan and Susan R. Loth
Department of Anthropology, Florida Atlantic University, Boca Raton, Florida 33431-0991

INTRODUCTION

Estimation of age is an essential part of reconstructing life from the skeleton. This determination is relatively straightforward during the developmental phase of human growth. These early years are characterized by definite, predictive sequences of tooth formation and eruption and epiphyseal closure in endochondral bones. However, once growth has ended and adulthood has been reached, age determination becomes much more difficult. One must recognize the more variable, less distinct changes produced by the process of remodeling to maintain the status quo and, later, the inevitable signs of deterioration. As Todd (1920) so aptly stated, "Many of these modifications which appear successively during adult age are on the border-line between the anatomical and the pathological."

Because the manifestations of age in the adult are so much less obvious than those characterizing the developmental years, it is necessary to carefully observe the bones in order to detect subtle variations in morphology. Furthermore, one must be able to discern where individual variation ends and universal age-related metamorphosis begins. Once promising sites have been isolated, the pattern, sequence, and rate of age-related change must be elucidated.

Every bone with an open end, such as epiphyseal regions, sutural borders, and articular surfaces, will show visible signs of aging. Furthermore, depending on its position, structure, and function, each part of the skeleton reflects different aspects of the aging process. In synovial joints, this process is more in the nature of wear and tear. In other areas, changes are specific to the nature of a particular type of articulation like that in the sternal end of the rib, symphyseal surface of the pubis, costal margins of the sternum, sutural edges of the cranial bones, vertebral bodies, and auricular surfaces of the ilium and sacrum. For example, in the vertebral column, age can be manifest by either osteophytosis or erosion. In the rib, the anatomic relationship between the bone and cartilage at the costochondral junction allows mineralization at the sternal extremity of the rib to extend over the costal cartilage. Yet, in spite of this plethora of potential skeletal age markers, attention has focused almost exclusively on the cranial sutures and pubic symphysis for age determination in the adult. This seems to have discouraged most physical anthropologists from initiating studies of other skeletal sites that can be equally significant, if not better, reflectors of age.

Thus, it is imperative to reexamine the past, illuminate the present, and contemplate the future of age assessment from the skeleton. The urgency of this exercise is underscored by the resurgence in the last few years of serious activity in this area, ranging from the modification of existing systems in the skull and pelvis to the introduction of the sternal extremity of the rib as an entirely new site. Therefore, the purpose of this chapter is to carry out a critical review and examination of the development and applicability of different techniques on diverse bones.

GENERAL ASSESSMENT OF AGING TECHNIQUES

Patterns of aging are detected on both the macroscopic (direct observation and radiological examination) and microscopic levels (Krogman and İşcan, 1986; Zimmerman and Angel, 1986; İşcan, 1989).

Direct Morphological Examination

The most traditional approach to skeletal age estimation has been the observation of changes in morphology detectable by the naked eye. Obviously, there are many advantages to this method since it is the most readily available and does not necessitate specialized technical equipment, specimen preparation, or complicated interpretation. However, like all anthroposcopic methods, direct analysis requires a sound knowledge of and familiarity with the skeletal system, its inherent variation, and the factors that can affect it.

Skull. Historically, the skull was the first part of the skeleton systematically investigated for the estimation of age at death. By the end of the nineteenth century, studies of cranial suture closure had been conducted by Broca (1861), Ribbe (1885), Schmidt (1888), Dwight (1890a), and Parsons and Box (1905).

These early researchers found a positive correlation with age commencing with basilar suture (synchondrosis) closure at 18–21 years followed by observations of the vault beginning endocranially anywhere between 25 and 40 years of age and continuing through the sixties. The general progression of sutural closure is depicted in Figure 1. However, the extreme variability in the order and timing of closure was noted (Dwight, 1890a). At the turn of the century, Frédéric (1906, 1909/1910) introduced a five-point rating scale (0–4) for both vault and

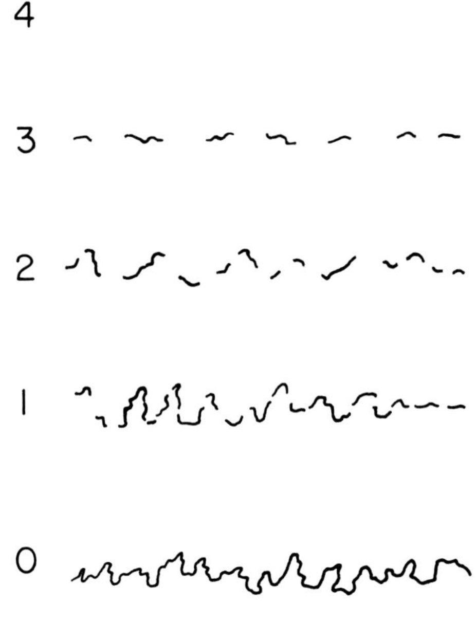

Fig. 1. Age changes in the cranial sutures are characterized by the gradual closure, sometimes leading to the complete obliteration of the suture lines of articulation between the bones of the skull. This process shows extreme variability in timing from one individual to the next, but all proceed in the indicated order through at least some of the stages illustrated above and described as follows: **0,** Open suture. A slight space can be detected between the edges of adjoining bones. **1,** Suture is closed, but clearly visible as a continuous, usually tortuous, line. **2,** Suture line becomes less distinct and complex with some disruptions created by areas of complete closure. **3,** Only scattered pits remain to indicate the location of the suture. **4,** Suture is completely obliterated with no recognizable evidence of its location. Modified from Perizonius (1984, Fig. 3).

facial sutures. Sex differences were characterized by later closure in females (von Lenhössek, 1917). The unreliability of this site for any precise estimation of age was emphasized.

The landmark studies of cranial suture closure in white and black American males were published by Todd and Lyon (1924, 1925a–c) using specimens from the Western Reserve University (now called the Hamann-Todd) collection. Their work differed fundamentally from that of previous investigators because they sought to "establish a definite age relationship in the closure of sutures" (Todd and Lyon, 1924). Ironically, they criticized their predecessors for using crania of unknown age and basing their conclusions strictly on a "general average," which they termed a "closure tendency," that would necessarily vary with each collection (Todd and Lyon, 1924).

Todd and Lyon used Broca's (1861) arrangement of the complication of sutures, degrees of closure, and subdivision of each suture, but followed Frédéric's (1906) inverted rating scale of 0–4 to denote the degree of obliteration. Thus, when applied to the three or four designated segments of each suture, their technique resulted in a closure formula for a given skull. Todd and Lyon found endocranial sutures more reliable than ectocranial sutures, which frequently exhibited lapsed union, but they too expressed serious reservations about the accuracy of age estimation by this method.

Wisely, Todd and Lyon (1924, 1925a–c) separated their specimens by race and sex. They had originally intended to include females of both races, but their sample was so decimated by the exclusion of what were considered to be anomalous skulls that this part of their project was abandoned.

When whites and blacks were compared, a number of interracial differences were found. Todd and Lyon (1925c) noted that individual variability was greater in blacks, and a significantly larger number of "abmodal" patterns, especially in the lambdoid suture endocranially and the coronal suture ectocranially, were encountered. These observations resulted in a rejection rate for black skulls that was three times higher than that for whites. While these authors speculated that the "large number of Negro rejects must however raise doubt as to whether [their] Negro graph is . . . the result of [their] subconscious prejudice in favor of the White type," they were convinced that their "method of rejection was exactly the same" for both races. In the end, despite obvious differences, Todd and Lyon (1925b) concluded that "there is one modal type of human suture closure . . . common to White and Negro Stocks" and separate standards were not necessary.

Following the work of Todd and Lyon, researchers began to examine the sutures and test their methods. Using 100 Argentine skulls, Cattaneo (1937) allowed that cranial suture closure was only a "suggestive indicator" of age. Hrdlička (1939) stated that ectocranial closure "could hardly be relied upon" to come within "10 years on either side of reality."

The major criticisms of Todd and Lyon were published by Singer (1953) and McKern and Stewart (1957). Singer (1953) analyzed Todd and Lyon's work and harshly condemned the way in which they handled and interpreted their material. Observations of extreme variability within the range of normalcy led him to state unequivocally that age determination from the cranial sutures is "hazardous and unreliable" (Singer, 1953). In 1957, McKern and Stewart warned that the onset and progress of sutural closure is so erratic that almost any pattern can be found at any age, rendering this site and technique "of little use" and "generally unreliable."

One might have thought the death knell had been sounded on this topic, but, despite these warnings, research on the sutures continued. In 1960, Nemeskéri et al. divided the vault sutures into 16 sections, evaluating the progress of each area using a five-phase assessment of obliteration. They concluded that sutural closure can be useful, but only as part of their "complex method." Perizonius (1984) applied the aforementioned method to 79 Dutch crania and advised that, while this site may still have potential, further investigation is needed to explain the underlying mechanism of sutural closure and its relationship to age.

A slightly different approach was taken by Meindl and Lovejoy (1985), who used a scale of 0–3 to judge closure at specified 1 cm sites (rather than along the entire suture) on all ectocranial sutures in 236 crania from the Hamann-Todd collection. They concluded that the lateral anterior points were more accurate than the vault sites, race and sex were not important, and the correlation with age was better than those obtained from the McKern and Stewart pubic symphysis components (when applied to Hamann-Todd specimens), but inferior to most other methods. Like Nemeskéri and associates (1960), these authors suggested that suture closure can be of value "when used in conjunction with other skeletal age indicators" (Meindl and Lovejoy, 1985).

One area of concern centers on the fact that Meindl and Lovejoy did not separate their samples by race and sex. It might have been a more prudent approach in light of significant racial and sexual variation in the aging process in suture closure, as noted by the researchers mentioned in this section, and in other parts of the skeleton (Hanihara, 1952; Gilbert, 1973; Gilbert and McKern, 1973; Burns and Maples, 1976; Zhang, 1982; İşcan et al., 1985, 1987).

Finally, Masset (1971, 1989) took a mathematical approach to this problem by tracing systematic statistical errors due to sex differences, the age structure of the reference population in relation to the unknown group, and "attraction of the middle." The "attraction" results from combining individual estimates into an age structure for a given population, in which case they tend to accumulate in the middle age range. While agreeing that the cranial sutures cannot be used for precise individual age estimation, he advocates their usefulness in revealing major demographic shifts over time in a particular cemetery. Masset (1989) suggests that statistical manipulations such as the probability vector method can eliminate many systematic errors, but cautions that the age distribution cannot essentially deviate from that of the reference population.

Thyroid cartilage. Because the thyroid cartilage is frequently missing from most archaeological and forensic skeletons, it is rarely thought of as a site for age estimation. However, a number of studies have associated age with the degree and progression of ossification of the thyroid cartilage (Yoshikawa, 1958; Vlček, 1980; Černý, 1983). The most notable of these was Vlček's presentation of nine phases of progressive ossification in males and their correlation with age from 15 to nearly 70 years. However, he noted that difficulties arose after age 50. Černý (1983) tested Vlček's method on five ossified cartilages and found that although it was fairly easy to classify a specimen of known age, this was not the case when he attempted to determine age from an unknown individual. He cautioned that lacunar resorption may result in a deceptively younger-looking bone and that damage can obscure the actual manifestations of age. Černý (1983) concluded that thyroid cartilage ossification might best be used as a complement to other methods.

Scapula and sternum. Two of the least-used bones for age estimation are the scapula and sternum. Aging in the adult scapula was investigated by Graves in 1922. Using the Hamann-Todd collection, he noted two "diametrically opposed" types of age-related manifestations: ossification and atrophy. He identified six loci undergoing postmaturity ossification, including lipping of the glenoid fossa, and four types of atrophic changes in the general character of the scapular bone. However, he did not associate them with specific ages. Graves used transillumination to pinpoint atrophic alterations in the bony tissue itself. He warned that race, sex, and disease may affect the manifestations of age at this site, but did not study them personally. Krogman (1949) later supplied age ranges for Graves's features. Basically, this method can only furnish a general delineation of open-ended intervals such as "under 25" or "over 50."

Stewart (1954) thought the sternum had the potential to be of value in age estimation despite the warnings of Dwight (1890b) and Todd (1920) to the contrary. Stewart associated five stages of metamorphosis in the sternal articular areas with concurrent epiphyseal closure and arthritic changes. However, he found these changes cease to be quantifiable by about age 35 and concluded that "although . . . it is impossible as yet to assign definite ages to developmental events . . . the association of these events with datable age changes in other bones should prove useful in assessing the age of skeletons."

The most recent study by Jit and Bakshi (1986) assessed the time of fusion of the mesosternum with the manubrium and xiphoid process on a sample of over 1,000 Indian males and females ranging in age from 5 to 85 years. They concluded that because sternal ossification proceeds so irregularly throughout life, it is not helpful for age estimation in males over 18 and females over 20.

Vertebral column. As early as 1943, Stewart noticed that osteoarthritic vertebral lipping increased with age. In 1958, he published the results of a study of both the Terry collection (N = 87) and Korean war casualties (N = 368) in which he quantified the degree of osteophytosis and attempted to correlate it with age. He rated these variables on an admittedly subjective scale of 0 to ++++, averaged the total for the cervical, thoracic, and lumbar regions separately, and then plotted the correlation of each region with age on graphs. Results indicated that during the first 50 years of life, the number, rather than the size of the osteophytes, increased. The first significant increase in osteophytic size was not observed until after age 51. Finally, some individuals did not show osteophytosis even into their eighties, in contrast to others in their forties who showed considerable lipping.

Although the general correlation of lipping with age is not disputed, Stewart concluded that "osteophytosis itself does not permit close aging of skeletons." He felt its value lies in allowing the assumption that the absence of any grade ++ lipping usually indicates age less than 30 years; conversely, specimens exhibiting grades ++ or +++ are over 40.

In 1965, Howells used Stewart's data to determine whether regression equations could be developed to allow practical application of osteoarthritic lipping for age estimation. He found that the highest correlation with age occurred in the cervical region, followed by the lumbar vertebrae. However, he agreed that "Stewart's pessimism . . . is justified, and regression formulae . . . are not likely to be worthwhile." Howells added that what is actually being assessed here is not "age," but the effects of "function and stress . . . the passage of time rather than a process of aging." In this vein, the vertebral column might be more useful as an evaluation of stress during an overall age evaluation. Without this consideration, the effects of extreme stress in a relatively young adult skeleton may likely result in that individual being "overaged."

Rib. The structure, position, and function of the rib make it a particularly good site from which to observe the effects of age. Kerley (1970) noted that the sternal extremity of the rib shows metamorphosis throughout life. Yet it was not until 1984 that we quantified the age-related changes at this site and introduced two techniques (component analysis and phase analysis) for precise age determination from the rib in white males (İşcan et al., 1984a,b). When the ribs of white females were found to age differently in onset, rate, and pattern, separate phase standards were introduced a year later (İşcan et al., 1985).

Based on a sample of 204 specimens from white males and females of documented age, sex, and race, the rib phase technique assigned changes observed in the pit shape, depth, rim configurations, and overall condition of the bone to nine phases (0–8) of progression spanning seven decades, from the teens through the seventies (İşcan et al., 1984a, 1985). The morphological features defining the phases are illustrated in Figure 2. Both male and female standards were blind tested by physical and forensic anthropologists (İşcan and Loth, 1986a,b). The phase method was shown to yield a reliable estimation of age in both sexes. Its application was minimally affected by interobserver error and negligibly by the relative experience and educational level of the tester. The overall test results were extremely encouraging because, despite the fact that only the photographic standards were used (without the written instructions and descriptions that normally accompany them) the phase estimations averaged within one phase of the chronological age.

Since the rib standards were based on whites, a sample of blacks of both sexes (N = 73) was collected to assess racial variation. Blacks were found to differ significantly both in size (Loth and İşcan, 1987) and morphological characteristics (İşcan et al., 1987). Furthermore, we determined that the aging process in the sternal extremity of the rib was sufficiently different in both rate and pattern to severely limit the use of white-based standards on blacks. Ossification was more pronounced in younger blacks, making them appear older than their white counterparts beginning in the late twenties. On the other hand, black bones retained a much more youthful firmness with ad-

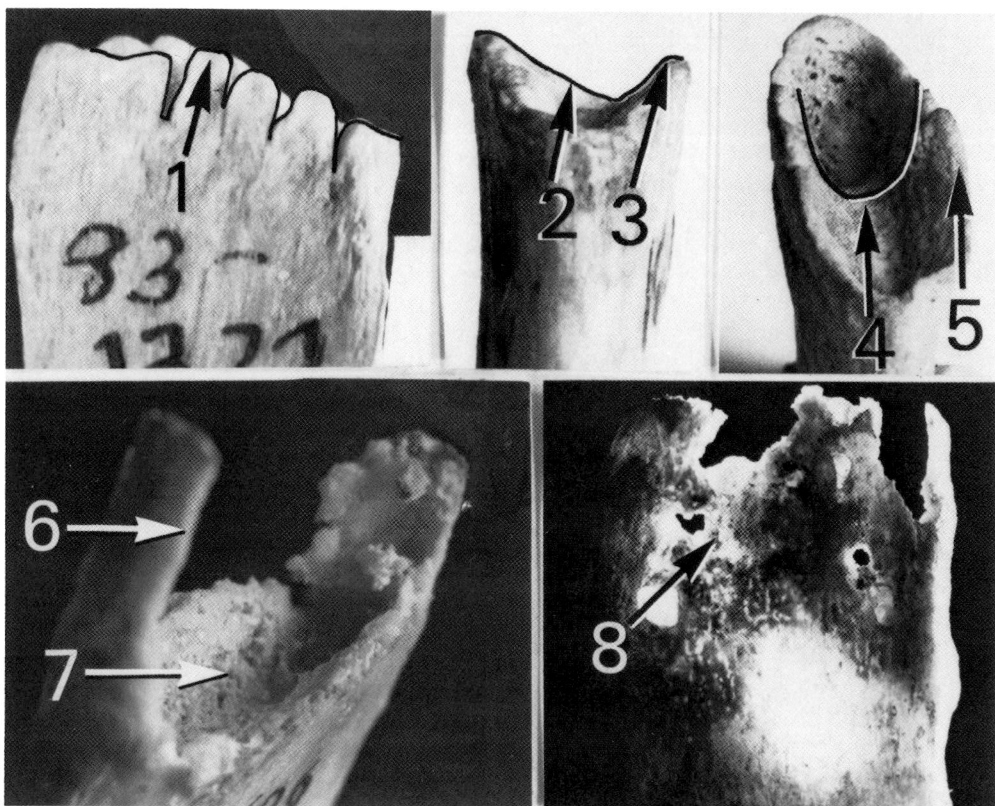

Fig. 2. At the sternal extremity of the rib, the smooth, dense, rounded regularity characterizing the teens and twenties is gradually metamorphosized over the years by the combined forces of endosteal resorption, intra-cartilagenous mineralization, and periosteal deposition to the sharp, porous, fragile irregularity of old age. Some of the features upon which the authors based the rib phase method to determine age from this site are illustrated above. **1**, Smooth, solid bone with scalloped edges. **2**, V-shaped pit with smooth, billowy walls (**3**). **4**, Transition to a U-shaped pit is complete along with early signs of porosity, yet the edges (**5**) are still rounded and regular. **6**, Superior/inferior projections accompanying a rough, porous pit with sharp erose edges (**7**). **8**, Backlighting clearly highlights the deteriorated, coarse, fragile texture, and extreme irregularity especially obvious in the periosteally deposited bone extending over the costal cartilage common in individuals over the age of 70 years. Modified from Krogman and İşcan (1986, Fig. 5.1).

vancing age. The preparation of black standards is currently underway (Loth, 1988).

The rib is a particularly advantageous site for a number of reasons. While there is always a certain amount of individual variation, this bone has shown much greater consistency and reliability than the cranial sutures. The costochondral junction is a relatively stable location and not directly subjected to the effects of weight bearing, locomotion, pregnancy, and parturition, as are the pubic symphysis, auricular surface of the ilium, and long bones. Therefore, it is more likely to meet Howells' (1965) criteria of reflecting age rather than the effects of "function and stress." Furthermore, the rib techniques for age determination are particularly effective since they are relatively easy to apply, are sex and race specific, and are drawn from a collection with precise documentation of age, as well as other demographic information.

In order to make a valid comparison of the accuracy of age estimation from the rib and pubic symphysis, the authors collected these bones from the same individuals in a sample of documented medical examiner's cases (N

= 80) (İşcan et al., 1989b). Before learning the actual age of the specimens, each site was assigned to age phases separately so that the appearance of one bone would not influence assessment of the other. This study revealed that the rib was judged to be in the correct age phase twice as often as the pubic symphysis in both males and females. Additionally, when the rib was in error, it was usually within one phase of "ideal" and reached a maximum of 2 phases in only a few cases. This contrasted sharply with results from the pubic symphysis where error ranged from 2 to 7 phases in about half of the sample.

The only real concerns expressed about the rib techniques stem from the fact that the standards were derived from the right fourth rib. While there is no evidence of side differentials (Loth, 1988), intercostal variation in the aging process among the lower ribs is known to exist (Semine and Damon, 1975). However, in the majority of cases examined to date, ribs 3, 4, and 5 have been assigned to the same phase (Loth, 1988; İşcan et al., 1989a).

Sacroiliac region. The effects of age can be seen in two ways at the sacroiliac joint: changes in the topography of the articular surfaces of the sacrum and ilium, and ankylosing of the joint itself. Brooke (1924) wrote that this joint does not show sex differences until puberty, at which time males "progress along lines of strength" and females sacrifice strength for mobility. When considering this region, it must be kept in mind that the pelvic structure is more influenced by sex-linked factors than any other part of the skeleton.

Nearly 60 years ago, Sashin (1930) associated regular changes in the sacroiliac joint with increasing age. Weisl (1954), in an attempt to correlate the shape of the articular surfaces with sacral movement, also noted that the height of craniad sacral elevations increased gradually in the first 30 years of life and became prominent in the third and fourth decades, with little change thereafter.

Lovejoy and associates (1985a) introduced a method to estimate age at death from changes in the auricular surface of the ilium. Using a mixed sex/race sample of 500 specimens from the Hamman-Todd collection, 250 archaeological remains from the Libben population, and 14 recent forensic cases, they classified changes at this site into eight phases spanning late adolescence to old age, paying particular attention to topography, marginal lipping, and porosity. Although this technique was offered as "unisex," they warned that certain features are accentuated in females with marked preauricular sulci. Therefore, the entire inferior demiface should be ignored in the assessment of these individuals. Tests indicated that the reliability of this method compared favorably with the other sites chosen in their multifactorial studies (Lovejoy et al., 1985b).

In a 1924 study, Brooke observed changes in the mobility of the sacroiliac joint and linked them definitively with sex and age. He noted that, in males, what little movement they have progressively decreases until the fifties, after which time (in most cases) complete ankylosing led to immobility. Not one of his female sample of the same size (N = 105) showed ankylosis. Stewart (1976) looked into this phenomenon by analyzing ankylosing spondylitis of the sacroiliac joint in various populations, including American whites and blacks and the Bantu of South Africa. He observed that the condition progressed fairly regularly with age, occurred more commonly on the right side, and intensified in the fifth decade. Statistically, almost 90% of cases were male, and ankylosing was found most frequently in American blacks, followed by Bantu, then whites. Recent studies (İşcan and Derrick, 1984; Andersen, 1986) confirmed that the tighter postauricular space between the sacrum and ilium in males probably predisposes them to ankylosis.

Pubic symphysis. Like the cranial sutures, the pubic symphysis has been the focus of a lion's share of the studies and methods for age estimation. As early as 1858, Aeby noted age-related change at this site. Although his studies focused on the soft tissues of this region, he did observe marked changes in the bony symphyseal face. The general progression of the aging process at this site is illustrated in Figure 3. As with cranial sutures, the pubic bone was formally ushered in as a locus for age determination by Todd (1920, 1921a,b) with the introduction of his developmental phases.

Using dissecting room specimens from the Western Reserve University (Hamann-Todd) collection, Todd analyzed a sample of 306 white males. With the aim of distinguishing

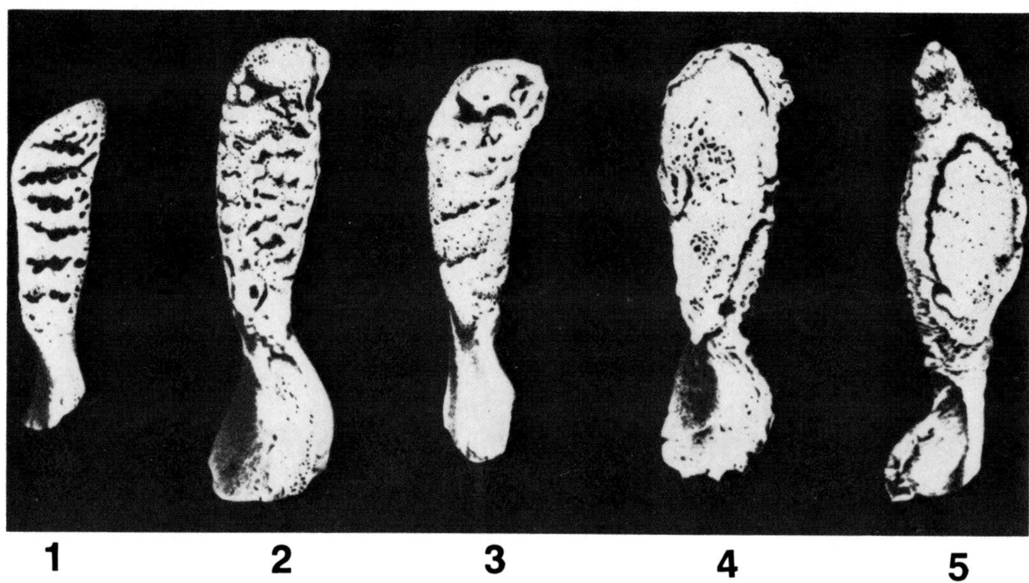

Fig. 3. At the pubic symphyseal face, the aging process is illustrated by the diminution and disappearance of youthful billowing, followed by the buildup of bony ramparts, and finally proceeding to rarefaction, erosion, and erratic ossification in individuals over 50. **1,** Convex face with pronounced horizonal ridges. **2,** Ridges flattening; dorsal and ventral rims forming. **3,** Ridges reduced to granular remnants. Note continuous rim and well-defined border. **4,** Symphyseal face is completely smooth; both margins sharply rimmed. **5,** The shrunken, porous, concave face is surrounded by fully developed dorsal and ventral rims. Modified from Acsádi and Nemeskéri (1970, Fig. 21).

"between metamorphosis and growth," he included only skeletons 18 years and older. Beginning with the "first post-adolescent phase," Todd described the appearance and changes manifested in the symphyseal face in ten phases ranging from 18 years to the fifties. Variation was coped with in two ways: for what he considered normal, moderate variation, the range was defined within each phase. Alternatively, all specimens showing more extreme variation were pronounced "anomalous" and were eliminated from the sample.

The following year, Todd (1921a) used white females and blacks from the same collection to check for sex and race differences. When black males were compared with whites, he observed that although blacks run through the same general phase metamorphoses, they tended to proceed more rapidly, especially over the age of 40. However, while "lipping of the dorsal margin" and "rarefaction and ventral erosion" tended to "commence some five years earlier" in black bones, they never reached the same advanced state of progression as their white counterparts.

Todd was aware of Aeby's (1858) findings of sex-related differences in the pubis. Yet his own investigation showed that "there are only a few differences in the expression of one or two . . . phases and these are of relatively minor consequence" (Todd, 1921a). Furthermore, he found no evidence of changes in the pubic symphysis that could be linked to pregnancy and parturition. He did admit to feeling hampered by his small sample size and suggested that further study was necessary.

With regard to race, Todd concluded that differences between the sexes were greater than those between races because, although they shared the variation found in black males, "in age relationship," black female pubes "agree with" white females rather than black males. Thus, while Todd did find definite variation by sex and race, he did not deem it significant enough to necessitate discrete sex- and race-specific standards.

Despite reservations by many members of the discipline, Todd's technique remained formally unchallenged for 35 years. In 1955, Brooks modified the age ranges for Todd's phases to account for the increased variation observed in individuals over 25. Two years later, the first major criticism of Todd's phase methodology was leveled by McKern and Stewart (1957). In their opinion, Todd's model was too static to adequately deal with the wide range of variation encountered at this site. Using a well-documented sample of Korean War dead, they developed a component analysis system to better assess individual variation in the male pubic symphysis by evaluating each morphological aspect as a separate entity, independent of the others.

It was not until over 40 years after Todd's work that discrepancies between the sexes were demonstrated at that site (Gilbert, 1973). Using their own documented collection, Gilbert and McKern (1973) followed McKern and Stewart's (1957) component analysis system to provide appropriate pubic symphyseal standards for females. While these methods have been generally accepted and widely used, questions have arisen about problems with interobserver error (Suchey, 1979) and the effects of pregnancy and parturition in females.

Research by Meindl and associates (1985) was undertaken to conduct a blind test of all pubic symphyseal methods (Todd, 1920; McKern and Stewart, 1957; Gilbert and McKern 1973; Hanihara and Suzuki, 1978). They attempted a "systematic correction of . . . standards in current use." Using a sample from the Hamann-Todd collection that was not separated by sex or race, Brooks's (1955) modifications of Todd's phases were found to be the most successful. Next, based on observations of a carefully selected mixed sex/race sample of skeletons from the same collection, Meindl's group condensed Todd's ten phases into "five major biological phases" with the aim of preserving the simplicity of Todd's method while better accounting for variation (Meindl et al., 1985). Their work is being called into question because despite their awareness that sex differences are very real, they chose to minimize them. Furthermore, this group did not investigate the effect of racial differences, except to speculate that they might exist. The problem of temporal differences in aging at the pubic symphysis was also not addressed.

What was really needed was a test of both Meindl's team's modifications and the traditional standards on modern, contemporary cases, because other investigators have found evidence that the older standards can no longer be successfully applied. Specifically, recent studies have revealed that the original pubic symphyseal standards of Todd (1920, 1921a) and McKern and Stewart (1957) have not been effective for contemporary males (Angel et al., 1986). Therefore, Suchey and coworkers (Angel et al., 1986) used a sample of 739 well-documented modern male forensic specimens to modify and condense Todd's ten phases into five to account for changes in the rate and pattern of aging prevalent today. In another 1986 study, Katz and Suchey recommended a six-phase system. Subsequently, the six phases were again modified and reintroduced as the Suchey-Brooks standards, in which each phase was divided into two stages. (These standards, however, have not been published in detail.) Statistical analysis revealed significant differences in the mean age at death among whites, blacks, and Mexican-Americans in their sample (Katz and Suchey, 1987). Since the sample was not analyzed separately by race, they admitted that the standards will have to undergo further modification to account for what they now recognize as noticeable racial variation.

With regard to females, Suchey's team attempted to establish contemporary standards using 369 accurately documented pubes from modern forensic cases. However, they found that extreme morphological variability "made the formation of an aging system virtually impossible" (Angel et al., 1986).

Radiography

Radiographic assessment of the skeleton has been a valuable tool in the study of developmental changes and has led to the publication of universally applied standards of growth during childhood and adolescence (Greulich and Pyle, 1959; Pyle and Hoerr, 1969). Standards from the wrist, hand, knee, and foot have enabled physical anthropologists to assess physiological growth and associate it with chronological age. X-rays also allow researchers to determine dates of appearance of the centers of ossification in living infants as well as the sequence of epiphyseal closure in adolescents (Francis et al., 1939; Francis, 1940).

The use of radiography to estimate age from the skeleton in adults has been attempted since the introduction of x-ray technology itself. However, it is infrequently used because of the need for specialized training to interpret radiographs, the difficulty of standardized filming, and the expense involved in obtaining equipment and film (Krogman and İşcan, 1986; Sorg et al., 1989).

Radiographic techniques can assess age by evaluating several forms of skeletal change, including the involution of epiphyses and other cancellous bone, mineralization, measurement of cortical thickness, and determination of bone density. Of these, the most common assessment technique is based on the progression of endosteal resorption of the cortex with concomitant expansion of the marrow cavity, as exemplified in Figure 4. This analysis focuses on alterations in trabecular patterns.

One of the earlier attempts at radiographic age estimation was made by Todd in 1930. He defined four phases of pubic symphyseal metamorphosis commencing with individuals up to age 25 in phase 1 and covering lustra of approximately 15 years through phase 4, which represented specimens over 55. Changes in bone texture and the appearance and progression of a "grey streak of compacta" after age 25 were Todd's markers.

Most investigators in this field have concentrated on transformations in the proximal end of long bones. Schranz (1959) reported that age-related changes in the internal structure of the humerus were first observed by Wachholtz (1894) and later by Poirier and Charpy (1931), who studied macroscopic sections of fresh bone. Schranz (1933) found inaccuracies in their work and began research in 1927 using both bone sections and radiographic films. His results were later confirmed by Bruno (1934), Berndt (1947), and Hansen (1953). In his 1959 article, Schranz presented a composite of all findings on the humerus arranged in a chronological sequence from age 15 to over 75 years and cautioned that there are differences between the sexes. He pointed out that "radiography of the upper humerus should be used as a method of age determination only when the bones are too valuable to be sectioned."

Although work on the femur did not show as distinctive age changes as the humerus (Hansen, 1953; Jacqueline and Veraguth, 1954; Schranz, 1959), Schranz stated that "more is likely to be learned by studying the two bones together than either one alone." Nemeskéri and associates (1960) also concluded that chronological age could be better assessed by using a number of bones and, as part of their "complex method," developed six phases of radiologically observable morphological changes in the proximal humerus (Figure 4) and femur "relying on the data of previous authors and [their] own observations" (Acsádi and Nemeskéri, 1970).

Bergot and Bocquet (1976) studied the effects of age on trabecular and cortical bone in the humerus and femur and presented six stages of change in the trabecular pattern. They noted that except for the trabecular structures of the femur, there were pronounced differences between the sexes, with females showing a greater loss of both types of bone, especially after age 50. Furthermore, they found that demineralization does not occur with equal intensity in different parts of the same bone.

The most recent radiographic study (Walker and Lovejoy, 1985) compared the clavicle, calcaneus, proximal humerus, and femur. The aging process in the clavicle and proximal femur were divided into eight descriptive phases covering an age range of 15 to 75 years. They found the clavicle to be by far the best site for age estimation by this method, regardless of sex. The humerus and femur were intermediate, and the calcaneus showed virtually no consistent age-related change. The authors' results agreed with Bergot and Bocquet (1976) that bone loss is "highly site specific." All of these research groups warned that the major sources of errors arose from improper development of the x-rays and inconsistencies of interpretation when the cortex was measured either by different people or different devices. They stressed that experience is very important to the success of this technique.

Radiological evidence of age-related change at the costochondral junction has been noted for more than 50 years (Michelson, 1934; Falconer, 1938; Fischer, 1955; Semine and Da-

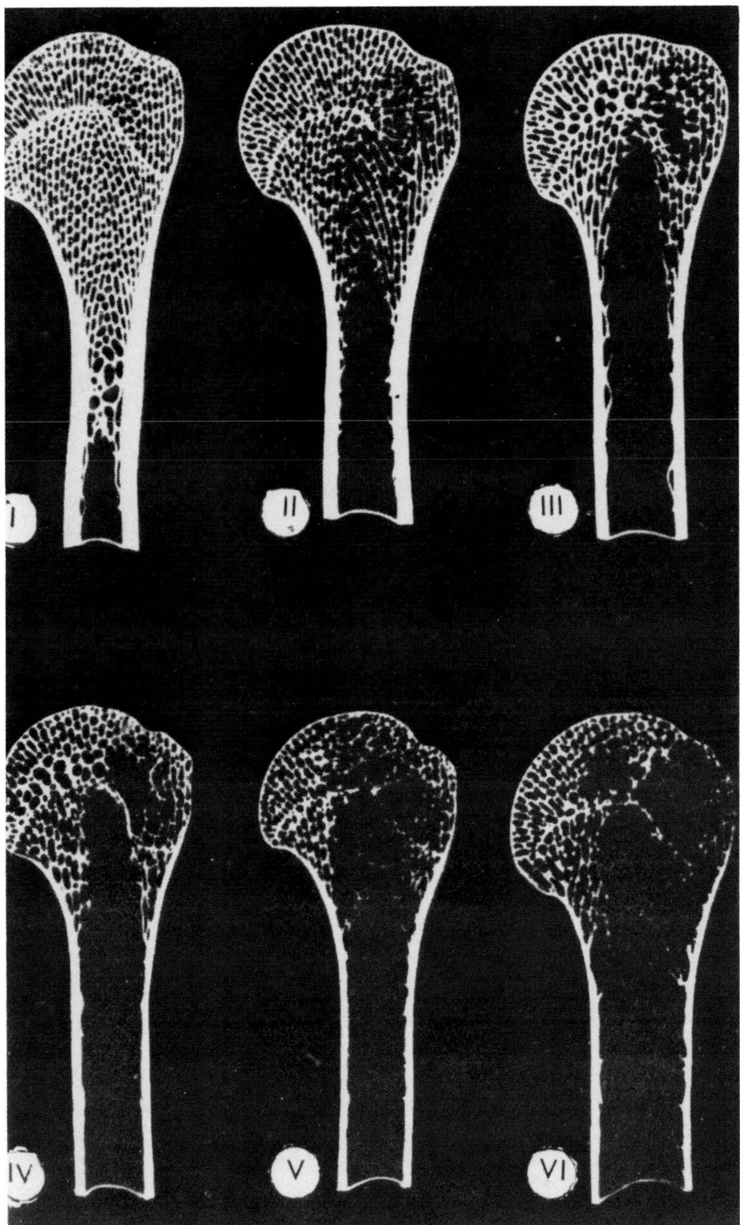

Fig. 4. Radiographically derived phases of structural changes in the spongy substance of the proximal epiphysis of the humerus illustrate the progressive loss of trabecular bone and cortical thinning, which first becomes noticeable after age 40. Changes between the ages of 41 and 62 proceed as follows: **I,** Medullary cavity apex below surgical neck; radial trabecular systems. **II,** Apex extends to surgical neck or above; trabecular systems more fragile. **III,** Apex extends to epiphyseal line; individual trabeculae thicken. **IV,** Apex extends to epiphyseal line or above; gaps appear in trabecular systems. **V,** Apex extends above epiphyseal line or above; lacunae form in major tubercle. **VI,** Trabecular system intensely rarified; cortex atrophied and fragile. Reproduced from Acsádi and Nemeskéri, 1970, with permission of Akadémiai Kiadó.

mon, 1975; McCormick and Stewart, 1988). However, these studies primarily focused on the rough correlation of age with mineralization of the costal cartilage. The most exhaustive of these studies was done by Semine and Damon (1975), who examined over 1,500 chest plates from five different populations. They obtained a linear correlation between increasing mineralization and age and uncovered interpopulational variation and definite sex differences. They concluded that "costochondral ossification has a close association with age and may well serve as an index of aging," but did not develop standards for this purpose (Semine and Damon, 1975).

Histology

Histological methods are based on age-related changes observable at the microscopic level. In bones, aging is monitored by histomorphometric quantification of the remodeling process reflected in the life cycle of the osteon. In the dentition, the emphasis shifts to a qualitative analysis of degenerative changes in the microstructure of the tooth.

Although histological assessment is more widely applied than radiography, it too is limited by the drawbacks of specialized equipment and the need for strict standardization of parameters (e.g., field size and tissue thickness). Microscopic examination also requires the destruction of bone and hours of complicated preparation necessary to produce the slides. Furthermore, even though this procedure is capable of giving a good estimation of age covering a long range, technical training is needed to become familiar with the nuances of bone histology in order to properly evaluate the sections. A detailed explanation and critique of histomorphometric techniques is provided by Stout (Chapter 4, this volume).

At present, two different sectioning techniques are used. The first was introduced by Kerley in 1965 and is based on the analysis of selected fields within a cross section of long bone. In order to reduce the destructiveness of obtaining an entire cross section, Thompson (1979) proposed a second method using a small diameter core of bone.

Histomorphometric aging methods have been developed for use on many different bones, including the femur, tibia, fibula, rib, clavicle, and mandibular ramus (Kerley, 1965; Ahlqvist and Damsten, 1969; Singh and Gunberg, 1970; Thompson, 1979; Stout, 1989). Like every other aging technique, it is affected by the physiological environment of the body. Histological methods do not account for individual variation arising from differences in endocrine function, physical activity, disease, trauma, and diet (Ortner, 1975; Stout, Chapter 4, this volume), and between and within the sexes (Ericksen, 1976).

Microscopy was first used to analyze dentition by Gustafson (1950), who cross-sectioned 37 teeth ranging in age from 11 to 69 years and observed progressive changes in six features of the dental microstructure: attrition, periodontosis, secondary dentin, cementum, root resorption, and root transparency. He ranked the status of each on a scale of 0–3, added the resultant scores, and used the total in a regression formula to obtain the age of the individual. Some problems with this method have been noted. Gustafson himself warned that poorly maintained teeth may look older, necessitating adjustment of the results. Others pointed out that sex and race should have been considered (Burns and Maples, 1976; Krogman and İşcan, 1986).

Twenty years later, Bang and Ramm (1970) studied a much larger sample (N = 158 males, 107 females) and found that one of Gustafson's criteria, root transparency, was adequate to use by itself. This feature was quantified by measuring the length of the transparent part of the root and developing three regression formulas based on these values. Although these authors separated their sample by sex, no significant differences were detected. They did note a tendency for older individuals to be underaged.

Another modification was attempted by Vlček and Mrklas (1975) using thin sections of single rooted teeth. While in general agreement with Gustafson's results, they did find that it was not possible to evaluate periodontosis and transparency in archaeological skeletal material.

Burns and Maples (1976) tested Gustafson's method and multiple regression formulas on a large sample (N = 355). They found the formulas somewhat more successful and concluded that sex, race, tooth position, and periodontal health status are significant variables in age estimation. A serial-sectioning technique was also introduced for undecalcified specimens that allowed analysis of asymmetrical and multirooted teeth.

Using the same sample, Maples (1978) tested various combinations of Gustafson's areas of change along with a consideration of tooth position using multiple regression statistics. He determined that the best results for aging were obtained from the "overall position weighted formula," which only necessitated the scoring of transparency and secondary dentin.

A comprehensive article covering dental histological aging from its inception to the most recent research was written by Kilian and Vlček (1989). In addition to the works of Gustafson (1950) and Maples (1978), these authors discussed and evaluated methods introduced by Johanson (1971), Falter (1974), Hiemer (1975), Pilin (1981), and Kilian (1986). They concluded that Kilian's method, which reported that over 75% of their estimates were within a range of ±5 years, has many advantages over the others, including the fact that an acceptable assessment can be obtained from only one tooth.

Tooth wear has been associated with age since Broca introduced his five-stage scale in 1897, and nearly all the succeeding works on this subject were modifications of his system (Lovejoy, 1985). Yamada (1931) suggested a macroscopic analysis of dental attrition for age estimation, but this concept was not actively pursued until nearly 20 years later when reviewed by Gustafson (1950). Detailed studies were performed by Hojo (1954) on the Japanese and Murphy (1959) on Australian aborigines (Brothwell, 1989). Probably the most commonly applied standards were charted by Brothwell (1981) and appear in his book *Digging Up Bones.*

With the exception of new standards derived from the archaeological Libben population by Lovejoy (1985), all of the post-1972 research in this area consisted primarily of tests of factors affecting dental attrition. Differences between the sexes ranged from nonexistent (Lunt, 1978) to slight but not statistically significant (Lovejoy, 1985). A number of studies have found that tooth wear rates and patterns vary widely among populations and can be affected by diet, jaw size, and chewing stresses (Miles, 1962; Lavelle, 1970; Molnar, 1971; Brothwell, 1981). Although significant correlations were made with other age indicators (Nowell, 1978; Lovejoy et al., 1985b), this method is not effective past age 50 (Miles, 1958). Finally, it should be pointed out that this type of analysis is better suited to archaeological remains, because the increased refinement of food minimizes wear in most contemporary populations.

A CAUTIONARY NOTE

The most fundamental priority in developing a reliable age estimation technique is the use of a skeletal assemblage for which there is dependable information on the age at death of the specimens. In their recent work on the Hamann-Todd collection, Lovejoy and associates (1985b) reminded us that the age assignation of these specimens was highly questionable. In the introduction to his work on the pubic symphysis, Todd (1920) addressed the problem of a lack of accurate age documentation in this collection. He stated that "for the vast proportion of skeletons . . . between 25 and 55, we have no reliable criteria of age and can make only the most hazardous guess even after long experience because experience without accurate data can result only in a quite general 'appreciation' of age." Information regarding the age of these individuals was either unreliable or nonexistent, and the ages of nearly all cadavera were estimated by Todd and other anatomists by comparing the often incorrectly stated age at death with a combination of external and skeletal characteristics. Although Todd (1920) was openly concerned about this problem and considered it very important to this type of research, he justified use of the collection on the grounds that "much greater confidence in the internal evidence of the skeleton itself upon the age problem" had been gained and no effort was spared "to obtain complete satisfaction in the question of age."

These concerns were extensively studied and discussed by Cobb (1952), who stated that the "existence of considerable dissatisfaction with the scientific validity and general utility of current methods of appraising age in the adult skeleton must be freely acknowledged." He further commented that the "lustral peaks of the . . . mortality curve . . . represent both antemortem subjective estimate as well as . . . postmortem objective guess," and "the skeletal assessment technique cannot purport to approximate the true age by more than seven years" in the adult and even more in old age (Cobb, 1952).

In their 1973 study on the female pubic bone, Gilbert and McKern pointed out that "estimations of the age of a great many individuals" in the Hamann-Todd collection "were rounded off to the nearest figure in five year periods." Lovejoy and associates (1985b) stated that only "three records were found to contain legal documentation of birth date," and, in most cases, the "stated ages were clearly gross approximations" with some screening by Todd and his coworkers until 1931. Lovejoy's group tried to minimize this problem by including only skeletons whose "stated age" and age observed by the anatomists were within ±5 years. They felt "confident that the great majority of specimens used in [the] tests had essentially known ages at death," although "a few represent approximations." However, Cobb's 1952 article stressed that in most cases, agreement between skeletal and stated ages, especially in individuals over age 60, resulted from the "inability of the skeletal appraiser to dispute them." This information, along with many other cogent revelations by Cobb, weakens any rationale for assuming "known age." Therefore, this situation must be carefully considered when assessing or applying age estimation techniques developed from the Hamann-Todd collection. Obviously, this caution also applies whenever a base sample is derived from or supplemented with undocumented specimens such as those obtained from archaeological populations.

SYNTHESIS

In this chapter, the advantages and disadvantages of numerous techniques and sites are discussed. For the most part, many researchers seem to have lost sight of the fact that each bone is only a single aspect of the skeleton and, by its nature, has a different function from all others. These functional differences no doubt affect the manifestations of age. Therefore, it has yet to be determined if one type of method and one region of the skeleton is best able to reflect correct chronological age or if a weighted combination will improve accuracy.

TABLE 1. Summary of Skeletal Regions Used To Assess Age-Related Changes

Skeletal regions	Assessment techniques: Morphology	Radiography	Histology
Cranium	Yes	No	Yes
Tooth	Yes	Yes	Yes
Clavicle	Yes	Yes	Yes
Rib	Yes	Yes	Yes
Auricular surface	Yes	Yes	No
Pubis	Yes	Yes	No

Three methodological approaches to the assessment of age in many parts of the skeleton are presented. Yet the intensity of specialization has precluded a comprehensive intermethodological comparison. Thus, the development of a new approach that will assess age-related changes in different parts of the human skeleton using combined analytical techniques is desirable.

The regions chosen for future study should include the rib, pubic symphysis, auricular surface of the ilium, clavicle, teeth, and cranium. They can be analyzed by gross morphological examination, radiographic observation, and histological techniques where appropriate. This study should reveal whether one particular part of the skeleton best reflects the actual age at death or whether a differential analysis involving two or more areas better accounts for individual and methodological variation (İşcan, 1986).

Table 1 summarizes these considerations by listing bones and recommended methods for evaluation and comparison in a study of this nature. In order for this or any other new method to lead to reliable and accurate results, its standards must be derived from a sample whose ages are precisely documented. In this regard, it is imperative to amass a modern skeletal collection with a carefully authenticated data base to serve not only for age assessment, but also for all other types of demographic determinations. Furthermore, because a number of studies have shown that the aging process is affected by sex and race, the specimens must first be separated by these variables.

Finally, the growth of our understanding of the aging process will advance with a better elucidation of the biological and cultural factors affecting it. Studies are needed to clarify the effects of genetics along with a host of internal and external influences, including disease, substance abuse, diet, endocrine function, physical activity, and mechanical and biological stresses. Only with this knowledge will we be able to separate the "normal" from the "abnormal" and actual aging from the highly variable effects of "wear and tear."

CONCLUSIONS

Since the beginning of serious study on age determination from the skeleton, experts have cautioned that several very important factors must be kept in mind. Despite Todd's warning in 1920 that "no individual part of the skeleton . . . is infallible, and the most accurate estimate of age can only be made after examination of the entire skeleton" and Graves's (1922) caution that a single bone "is only one of many skeletal features showing the ravages of time. Therefore, [an individual bone's] worth as a 'time-marker' should only be evaluated in connection with other bones . . . ," there has been a natural tendency toward a singular "tunnel vision" approach to age assessment. With few exceptions (Nemeskéri et al., 1960), the skeleton continues to be viewed as a disjointed collection of bones rather than an integrated system with each part showing the signs of age a little differently within the same individual. While there have been numerous efforts made to estimate age from several regions of the skeleton, many researchers continue to assume that each site equally reflects chronological age.

Skeletal perspective is not the only issue that must be entertained. A particularly important matter of which the profession has long been aware is the existence of inherent differences among individuals and populations. Yet these have been downplayed, if not ignored completely. Another dilemma arises from the passage of time, with its cultural and environmental changes. Schranz (1959) pointed out that when addressing the question of using recent standards on ancient man, "chronological and physiologicobiological ages are not identical. This difference may increase as we go back in time, just as today it varies among peoples living under different circumstances." Although it is only logical that these factors will affect the manifestations of the aging process, few have considered their importance when developing and applying aging techniques.

Currently, most conscientious practitioners assess age from several regions and informally "average" them out based on experience. However, these evaluations are derived from a collection of techniques developed from different individuals and populations rather than a set of multiregional and multimethodological standards from several parts of the same skeleton (İşcan, 1986). The latter approach could bring about a better understanding of the aging process itself in different parts of the body, as well as revealing whether any one site more consistently and accurately reflects chronological age.

The future lies in a multiregional approach—the intensive analysis and comparison of many sites on each individual skeleton to establish and quantify the relationship between the physiological and chronological manifestations of age. In this way, we will be able to find the best possible technique and bone for precise age determination and have a much better understanding of individual and intraskeletal variation in the aging process itself.

REFERENCES

Acsádi G, and Nemeskéri J (1970) History of Human Life Span and Mortality. Budapest: Akadémiai Kiadó.

Aeby C (1858) Über die symphyse ossium pubis des menschen nebst beiträgen zur lehre vom hyalinen knorpel und seiner verknöcherrungen. Z Rationelle Med, Series 3, 4:1–77.

Ahlqvist J, and Damsten O (1969) A modification of Kerley's method for the microscopic determination of age in human bone. J Forensic Sci 14:205–212.

Andersen BC (1986) Parturition scarring as a consequence of flexible pelvic architecture. Ph.D. dissertation, Simon Fraser University, Burnaby, B.C., Canada.

Angel JL, Suchey JM, İşcan MY, and Zimmerman MR (1986) Age at death from the skeleton and viscera. In MR Zimmerman and JL Angel (eds): Dating and Age Determination in Biological Materials. London: Croom Helm, pp 179–220.

Bang G, and Ramm E (1970) Determination of age in humans from root dentin transparency. Acta Odontol Scand 28:3–35.

Bergot C, and Bocquet J-P (1976) Étude systématique en fonction de l'age de l'os spongieux et de l'os cortical de l'humérus et du fémur. Bull Mem Soc Anthropol Paris 3 (Serie 13):215–242.

Berndt H (1947) Entwickelung einer röntgenologischen altersbestimmung am proximalen humerusende, etc. Z Gesamte Inn Med 2:122.

Broca P (1861) Sur le volume et le forme du cerveau suivant les individus et les races. Bull Soc Anthropol Paris II:139–207.

Brooke R (1924) The sacro-iliac joint. J Anat 58:299–305.

Brooks ST (1955) Skeletal age at death: Reliability of cranial and pubic age indicators. Am J Phys Anthropol 13:567–597.

Brothwell DR (1981) Digging Up Bones. Ithaca: Cornell University Press.

Brothwell DR (1989) The relationship of tooth wear to ageing. In MY İşcan (ed): Age Markers in the Human Skeleton. Springfield, IL: Charles C Thomas (in press).

Bruno G (1934) Über senile strukturveranderungen der proximalen humerusepiphyse. Fortschr Rontgenstr 50: 287.

Burns KR, and Maples WR (1976) Estimation of age from adult teeth. J Forensic Sci 21:343–356.

Cattaneo L (1937) Las suturas cranean en la determinacion de la edad. Examen de 100 craneos. Rev Assoc Med Argent 50:387–397.

Černý M (1983) Our experience with estimation of an individual's age from skeletal remains of the degree of thyroid cartilage ossification. Acta Univ Palacki Olomuc Fac Paedagogica Biologica 3:121–144.

Cobb WM (1952) Skeleton. In AI Lansing (ed): Cowdry's Problems of Ageing. Baltimore: Williams and Wilkins, pp 791–856.

Dwight T (1890a) The closure of the sutures as a sign of age. Boston Med Surg J 122:389–392.

Dwight T (1890b) The sternum as an index of sex, height and age. J Anat Physiol 24:527–535.

Ericksen MF (1976) Cortical bone loss with age in three native American populations. Am J Phys Anthropol 45: 443–452.

Falconer B (1938) Calcification of hyaline cartilage in man. Arch Pathol 26:942–955.

Falter G (1974) Altersbestimmung an Zähnen zur Identifizierung unbekennter Toter. Medical Dissertation München.

Fischer E (1955) Verkalkungsformen der rippenknorpel. Fortschr Geb Rontgenstr Nuklearmed 82:474–481.

Francis CC (1940) The appearance of centers of ossification from 6–15 years. Am J Phys Anthropol 27:127–138.

Francis CC, Werle PP, and Behm A (1939) The appearance of centers of ossification from birth to five years. Am J Phys Anthropol 24:273–299.

Fréderic J (1906) Untersuchungen über die normale obliteration der Schädelnahte. Z Morphol Anthropol 9:373–456.

Fréderic J (1909/1910) Die obliteration der nähte des gesichtsschadels. Z Morphol Anthropol 12:371–440.

Gilbert BM (1973) Misapplication to females of the standard for aging the male os pubis. Am J Phys Anthropol 38:39–40.

Gilbert BM, and McKern TW (1973) A method for aging the female os pubis. Am J Phys Anthropol 38:31–38.

Graves WW (1922) Observations on age changes in the scapula. Am J Phys Anthropol 5:21–33.

Greulich WW, and Pyle SI (1959) Radiographic Atlas of Skeletal Development of the Hand and Wrist. Stanford: Stanford University Press.

Gustafson G (1950) Age determinations on teeth. J Am Dent Assoc 41:45–54.

Hanihara K (1952) Age changes in the male Japanese pubic bone. J Anthropol Soc Nippon 62(698):245–260.

Hanihara K, and Suzuki T (1978) Estimation of age from the pubic symphysis by means of multiple regression analysis. Am J Phys Anthropol 48:233–240.

Hansen G (1953) Die alterbestimmung am proximalen humerus und femurende in rahmen der identifizierung menschlicher skelettreste. Wissenschaftliche Zeitschrift der Humboldt-Universität zu Berlin, Mathematisch-naturwissenschaftliche Reihe 3(1):1–73.

Hiemer R (1975) Untersuchungen zur Altersbestimmung an Zähnen. Medical Dissertation München.

Hojo M (1954) On the pattern of the dental abrasion. Okajimas Folia Anat Jpn 26:11–30.

Howells WW (1965) Age and individuality in vertebral lipping: Notes on Stewart's data. In Homenaje a Juan Comas en su Aniversario, Mexico, Vol. II, pp 169–178.

Hrdlička A (1939) Practical Anthropometry. Philadelphia: Wistar Institute.

İşcan MY (1986) Future directions in research on ageing: One method one bone or many methods and many bones. Am Acad Forensic Sci Program 1986, p 102 (abstract).

İşcan MY (ed) (1989) Age Markers in the Human Skeleton. Springfield, IL: Charles C Thomas (in press).

İşcan MY, and Derrick K (1984) Determination of sex from the sacroiliac joint: A visual assessment technique. Fla Sci 47:94–98.

İşcan MY, and Loth SR (1986a) Determination of age from the sternal rib in white males: A test of the phase method. J Forensic Sci 31(1):122–132.

İşcan MY, and Loth SR (1986b) Determination of age from the sternal rib in white females: A test of the phase method. J Forensic Sci 31(3):990–999.

İşcan MY, Loth SR, and Scheuerman EH (1989a) Assessment of intercostal variation on the estimation of age from the sternal end of the rib. Am J Phys Anthropol 78(2):245 (abstract).

İşcan MY, Loth SR, and Wright RK (1984a) Metamorphosis at the sternal rib end: A new method to estimate age at death in white males. Am J Phys Anthropol 65(2):147–156.

İşcan MY, Loth SR, and Wright RK (1984b) Age estimation from the rib by phase analysis: White males. J Forensic Sci 29(4):1094–1104.

İşcan MY, Loth SR, and Wright RK (1985) Age estimation from the rib by phase analysis: White females. J Forensic Sci 30(3):853–863.

İşcan MY, Loth SR, and Wright RK (1987) Racial variation in the sternal extremity of the rib and its effect on age determination. J Forensic Sci 32(2):452–466.

İşcan MY, Scheuerman EH, and Loth SR (1989b) Assessment of age from the combined use of the sternal end of the rib and pubic symphysis. Am Acad Forensic Sci Program 1989, p 116 (abstract).

Jacqueline F, and Veraguth P (1954) Étude radiologique de la tête fémoral du sujet agé. Rev Rheumatism 21:237.

Jit I, and Bakshi V (1986) Time of fusion of the human mesosternum with manubrium & xiphoid process. Indian J Med Res 83:322–331.

Johanson G (1971) Age determination from human teeth. Odontologisk Revy 22 (Suppl 21):1–126.

Katz D, and Suchey JM (1986) Age determination of the male os pubis. Am J Phys Anthropol 69:427–435.

Katz D, and Suchey JM (1987) Determination of age in the male os pubis: Consideration of the race variable. Am Acad Forensic Sci Program 1987, p 122 (abstract).

Kerley ER (1965) The microscopic determination of age in human bone. Am J Phys Anthropol 23:149–163.

Kerley ER (1970) Estimation of skeletal age: After about age 30 years. In TD Stewart (ed): Personal Identification in Mass Disasters. Washington, DC: National Museum of Natural History, pp 57–70.

Kilian J (1986) Urcování veku dospelých osob podle chrupu. Doktorská disertacní práce, Plzen.

Kilian J, and Vlček E (1989) Age determination from teeth in adult individuals. In MY İşcan (ed): Age Markers in the Human Skeleton. Springfield, IL: Charles C Thomas (in press).

Krogman WM (1949) The human skeleton in legal medicine: Medical aspects. In SA Levinson (ed): Symposium on Medicolegal Problems. Philadelphia: Lippincott, pp 1–92.

Krogman WM, and İşcan MY (1986) The Human Skeleton in Forensic Medicine. Springfield, IL: Charles C Thomas.

Lavelle CLB (1970) Analysis of attrition in adult human molars. J Dent Res 49:822–828.

Lenhössek M von (1917) Über Nahtverknocherung im Kindesalter. Arch Anthropol N F 15:164–180.

Loth SR (1988) Analysis of Terry Collection black ribs. Presented at the 12th International Congress of Anthropological and Ethnological Sciences, Zagreb, Yugoslavia, July 21–31. Collegium Antropol 12 (Suppl):300 (abstract).

Loth SR, and İşcan MY (1987) The effect of racial variation on sex determination from the sternal rib. Am J Phys Anthropol 72(2):227 (abstract).

Lovejoy CO (1985) Dental wear in the Libben population: Its functional pattern and role in the determination of adult skeletal age at death. Am J Phys Anthropol 68:47–56.

Lovejoy CO, Meindl RS, Pryzbeck TR, and Mensforth RP (1985a) Chronological metamorphosis of the auricular surface of the ilium: A new method for the determination of age at death. Am J Phys Anthropol 68:15–28.

Lovejoy CO, Meindl RS, Mensforth RP, and Barton TJ (1985b) Multifactorial determination of skeletal age at death: A new method with blind tests of its accuracy. Am J Phys Anthropol 68:1–14.

Lunt DA (1978) Analysis of attrition in adult human molars. In PM Butler and J Joysey (eds): Development, Function and Evolution of Teeth. London: Academic Press.

Maples WR (1978) An improved technique using dental histology for estimation of adult age. J Forensic Sci 23:747–770.

Masset C (1971) Erreurs systématique dans la détermination de l'âge par les sutures crâniennes. Bull Mem Soc Anthropol Paris 7:85–105.

Masset C (1989) Age estimation on the basis of cranial sutures. In MY İşcan (ed): Age Markers in the Human Skeleton. Springfield, IL: Charles C Thomas (in press).

McCormick WF, and Stewart JH (1988) Age related changes in the human plastron: A roentgenographic and morphological study. J Forensic Sci 33:100–120.

McKern TW, and Stewart TW (1957) Skeletal age changes in young American males. Analysed from the standpoint of age identification. Environmental Protection Research Division (Quartermaster Research and Development Center, U.S. Army, Natick, MA), Technical Report No. EP-45.

Meindl RS, and Lovejoy CO (1985) Ectocranial suture closure: A revised method for the determination of skeletal age at death and blind tests of its accuracy. Am J Phys Anthropol 68:57–66.

Meindl RS, Lovejoy CO, Mensforth RP, and Walker RA (1985) A revised method of age determination using the os pubis, with a review and tests of accuracy of other current methods of pubis symphyseal ageing. Am J Phys Anthropol 68:29–45.

Michelson N (1934) The calcification of the first costal cartilage among whites and negroes. Hum Biol 6:543–557.

Miles AEW (1958) The assessment of age from the dentition. Proc R Soc Med 51:1057–1060.

Miles AEW (1962) Assessment of the ages of a population of Anglo-Saxons from their dentitions. Proc R Soc Med 55:881–886.

Molnar S (1971) Human tooth wear, tooth function and cultural variability. Am J Phys Anthropol 34:175–190.

Murphy T (1959) The changing pattern of dentine exposure in human tooth attrition. Am J Phys Anthropol 17:167–178.

Nemeskéri J, Harsányi L, and Acsádi G (1960) Methoden zur diagnose des lebensalters von skelettfunden. Anthropol Anz 24:70–95.

Nowell GW (1978) An evaluation of the Miles method of ageing using the Tepe Hissar dental sample. Am J Phys Anthropol 49:261–276.

Ortner DJ (1975) Aging effects on osteon remodeling. Calcif Tissue Res 18:27–36.

Parsons FG, and Box CR (1905) The relation of the cranial sutures to age. J R Anthropol Inst 35:30–38.

Perizonius WRK (1984) Closing and non-closing sutures in 256 crania of known age and sex from Amsterdam (A.D. 1883–1909). J Hum Evol 13:201–216.

Pilin A (1981) Stomatologicka identifikace a moznosti urceni veku podle zubu. Kandidatska disertace, Praha.

Poirier P, and Charpy A (1931) Traite d'Anatomie Humaine. Paris: Masson.

Pyle SI, and Hoerr NL (1969) A Radiographic Standard Reference for the Growing Knee. Springfield, IL: Charles C Thomas.

Ribbe FC (1885) L'ordre d'oblitération des sutures du crâne dans les races humaines. These, Paris.

Sashin D (1930) A critical analysis of the anatomy and pathologic changes of the sacro-iliac joints. J Bone Joint Surg [Am] 12:891–910.

Schmidt E (1888) Anthropologische Methoden: Anleitung zum Beobachten und Sammeln für Laboritorium und Reise. Leipzig: Veit Co.

Schranz D (1933) Der oberarmknochen und seine gerichtlich-medizinische beteutung aus dem gesichtspunkte der identität. Deutsche Z Gesamte Gerichtl Med 22:332–361.

Schranz D (1959) Age determination from the internal structure of the humerus. Am J Phys Anthropol 17:273–278.

Semine AA, and Damon A (1975) Costochondral ossification and aging in five populations. Hum Biol 47:101–116.

Singer R (1953) Estimation of age from cranial suture closure: A report on its unreliability. J Forensic Med 1:52–59.

Singh IJ, and Gunberg DL (1970) Estimation of age at death in human males from quantitative histology of bone. Am J Phys Anthropol 33:373–383.

Sorg MH, Andrews RP, and İşcan MY (1989) Radiographic aging of the adult. In MY İşcan (ed): Age Markers in the Human Skeleton. Springfield, IL: Charles C Thomas (in press).

Stewart TD (1954) Metamorphosis of the joints of the sternum in relation to age changes in other bones. Am J Phys Anthropol 12:519–536.

Stewart TD (1958) The rate of development of vertebral osteoarthritis in American whites and its significance in skeletal age identification. Leech 28(3,4,5):114–151.

Stewart TD (1976) Sacro-iliac osteophytosis. Am J Phys Anthropol 44:210 (abstract).

Stout SD (1989) The use of cortical bone histology to estimate age at death. In MY İşcan (ed): Age Markers in the Human Skeleton. Springfield, IL: Charles C Thomas (in press).

Suchey JM (1979) Problems in the aging of females using the os pubis. Am J Phys Anthropol 51:467–470.

Thompson DD (1979) The core technique in the determination of age at death in skeletons. J Forensic Sci 24:902–915.

Todd TW (1920) Age changes in the pubic bone: I. The male white pubis. Am J Phys Anthropol 3:285–334.

Todd TW (1921a) Age changes in the pubic bone: II. The pubis of the male Negro-white hybrid; III. The pubis of the white female; IV. The pubis of the female Negro-white hybrid. Am J Phys Anthropol 4:1–70.

Todd TW (1921b) Age changes in the pubic bone: VI. The interpretation of variations in the symphyseal area. Am J Phys Anthropol 4:407–424.

Todd TW (1930) Age changes in the pubic bone: VIII. Roentgenographic differentiation. Am J Phys Anthropol 14:255–271.

Todd TW, and Lyon DW Jr (1924) Endocranial suture closure, its progress and age relationship: Part I. Adult males of white stock. Am J Phys Anthropol 7:325–384.

Todd TW, and Lyon DW Jr (1925a) Cranial suture closure, its progress and age relationship: Part II. Ectocranial closure in adult males of white stock. Am J Phys Anthropol 8:23–45.

Todd TW, and Lyon DW Jr (1925b) Cranial suture closure: Its progress and age relationship: Part III. Endocranial closure in adult males of Negro stock. Am J Phys Anthropol 8:47–71.

Todd TW, and Lyon DW Jr (1925c) Cranial suture closure: Its progress and age relationship. Part IV. Ectocranial closure in adult males of Negro stock. Am J Phys Anthropol 8:149–168.

Vlček E (1980) Odhad stári jedince stanovený na kosternim materiálu podle stupne osifikace chrupavky stitné. Soud Lek 25(3):45.

Vlček E, and Mrklas L (1975) Modification of the Gustafson method of determination of age according to teeth on prehistorical and historical osteological material. Scripta Medica (Brno) 48:203–208.

Wachholtz L (1894) Über die altersbestimmung an leichen auf grund des ossificationsprozesses im oberen humerusende. Friedreichs Blatter Gerichtl Med 45:210.

Walker RA, and Lovejoy CO (1985) Radiographic changes in the clavicle and proximal femur and their use in the determination of skeletal age at death. Am J Phys Anthropol 68:67–78.

Weisl H (1954) The articular surfaces of the sacro-iliac joint and their relation to movements of the sacrum. Acta Anat 22:1–14.

Yamada E (1931) On the relation of age to the abrasion of teeth in the Japanese. Juzenkai Z 36:456–468.

Yoshikawa E (1958) Changes of the laryngeal cartilages during the life and their application for determination of the probable age. Jpn J Legal Med (Nihon Hoigaku Zassi) 12: 1–40.

Zhang Z (1982) A preliminary study of estimation of age by morphological changes in the symphysis pubis. Acta Anthropol Sinica 1:132–136 [in Chinese].

Zimmerman MR, and Angel JL (eds) (1986) Dating and Age Determination in Biological Materials. London: Croom Helm.

Reconstruction of Life From the Skeleton

Chapter 4

Histomorphometric Analysis of Human Skeletal Remains

Sam D. Stout
Department of Anthropology, University of Missouri, Columbia, Missouri 65211

INTRODUCTION

Bone is not the relatively inert material it was once believed to be. It is, in fact, a dynamic tissue that is capable of responding to a broad range of stimuli, ranging from environmental and hereditary stresses to mechanical usage. In addition, unlike other tissues of the body, bone possesses the unique property of providing a "living, dynamic and durable record" of past metabolic events (Pirok et al., 1966).

Since 1960, the growth in our understanding of mammalian skeletal physiology has provided the means for extraction of the biological information encoded in the structure and composition of bone. A major factor leading to this new understanding was the recognition of a skeletal intermediary organization (IO) analogous to that existing in other organs of the body, such as the nephron of the kidney (Frost, 1983). In bone, the IO occupies the tissue level of organization, which bridges the gap between unassociated cells and intracellular materials and the organ level of bone structure (Fig. 1). Its major functions involve growth, modeling (changes in the geometry of bones), remodeling, repair, and homeostasis. The IO provides a basis upon which nonartifactual features of bone that are capable of being defined in skeletal remains can be interpreted as they relate to cellular activity (Frost, 1985b). This new understanding, sometimes referred to as the "new bone," has been reviewed by a number of authors (Frost, 1983, 1985a; Recker, 1983; Jaworski, 1984; Parfitt, 1984).

One area in which knowledge of the skeletal IO has expanded significantly is histomorphometry (quantitative histology). Because it has been demonstrated that histomorphology is often preserved in bone of considerable antiquity (Aeby, 1878; Graf, 1949; Ascenzi, 1955; Race et al., 1966; Stout and Teitelbaum, 1976a; Stout, 1978, 1983; Thompson and Trinkaus, 1981), paleohistology holds considerable promise for the field of anthropology. The purpose of this chapter is to discuss the use of bone histomorphometry for the analysis of human skeletal populations. In order to fully understand the uses and limitations of histomorphometric analysis, it will be necessary to first review some of the underlying histomorphometric principles.

The bone composing the skeleton of higher vertebrates is in a constant state of turnover, referred to as "remodeling." Bone remodeling responds to a number of factors—microdamage, mechanical usage, nutrition, hormones, and others, some yet to be identified (Frost, 1985b) (Table 1). The turnover occurs through the sequential removal (resorption) of packets of relatively constant bone volume through the activity of specialized cells called osteoclasts, followed by replacement of most, but not all, of the bone by osteoblasts (Fig. 2).

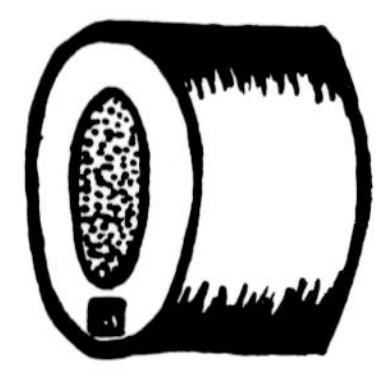

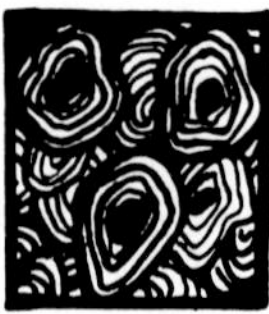

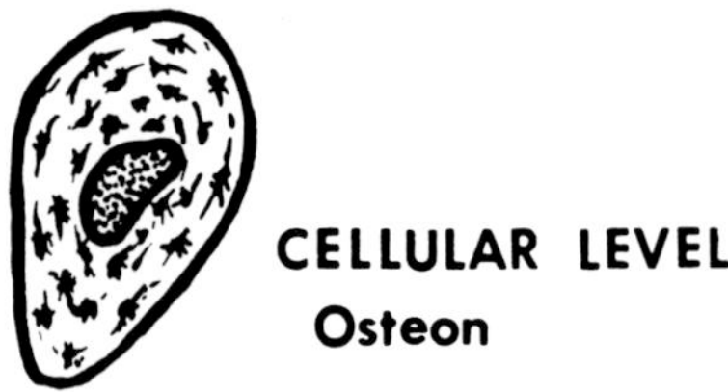

Fig. 1. Three levels of metabolic activity in bone remodeling (based on Frost, 1969).

In cortical bone, the packets of bone representing foci of remodeling activity are observable as discrete, quantifiable, and measurable structures (Figs. 2, 3). When viewed in a two-dimensional transverse cross section, the resorptive phase of remodeling activity is indicated by the presence of resorptive bays or cutting cones. These are clearly distinguished by the presence of scalloped borders resulting from the presence of Howship's lacunae. Resorption is followed by an inactive phase during which a dense irregular reversal line is laid down. The centripetal bone formation that follows next proceeds until all but a small central haversian canal remains, resulting in a completed haversian system or osteon. These are the basic structural units of cortical bone remodeling. Similar structural units probably also occur in trabecular and endosteal bone, but the complex nature of the geometry of these types of bone makes their measurement essentially impossible. For this reason, most of the methods of static histomorphometry, and those that are applicable to skeletal remains, relate to cortical bone.

The term "remodeling" has also been used to include bone formation and resorption drifts that are related to growth. This separate process, which has more recently been termed "modeling" (Frost, 1985b), involves the same kinds of cells as remodeling, but is distinct in several important aspects. Modeling serves to size and shape intact bones and modify the amount of bone in them to meet the needs of their typical peak mechanical loads (Frost, 1985b). Whereas remodeling continues throughout the life of the individual, modeling activity essentially stops once the bones of the skeleton reach their adult size and shape. Further, unlike remodeling, in which resorption and formation are coupled and occur in predetermined packets of bone, resorption and formation in modeling are independent and variable in duration. Except for the extent to which prior modeling activity is an important factor in the histomorphometrics of bone remodeling, it will not be discussed further here. For a review of the relation between biomechanical factors and bone geometry and histomorphology, the reader is referred to Burr (1980), Bouvier and Hylander (1981), Ruff and Hays (1983), Currey (1984), Schaffler and Burr (1984), and Frost (1985b). For excellent reviews of current histomorphometric methods, Anderson (1982) and Recker (1983) are recommended.

SAMPLE PREPARATION AND EQUIPMENT

Adequate sample preparation is essential to histological analysis. Every minute spent to im-

TABLE 1. Factors Known to Influence Osteonal Remodeling and Accumulated Osteon Populations

Age, chronologic	Regional trauma
Life span	Paralysis
Sex	Mechanical usage
Maturation, skeletal	Acute mechanical disuse
Species	Nutrition
Hormones	Metabolic alkalosis
Electrolyte disorders	Metabolic acidosis
Metabolic	Vitamins
Genetic disorders	Genetic structural disorders
Toxic agents	Microdamage
Radiation damage	Drugs
Bone growth	Mean tissue age
Bone remodeling patterns	Mechanical strain

Reproduced from Frost, 1985b, with permission of Yearbook of Physical Anthropology.

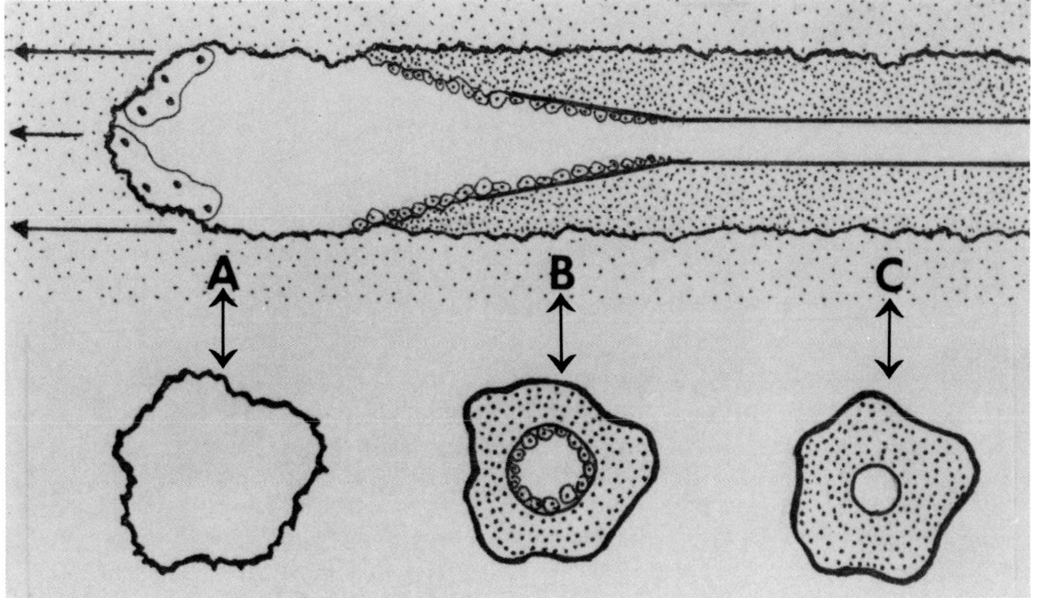

Fig. 2. A schematic illustration of the sequential processes involved in cortical bone remodeling that result in the production of an osteon or haversian system, as viewed both longitudinally and transversely. **A** represents the resorptive phase as indicated by the presence of a resorptive bay, **B** is illustrative of the formation phase, and **C** represents a completed osteon.

prove the quality of the microscopic section is repaid tenfold in ease of analysis and accuracy. Stout and Teitelbaum (1976a,b), Ubelaker (1978), and Anderson (1982) describe the preparation of undecalcified sections of bone. Following is a discussion of the aspects of sample preparation that relate specifically to the use of archaeological and paleontological material.

Because of the friability that often occurs in nonrecent bone, embedding is usually required to maintain the integrity of the sample during sectioning and grinding. There are a number of embedding compounds available commercially that are suitable for working with undecalcified bone, e.g., Castolite (Buehler), Bioplastic (Ward), and methylmethacrylate. Vacuum impregnation is advisable.

The exact procedures used to prepare nondecalcified thin sections vary according to the equipment and facilities available to the researcher. Initial removal of a section can be accomplished with a wide range of instruments, from geological rock saws to sophisticated thin-sectioning saws with diamond embedded blades.

Final section thickness for most purposes should be in the range of 50 to 100 μm, thin enough to permit microscopic analysis, yet thick enough to maintain structural integrity. In order to achieve the proper thickness, grinding is required; this can be accomplished manually with a minimum of equipment (Frost, 1958) or with the aid of automated grinders and petrographic slide holders, which ensure parallel surfaces and consistent section thicknesses.

The sections should be cleaned, cleared, mounted, and coverslipped as in standard histological procedures. Surface quality is considerably enhanced if the sections are allowed to soak in xylene overnight and then mounted without allowing them to dry. This procedure usually removes much of the cloudiness that often obscures histological features in archaeological specimens. Alternatively, a number of researchers use microradiographs, which are high-resolution x-rays of the bone section (Jowsey et al., 1965; Pankovich et al., 1974;

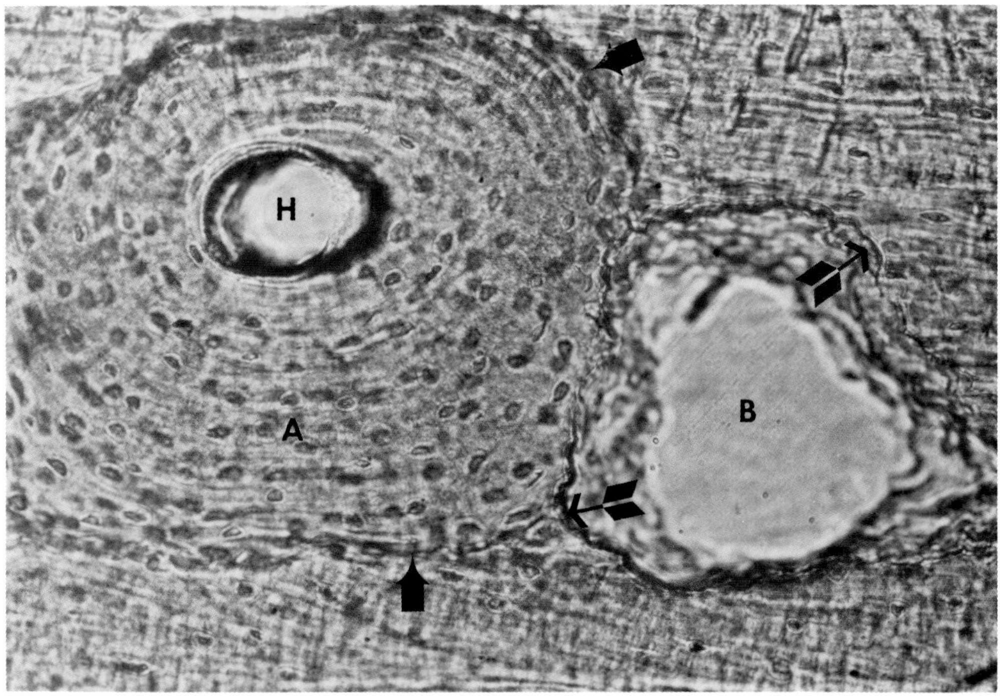

Fig. 3. Photomicrograph of both a completed osteon (A) and a resorptive bay (B). An haversian canal (H), cement line (darts), and scalloped border due to Howship's lacunae (arrows) are identified. Unstained ground section, magnification approximately ×20.

Richman et al., 1979; Martin, 1983). Microradiography provides the advantage of differentiating osteons in various states of maturity on the basis of their degree of mineralization (Fig. 4).

Histomorphometric analysis requires a relatively high-quality binocular research microscope, fitted with a suitable integrating eyepiece system that enables the measurement of field sizes and cross-sectional areas (Fig. 5). Descriptions of the use of integrating eyepieces can be found in Anderson (1982) Kimmel and Jee (1983).

METHODS

When undertaking histomorphological analysis, it is important that the researcher follow the definitions of variables as described for each particular method. Three commonly encountered definitions for complete secondary osteons, for example, are unremodeled systems (Wu et al., 1970), those systems in which 80% or more of their area is intact (Kerley, 1965), and those in which the haversian canal remains intact (Stout and Teitelbaum, 1976b). Fragmentary osteon definitions are, of course, complementary to the definition of complete osteon that is being used. It would be extremely useful if commonly agreed-upon definitions were established by histomorphometrists.

Use of Bone Histomorphometry to Estimate Age

Perhaps the most well-known use of histomorphometry in anthropology has been to estimate age at death for skeletal remains. The continuous bone remodeling from birth to death in the human is responsible for the observed association between number of osteons and chronological age (Amprino and Bairatti, 1936; Jowsey, 1960; Currey, 1964) and is the primary basis for histological age-predicting methods.

Currently, there are a number of histological age-estimating methods available; most are pri-

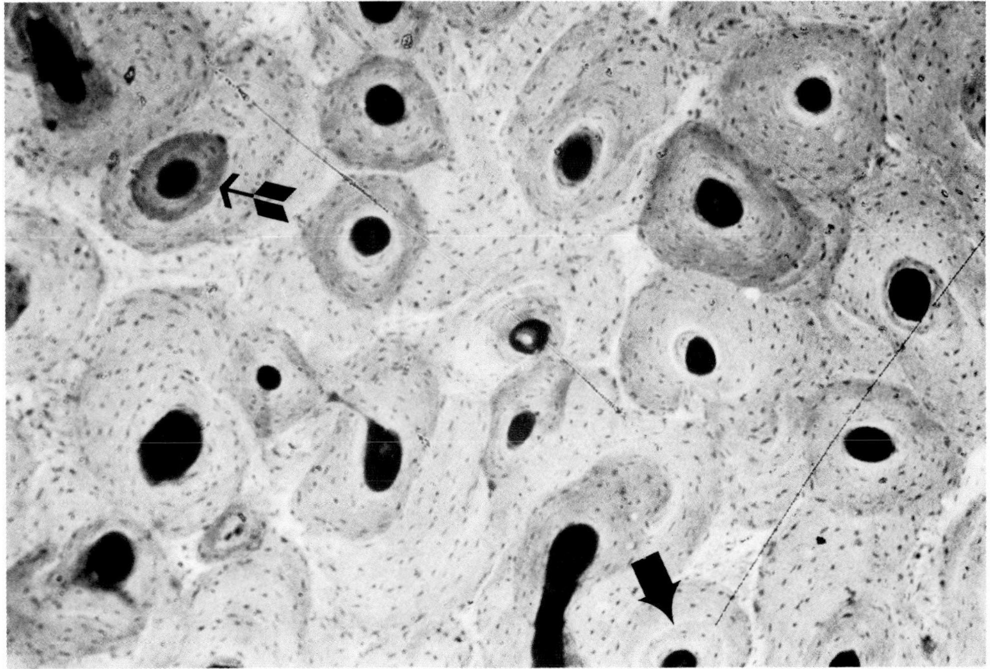

Fig. 4. Photomicroradiograph of a transverse section from a prehistoric Nubian femur. The arrow indicates a type II osteon, and the dart denotes the arrest line of a double zone osteon. (Photo courtesy of Dr. Debra Martin, Hampshire College.)

marily modifications of the original method introduced by Kerley (1965), as modified by Kerley and Ubelaker (1978). The various methods primarily provide predicting equations that are based upon different bones and/or microscopic field locations. Kerley's method (Kerley and Ubelaker 1978) utilizes complete transverse cross sections from the midshaft of the femur, tibia, and fibula. Histomorphological variables are quantified in four equidistant microscopic fields (anterior, posterior, medial, and lateral) tangential to the periosteal surface. In order to obviate the problem of distinguishing between complete and fragmentary osteons, Ahlqvist and Damsten (1969) have developed a method that is simply based on percent haversian bone measured in four fields in transverse cross sections from the midshaft of the femur. In addition, microscopic fields are chosen that are approximately midway between those required by Kerley's method in order to avoid the linea aspera region.

Comparisons of the above histological methods suggest that precision and accuracy differ among them. Bouvier and Ubelaker (1977) compared Kerley's (1965) method for the femur with that of Ahlqvist and Damsten (1969) and found Kerley's method to be more accurate. Stout and Gehlert (1980) tested the relative accuracy and reliability among Kerley's profile method (Kerley, 1965), all revised osteonal age-predicting equations (Kerley and Ubelaker, 1978), and Ahlqvist and Damsten's (1969) method, using an independent sample. It was concluded that averaging the ages resulting from Kerley and Ubelaker's (1978) regression equations provides the greatest accuracy and reliability (Table 2). In addition, research in the author's laboratory has found that although osteon counts exhibit a relatively strong age correlation, it is often not significantly different from zero for percent haversian bone. For a more detailed review of the use of histomorphology to estimate age at death, see Stout (1989).

There are also a number of other methods that are available; they have not yet been adequately tested on independent samples, how-

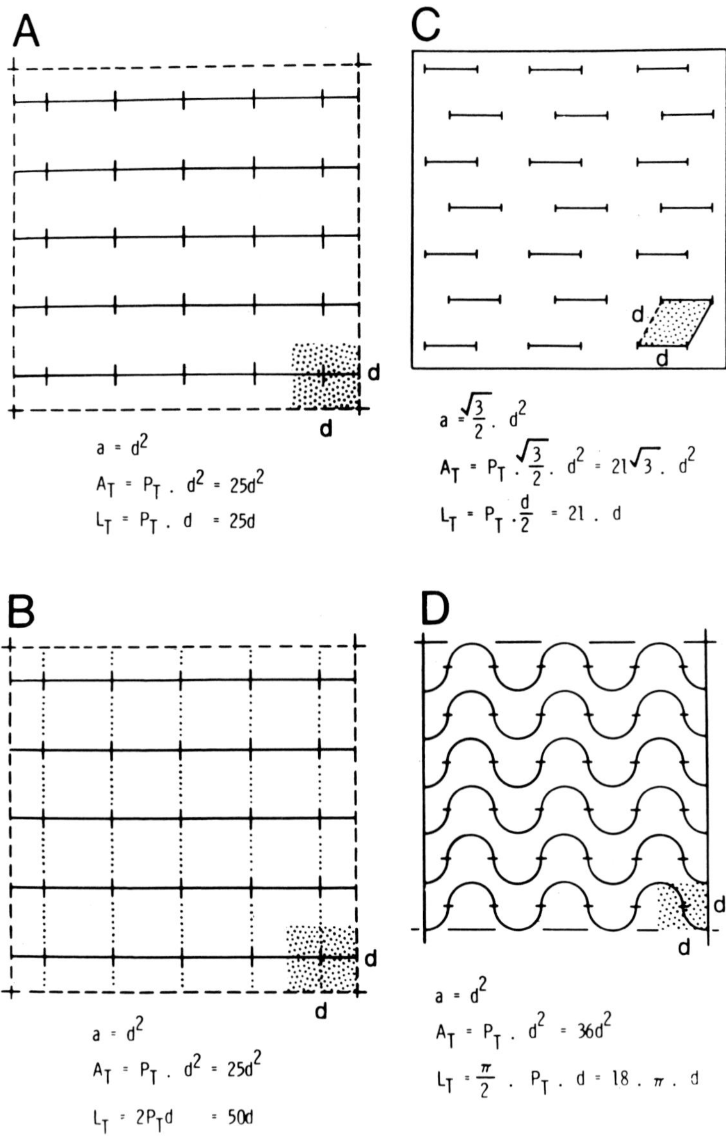

Fig. 5. Illustration of several types of integrating eyepieces used in histomorphometry. **A:** Zeiss Integrationsplatte II; **B:** same, with interpolated vertical as well as horizontal lines; **C:** Weibel grid; **D:** Merz grid. (Reproduced from Parfitt, 1983, with permission of CRC Press.)

ever they do offer certain advantages that make them worth considering. Singh and Gunberg (1970) have developed a method that employs multiple linear regression using three histomorphological variables: number of complete osteons, average number of lamellae per osteon, and average haversian canal diameter. They provide predicting equations for various combinations of the three variables determined from two randomly chosen microscopic fields located in the anterior midshaft of the femur and tibia and the posterior border of the mandibular ramus. The authors claim an accuracy of within six years of the true value in 95% of human males. It should be noted that Singh and Gunberg's (1970) method is based on a sample that consisted exclusively of adult males.

TABLE 2. Ranking of Histological Aging Methods on the Basis of Both Accuracy and Reliability[a]

1. Mean regression[b]
2. Femur osteon fragments
3. Femur intact osteons
4. Profile method of Kerley (1965)
5. Tibia intact osteons
6. Modified method of Ahlqvist and Damsten (1969)
7. Fibula osteon fragments
8. Fibula intact osteons
9. Tibia osteon fragments

[a] Independent sample of 13 cadavers with an age range of 13 to 102 years. Accuracy and reliability were based on mean differences between predicted and known age and predicted ages by two observers, respectively. Based on Stout and Gehlert (1980) and Stout (1989).
[b] Age estimated by averaging the results by the regression equations of Kerley and Ubelaker (1978).

Thompson (1979) has developed a core technique that employs multiple regression for combinations of a relatively large number of variables (19), e.g., osteon area, cortical thickness, osteon counts, osteon size, and cortical bone density. Contrary to the independent comparisons among methods discussed above, Thompson (1979) found osteon area to be the best single predictor of age. Since it employs only a 0.4 cm diameter core of bone from the anterior midshaft of a long bone, this method has the advantage of being less invasive than other methods that require complete cross sections of bone. In addition, Thompson (1979) provides formulas applicable to bones of the upper extremity. The use of only a single small core, however, raises the question of sampling error, particularly that due to incoherence, described by Frost (1969) as random variation of one unit of tissue to an adjacent comparable unit.

In response to the need for a method with which to estimate age when no long bones are available, a histomorphometric age-predicting technique that utilizes the middle third of the sixth rib and midshaft of the clavicle was developed in the author's laboratory (Paine, 1983; Stout, 1986). Because biomechanical factors have been shown to affect cortical bone remodeling (Bouvier and Hylander, 1981; Lanyon et al., 1982; Stout, 1982; Schaffler and Burr, 1984), the use of non-weight-bearing bones such as the rib and clavicle should be further explored. There are several additional advantages to this method. Entire cross sections are read, thus avoiding the problem of field location. Values from at least two sections per bone are used in order to minimize sampling error. Osteon counts are expressed in terms of number per unit area, which, along with the reading of the entire cross section, eliminates the problem of field size corrections. Finally, intact and fragmentary osteon densities are summed to produce total visible osteon density, thus minimizing errors due to different interpretations of what constitutes a complete or fragmentary osteon. Table 3 presents the results of a test of this method for the rib.

Histomorphometric Measurement of Bone Remodeling Dynamics in Ancient Skeletal Populations

As noted above, bone remodeling is affected by a number of factors other than chronological age (Table 1). A number of researchers have begun to apply our new understanding of bone remodeling dynamics to estimate several parameters of bone remodeling activity in extinct human populations, leading toward the realization of what might be called paleophysiology.

Ericksen (1973) compared patterns of age-associated changes in the cortical bone histomorphology of three aboriginal American skeletal populations (Eskimo, Arikara, and Pueblo) to investigate possible effects of environmental and genetic factors on intracortical remodeling. The methodology employed was a modification of that reported by Kerley (1961, 1965). It should be noted that the modifications were significant. The bone samples consisted of 1.27 cm cores from the anterior midshaft of the femurs, rather than complete transverse cross

TABLE 3. Test of New Rib Age-Predicting Formula Using Mean Total Visible Osteon Densities and Known Mean Ages Reported by Wu et al. (1970)

Total visible osteon density	Age	Predicted age[a]
9.8	15.8	15.8
12.7	23.2	24.1
17.4	36.0	37.6
19.3	46.1	43.1
21.1	53.7	48.3

[a] Predicting formula is age (yrs) = −12.3490 + 2.87351 (total visible osteon density), N = 63, $r = 0.68244$.

sections, and the definitions of complete and fragmentary osteons were different from those used by Kerley (1965).

Ericksen found that the patterns of age-associated remodeling in the archaeological populations were comparable to those of modern samples reported by Kerley (1965). Contrary to the findings for modern skeletal samples, however, a difference between sexes was found. While the relative magnitudes of remodeling for males, as reflected in osteon counts, did not differ among the populations, those for females did. Eskimo females exhibited the highest density of osteons per unit area, and Pueblo females the lowest. The Arikara females generally fell into an intermediate category, although some anomalies in the sample made their comparison tentative. Ericksen suggests that the observed differences reflect dietary and/or physical activity differences among the populations, specifically the high-protein diet of the Eskimo and low-protein diet of the sedentary Pueblo populations. Two additional indicators of cortical bone remodeling—type II and zonal osteons—have been described by a number of authors (Jaworski et al., 1972; Ortner, 1974; Pankovich et al., 1974; Richman et al., 1979) employing microradiography (Fig. 4). Type II osteons have been reported to represent evidence of intraosteonal remodeling in response to the demands of mineral homeostasis (Richman et al., 1979; Martin, 1983), whereas zonal osteons represent recovery and resumption of normal growth after a severe stress (Stout and Simmons, 1979). Stout and Simmons (1979) suggested that zonal osteons represent growth disturbances affecting the centripetal radial closure rate of bone formation and are comparable to Harris lines. Therefore, they should show a relative increase in individuals with nutritional deficiencies.

Richman et al. (1979) compared the relative incidences of type II structures in the femur among the same three aboriginal American populations used in the study by Ericksen (1973) discussed above. The Eskimo, considered to have a high-protein diet, exhibited the highest degree of type II remodeling. These authors suggested that this might be due to the accelerated mobilization of calcium in a high-protein diet, which is characterized by metabolic acidosis, bone loss, and hypercalciuria. In contrast, the Pueblo population, with a low-protein diet, as lowest in type II structures. Unlike the findings by Ericksen, no interpopulational difference was found for the frequency of type I osteons, and no difference was observed between the sexes.

In a recent study of the intraskeletal variability of type II and zonal osteons using modern cadaver samples, Kidder and Stout (1986) found a significant association between type II osteons and a disease classification that included diseases such as cancer, diabetes mellitus, immobilization, senile osteoporosis, and heart condition. However, no association was found between disease and zonal osteons.

Wu et al. (1970) described a methodology by which cortical bone formation rates could be estimated for the human rib without the use of tissue time markers and further suggested that it should be applicable to ancient bone. The method is primarily based on the physiological basis of cortical bone histomorphometry as described above. Since some of the underlying principles may be arcane to non-histomorphometrists, a brief summary of the method follows.

Total visible osteon density, the sum of the intact and fragmentary osteon population densities, represents all visible remains of past cortical remodeling activity in a given cross section of bone. Total osteon creations, an indirect measurement of the actual total number of osteons created throughout the life span of the individual, must be derived. It takes into account those osteons that were created in the past but have been totally obliterated by subsequent remodeling activity. This parameter is determined from Figure 6, which graphically presents the relation between total osteon creations and total visible osteon density for the middle third of the human sixth rib based on in vivo labeling studies. It assumes a mean osteonal cross-sectional area of 0.037 mm^2. For those individuals in whom the measured mean osteonal area does not equal 0.037 mm^2, total visible osteon density is multiplied by a correction factor determined by dividing observed mean osteonal cross-sectional area by 0.037 mm^2. Total osteon creations are then determined from Figure 6 using this derived value for total visible osteon density. Frost (1987) has recently proposed a means by which this relation can be more accurately defined by taking into account perturbations due to adult-life

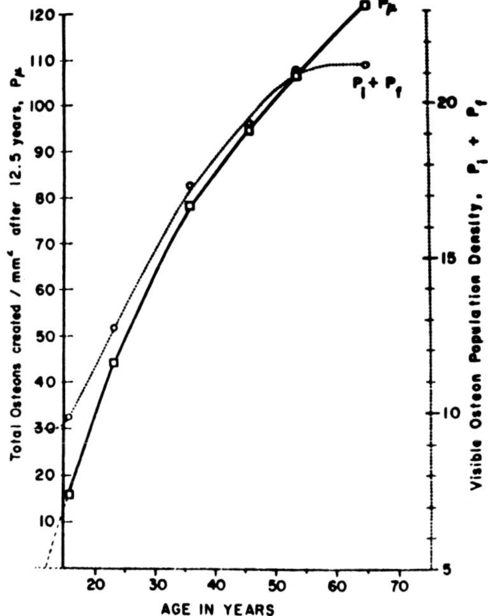

Fig. 6. Graph illustrating the relation between total visible osteon number and actual total osteon creations (reproduced from Wu et al., 1970, with permission of Calcified Tissue Research).

modeling drifts and a cortical thickness/osteon diameter effect.

Mean annual osteon creation frequency, the total osteon creations determined for an individual rib divided by the effective age of adult compacta is next calculated. It is the average annual rate at which osteon creations, and thus basic structural units of remodeling, occurred. Effective age of the adult compacta is used rather than chronological age because the increase in cross-sectional diameter of long bones and transverse cortical drifts, which occur during the growth period, rapidly remove evidence of remodeling activity (Fig. 7). The earliest age at which histomorphological features observed in the middle third of the sixth rib in the human adult could have been created has been determined to be approximately 12.5 years (Wu et al., 1970). Effective age of the adult compacta, therefore, is chronological age minus 12.5 years. Mean annual haversian bone formation rate is finally determined by multiplying the mean annual osteon creation frequency for an individual by the mean osteonal cross-sectional area, which represents the amount of bone added with each new osteon creation.

Stout and Teitelbaum (1976b) have adapted and applied this method to archaeological skeletal material. Mean annual osteon creation and bone formation rates determined for a midwestern Late Woodland population compared favorably with values for an age-matched modern sample. The authors concluded that these two parameters of bone remodeling can be reliably determined for nonrecent skeletal remains.

Using this same methodology, Stout (1983) compared the bone remodeling dynamics of several ancient New World populations, including the Middle Woodland Gibson and Ray sites and Late Woodland Ledders site from Illinois, and the Archaic Peruvian site of Paloma, which is dated at between 7700 B.P. and 5000 B.P. Although all histomorphometric values for the populations fell within the ranges reported for modern hospital and cadaver samples, one population—Ledders, the only maize agricultural population in the study—exhibited consistently higher cortical bone remodeling rates

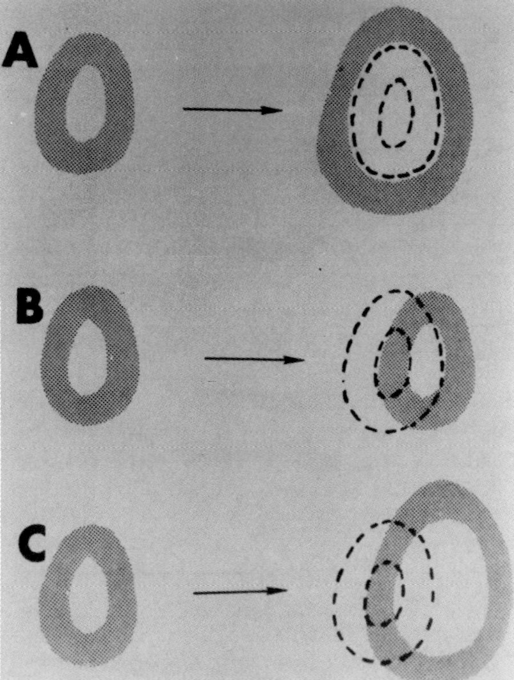

Fig. 7. Illustration of the effect of growth (**A**) and cortical drift (**B**) on the cross section of a bone. **C** illustrates the combined effects of A and B (redrawn from Frost, 1973).

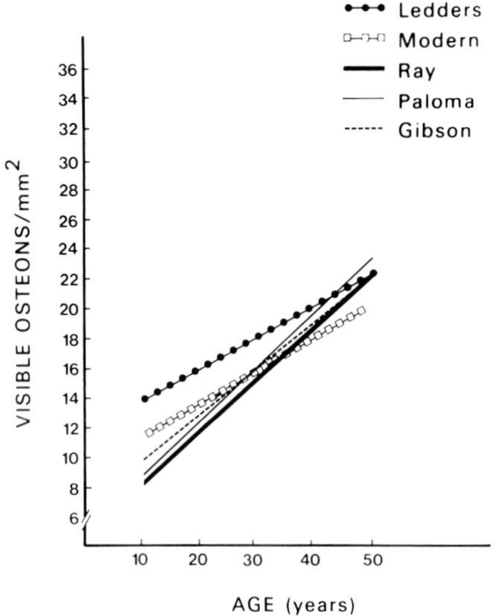

Fig. 8. A comparison of age-associated total visible osteon counts for the rib among four archaeological populations—the Archaic Paloma site, Peru; Middle Woodland Ray and Gibson and Late Woodland Ledders sites from southern Illinois—and a modern cadaver sample (reproduced from Stout, 1983, with permission of Anthropos (Greece)).

(Fig. 8). These findings might reflect dietary differences because maize is poor in calcium and high in phosphorous, a combination which, if relied upon heavily, could lead to reduced serum calcium levels and thus induce increased levels of parathyroid hormone. Parathyroid hormone is known to be a general stimulator of bone remodeling.

The extensive collaborative work on prehistoric Nubian skeletal remains provides an example of the combined use of several of the above histomorphometric parameters. The relation between histomorphometric indicators of bone turnover and the age of onset, patterning, and frequency of cortical bone loss as a function of sex was examined by Martin and Armelagos (1979) and Martin et al. (1981). They reported that a greater loss of cortical bone in females, particularly in the third decade, is associated with higher frequencies of resorptive spaces, suggesting increased resorption (or activation frequencies) and higher frequencies of forming osteons, a possible indication of decreased osteonal bone formation rates. After the third decade, no difference in frequencies was found between the sexes. In a more recent study, Martin (1983) reported finding evidence for different mechanisms underlying bone loss in young adult and postmenopausal females. While postmenopausal females exhibit the classic picture of reduced turnover, young adult females appear to have accelerated turnover. It was further noted that individuals with reduced cortical bone mass also exhibited reduced frequencies of double zone osteons and increased frequencies of type II osteons. Martin (1983) concluded that the females of this population are reflecting reduced calcium levels due to nutritional stress exacerbated by pregnancy and lactation.

A study of the effects of long-term immobilization on the histomorphology of human cortical bone serves as a final example of the uses of histomorphometrics for the analysis of human skeletal remains (Stout, 1982). A comparison was made of the osteon population densities for the major long bones and sixth ribs of two individuals with neurological deficits. One was a multiple sclerosis patient who had been in a wheelchair for 15 years; the other was a quadriplegic for 26 years as a result of bulbar poliomyelitis. Significantly lower osteon population densities were observed for most of the quadriplegic's bones when compared to age-matched values. Values for the M.S. individual were not significantly different from normal. These findings are explained by the fact that the quadriplegic represents true disuse osteoporosis, whereas the individual with M.S. had impaired control of the limbs, which were most likely spastic, and therefore retained a degree of mechanical loading of bones by muscle contraction. Most interesting was the observation that those bones that were not significantly different in the quadriplegic were those of the right arm, the limb for which the individual had retained some use (Fig. 9).

CONCLUSIONS

In conclusion, histomorphometric analysis of archaeological skeletal populations can reveal valuable information concerning the health and disease of individuals in extinct populations. The population-level histomorphometrics provides a measure of health that can be compared among populations with various genetic backgrounds, diets, and life-styles. Such comparisons can point to factors that affected health and disease in past populations

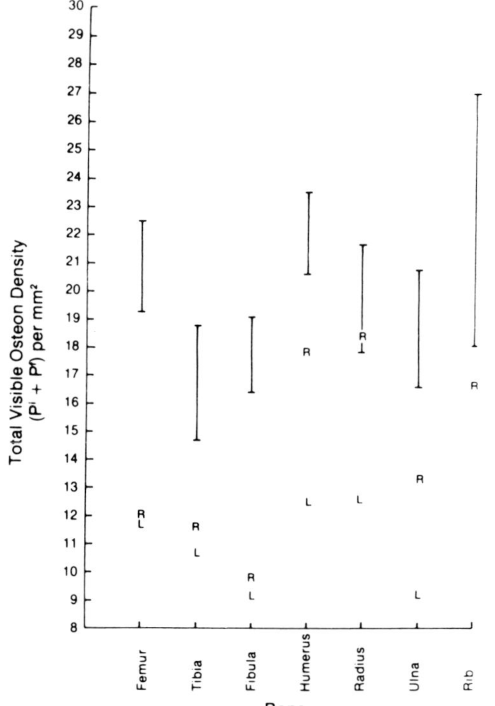

Fig. 9. Total visible osteon creations (intact plus fragmentary osteon densities) for a 51-year-old quadriplegic, compared to an age-matched nonimmobilized sample. Bars represent the 95% confidence limits for the mean value for each bone in the age-matched sample (reproduced from Stout, 1982, with permission of Calcified Tissue International).

and that might be worth closer investigation today. At present, the identification of relatively specific factors that may account for observed population differences in bone remodeling dynamics, although thought-provoking, must remain highly tentative. This is because bone remodeling provides a common pathway that satisfies many needs (Frost, 1985b). The future lies in basic research that will allow us to distinguish among specific factors that can be demonstrated to affect bone remodeling and become encoded in its histomorphology. Only then will the potential of histomorphometry be fully realized.

ACKNOWLEDGMENTS

The author is grateful to Mr. Mark Jones for the original art work for Figure 2 and to Dr. James Gavan for his critical reading of the manuscript and helpful comments. Dr. Harold Frost has been a major influence in the uses of bone histomorphometry and continues to provide encouragement and direction for the future. Finally, the author is indebted to Drs. İşcan and Kennedy for the opportunity to discuss the use of histomorphometry for the analysis of skeletal remains.

REFERENCES

Aeby C (1878) Das histologische verhalten fossilen knochen-und-zahngewebes. Arch Mikrosk Anat 15:371–382.

Ahlqvist J, and Damsten O (1969) Modification of Kerley's method for the microscopic determination of age in human bone. J Forensic Sci 14:205–212.

Amprino R, and Bairatti EA (1936) Processi di ricostruzione e di riassorbimento nella sostanza compatta delle osa dell nomo. Richerche see cento soggetti della nascita sino a tarda eta. Z Zellforsch Mikrosk Anat 24:439–511.

Anderson C (1982) Manual for the Examination of Bone. Boca Raton, FL: CRC Press.

Ascenzi A (1955) Some histological properties of the organic substance in Neanderthal bone. Am J Phys Anthropol 13:557–566.

Bouvier M, and Hylander WL (1981) The effect of bone strain on cortical bone structure in macaques (*Macaca mulatta*). J Morphol 167:1–12.

Bouvier M, and Ubelaker D (1977) A comparison of two methods for the microscopic determination of age at death. Am J Phys Anthropol 46:391–394.

Burr D (1980) The relationships among physical, geometrical and mechanical properties of bone, with a note on the properties of nonhuman primate bone. Yrbk Phys Anthropol 23:109–146.

Currey JD (1964) Some effects of aging in human haversian systems. J Anat 98:69–75.

Currey JD (1984) The Mechanical Adaptation of Bones. Princeton: Princeton University Press.

Ericksen MF (1973) Age-related bone remodeling in three aboriginal American populations. Unpublished Ph.D. dissertation, George Washington University, Washington, DC.

Frost HM (1958) Preparation of thin, undecalcified bone sections by a rapid manual method. Stain Technol 33: 272–276.

Frost HM (1969) Tetracycline-based histological analysis of bone remodeling. Calcif Tissue Res 3:211–237.

Frost HM (1973) Bone Remodeling and Its Relationship to Metabolic Bone Diseases. Springfield, IL: Charles C Thomas.

Frost HM (1983) The skeletal intermediary organization. A review. J Metab Bone Dis Rel Res 4:281–290.

Frost HM (1985a) The Skeletal Intermediary Organization. Boca Raton, FL: CRC Press.

Frost HM (1985b) The "new bone": Some anthropological potentials. Ybk Phys Anthropol 28:211–226.

Frost HM (1987) Secondary osteon populations. An algorithm for estimating the missing osteons. Ybk Phys Anthropol 30:239–254.

Graf W (1949) Preserved histological structure in Egyptian mummy tissues and ancient Swedish skeletons. Acta Anat 8:236–250.

Jaworski ZFG (1984) Lamellar bone turnover system and its effector organ. Calcif Tissue Int (Suppl) 36:546–555.

Jaworski ZFG, Meunier P, and Frost HM (1972) Observations on two types of resorption cavities in human lamellar cortical bone. Clin Orthop 83:279.

Jowsey J (1960) Age changes in human bone. Clin Orthop 17:210–218.

Jowsey J, Kelly PJ, Riggs BL, Bianco AJ, Scholz DA, and Gershon-Cohn J (1965) Quantitative microradiographic studies of normal and osteoporotic bone. J Bone Joint Surg [Br] 47:785–872.

Kerley ER (1961) The microscopic determination of age in human bone. Unpublished Ph.D. dissertation, University of Michigan, Ann Arbor.

Kerley ER (1965) The microscopic determination of age in human bone. Am J Phys Anthropol 23:149–164.

Kerley ER, and Ubelaker DH (1978) Revisions in the microscopic method of estimating age at death in human cortical bone. Am J Phys Anthropol 49:545–546.

Kidder L, and Stout SD (1986) The intraskeletal variability of type II and double zone osteons. Unpublished manuscript.

Kimmel DB, and Jee SS (1983) Measurements of area, perimeter, and distance: Details of data collection in bone histomorphometry. In RR Recker (ed): Bone Histomorphometry: Techniques and Interpretations. Boca Raton, FL: CRC Press, pp 89–108.

Lanyon LE, Goodship AE, Pye CJ, and MacFie JH (1982) Mechanically adaptive bone remodeling. J Biomech 15: 141–154.

Martin DL (1983) Paleophysiological aspects of bone remodeling in the Meroitic, X-Group and Christian populations from Sudanese Nubia. Unpublished Ph.D. dissertation, University of Massachusetts, Amherst.

Martin DL, and Armelagos GJ (1979) Morphometrics of compact bone: An example from Sudanese Nubia. Am J Phys Anthropol 51:571–578.

Martin DL, Armelagos GJ, Mielke JH, and Meindl RS (1981) Bone loss and dietary stress in an adult skeletal population from Sudanese Nubia. Bull Mem Soc Anthropol Paris 8(13):307–319.

Ortner DJ (1974) Aging effects on osteon remodeling. Calcif Tissue Res 18:27–36.

Paine RR (1983) Histological aging utilizing clavicles and ribs. Unpublished MA research paper, Department of Anthropology, University of Missouri, Columbia.

Pankovich AM, Simmons DJ, and Kulkarmi VV (1974) Zonal osteons in cortical bone. Clin Orthop 100:356–363.

Parfitt AM (1983) Stereologic basis of bone histomorphometry; theory of quantitative microscopy and reconstruction of the third dimension. In RR Recker (ed): Bone Histomorphometry: Techniques and Interpretation. Boca Raton, FL: CRC Press, pp 53–87.

Parfitt AM (1984) The cellular basis of bone remodeling. The quantum concept reviewed in the light of recent advances in the cell biology of bone. Calcif Tissue Int (Suppl) 36:538–545.

Pirok DJ, Ramser JR, Takahashi H, Villanueva AR, and Frost HM (1966) Normal histological tetracycline and dynamic parameters in human mineralized bone sections. Henry Ford Hosp Med Bull 14:195–218.

Race GJ, Fry EI, Mathews JL, Martin JH, and Lynn JA (1966) The characteristics of ancient Nubian bone by collagen content, light and electron microscopy. Clin Pathol 45:704–713.

Recker RR (1983) Bone Histomorphometry: Techniques and Interpretation. Boca Raton, FL: CRC Press.

Richman EA, Ortner DJ, and Schulter-Ellis FP (1979) Differences in intracortical bone remodeling in three aboriginal American populations: Possible dietary factors. Calcif Tissue Int 28:209–214.

Ruff CB, and Hays WC (1983) Cross-sectional geometry of Pecos Pueblo femora and tibia—a biomechanical investigation: Method and general patterns of variation. Am J Phys Anthropol 60:359–381.

Schaffler MB, and Burr DB (1984) Primate cortical bone microstructure: Relationship to locomotion. Am J Phys Anthropol 65:191–197.

Singh IJ, and Gunberg DL (1970) Estimation of age at death in human males from quantitative histology of bone fragments. Am J Phys Anthropol 33:373–382.

Stout SD (1978) Histological structure and its preservation in ancient bone. Curr Anthropol 19:601–603.

Stout SD (1982) The effects of long-term immobilization on the histomorphology of human cortical bone. Calcif Tissue Int 34:337–342.

Stout SD (1983) The application of histomorphometric analysis to ancient skeletal remains. Anthropos (Greece) 10:60–71.

Stout SD (1986) The use of bone histomorphology in skeletal identification: The case of Francisco Pizarro. J Forensic Sci 31(1):296–300.

Stout SD (1989) The use of cortical bone histology to estimate age at death. In MY İşcan (ed): Age Markers in the Human Skeleton. Springfield, IL: Charles C Thomas.

Stout SD, and Gehlert SJ (1980) The relative accuracy and reliability of histological aging methods. Forensic Sci Int 15:181–190.

Stout SD, and Simmons DJ (1979) Use of histology in ancient bone research. Ybk Phys Anthropol 22:228–249.

Stout SD, and Teitelbaum SL (1976a) Histological analysis of undecalcified thin sections of archaeologic bone. Am J Phys Anthropol 44:263–270.

Stout SD, and Teitelbaum SL (1976b) Histomorphometric determination of formation rates of archaeological bone. Calcif Tissue Res 21:163–169.

Thompson DD (1979) The core technique in the determination of age at death in skeletons. J Forensic Sci 24(4): 902–915.

Thompson DD, and Trinkaus E (1981) Age determination for the Shanidar 3 Neanderthal. Science 212:575–577.

Ubelaker DH (1978) Human Skeletal Remains: Excavation, Analysis, Interpretation. Chicago: Aldine.

Wu K, Schubeck EE, Frost HM, and Villanueva A (1970) Haversian bone formation rates determined by a new method in mastodon, and in human diabetes mellitus and osteoporosis. Calcif Tissue Res 6:204–219.

Reconstruction of Life From the Skeleton

Chapter 5

Determination of Sex and Race: Accuracy and Assumptions

Lucile E. St. Hoyme and Mehmet Yaşar İşcan
Department of Anthropology, Smithsonian Institution, Washington, D.C. 20560 (L.E.S.); Department of Anthropology, Florida Atlantic University, Boca Raton, Florida 33431 (M.Y.İ.)

INTRODUCTION

Fifty years ago, listing sex and race identifiers would have been less complicated than it is today. The American "melting pot" had been simmering sedately for a century, and technological advances had not yet upset a fairly stable life-style. For those of us who were adults in 1950, the old criteria probably still apply. For those born between 1940 and 1970, modifications are probably needed. For those of us born since 1970, the nature and degree of change is mostly unknown, but the probability of change is almost certain.

If World War II is taken as a turning point, much has changed. Immigration from new sources has altered the racial profile of the United States (and other countries), while changes in diet, environment, customs, and mores have been equally important. Politics and law have realigned and renamed racial, national, and social boundaries. These changes will continue and probably accelerate.

A new approach to race and sex identifiers is needed. The traditional characters are probably applicable to those who reached adulthood in relatively unaltered environments. For those who reached, or will reach, adulthood in changed environments—the New Americans—these criteria will have to be adjusted. When Boas (1912) studied the descendants of an earlier immigrant wave, changes had already occurred. There has not yet been enough time to study the New Americans, but comparable changes are to be expected. Until new data are available, we must make do with the old.

If we are to adapt race and sex criteria to new circumstances, we need to know which are genetic or hormonal and which are cultural or functional. We need to know how they interact with both nongenetic and environmental factors. Our theories of race formation will influence our concept of environmental interaction, and our knowledge of legal and bureaucratic race classification must work with our zoological taxonomy.

Relations Between Sex and Race Characters

Some characteristics, such as the preauricular sulcus, were first introduced as race markers (Zaaijer, 1893). It was later decided that these are primarily sex indicators, resulting either from growth or childbearing (Kelley, 1979a) or both (St. Hoyme, 1984). Other physical features—height, brow ridges, chin shape, body build, septal apertures of humeri, to list a few—have been used as criteria of sex or race or both. Such features are usually polygenic and are frequently modified by environment. Many visible race/sex traits are absent in infancy and childhood, developing fully about puberty, apparently by endocrine stimulus. Other traits are clearly the result of habitual activity. Some features, such as pelvic enlargement for childbearing, have a clear logic for their existence; but for others, such as large brow ridges, there is no reasonable functional explanation. Some traits are bilaterally symmetrical; others show marked side incidence. Some occur with fair constancy from population to population; others range from absent to nearly universal within genetically related populations. If visible external characters vary in these ways, we can reasonably assume that skeletal characteristics also vary in this way.

Biological sex is fixed by the X and Y chromosomes, but its phenotypic expression is modified by local customs and environment, along with the individual's health, heredity, and activities. Much the same may be said for race.

We know that growth rates and the timing and sequence of epiphyseal appearance and closure differ by both sex and race (Stevenson, 1924; Stewart, 1934; Greulich and Pyle, 1959). It is natural to presume that both sex and race differences are controlled by inherited hormonal or endocrine growth regulators. Working together, these produce adults of varying sizes and shapes. Even before birth, the rates of growth for head, trunk, and distal and proximal limb segments vary, both by sex and by race. Girls, in general, grow more rapidly than boys and cease growth sooner. Thus women differ from men in size and body proportions. Similarly, people of different races vary in size and shape. Because related growth regulators and mechanisms are involved, some physical characteristics reflect both race and sex.

Portraits of the Living in Skeletal Identification

Our choice of diagnostic characters and how we use them will depend, more than we think, on our preconceptions regarding the nature of populations. All Vietnamese are not short, nor are all Scots tall. Lacking atlases of crania or bones for most skeletal populations, familiarity with the real range of variation should be refreshed by looking at copiously illustrated books such as Hoffman (1936), Coon (1939), and Coon and Hunt (1965), which show pictures of peoples from many parts of the world. Back issues of *National Geographic,* and even old anthropology texts such as Deniker (1900, 1926) or field anthropometry reports, will have realistic enough portraits of the living to provide a basis for visualizing the underlying skull and bones.

Concepts of Race

Our choice and use of diagnostic features depend upon theories of the origin and significance of race and sex differences; a brief review of race theories is therefore needed.

Earliest theories of race often posited three, four, or five original races, descended from Noah's three sons perhaps, but dispersed to the continents where they were resident when historical records began. Until they migrated, or mixed, they were "pure," and by diligent research anthropologists might discover their original state. Monogenists claimed a single origin for mankind at a single time, either from Adam or a single primate taxon. Polygenists put the separation of human races farther back in time: perhaps each human race had descended from a different primate type, some perhaps more ancient than others.

Darwinian theory did little to upset these views. It was obvious that some peoples were more "primitive" or "apelike" than others. "Primitive" types included Lapps, all blacks, fossil specimens, the western Irish, and Australian aborigines. The laboring classes, at home or in the colonies, were not much more advanced. Vogt (1865) considered women and especially children to be more apelike than the "lower races." Verneau's (1875) study on the human pelvis, as with much other research, was aimed at ranking relative racial advancement. If you were a male WASP (white Anglo-Saxon Protestant), it was comforting to know that the secondary status enjoyed by women and lower races was divinely ordained.

Other early anthropologists worried less about the origin of races than about their current status and distribution. Good descriptions might allow better racial phylogeny and taxonomy. Accordingly, von Eickstedt (1937) and other typologists named a large variety of races of the world. Coon (1939) listed some 40 races for Europe, and Neumann (1952), seven for Amerindians.

All continents seem equally well provided with races. Buxton (1925) and Bowles (1977) describe peoples of Asia, while Oschinsky (1954) and Hiernaux (1975) describe variation in African populations. Australian aborigines seem to have come in several geographic varieties, as do Eskimos (Oschinsky, 1964).

Genetically associated racial "packages" of characteristics are frequently identified by terms ending in "id" (e.g., Iswanid), "omorph" (e.g., Bantutomorph), or a similar suffix. The unspoken implication seems to be that these traits do not "assort independently." One does become aware, in some parts of Europe especially, of recurring hair form, eye color, and face shape combinations. For some anthropologists, a description of a race or variety is simply a list of the means or modes of physical characters, without implying anything more than high frequency within a population. Other racial exemplars resemble the zoologists' type specimens. Any or all of the above were useful ways of viewing race, but they will influence interpretation of evidence in the skeleton.

Hormonal Theories of Race

About 1909, Sir Arthur Keith (1919) began speculating that race characters might result from inherited differences in endocrine activity. By the time Keith (1948) published *A New Theory of Human Evolution,* endocrine mediation of growth and physique was generally accepted by biologists as one mechanism of evolution.

Basically, hormonal theories have evolved into several groups. By 1950, biological theory had modified a strict "ontogeny recapitulates phylogeny" to include neoteny, in which the juvenile form in one species resembles the sexually mature form of a closely related taxon. If species and genera do this, why not human races? For example, among humans, Asiatics may be considered pedomorphic, because of sparse body hair, small brow ridges, and "infantile" body form (i.e., relatively short limbs and long trunk). But these mongoloid traits are also feminine. Similarly the hairier Europeans are both gerontomorphic and masculine. Perhaps pedomorphs and gerontomorphs are produced by altered androgen/estrogen balance (R. Marett, 1935; J. Marett, 1936). Unfortunately, regardless of its biological merits, this theory lends itself too easily to racist/sexist misuse. Are women pedomorphic? Childish? Are pedomorphs feminine? Wimps? Describing Genghis Khan as childlike or effeminate is incongruous. A more serious problem arises from the fact that a group pedomorphic in some respects is often gerontomorphic or neutral in others.

A second group of hormonal race theories might include the geneticists' "one gene, one enzyme" theory. Most genetic anthropologists, for example Boyd (1950), recognized the complex interactions of environment and growth regulators on body form and preferred to simplify racial comparisons by using traits apparently controlled by single genes such as blood groups. At that time, these characters were believed not to be modified by age, sex, or environment, nor subject to selection. Their study required minimal equipment and/or training. This was significant in the period immediately after World War II, when newly established anthropology departments lacked skeletal collections and the instruments to measure them.

Germ layer theories, such as Sheldon's concept of somatotypes (Sheldon et al., 1954), might be regarded as a third type of hormonal approach. Correlations between physique, personality, and health are attributed to differential development of embryonic ectodermal, mesodermal, and endodermal germ layers. Although these correlations are used more for predicting individual psychosomatic patterns, their incidence varies with race and sex (Roberts and Bainbridge, 1963).

While one may disagree about details, genetically mandated endocrine levels are the only conceivable basis for differentiating growth. Endocrine levels control the use of minerals, amino acids, and other dietary components in an environment of varying day length, temperature, humidity, and so forth. "And so forth" could include barometric pressure, angle of solar insolation, and other factors whose biological effects are still largely unexplored.

Ecological Theories of Race

A second group of theories flourishing since the 1950s attributes the formation and distribution of races and their physical features to climatic stresses.

Coon and associates (1950) attributed a major role in race formation to selection of physique by climatic factors. For example, the same "short limb, long trunk" Asian body build postulated by the hormonal theories also fits this model. Here the explanation is that a low surface:volume ratio, by conserving body heat, would be advantageous in cold climates. The world distribution of relative sitting height indices suggests and seems to support this hypothesis.

Alternative ecological hypotheses can also produce similar end results. The more calories an infant or child uses to maintain body heat, the less that is available for growth. Climate may also influence physique indirectly, just as day length, rainfall, and length of growing season influence the quantity and quality of food produced.

Because Coon and his coauthors (1950) speak of "race formation," one assumes that they refer to genetic selection rather than to temporary ontogenetic modifications to meet transient environmental stresses. Plant biologists recognize ecotypes and ecospecies as valid, albeit impermanent, expressions of genotypes in particular environmental settings. Immigrant human groups raise the question, To what extent are racial characters labile ecotypes?

Taxonomic and Political Theories of Race

Beginning around 1950, anthropologists had to contend increasingly with political implications of race. Racists, for centuries, had been using race as a justification for a wide range of injustices. For 15 years, Nazi Germany compiled anthropometric data to justify exterminating "degenerate races" in favor of an Aryan superrace. In an understandable reaction to a half century of genocide, there were a spate of declarations, resolutions, and legal actions on "race" from a multitude of sources. Resolutions, such as the UNESCO (1952) *Statement on Race,* held that physical differences were not related to differences in abilities or human worth and should not be used as a basis for discrimination. Such statements were often accompanied by action. Many of the war crimes prosecuted at Nuremberg after World War II involved genocide.

In the United States, long overdue corrections were begun at this time. Over 1 million black Americans, men and women, had served in the Armed Services in World War II. In 1948, three years after the war ended, President Truman outlawed discrimination in the military. In the next decades, new civil rights laws were passed and old Supreme Court decisions were overturned. Photographs were no longer required with job applications, and it became illegal to discriminate in education. In that climate, fears that anatomical race differences could be construed as signs of inferiority and might thus support discrimination discouraged both granting agencies and researchers. The need for forensic identification data had not yet burgeoned. One could safely study adaptation and selection in skeletons of fossil humans, but not in contemporary humans.

Bureaucratic Approach to Race

Biological anthropologists who examine human bones must communicate with law enforcement personnel, students, and the general public. The anthropologist is trying to identify and quantify the major racial (i.e., genetic) components contributing to the person's appearance. The police officer, official, or witness must fit this biological description into the current, local, legal, or social definition of race, which may have little to do with biology. It is essential that they understand each other. Occasionally, there is confusion about the sex of an adult. Race is often more complex.

Race has long been a concern of politics. In the 1950s, the school system in Washington, D.C., decided that local Negro children, regardless of skin color or hair form, should go to "colored" schools, while the children of African diplomats could attend "white" schools. Similar convoluted reasoning attended other aspects of public accommodation in many parts of the country, even after the passage of civil rights legislation. Meanwhile, there are 50 states, and just as many legal definitions as to who is black, Indian, white, or "other" and how race is determined. A person who is black in one state may be legally or socially white or Indian (or vice versa) in another. Some blacks who could "pass" for white do so; others prefer, for political, economic, or other reasons, not to pass. How Amerindians, Hispanics, Asiatics, and people of mixed ancestry are categorized depends on local law or custom. State laws and customs vary; so do national laws.

The 1911 Immigration Commission handbook (Folkmar, 1911) spelled out nationality and race, ignoring admixture. Asiatic Indians were listed among Europeans. About this time, census definitions recognized that a nationality might include people of several races and/or languages, but they, too, ignored admixture. Dealing with di-, tri-, and multihybrid crosses would have been impossible in an era when census data were computed largely by hand.

More recently, Wallman and Hodgdon (1977) prepared *Race and Ethnic Standards for Federal Statistics and Administrative Reporting* for the Office of Management and Budget, revising an earlier set of standards. The authors state specifically that "these classifications should not be interpreted as being scientific or anthropological in nature. . . . They have been developed . . . to provide for the collection and use of compatible, nonduplicated, exchangeable racial and ethnic data by Federal agencies."

Wallman and Hodgdon's five basic categories are as follows:

1. *American Indian or Alaskan native:* A person having origins in any of the original peoples of North America and who maintains cultural identification through tribal affiliation or community recognition.

2. *Asian or Pacific Islander:* A person having origins in any of the original peoples of the Far East, Southeast Asia, the Indian subcontinent, or the Pacific Islands. This area includes, for example, China, India, Japan, Korea, the Philippine Islands, and Samoa.

3. *Black:* A person having origins in any of the black racial groups of Africa.

4. *Hispanic:* A person of Mexican, Puerto Rican, Cuban, Central or South American or other Spanish culture or origin, regardless of race.

5. *White:* A person having origins in any of the original peoples of Europe, North Africa, or the Middle East.

The category that most closely reflects the individual's recognition in the community should be used for purposes of reporting on persons who are of mixed racial and/or ethnic origins. The directive adds that "Other (specify)" may be used to increase compliance, but only where the agency can restate the information in one of the above five categories. The definitions have some further clarifications: e.g., non-Spanish speakers from Latin America (from Brazil, Haiti, Trinidad, etc.) are to be classified by their race and "would not necessarily be included in the Hispanic category" (Wallman and Hodgdon, 1977).

Because of the number of government agencies involved in devising these unified, simplified standards, it is likely that any racial data in an official description of a missing person will be in terms of his "bureaucratic" race. As long as the anthropologist understands the meaning of these official terms, it should be possible to communicate with law enforcement personnel.

Population Changes

Over the last 50 years especially, immigration has notably extended the range of people with diverse physical features that might be expected to appear in the anthropologist's laboratory. Since 1960, 3,723,600 Asiatics, 225,300 Africans, 1,681,000 people from the Caribbean, 390,600 Central Americans, and 739,000 South Americans have come to the United States. According to the U.S. Bureau of the Census (1988), these 6.76 million immigrants are a minor addition to the total U.S. population of over 242 million. Like earlier immigrants, they have tended to congregate near large cities (Allen and Turner, 1988). Students prefer to attend colleges where countrymen are already on campus, service wives live near military bases, and newcomers, near relatives. Some enclaves seem exotic: Druzes in West Virginia, Samoans in inland Alaska, and Assyrians in Modesto, California. There is a 7′6″ Dinka playing professional basketball in Washington, D.C. Trying to guess the race or nationality of the person at the next table in the student union or behind you in the supermarket should sober an anthropologist. Familiarity with the range of physical features to be found in any of the references to "races of the world" or area handbooks is essential preparation for skeletal identification. Equally valuable is familiarity with current Standard Metropolitan

Statistical Area Census data on the national origins of the population of the area.

When the Supreme Court outlawed antimiscegenation laws in 1967, 16 states still forbade interracial marriages. Census data (U.S. Bureau of the Census, 1988) reports that interracial marriages have increased from 310,000 in 1970 to 827,000 in 1986. Many of these are black-white marriages; others are servicemen who married women living near overseas bases. In addition to children born to these marriages, many families have adopted Asian-American and other infants of mixed ancestry since World War II. In addition, informal arrangements outside of marriage have always existed and will continue. In short, for a variety of reasons, the number of Americans of newly mixed ancestry is likely to continue to increase.

Older mixed populations have long existed in the United States; these include Jackson Whites, Brass Ankles, Melungeons, Moores, and many others (Weslager, 1943; Berry, 1963). Many of these are trihybrid groups; some have established an Amerindian identity, while others have not. There have been a few blood group studies of these people and some vernacular descriptions of the living, supplemented with photographs. Nothing exists that would be directly useful in studying their skeletons.

There are a few older anthropological studies of living racially mixed populations, notably Fischer's (1913) Rehobother Bastards. Eugenically oriented studies often report evidence of physical degeneration, not always separating genetic factors from economic effects of the social opprobrium experienced by mulattos, mestizos, cafusos, creoles, and even octaroons. One of the better studies was Davenport and Steggerda's (1929) *Race Crossing in Jamaica.* There are a few recent studies such as one by Kimura (1976) on growth of children of Japanese-American parents, but very little descriptive anthropometry is included.

Diet, Environment, and Lifeways

Over the last hundred years, and especially within the last 50 years, diets and living conditions have changed substantially. New wartime technology for preserving, transporting, and storing perishables has enriched the diets of many nations. Since the 1950s especially, the introduction of new foods and changes in eating habits have produced marked physical changes in many populations. Goldstein (1943) has described such changes in Mexicans, Damon (1965), in Italians, and Greulich (1976), in Japanese children. Meredith (1976) has assembled data on children of many national backgrounds. Ohyama et al. (1987) have reported changes in height and body proportions in Japanese medical students.

Migration to a new home usually means a new environment, with nongenetic changes in the children of existing marriages. Appleton (1927) was one of the earliest to report on the differences in growth patterns between Chinese in Hawaii and China. The Southeast Asian Hmong surely find the icy winters and hot summers of Missoula, Montana, to be a striking contrast to their former home. Activities, child care, and public health concepts also are different. Physical changes, whether purely secular or involving migrations, may make old data inapplicable to present populations.

New occupations, a new emphasis on professional sports, and new specializations have proliferated in the last 30 years. Some of these involve different—not necessarily more healthful—working conditions; others primarily affect activities. Even the air around us has changed. Filters attempt to remove pollutants, while room air conditioners mitigate the worst of a Washington summer. A few studies of physical differences marking occupational groups (Bayer and Gray, 1934; Damon and McFarland, 1955; Damon and Crichton, 1965) or, in Europe, athletes specializing in particular sports (Eiben, 1981) provide current data for nonathletic controls.

Forensic Studies of Human Remains

Fifty years ago, most forensic skeletons were those of adult males. The number of women, adolescents, and young children whose bones reach the forensic anthropologist today has increased steadily over the last two decades. Data regarding the age at which physical characters become reliable sex and race indicators are urgently needed, as are data on new populations in the vicinity. At present, we can only make inferences regarding the skeleton from inadequate data on the living.

Fifty years ago, too, mixture of remains was less of a problem. The anthropologist has always been confronted by the isolated bone or incomplete skeleton, or an ossuary or carelessly curated collection. Now plane crashes and other mass disasters (Stewart, 1970) create new problems. The hundred or more passengers carried on even local flights may be of any race, sex, or national origin.

In the past, the anthropologist could usually assume that specimens came from someone "normal," i.e., whose growth and development were probably unaltered by complex medical intervention or ecological contamination. Increasingly, hormones have been used for treating acne, wrinkles, and morning sickness. They have been issued to teenagers for contraception and improving sports performance and to farmers for increasing meat production. A variety of growth regulators serve as antibiotics, pesticides, or herbicides, and soil and water chemistry have been greatly altered. The effects of these environmental alterations on growth, maturation, skeletal proportions, or other race or sex characters is still largely unknown. Increased cancer rates associated with such pollutants are being reported.

Etiology of Sex and Race Differences

When we generalize that "women are shorter than men," we forget that for most physical characteristics, both sexes share about 95% of the total range of variation. This range is further shifted by a relatively fixed racial genome and modified still further by inconstant environmental factors and by the individual's health, diet, and life-style. Age may also modify the expression of sex. Biological sex and genetic and/or racial heritage are about the only constants in this complex equation.

There are four basic groups of sex indicators. Except for pelvic changes associated with reproduction, race characteristics fall into much the same groupings. To be useful, sex and race indicators must be easy to recognize and have statistically distinct distributions. Their etiology should be known if they are to be properly applied.

1. Under hormonal influence, at puberty, pelvic changes preparatory for childbearing occur. Other hormonally mediated changes in body size and shape, of less obvious rationale, also occur. These include traits often associated with race.

2. "Scars" reflecting parturition (Putschar, 1976), occupation, or other events, are acquired. These may be the most useful sex/race identifiers. They are highly significant if present, but inconclusive if absent.

3. Underlying all this is a basic body size difference, which must be evaluated separately, along with body proportions. Unfortunately, we are not always certain which changes in proportion are sequelae of size or originate from other causes.

4. Some traits that once were manifest frequently no longer exist. These include pipe-smoker grooves. The clay stems that produced them have largely been replaced by softer plastic. Other traits never existed, but logic or tradition suggests their existence.

Not all skeletal clues to sex and race are of equal value. Sometimes a clear cultural clue or activity scar is more useful than an unclear biological indicator. For example, a bound foot is an excellent sign of female sex in a "Chinese" skeleton provided that the individual 1) lived at the proper time, 2) was of the proper social class, 3) came from a region where this custom prevailed, and 4) was indeed Chinese. Similarly, a deformed skull may point to time, people, and place. One must recognize the nature of the deformity and whether it took place in life or after death. Interpreting the evidence is not always easy. Negative evidence does not necessarily lead to a negative conclusion; but even positive evidence may sometimes mislead.

To properly utilize osteological clues to sex or race, we need to know, for each clue:

1. Its basic etiology: whether it is primarily biochemical, hormonal, or activity related, so that we may predict its pattern of variation.

2. Its range of variation by sex in various racial/ethnic groups.

3. Its manifestation by age: the age at which it appears and its pattern of change from childhood to old age.

4. How it is influenced by health, nutrition, occupation, or other circumstances of an individual's life.

5. Whether there have been secular changes in its expression.

6. Most important, whether the characteristic is real, but temporary.

Race and sex identifiers may be viewed in many ways, for example:

1. Permanence: Is the trait temporary (i.e., cultural or environmental) or relatively stable? This could include scars of pregnancy, tribal tooth filing, and squatting facets, all of which reflect an individual's participation in a group's activities. Some of these traits disappear in new circumstances—new way of life, new diet, new climate, or any combination of these. This does not diminish their usefulness, but does affect their interpretation.

2. Type of variable: Metric (continuous) variables can be manipulated statistically; morphological (discontinuous) traits must be counted and expressed as percentages. Are the differences large enough to be useful?

3. Real or imaginary: Some of these are traditional folk wisdom, still widely accepted by many. There may be honest confusion as to why the anthropologist has "overlooked" these clues.

4. Are they useful? If bones or crucial parts are too fragile to survive, if landmarks are hard to locate consistently, if measurements cannot be taken reliably, or if differences are too small to matter, their effectiveness is questionable.

SKELETAL SOURCES FOR RACE AND SEX STUDIES

Data on sex and race are no more reliable than their sources. Equally important are the methods for evaluating these data. Although the following comments apply primarily to data from U.S. collections, they apply equally to collections from other sources. Some European churchyards have yielded series of known age and sex. A few dissecting room series have been used. But undocumented archaeological series and the lack of identified subadults are a universal problem.

Ideally, the nature and range of variation of sex and race characteristics are determined from large skeletal collections of known age, sex, and race. All biographical information is useful: date and place of birth, occupation, place and cause of death, parity (if a woman), medical history, nationality/ethnicity of parents, language spoken, socioeconomic status (especially in childhood), and so forth. Occupational scars may be useful in interpreting sex or race. Even data on parents is useful.

In the United States, a few skeletal collections with known age and sex are available. Most of these came originally from anatomy dissecting rooms. Although cadaver "heights" differ sensibly from living stature, these and other measurements allow calculation of height reconstruction formulas and other formulas relating to body proportions. Trunk height, span, and chest and hip proportions also provide a basis for interpreting bone dimensions.

The Terry collection includes some 1,600 U.S. white and black adult skeletons. These came from bodies received by the Anatomy Department, Washington University Medical School, St. Louis, MO, from about 1920 to 1965. Some persons were born as early as the 1840s; dates of death range to the 1960s. Secular changes in height have been noted (Trotter and Gleser, 1951). Ages at death range from mid-twenties to nineties. Photographs, death masks, and hair samples may be useful in estimating the relative racial components. "Whites" are frequently Old Americans or from Germanic groups settling in the St. Louis area. The "blacks" have variable white ancestry. These skeletons are now in the Anthropology Department, U.S. National Museum of Natural History, Smithsonian Institution, Washington, D.C. They are the basis for the height reconstruction formulas of Trotter and Gleser (1952, 1958, 1977).

The Smithsonian also houses the D.S. Lamb and F.P. Mall collections, which consist of about 300 white and black fetal and infant skeletons from Washington, D.C., and Baltimore, MD, gathered around 1910. Sex, race of mother, and crown-rump lengths or other age data are given for most. There is a similar collection of fetal and infant skeletons in the Department of Anthropology, Cleveland Museum of Natural History.

The Huntington collection came from the dissecting rooms of the College of Physicians and Surgeons, Columbia University, and includes many immigrants who died in New York City between 1890 and 1920. Ancestry or country of birth is usually given. Many are from the British Isles, along with some Germans, Italians, and other Europeans. Ages at death begin in the late teens. However, few skeletons are complete enough to study. There is some information on occupation and cause of death. Many of Hrdlička's early studies of shape of shaft, and of femur, tibia, and other long bones were based on these skeletons.

The Cobb collection at Howard University, Washington, D.C., has about 600 skeletons of blacks from the Washington, D.C., area. Sex, approximate age, cause and date of death, occupation, and some other data are known.

The Hamann-Todd collection, from the Western Reserve University Medical School dissecting rooms, consists predominantly of U.S. whites and blacks who died from about 1925 to 1940. It is now in the Cleveland Museum of Natural History. Todd and his associates (e.g., Todd and Lindala, 1928; Todd, 1929; Todd and Tracy, 1930) published a series of studies on black-white differences based on this collection.

From these brief descriptions, the limitations of these collections are obvious. Except for infants, most individuals are over 25 years of age. Only "whites" and "blacks" are represented. These racial terms are social or legal, not biological, assessments, based on local custom. Percentage of ancestry in "blacks" is not known, but may be estimated from photographs or other accompanying data. Several studies (e.g., Saksena, 1974) have attempted to estimate admixture. Amerindian ancestry is probably frequent, especially in blacks, but not recorded. Admixture with other racial groups is not stated, but is unlikely.

Dissecting room populations are usually of below average socioeconomic status. Older women, particularly in dissecting room populations, frequently have had minimal health care and diet, possibly even since childhood. There is, therefore, the possibility of mistaking results of rickets, scurvy, or other stigmata of poverty for normal expressions of sex or race. For both sexes, occupations probably involved hard physical labor.

Recently, an increase in willed bodies has provided a small group of younger, healthier, more affluent individuals. These offer an opportunity for checking supposed race and sex characters, seen in usual dissecting room populations, against a group from a higher socioeconomic background.

Secular changes in physique, especially in height, are well known. Distributions of sizes and shapes within contemporary populations have changed over the last 140 years. Data based on older or sedente cohorts should be used with care in dealing with members of younger or migrant groups.

For many characteristics, for many age groups, for many racial groups, we will simply have to interpolate on the basis of studies of the living.

Some museums have large collections from old, unmarked burial grounds. They are limited, obviously, by lack of information on sex, age, race, or life history. Although some anthropologists have advocated measuring stature or sitting height before the skeleton is removed from the ground or articulating the spine (allowing for intervertebral discs), this is rarely done and is not very accurate. Unless appropriate information for a closely related living group is available, body build reconstructions are questionable.

Sometimes these bones were recovered as individual burials. Often, however, burials have become commingled, or records lost. Although they are less than ideal, these collections are our only source of biological information about these populations.

Archaeological data, if not separated from the bones, may provide useful information. Burial customs and grave goods vary, and suggested sex and race should be confirmed by other evidence. We assume, probably safely in most cases, that these are not admixed, even with other tribes. Adoption of captives is well known, and contemporary burials of foreigners in native sites is a possibility. We forget, too, that explorers and traders often antedated settlers in an area by several decades. Intrusive burials of later whites or blacks in Amerindian sites are usually fairly easy to identify by stratigraphy, morphology, or grave goods and are not likely to confuse the data.

Because of the practical, religious, and social obstacles to the study of juvenile skeletons of known sex, our major sources of information must be studies of the living and judicious use of archaeological material. Another contributing problem is that deaths in most groups are usually, at a minimum, in the 2–16 year age range. Probably we will never have enough identified skeletal remains of children between infancy and late adolescence to allow direct studies of sex and race differentiation and of the age at which various sex and race features appear.

While "statistically significant" differences in many skeletal dimensions exist even in fetal life and infancy, the great overlap in their distributions makes them nearly useless for identification purposes. There are also the practical problems of locating landmarks accurately and of handling fragile bones.

Where firm age information is not available, e.g., in runaways or archaeological populations, one can arrange skeletons by size, dental or epiphyseal stage, or some other index of physiological age and get some idea of the sequence and timing of bony changes. This is essentially the procedure used by Johnston and Snow (1961) to reassess the age and sex of the juvenile Indian Knoll, KY, Archaic skeletons and by y'Edynak (1976) for Alaska long bones. Previous studies by Stevenson (1924) and Stewart (1934) had examined race differences in sequence of epiphyseal closure in Chinese and prehistoric Amerindians.

Radiographic studies of living children usually show sex differences in mean ages for epiphyseal and dental development. Hunt and Gleiser (1955) and Bailit and Hunt (1964) used discrepancies between dental age and epiphyseal age as a clue to sex in U.S. children of normal nutrition and health. However, developmental stages are of variable duration, and the ages at which they begin and end both vary. McKern and Stewart (1957) report an age range of several years in young adults for most maturation stages in most bones. Age variability for all processes from tooth formation to suture closure seems to be the rule. Despite this variation, such information may be helpful in confirming a tentative identification; but when the sex of a child's skeleton is unknown, its age and race are equally dubious.

Studies of living children may provide some guidance on dimensions of head, face, limbs and their segments, and height. However, living segments cannot be directly compared with x-rays, because tube-film distance variation distorts dimensions, or either of these with bones whose epiphyses are not yet attached. For the time being, the sex and race of juvenile bones, under 12–16 years of age, should be approached with extreme caution. In a few skeletons, there may be traits clearly indicating race or sex. These should be described carefully, and their possible significance considered in detail.

RACE AND SEX DATA ON THE LIVING

The year 1950 marks the virtual cessation of anthropological studies of race differences in the human skeleton, at least in the United States. Most American studies since that period are elaborate statistical treatments of data on sex, reports of biochemical differences, mostly in remote tribes, and studies of long-dead peoples. It is ironic that the increased need in forensic anthropology for more reliable data on race and sex differences in the skeleton has come at the time when fear of racial discrimination has made funding for racial studies nearly impossible to obtain. Whatever the cause, in the last 30 to 40 years, there have been very few publications reporting new skeletal characteristics associated with human geography. Most of these have appeared in forensic media, rather than in primarily anthropological journals (Krogman and İşcan, 1986).

While the nineteenth-century anthropologists were preoccupied with the nature and causes of race (and sex) differences, in the twentieth century it is primarily the politicians who focus on these problems. If racial biology is approached, it is usually obliquely, by studies of selectivity for biochemical factors or micro- or macroevolutionary problems such as evolution from *Australopithecus* to *Homo*.

The largest body of data on human geographical variation comes from older studies antedating current political taboos. Many such studies investigated currently unfashionable hypotheses, such as relative evolutionary advancement. Yet the data usually validly describe those measured and have the additional virtue of being from populations probably relatively less admixed with foreigners.

"Relatively less mixed" is relative indeed. It is unlikely that any populations are "pure" or unmixed. Caesar's military policy, 2,000 years ago, was to send foreign troops to occupied countries, both to ensure an unsympathetic occupation army and to better control the conquered. Long before that, the Babylonians systematically repopulated conquered countries. The technique is as old as war. During World War I, Southeast Asian and North African troops were stationed in France; there were some 30,000 German infants of American white and black parentage after World War II; and, more recently, at least 20,000 infants of American white and black ancestry have created problems in Vietnam, Japan, and other Asian countries. Most armies of occupation have taken advantage of available opportunities.

Add to war the migrations by peoples in search of food: Israelites to Egypt 4,000 years ago, Irish to the United States during the potato famine, and Germans to the Ukraine and Koreans to central Asia during the nineteenth century. Most immigrants to the United States came for religious or political freedom, economic advantage, curiosity, or simply personal preference. Some moves involved only a few families; others have involved millions. Although we are most aware of our own anthropological history, similar movements have enriched other modern nations.

Trade produces even more distant contacts. In Bronze Age times, Mediterranean traders visited southern England and Ireland to bring back tin. Trade along the Silk Route, from Turkey to China, surely exchanged genes as well as goods. In A.D. 1200, Chinese junks, carrying 500 to 600 passengers, visited Japan, Annam, Malaya, South India, and the African coast (Gernet, 1962). Arab and Persian merchants had been trading regularly between the Persian Gulf and Canton and Fuchow for several centuries. Goods and genes were not restricted to the coast. Canals linked major rivers to the Yangtze, which was navigable for 2,000 miles, as far inland as western Szechuan province. Thus Hangchow, on the east coast, was the hub of a network of inland trading centers. By 1276, the time of the Mongol invasions, Hangchow was the largest and richest city in the world. It had large foreign quarters: Jews, Muslims from central Asia, Syrians, etc. Sung coins and ceramics of this period have been found from Cairo to Zanzibar, to the Philippines and Java. Such extensive contact is not unique. Coon (1981) tells of Arabic sailors from the Red Sea bringing back wives from South India, Indonesia, and other ports of call.

One unusual genetic interchange merits mention. In July 1987, the Greenland Eskimo son of Matthew Henson, a U.S. black member of the 1904 Peary expedition, visited his father's grave in Washington, D.C. (Stafford and Counter, 1988). He was accompanied by Peary's Eskimo son, born at the same time. Other equally unexpected combinations may have occurred.

In the century of colonialization ending with World War I, administrators preceded businessmen, troops, and travelers into the South Seas: Germans occupied the Bismarck Archipelago, the Dutch, most of Indonesia, and the French were in Indochina. The British and Spanish had been in Australia and the Philippines long before.

Memories are short, but gene pools remind us of the past. Visitors have been contributing to gene pools for millenia. Still, it is likely that pre-nineteenth-century residents of inland areas had fewer opportunities to acquire foreign genes; pre-eighteenth-century mixtures were even less frequent and less exotic. In the last century, we have seen Italians in Eritrea, Belgians in the Congo, the English in Africa and India, and Cubans in Angola. It may be possible to recognize the heritage of individuals of recent mixture. The North African genes left in the British Isles by the ancient tin traders (Mourant, 1959) are surely scattered randomly throughout the population. In the United States, mixture has been mostly confined to the past 450 years in the Southwest and 350 years in the South and East. Meier (1949) estimated that although 50% of his sample had dark skin, 70% of the Mississippi college Negroes he studied had white ancestry, and 75% claimed Indian ancestors. He expected these percentages to increase as genes were further dispersed by marriage. As for American Indians, comparable figures may be available for some groups, because participation in certain government benefit programs depends on ancestry, as recorded in official tribal rolls. Nevertheless, "fullblood" frequently refers to Amerindians who are "traditional and unacculturated to White ways," rather than to those without non-Indian ancestry (Allen and Turner, 1988).

The data summarized by Martin (1928) purport to represent relatively "pure" populations. These samples were collected well before World War II (some much earlier) and frequently represented residents of a colony administered by the anthropologist's government. Under such circumstances, the anthropologist would be acutely aware of the racial status of individuals in the samples and would take pains to eliminate the atypical. On the other hand, an anatomist working on dissecting room populations may have accepted the social race of the cadaver or gone by its appearance, especially if its ancestry were not crucial to his problem.

In his summary tables, Martin rarely gives sample size or standard deviation, limiting himself to the names of the author, the group, and any geographical data needed to distinguish them from a related group. In abridging these tables for each area, groups meeting the following criteria were selected: 1) those with highest and lowest values, 2) those with both male and female data, where possible, 3) those with greatest climatic diversity, and 4) those that appear most often in other tables. Except for a few obvious names, no attempt was made to anglicize or standardize the names used in Martin's (1928) tables.

Martin's data, for all dimensions and indices, suggest the same conclusions regarding their usefulness for identifying race and sex. Relative sitting height is a good example (Table 1).

TABLE 1. Sitting Height:Stature

Population	Male	Female
Europe		
Jews, Ukraine	51.4	—
French	51.9	53.6
German	52.0	52.9
Belgians	52.2	53.4
Albanians	52.6	—
Balkan Tatars	52.6	53.5
Norwegians	52.8	53.3
Jews, Russian	53.0	53.7
Lapps	53.1	—
Africa		
Masai	48.9	—
Bushmen	49.5	50.5
M'Baka	50.4	50.6
Somali	51.0	—
Fan	51.3	50.4
Kharga Oasis	51.3	—
Batwa	51.8	52.5
Togo	51.9	—
Babinga	54.0	—
Asia		
Malser	50.8	—
Cambodians	—	51.7
Annamites	—	51.9
Toda	51.5	—
Kalmucks	52.7	52.7
Yakuts	53.0	—
Tibetans	53.2	54.3
Armenians	53.6	—
Kubu	53.9	54.0
Aino, Shikotan	54.8	54.6
Americas		
Trumai	50.6	51.1
Eskimo	50.6	51.1
Nahuqua	51.8	52.2
Shoshone	52.2	52.7
Polar Eskimo	52.5	53.7
Pima	52.9	—
Apache	53.2	—
Kukpagmiut	53.5	—
Oceania		
Australians	46.5	48.4
Mid-mean: 52.1—Key-sigma: 2.1		

From Martin (1928, p. 339).

1. Variation within each continent covers about the same range. European male means range from 51.4 to 53.1; Asiatics, 50.8–54.8; Africans, 48.99–54.0; and New World peoples, 50.6–53.5, with an average, or mid-mean, of 51.85. The range of 5.9 between highest and lowest male mean is approximately 11% of the mid-mean, which suggests rather high variability. Still, if we estimate a standard deviation, of "key-sigma" using 4% of the mean, only the populations at the extreme ends of the ranges are likely to differ significantly from the average series and from each other. Their ranges will undoubtedly show the usual overlap. In short, intrapopulation variability is nearly as great as interpopulation variability.

2. Climatic contrasts within a geographic unit do not necessarily produce postulated physical contrasts. Southeast Asians, such as Toda (Nilgiri Hills, South India) and Cambodians, with relative sitting height means of 51.5, do not differ greatly from Siberian Kalmucks (52.7), Lena River Yakuts (53.0), or Tibetans (53.2). In Africa, Masai (equatorial highlands, East Africa) and Bushman (Kalahari Desert) means do not differ greatly (49.0), nor do Fan means (Ogowe Basin) differ greatly from those of Kharga Oasis Egyptians or Batwa (all 51.3). The latter are close to Eskimo (51.4) and French (51.9) indices.

3. Sex differences, regardless of area, are neither great nor consistent. The exceptions to this

TABLE 2. Other Body Proportions in the Living

	Upper arm:Stature	Forearm:Stature	Upper:Forearm
Europe	18.5–19.8	14.3–15.9	75.4–80.7
Africa	18.0–20.2	14.2–17.7	76.9–88.1
Asia	16.9–20.1	13.7–16.3	75.8–86.0
Americas	18.5–20.9	14.1–15.6	76.2–85.0
Oceania	19.2–19.7	14.6–15.4	76.2–84.6
Mid-mean	18.9	15.5	80.0
Key-sigma	0.8	0.6	3.2

	Thigh:Stature	Calf:Stature	Thigh:Calf	Arm:Leg
Europe	27.1–27.2	22.2–24.5	82.0–88.9	68.0–73.6
Africa	25.6–30.8	21.8–28.0	. . .	70.9–72.2
Asia	23.3–27.8	21.9–24.1	72.0–88.6	67.1–73.6
Americas	. . .	22.2	. . .	74.4
Oceania	26.7	. . .	. . .	70.9–72.2
Mid-mean	26.6	24.8	83.9	70.1
Key-sigma	1.1	0.9	3.3	2.8

From Martin, 1928.

are indices comparing hip breadth to stature or shoulder breadth.

Examinations of body proportion data show that for ratios of upper arm, forearm, thigh and calf to stature, and for brachial, crural and intermembral indices in the living, ranges of variation are almost identical by continent; with no consistent sex differences (Table 2). Some of the Asiatic series seem to have unusually short distal limb segments, while some of the Africans seem to have unusually long distal limb segments. But intraseries variability in all races seems so great that the anthropologist should not depend too heavily on body proportions for his decisions.

RACE AND SEX IN THE SKELETON AS A WHOLE

In modern humans, adolescence in boys occurs about 10% later than in girls, allowing a longer growing period. We can expect male size averages to be 5–10% larger than those for females. However, as we have seen, size alone is a dubious sex criterion because of the 95% overlap in ranges. Sex ratios for long bone dimensions are too variable to be genetic, suggesting culture and environment as more likely agents. Tables 3–6.

Customs affect quantity and quality of food available to infants, children, adolescents, and adults. Dietary restrictions on pregnant women affect unborn infants of both sexes. Status, fads, economic depression, war, famine, migration, population fluctuation—in short, almost any change in living conditions—all change the kind, amount, and distribution of food available and, ultimately, sex:size ratios.

Female long bone lengths and diameters as a percentage of those of the male (male = 100%) vary considerably (Hrdlička, 1944, 1945) between and within groups. This inconstancy reflects economics or custom rather than biology. Studying secular variations in long bone length at Amerindian sites, Hamilton (1975) reported that in times of plenty, both sexes were taller; in times of severe shortage, both were shorter; but during uncertain times, males were disproportionately taller than females. The boys, as future hunters and defenders, might get more food as a means of ensuring group survival. St. Hoyme and Gindhart (1978) note a similar shifting size dimorphism in recent U.S. black populations. Because of this inconstancy within populations, generalizations about other populations, in time and space, are not advisable. Since male bones are larger, it is not surprising that they are usually heavier (Vallois, 1957).

Bones as well as bodies vary in proportions. Arm and leg bones from Arnhem Land natives, in northern Queensland, Australia, are unusually long, slender, and heavy, as compared with Amerindian and other bones (Burkitt, 1924).

TABLE 3. Brachial Index (Radius:Humerus)

Population	Male	Female
Europe		
French, Paris	71.3	74.3
Europeans	72.5	72.4
Europeans	73.9	71.8
Swabia, Alamannen	74.3	76.7
Tyrol	74.5	76.5
Neoanderthal	75.0	—
Bohemia, Neolithic	76.5	75.7
Africa		
"Neger"	78.0	76.8
Bushmen	78.3	—
Naqada Egypt	78.8	78.1
"Neger"	79.0	78.3
Masai, Jaunde	79.5	76.4
"Neger"	80.1	77.7
Asia		
Chinese	75.4	73.4
Japanese	75.6	73.9
Aino	77.6	77.0
Negrito	78.3	78.2
Andamanese	80.5	79.7
Vedda	79.8	78.8
Chinese	—	77.4
Cambodians	—	77.0
Annamites	—	86.7
Americas		
"Indians"	76.3	75.4
Paltacalo	77.3	76.4
Eskimo	79.4	71.4
Fuegian	80.6	76.3
Baja California	81.5	76.2
Salado	81.5	78.8
Oceania		
Australian	76.9	78.5
Maori	77.8	—
New Hebrides	80.5	76.6
Mid-mean: 77.8—Key sigma: 3.2		

From Martin (1928, p. 395).

X-rays of the shaft seem in accordance with usual medulla:cortex ratios, so the heaviness may reflect density rather than cortical thickness. Unfortunately, the Smithsonian collection from this area consists of isolated bones rather than individual burials, so that nothing can be said of their intraskeletal proportions.

Robusticity is a popular sex character. The term may refer to 1) several indices of width/circumference to length, 2) muscular markings, 3) cortical thickness, 4) bone weight (absolute or relative to size), or 5) any combination of these. Authors frequently do not specify which definition they mean. To a lesser extent, robusticity has also been a racial, social, and status character.

Our Victorian predecessors valued "delicacy" and "refinement." For them, a proper lady was delicate, enjoying poor health; gentlemen were often healthy. But the laboring classes, including housemaids, porters, and cabmen, possessed both rude good health and crude manners. It is often hard to say whether the delicacy attributed to upper-class women was valued as a status symbol or as an excuse for overprotective contempt.

Analogous notions of race and class were equally common. At least one nineteenth-cen-

TABLE 4. Crural Index (Tibia:Femur)

Population	Male	Female
Europe		
Lapps	77.3	—
Bajuvaren	80.5	79.2
Alamannen, Swiss	80.6	81.7
Merovingian	80.8	81.5
French	81.1	80.8
Tirol	82.2	79.0
Mediaeval French	82.4	—
Neolithic Bohemia	83.4	83.3
Africa		
Ancient Egyptian	82.4	—
"Neger"	82.9	84.4
Berber	83.0	—
"Neger"	84.1	85.6
Bushman	84.1	—
Canary Islands	84.4	—
Congo Negro	84.8	—
Masai	85.3	85.0
Asia		
Japanese	80.4	79.8
Indochinese	82.4	—
Negrito	84.3	—
Andamanese	84.5	—
Malays	84.9	—
Vedda	85.2	83.8
Chinese	—	83.5
Annamite	—	89.6
Cambodian	—	90.7
Americas		
Eskimo	78.9	—
Fuegian	83.0	81.5
Californian	84.0	—
Paltacalo	84.1	83.7
Ancient Peruvian	84.7	85.1
Patagonian	84.8	—
Salado	85.0	83.1
Baja California	86.6	84.2
Oceania		
Polynesian	83.3	—
Australian	84.4	—
Melanesian	85.6	—
Mid-mean: 83.0—Key sigma: 3.4		

From Martin (1928, p. 418).

TABLE 5. Femur:Humerus Length Index

Population	Male	Female
Europe		
Bajuvaren	71.0	73.1
Alaman, Swiss	71.1	70.9
Tirol	71.6	70.4
Italians	72.9	72.1
Africa		
Neger (Broca)	69.0	68.9
Fan	69.8	68.8
Bushman	70.0	—
Masai	71.0	69.0
Naqada	71.0	70.1
Fiot	72.6	—
Asia		
Andaman	68.8	—
Senoi	69.9	—
Hindu (Turner)	70.5	—
Vedda	71.2	69.1
Aino	72.4	71.7
Americas		
Fuegians	69.8	—
Baja California	70.6	71.1
Salado	72.6	72.2
Oceania		
Australian	71.4	—
Mid-mean: 71.1—Key sigma: 2.9		

From Martin (1928, p. 429).

tury British anthropologist (Beddoe, 1870, 1885) explained that university students, descended from the Norman conquerors, were, naturally, taller than factory boys, whose Saxon and Celtic ancestors had been subjugated. Cultured races and persons were thought to have gracile skeletons, slender hands, pale skins, and other evidences of refined breeding. The stigmata betraying the primitive origins of the lower races/orders usually included dark skin, coarse hair, brute strength, and other apelike features. The earliest race (and sex) trait lists are more likely to reflect popular prejudices than objective investigations. However, most of our useful data on race and sex differences were collected in studies for ranking racial groups from most apelike to most advanced. Unfortunately, real differences that did not fit preconceptions were overlooked (Verneau, 1875; Hoyme, 1957).

"Robusticity" is usually described metrically by midshaft:length or epiphyseal width:length indices (Dorsey, 1897; Dwight, 1904/05) or simply by diameter (Garn et al., 1972; İşcan and Miller-Shaivitz, 1984b). Hrdlička (1939), after examining skeletons for more than 40 years, included both muscularity and indices among his sex identifiers. In his books on the Kodiak and Aleutian skeletons, Hrdlička (1944, 1945) gives means and ranges for long bone indices for Alaskan natives and related populations. Not surprisingly, his "females" were usually less robust than his "males." Ranges overlapped considerably and varied from one population to another, due more to population variation in time and space than to inconsistency. Means for right and left bones vary irregularly, as do means for populations. Activity, or handedness, seems to have contributed more to final form than has biochemical race or sex.

A combination of size and robusticity can be effective when used by an experienced osteologist. Hrdlička usually worked with femora, tibiae, or other isolated bones and less frequently with complete skeletons. His sex assessment of individual long bones, jaws, and skulls was re-

TABLE 6. Intermembral Index (Humerus + Radius:Femur + Tibia)

Population	Male	Female
Europe		
Tirol	68.6	69.4
European	69.1	68.0
Neolithic Bohemian	69.3	68.8
Schwaben and Alamannen	69.5	71.4
Bajuvaren	69.7	71.1
Europeans	70.0	69.3
Africa		
Bushman	68.1	—
"Neger"	68.3	67.7
"Neger"	68.4	68.1
Naqada Egypt	69.5	68.6
Asia		
Chinese	68.5	68.4
Vedda	68.7	—
Senoi and Semang	68.9	—
Negrito	69.0	—
Andamanese	69.5	—
Americas		
Baja California	68.6	68.0
Eskimo	68.7	—
Paltacalo	68.9	69.7
Fuegians	69.5	68.6
Salado	71.3	70.5
Oceania		
Australian	68.7	—
New Caledonia	70.1	70.1
Mid-mean: 69.7—Key sigma: 2.8		

From Martin (1928, p. 428).

markably consistent. Very rarely did he assign a femur to one sex and the corresponding tibia to the other. Most such cases occurred in mixed lots. It should be noted that for the pelvis, Hrdlička used general shape and size rather than an ischium:pubis index, which came into general use only some ten years after his death. Despite his apparently unstandardized methods, those working with his materials have seldom disagreed with Hrdlička's sex assignments.

Mean indices of robusticity, in which shaft or articular widths are divided by length, are generally higher in males. As Thompson (1917), following Galileo, pointed out, while height increases arithmetically, body weight increases geometrically. Therefore the width and thickness of a supporting structure must increase more rapidly than its length, producing an Eiffel Tower taper. One would expect to see this more clearly in leg bones than in arms. (In estimating body build, it would be useful to know whether weight also widens lower limb joints. We do not know whether the greater male thickness is hormonal or simply a function of a larger body. Unfortunately, widths of some epiphyses, especially of the lower tibia, increase with age, camouflaging differences due to sex.)

Morphological robusticity usually refers to prominence and clarity of muscular markings, but often includes general size. Unfortunately, there is as yet no scale of "very large" . . . "very small" to standardize recording these markings. Nor has anyone recorded the frequency of "trace" . . . "well developed" by sex or race. Are all areas of a bone, or skeleton, equally developed? Is an "indeterminate" bone "intermediate," a mosaic, or a little of both? Hrdlička and others have noted that ranges overlap, assuming that this overlap occurs in the "medium" area. Are the expected distributions and differences in robusticity real or simply expected? Without better evidence, we cannot assume that "muscularity" reflects hormones or genes rather than activity.

As to "muscularity," considering the strenuous lives of most women—including modern American city dwellers—there is little justification for the epithet "weaker sex." Anyone who has seen Third World women carrying heavy loads, cultivating fields, and processing hides will recognize this stereotype as a caricature. In the Third World, the major exceptions would be wealthy men's women, whose conspicuous obesity and idleness make them male status symbols. The Victorians, with whom our concepts of skeletal sex differences probably originated, were undoubtedly thinking of ladies—their wives or sweethearts or other imaginary females—rather than the maids, hired girls, and other hardworking women in the real world.

Indeed, the average "nonworking" American housewife, who carries in the groceries, wrestles with heavy, awkward appliances, and lifts 35–40 lb children, does a job as physically demanding as that of any supermarket bagger, waitress, or bus driver. Some pink-collar jobs are not strenuous. But most "unskilled" women's work today, as always, is hard labor, such as scrubbing floors, doing laundry, or caring for the sick. Even before Rosie the Riveter in World War II, many American women had been working on farms, in factories, and at other physically rough jobs. If these women have not acquired "strong muscle markings," it would be surprising. Conversely, one wonders about the muscle markings of chair-borne lawyers, accountants, and executives of either sex.

The ultimate silliness in sex identification by robusticity is Hooton's (1930) explanation that archaeologists recover fewer female skeletons because they are fragile and tend not to be preserved yet fetal bones survive. Culture is more likely than bone structure to explain why females are underrepresented in some skeletal series. A site with "too few" women or children may indicate a special activity site rather than a village burial area (Hoyme and Bass, 1962; Hoyme, 1963b). Complete accession lists are essential for demographic studies. The problems are compounded if a student, unfamiliar with culture and burial practices or collection methods, attempts to "correct" a site's demographic statistics by reevaluating skeletal sexing (e.g., Weiss, 1972).

But perhaps Hooton was thinking of demineralized bones of postmenopausal women. Despite the studies of Ericksen (1978, 1982), and others, much of our information on osteoporosis is ethnocentric. We do not know how universal osteoporosis is in older women, at what age it commences, why, or the degree to which men and women of other cultures are affected.

In aged individuals, bony muscle markings are said to become less clear; this may reflect diminution of hormonal levels, decreased physical activity, or nutritional problems. We do not know at what age or in how many older people this change occurs. We may need to allow for age in interpreting robusticity. But "decreased robusticity" may be related less to reality than to common stereotypes about "sexless," retired (i.e., idle) senior citizens.

One cannot expect muscular markings on long bones to be a useful sex identifier in subadults. Tanner (1962) reports that at about 7 to 8 years of age, a year or two before girls abandon boys' games, boys' calf x-rays begin to show higher muscle:bone:fat ratios. This suggests that hormones, rather than activity, are involved. However, clear muscle markings seem rare in preadolescent or even in older preadult bones. In bone that is growing both in length and diameter, rapid periosteal changes may obscure surface markings (Hoyte and Enlow, 1966). Perhaps, however, not expecting their presence, we have assumed their absence.

Sex and race differences in height: and trunk: limb ratios in the living have been cited. In working with the skeleton, it is unwise to attempt to reconstruct sitting height by articulating vertebrae. Even if all vertebrae are present, thickness of intervertebral disks is so variable that an accurate reconstruction is unlikely. Similar cautions apply to attempting to reconstruct pelvis, chest, span, or other measurements, including variable soft parts. Skeletal evidence for body proportions is thus restricted to long bone length ratios. Data on long bone lengths is rare for most populations, but reasonableness of estimated skeletal proportions can be checked against Martin's (1928) data on living series from a given population (cf. Tables 1–2).

Trotter and Gleser's (1952, 1958, 1977) stature reconstruction formulas (based primarily on the Terry collection) reflect differences in long bone indices. Both U.S. white and black females seem to have shorter forearms than males, especially when the corrected black female data are used. In blacks of both sexes, tibiae, fibulae, radii, and ulnae are longer, compared to femora and humeri, than in whites. Genovés' (1967) data on Mexicans suggests that Amerindian skeletons have somewhat different long bone proportions. Stature estimation formulas are available for other populations, including South African blacks (Lundy, 1983), Czechs (Černý and Komenda, 1982), and Chinese (Mo, 1983; Peng and Zhu, 1983). Steele and McKern (1969) and Sonder and Knussmann (1985) suggest how to estimate lengths of damaged long bones, and it may be possible to derive indices if bones are not too fragmentary. These and similar stature reconstruction formulas can be used, in the absence of better data, to assess relative bone length to supplement other sex and race data.

If all major long bones are present and there is no question of mixture of parts, brachial, crural, and intermembral indices may suggest race or sex. Yet we are told that body proportions are, at least in part, the result of climatic selection (Coon et al., 1950). If so, will children of Southeast Asian immigrants, now growing up in Alexandria, Virginia, or Missoula, Montana, follow their new ecology or their old genes?

Sex and race differences in children's arm:leg and other body proportions appear as early as fetal life. Most growth studies, particularly those that report length of limb segments, show age-modified sex and race differences. However, body proportions change rapidly during childhood. The age at which a child attains an adult configuration probably varies widely. On the average, girls are more mature than boys of the same age in tooth formation and eruption and in epiphyseal appearance and fusion (Hunt and Gleiser, 1955; Bailit and Hunt, 1964). But without age information, these sex/race indicators are useful only in evaluating a particular skeletal identification. Otherwise, normal variability, together with modifications reflecting health, race, or other considerations, may mask the sex factor.

THE SKULL: VAULT, FACE, JAW, AND TEETH

Many authors, including Hrdlička (1919a–d, 1939), feel secure in claiming 80% accuracy for sex identification from the adult skull alone, increasing this to 90% if the lower jaw is included. Others are even more confident, though few claim omniscience. A few anthropologists have suggested that some crania—perhaps up to 10%—cannot be sexed by any method or combination of methods. In short, the problem lies with the skull rather than with the expert or method. Race, judging from variation in the living, should be equally difficult. Although most experienced anthropologists have encountered skulls (and other skeletal parts) whose sex was unclear, there are no good data on whether sex traits in these individuals are 1) "intermediate," 2) a mosaic of male and female (i.e., some traits less well developed than others), or 3) both. Variations in hormone levels at different stages of development could produce either effect. Nor have we any idea of how frequent these individuals are, or whether uncertainty in one part of the skeleton is accompanied by like uncertainty in another.

The same limitations probably apply to race identification. It is likely that characteristics reflecting customary activities may be more useful as clues to race.

Of the skull parts, probably more usable sex and race traits are concentrated in the face and jaw than in the braincase. Unfortunately, like sex characters, racial identifiers seem not to develop until after adolescence. This may in part be an artifact of the limited number of identified juvenile crania available for study, or it may be because most studies of juvenile crania are concerned with growth rather than with race or sex differences. Either way, little is known about race and sex differences in the juvenile skull. Without clear supporting evidence, it would seem imprudent to be too positive on racial or sex identification until at least the teens.

In late adolescence, the boy's face elongates, the brow ridges (with the underlying frontal sinuses) enlarge, and the chin becomes more prominent. Enlarging the male brow ridges decreases orbital height slightly and lowers the orbital index. At the same time, the upper orbital margins become thicker and blunter, and apparent orbital shape becomes squarer. The supraorbital notch becomes deeper and may close into a foramen. These changes in brow ridge size also change the apparent nasal bridge profile rather than its actual shape.

So far, no reliable way has been found to distinguish skulls of preadolescent girls from those of boys. Change at adolescence is apparently restricted to boys, with females retaining the more or less juvenile form. Apparently these craniofacial changes are mediated by hormones, acting on a genetic substrate, for what is "large" in one race is average or "small" for another. Unless the individual is at least 16–17 years of age, i.e., old enough for adolescent sexual metamorphosis to have begun, it would seem foolhardy to insist on female sex without confirmation elsewhere in the skeleton.

Race differences in the skull are most evident in the face. Facial bones differ, particularly in their relative length, width, and projection. In human ontogeny, the facial structures seem to develop as the increasing number of teeth requires greater facial projection. In early life, children of all races have short, wide faces, short, wide noses, and rounded chins. Their skulls seem, to us at least, to look pretty much alike. Somehow, at adolescence, by differential growth, racial characteristics develop. But although the same structures are involved, racial differentiation in the growing face differs greatly from sexual metamorphosis. Because so few juvenile skulls from different races are available, little is known about what diagnostic characters are present or about the age at which they appear. Unless the child is old enough for some clear diagnostic evidence to have appeared, it is wiser to reserve judgment, not only on sex but also on race.

In general, adult male skulls are larger than those of females. Part of this size difference is due to the larger male brow ridges, which increase cranial length and slightly change sex means for cranial indices. Whether male cranial capacity (brain size) is also disproportionately larger is uncertain. In general, brain size and general body size are correlated. The degree of overlap in cranial capacity range is uncertain. Truncated but almost normal distributions of vault dimensions and cranial capacity estimates suggested to Stewart (1943) and to Howells (1943) that, in sexing skulls, Hrdlička and others relied unduly on size. Race differences in skull size seem to follow body size differences.

Cranial vault bone averages a fraction of a millimeter thicker in males and in blacks (Todd and Lindala, 1928). These sex and race differences are statistically significant. But the ranges of overlap and regional variation are too great for vault thickness to be useful for identification. "Hardness" or density of vault bone is probably related to thickness; both are popularly equated with stupidity. Inspired by tales of "nulla-nulla," in which it is said that Australian aboriginal women settle disputes by hitting each other on the head with long wooden poles, F. Ivaniček (unpublished report, ca. 1952) obtained a grant and permission to sample about 200 human parietal bones in the U.S. National Museum. Measuring total thickness as well as relative thickness of outer and inner tables and diploe, he found no structural differences that would substantiate this tale.

Generally, muscle markings on the occipital (nuchal crest), temporal (around zygomatic roots), and parietal (temporal crest) bones are larger and heavier in males. No consistent studies on relative racial development are available. In a few males, muscularity of the nuchal crest results in hooks or depressions at inion.

Heavier brow ridges, zygomata, malars, and temporal lines may reflect greater male robusticity, as seen elsewhere in the skeleton. Along with these, heavier nuchal crests and jaws may provide stronger muscular attachments for chewing. Yet, are male and female diets so different? Examining many mandibles, one has the impression that gonial angle eversion is greater in males, whereas slight inward turning is more characteristic of females. Angel and Kelley (1986) suggested that this might be a race rather than sex trait. The sex and race distribution and functional significance, if any, are yet to be investigated. Indeed, most of the group differences in the skull and mandible seem to be associated with general size and muscularity and seem to have no other functional rationale. Their distribution, in most cases, has never been reported for skulls of known sex or race and may simply reflect our stereotypes.

Brow ridges are part of the frontal bone, although they affect facial appearance. Sexual dimorphism in brow ridges seems to be a primate character, developing at adolescence. Why are large brow ridges "advantageous" to males? Undermined by frontal sinuses, brow ridges cannot provide much protection in a fight. The frontal sinuses have also been credited with increasing vocal resonance, thereby enhancing the male's sex appeal; more practically, they enhance communication between separated hunters. (Don't women call to children?) But if all males have large brow ridges and deep voices, who is impressed? Race differences in brow ridge development are striking. Brow ridges are usually smallest in Asiatics and blacks, with whites intermediate, and largest in Melanesians and Australian aborigines.

Cranial deformity, if present, is a useful index of race, whether intentional or accidental. One thinks first of the more spectacular Amerindian cradleboard deformity found almost entirely in archaeological crania; but child-care customs in modern European groups can also influence skull shape: traditional cradles used by Boston families of Middle Eastern origin (Ewing, 1950) account for the so-called Armenoid head shape. Similarly, pillows and bedding used in some central European areas could have contributed to the nearly spherical skull shapes sometimes found there. Tight crocheted caps, worn by some Puerto Rican infants for protection against malign influences (M. Moss, personal communication), may also influence later skull shape. Traces of these cultural practices may be subtle, amounting only to a slight occipital flattening, but can be useful indicators of nationality and/or race.

"Inca" bones were first observed in deformed Peruvian crania (Dureau, 1873). As cranial information increased, these extra sutural bones were found in other races. The frequency and size of Inca bones seem correlated with the type and severity of artificial cranial deformity rather than with biological race.

Metopic sutures, reflecting delayed closure in the frontal suture (which usually closes by the first year of life), occur in most racial groups (Bolk, 1917; Woo, 1949; Torgersen, 1951). Regardless of race, they seem more common in urban crania than in crania from rural settings.

A bulging forehead, with some constriction near the coronal suture, is said to have been typical of Negro crania. Whether this is African or Afro-American is uncertain. At least some crania of this shape suggest childhood malnutrition (subclinical rickets?) rather than a genetic basis.

Scaphocephaly, an uncommon pathology of unknown cause, seems to occur more frequently in American blacks. Vault sutures are obliterated, the skull vault is long with bulging frontal and occipital areas, and cranial texture seems denser than normal. The abnormality in itself is so striking that racial identification is almost an afterthought.

Eskimo crania are typically long, high, and narrow, with wide, long faces, long noses, wide zygomatic arches, and wide gonial flare. Temporal lines may be high, barely an inch from the sagittal suture. The general shape of both vault and face is nearly the opposite of that prescribed by Coon and coworkers (1950) as optimum for minimizing heat loss from the head and reduction of exposed facial surface.

A rounded, protruding "occipital bun" is often listed as characteristic of Algonquin Indians, but is often a feature of Neanderthal crania. The etiology is unclear.

Mastoid processes are both a sex and race character. They are largest and most prominent in males and Europeans and Amerindians, smallest in females and Africans.

With few exceptions, most vault shapes occur in most populations, so that few can be considered "typical" of any particular group.

Upper Face

Nasal bones may be lacking in some South Pacific peoples and occasionally in other Polynesians (Snow, 1974). Whether these are actually absent, merely reduced, or simply covered by the nasal processes of the malar bones is not certain. Morphology may vary from skull to skull. Width of the piriform aperture does not seem to be affected by this variant.

Nasal bridge width, flatness, and contour vary (Goldstein, 1939; Hartle, 1962). A narrow bridge is characteristic of Europeans and many Amerindians and Eskimos. Wide, flat bridges characterize African and Pacific (i.e., Melanesian) peoples. Projection of the bridge area above a plane defined by the anterior orbital edge of the frontomalar sutures also varies. It is greatest in Europeans, medium in Africans, and least in Asiatics, especially Eskimos. Nasal bridge projection can be traced with contourometers or measured by a simotic index (width between fmo-fmo/arc fmo-fmo).

Although cranial nasal indices vary from about 40 to 60, absolute nasal widths vary only slightly. This is in part because the incisive bone (= premaxillary = intermaxillary), which bears the incisors, forms the anterior floor of the nasal passage. The major variable is the height from nasion to some subnasal point. The location of nasion itself varies. The upper margin of the nasal bone lies atop the lower ends of the frontal, forming a sort of squamous suture. Connolly (1926) observed gradual upward displacement of the tips of the nasalia with aging. Eskimo nasal indices are quite "narrow," while indices for some other peoples suggest that noses are "wide."

Nasal shape is further complicated by nasal prognathism. This can be measured 1) as the angle from nasion to subnasal point to basion or 2) as the angle between the nasion-subnasal point axis and the Frankfort horizontal. A third way to visualize prognathism is to drop a perpendicular from nasion to the Frankfort horizontal, to see which parts of the face project in front of this plane. Using the Frankfort plane as a baseline, Mongoloid faces are remarkably vertical, the upper part of European faces projects, whereas prognathism of black faces is seen to be primarily alveolar.

Subnasal margins may be either blunt, sharp, or grooved. Deep pits, about 1 cm wide and up to 0.5 mm deep, occur in many prehistoric Hawaiian crania at the subnasal margin, above the incisor root tips. If these are genetic in origin, they may occur in their modern descendants. The cause of these pits is unknown.

The floor of the nose may be so smooth that the subnasal margins are difficult to locate and nasal height difficult to measure. Distinct subnasal margins are more common in Europeans and Asian skulls; those that are smooth, rounded, or depressed are more common in African or some Afro-American crania. Prominent, sharp subnasal spines, up to 1 cm long, are characteristic of European or Asiatic crania. There is great variation in shape and size. Shorter, blunter, smaller spines are more characteristic of blacks.

Nasal indices were claimed by a number of anthropologists (Weiner, 1954; Wolpoff, 1968) to be correlated with ambient temperature and humidity. By this theory, a narrow nose is useful in cold, dry parts of the world for warming and moistening inspired air and recovering heat and moisture from expired air. In hot, humid climates, a wide, open nose is adequate. If the geographical distribution of living nasal indices is plotted on maps, wide noses do seem to be tropical.

If we look at cranial measurements, rather than indices, a different picture emerges. The "low" Eskimo index is the result of a very high nose of average width, with a large estimated cross-sectional area. Similarly, the "wide" tropical noses are about the average width, but of very low height. Nasal height, incidentally, correlates strongly with upper facial height. None of these external measurements conveys any concept of the amount of turbinate area exposed within the nasal passage for temperature and moisture transfer, nor is the depth of the nasal passages usually considered. Width of the piriform aperture is about the same in most populations; nasion-subnasal height is the major variable. In adults, the greatest heights are found in Europeans and Mongoloid Asiatics; this feature is lowest in African, Melanesians, and other tropical peoples.

Orbital size seems proportional to general face size in most human groups. Enlargement of brow ridges, especially in males, seems to lower upper margins and to decrease orbital heights and indices, but actual capacity of the orbital cavity is not altered. Horizontal orbital axis inclination seems greatest in European crania, and especially in those from the British Isles. Because this seems to vary from sample to sample, it is more likely to be nutritional than genetic.

The width and shape of the malar bones show clear racial distinctions. In whites and blacks, the width of the malar bone at the frontomalar suture is minimal, gradually increasing toward the temporal process, so that the area is a slender triangle. In Asiatics and Amerindians, the width increases rapidly, so that the posterior margin of the orbit projects and the area is rectangular. Hartle (1962), who first described this, found some bilateral asymmetry in size and shape. The process is best developed in Mongoloids, but occurs occasionally in contiguous peoples. Its anatomical basis is not known.

Cameron (1920) devised an "indexometer" for indicating the relative positions and sizes of orbits and nose in the face. Although he supplemented his diagrams with measurements and indices, the indexometer gives a much more easily grasped impression of these relationships and the shapes and proportions of the face in various races.

Folklore speaks of the "high cheekbones" of Asiatics and Amerindians, but does not specify whether this refers to 1) malar or bizygomatic width, 2) anterior projection of the malars in relation to some vertical facial plane, or 3) relatively great upper facial height, with greater-than-usual distance from alveolar point to the lower orbital margins. Any of these could be described by this phrase.

The widest faces, in terms of bizygomatic widths and indices, and frequently also bijugal, are found in Asiatic crania and, to a slightly lesser extent, in Amerindians. Often bizygomatic width is considerably greater than upper facial width, measured at the frontomalar sutures or above, as minimum facial width. Most Asiatic faces are extremely long, wide, flat, and large. Coon et al. (1950) described the Mongoloid face as "cold screened," with projecting parts reduced so as to reduce danger from frostbite. Roughly estimating area by multiplying face height by bizygomatic breadth results in some of the largest cranial faces known.

Malars in some Mongoloid crania are so deep that they are divided by a horizontal suture. The resulting "os japonicum" is not confined, of course, to Japanese crania (Woo and Morant, 1934; Woo, 1937).

Oschinsky (1962) and Oschinsky and East (1964/65) contrast midfacial flattening in the Eskimo and Mongoloid face with Polynesian facial morphology. Viewed from below, the Eskimo malars are separated from the nasal area by fossae; from the side, they are seen to slant backward. Even so, when bijugal width is measured with coordinate calipers, the Eskimo nasal spine is seen to be less elevated than that in non-Mongoloids. With Eskimo facial morphology at the extreme of flatness, European prognathism tends more to the midface.

The smallest facial widths, heights, and areas, absolutely and relatively, are found in blacks and some Pacific peoples. Facial shortness and narrowness in these groups are often accompanied by considerable alveolar and dental prognathism.

Palate shape ranges from shallow to rather long and narrow, corresponding to some extent with prognathism. The frequency of maxillary hyperostoses, usually found on the external palatal margins above the molars, fits a pattern more suggestive of a pathological response than a racial character. Midpalatal tori (Woo, 1950) seem to vary genetically by race and to be more common in women. Mandibular hyperostoses on the anterior lingual mandibular surfaces are frequent in Aleutian, Eskimo, and Icelandic (Hooton, 1918) peoples. The high incidence in maritime peoples, regardless of race, suggests a response to some environmental stimulus rather than genetics. These benign bony tumors also occur in city-dwelling whites and blacks and probably have no real racial significance. Their ecological significance is still uncertain.

Mandible

Small, rounded chins are typical of female sex; square, heavier chins ("Dick Tracy" type) are found in many males. Children up to puberty have small, rounded chins, so that alternative forms appear in males at adolescence. At the same time, changes in the angle of the ramus and mandibular body also occur. Chin shape and projection are also racial characters. Projecting chins are found in Europeans and some Asiatics. Rounded, almost receding chins are found in Australian aborigines and in some South Pacific Islanders. Most African and Afro-American chins are intermediate.

General jaw shape corresponds reasonably with general skull shape: prognathous palates are associated with long, narrow mandibles with low rami; great bizygomatic width with wide mandibles with deep rami is associated with considerable gonial flare. In addition to general mandibular width, great gonial flare may increase apparent mandibular width. Greatest eversion is found in Eskimos and Amerindians. Angel and Kelley (1986) observed that flare, vs. inturning of gonial angle, was a racial trait. Koritzer and St. Hoyme (unpublished data) consider it to be a sex character, with flare suggesting a male. Until observations on larger series are available, it seems most likely that it is environmental, possibly associated with poor nutrition, rather than genetic.

Rocker jaws (Snow, 1974; Houghton, 1977) seem associated primarily with Hawaiian crania. If the jaw is placed on a flat surface and a condyle tapped, the jaw "rocks" like a rocking chair.

Dentition

There is a great deal of folklore regarding teeth: men have bigger teeth than women, teeth of black people are larger and whiter than those of whites, and so forth. The range of overlap in size, shape, and color is such as to make these features of dubious value for establishing race or sex.

The most usable racial clue relating to teeth is the "shovel-shaped incisors" found in most Asiatic Mongoloids and Amerindians. In the upper central and lateral incisors, the lateral margins fold sharply backward, so that the tooth resembles a miniature scoop. Unless the crown is badly worn, traces of this form can usually be observed. Hrdlička (1920) seems to have been one of the first to describe these teeth. Riesenfeld (1956) has reported their occurrence in Pacific peoples.

Dental decay and occlusal problems are not exclusive to modern whites. There is a common belief that Amerindians did not have cavities or other dental problems until they began to eat the white man's food. Both occlusal and root caries are found in teeth from pre-Columbian sites. Far more common, however, is heavy wear, followed by pulp cavity destruction and ensuing apical abscesses.

Increases in decay seem to accompany a shift from hunting/gathering to settled village life in Amerindians, associated with increased carbohydrate and other dietary change. Yet in some Southeast Asian peoples, where rice is a large part of the diet, caries seem to be rare. In the teeth of ancient Hawaiians, for whom taro, yams, and other carbohydrates were common, dental crowns are usually caries free, with much calculus formation, alveolar resorption, and root caries undermining the crowns. This distinctive pattern may be dietary rather than genetic.

Cultural usages are often useful in estimating race from dental evidence. Black stains from the betel nut are frequent in Indonesia and other parts of Southeast Asia, where this trait also indicates socioeconomic status. Teeth with excessive slanted wear, resulting from pulling fibrous, siliceous fern fronds between the teeth, are more likely to have come from South Pacific areas. Excessive wear, so that the pulp cavity is exposed, is more characteristic of ancient Amerindians. Heavy wear is uncommon in most contemporary peoples.

Removal or decoration of anterior teeth can also provide indicators of race or sex. In affluent U.S. families, usually white, removal of one premolar on each side or in each quadrant usually indicates orthodontic treatment to increase space for erupting teeth. Some groups are more careful of their daughters' teeth than their sons'. Many African tribes still knock out central, and sometimes also lateral, incisors as a tribal initiation rite at puberty.

Decoration of teeth can range from betel nut staining to filing, inlays, or crowns. Ortner (1966) describes the skull of a contemporary young African woman, later identified, whose front teeth had been filed in a traditional pattern. Grooved, notched, inlaid, and otherwise decorated teeth are more likely to be from archaeological contexts than contemporary populations. Hypoplastic grooves sometimes resemble filing, so they should be examined with a hand lens. Occasionally, evulsed teeth that have dried out or been carelessly stored become nicked and are described as artificially notched.

A gold crown or gemstone inlay on an anterior tooth may serve as a status symbol. Such decorative dental work was more common at the turn of the century, but modern dentists still have requests for such conspicuous restorations. "Occupational use" of teeth includes bobby pin chipping. Although bobby pins were nearly ubiquitous from 1930 to 1950, they have largely fallen into disuse, and teen-age girls no longer chip their incisor margins opening them. Fewer women do extended hand sewing, and thread quality has changed, so that seamstress' notched incisors are nearly extinct, or may now characterize male tailors.

Similarly, pipe-smoker grooves, formerly frequent in older (especially black) women, have disappeared as plastic has replaced clay pipe stems and cigarettes have replaced pipes. These grooves were usually about 1 cm in diameter and between the upper canine and premolar and the lower premolar. A piece of chalk would fit into the groove quite nicely. If the pipe was habitually held in the left hand, the groove would also be on the left, leaving the right hand free for work.

Styles in dental decoration and repair may also vary from time to time, not only as status symbols but as sex indicators. In each culture the need for dental care and restoration varies with sex and occupation, as well as with socioeconomic status. An experienced dentist can often recognize the country or situation—military service, jail, dental school clinic—in which dental restorations were done. This can be an additional clue to nationality and race.

THORAX AND PELVIS

Occasionally, skeletons are found in which the thyroid cartilages (Adam's apple) have ossified; these are generally older males. These bony plates are thin, very fragile, and likely to be overlooked by the collector, unless one is alert to the possibility of their presence.

Dwight (1881, 1890), Fawcett (1937), and Jit et al. (1980) have postulated sex differences in the sternum, i.e., that the female sternum should be longer and more slender than that of the male. Such differences have not yet been demonstrated. One practical problem with the sternum is that it is primarily cancellous bone and is rarely recovered intact. In dissecting room skeletons, this bone and the ribs are often cut in opening the chest cavity.

Schultz (1930) reports that about 10% of human skeletons have other than the standard 12 pairs of ribs. In about 5% of otherwise normal individuals, the last thoracic vertebra is "transitional," i.e., one costal process has fused to the vertebral body, while the other is free. These unfused costal processes vary from so short as to resemble a distal phalanx to 2 or 3 inches long. But they will have riblike heads with proper articular facets on the vertebral body. If this fairly common anomaly shows on a chest x-ray, it may be useful for individual identification. There is inadequate data regarding its incidence by side or sex. It is not an indicator of male sex. Allbrook (1955) reports similar numerical variation in East African spines.

There is also no evidence that the weight of the breasts of some "well-endowed" women flattens their ribs. Less legendary, but still of limited use, are the deformed ribs produced by tightly laced corsets (Imbelloni and Dembo, 1938). A complete or nearly complete rib cage would be needed to identify the ribs affected and to estimate the degree of deformity. A knowledge of the culture would be equally necessary, for both men and women have followed this fashion at times. Tight lacing would be limited to those affluent enough to afford this luxury. Working men and women need to breathe. Whether surgical scars associated with mastectomies might appear in the rib cage is as uncertain as the presence of other sex-associated pathologies.

The adult pelvis has the best-known and most reliable sex identifiers. In addition to traits reflecting body size, the pelvis has two additional kinds of sex character. At adolescence, the female pelvis enlarges preparatory to child bearing, with alterations in the size and shape of many parts. To the extent that this metamorphosis is complete, these areas are trustworthy indicators. Agreeing with the smaller body size of females, the length of the pubic bone, and indeed the entire pelvis, is generally lighter and more slender. The female pelvis appears to be longer horizontally and lower vertically than that of the male, as indeed it is.

Measurements of U.S. blacks, living and dead, indicate that for both sexes, blacks have narrower pelves than whites. It is not clear whether this decreased intercristal breadth results from greater innominate curvature, a change in bone dimensions, or in inclination in iliac blade. All of these are difficult to evaluate in an isolated innominate or even in an articulated pelvis.

Up to adolescence, the pelvic girdle is much the same size and shape in boys and girls (Reynolds, 1947). The adult male pelvis is basically an enlarged juvenile form. The age at which the pelvis begins to widen in girls varies. Typically, female pubic symphyses are sometimes seen in girls with a dental age of 8–9 years, but are not common until about 14–15 years of age (i.e., when acetabular fusion has commenced and the second permanent molars have erupted). Greulich and Thoms (1939) showed by serial x-rays that this period of growth usually spanned about 18 months and was usually completed by the mid-teens.

Sex differences in the anterior pelvis are usually clearly seen because only the medial ends of the pubic bones are involved. In the posterior pelvis, enlarging growth at the sacroiliac joint involves both ilia and sacrum, and the changes are more variable (Hoyme, 1963a; St. Hoyme, 1984).

Extra growth on the medial surface of the pubic symphysis enlarges the birth canal in girls and widens and rounds the subpubic arch. Indeed, after the fusion of the ischiopubic rami (usually at 7–8 years), there is no other growth site in the anterior pelvis to accomplish this. There is no evidence for elongation at the acetabular end of the pubic bone, which has often begun fusion with the ilium and ischium by this age.

Morphological evidence for this growth appears in the rounded subpubic arch (which remains a narrow V in males), the projecting squarish female symphysis, with a small triangular area of added bone on its lower anterior margin (Phenice, 1969), and an apparent flattening of the anterior ramus. The male symphysis appears thicker, shorter, and more triangular.

The triangular obturator foramen, said to characterize females, is most common in older women. It seems to result from resorption of the medial border of the foramen, rather than from pubic elongation. If the anterior pelvis as a whole were stretched horizontally, this shape could result. The drawings in older texts suggest such a process, rather than growth localized at the symphyseal face.

The usual metric evidence for pubic growth is an index combining pubic length (with or without acetabulum width) with a dimension correlated with body size, such as ischial height or acetabular diameter. A variety of indices have been reported by Washburn (1948, 1949), St. Hoyme (1982, 1984), Schulter-Ellis and Hayek (1984), and others. The resulting ischium : pubis indices are usually useful for sex discrimination. In most populations reported to date, the difference between male and female means is about one standard deviation, and distributions usually show only a small overlap.

As early as 1931, Putschar (1976) described pits on the inner surface of the pubic bone caused by subperiosteal hematomata following childbirth. Stewart (1957) suggested that these and other irregularities in the symphyseal surfaces might lead to errors in estimating age. Whether or not one can estimate the number of children borne, these pits are distinctive in size and position (Angel, 1969). If present, they are clear evidence for female sex. Their absence says nothing. Census data suggest that fewer than 10% of modern American women over the age of 50 have never borne children (U.S. Bureau of the Census, 1988), the probability of having had children increasing with age after adolescence. The frequency of pubic pits in the 90% of women who have had at least one child is unknown, nor do we have comparable figures for estimating the frequency of these pits in other populations.

The acetabulum and ischium are the major features of the lateral pelvis. Neither is affected by growth enlarging the pelvis. Thus they provide convenient body size comparators for use in indices. Acetabular diameters are as effective sex discriminators as femoral head diameters.

The sacroiliac joint surfaces are the site of enlarging growth in the posterior pelvis. Small bony nodules, similar to those on the acetabular margins, may be seen occasionally on these surfaces, especially along their edges. This growth may be predominately on the sacral margins, widening the sacrum; on the iliac auricular surface, widening the sciatic notch and elongating the iliac blade; or divided between the two surfaces in varying proportions. Again, this growth may be described both metrically and morphologically. Patterns vary by race, judging from variation in sacral andilia indices (Derry, 1909, 1912, 1923; Trotter, 1926). As a consequence, interpreting evidence as to sex is not so easy as at the pubic symphysis. A wide female sacrum may accompany a narrow iliac blade, or a wide iliac blade may be associated with a narrow, male-looking sacrum.

Usually the male iliac blade is higher and narrower than that of the female (Straus, 1927). However, the position of the auricular surface varies considerably. Both surfaces of the iliac blade should be examined.

If posterior pelvic enlargement takes place by growth at the sacroiliac joint, the following changes should be seen in the female pelvis:

1. Enlargement of brim circumference causes the position of the auricular surface to be displaced posteriorly on the iliac blade. This might leave traces that could mimic a preauricular sulcus.

2. Growth on the surface should elevate it above the surrounding iliac bone, producing a variety of circumauricular grooves.

3. Elevating the surface on even a slight pedestal could contribute to joint instability and increased possibility of arthritic changes with each pregnancy.

Many of the sex indicators in the bone around the sacroiliac joint seem to be responses to these predictions.

Examination of the auricular surface and the area around it may show several characteristics associated with sex (İşcan and Derrick, 1984; St. Hoyme, 1984) (Table 7).

Derry (1923) showed increased iliac breadth, especially at the arcuate line, suggesting growth at the sacroiliac margins. He pointed out that his chilotic and chorematic indices both indicated growth between the anterior auricular point and the area just above the acetabulum. He also noted differences between populations, which he suggested were genetic or racial in origin.

The posterior ischial spine, which is connected by a ligament to the lower border of the sacrum, is usually larger and heavier in males. When the spine projects and the sciatic notch is narrow, it can resemble a narrow closed loop (Sauter and Privat, 1954). The shape of the notch can be deceiving. Viewing only the iliac blade, it may appear narrow. But when the sacrum, which is its posterior border, is articulated, its true width is evident. A wide notch, which may widen even further if the sacroiliac joint is mobile, is of obvious value in childbearing (Cave, 1937). Letterman (1941) reports race differences in shape.

The preauricular sulcus, which is narrow and shallow in children and males, represents a growth scar. Its greater width and depth in adult women, along with structural details, suggests that it represents the site of posterior iliac widening. Houghton (1975) and Kelley (1979a) have demonstrated changes, including increased width, in multiparas. If the sacroiliac joint is more movable in women, it is reasonable to expect the stresses of pregnancy to enlarge or alter not only the auricular surface but the bone around it.

The sacrum is a complex of four, five, or six segments at the end of the spine, wedged be-

TABLE 7. Sex-Related Characteristics of the Auricular Area

	Female	Male
Iliac auricular surface	Raised, narrow	Depressed, wide
Arthritic changes	Common in older women	Rare
Preauricular sulcus	Wide, deep	Narrow, shallow
Sciatic notch	Wide, shallow	Deep, narrow
Iliac blade	Wide, low	High, narrow
Postauricular area	Thin, smooth	Thick, rough
Groove	Common	Rare
Center	Knob, bar, etc.	Thick, rough
Postauricular space	Wide, loose	Narrow, tight

tween the ilia. Each of these segments is composed of a body, two costal processes, and two neural arch processes. By early adolescence, the lateral parts have become partially united with the body of the sacrum, and longitudinal fusion is proceeding. At this age, the only site for increasing posterior pelvic width, and widening the sacrum, is at the sacral alar surfaces. The presence of epiphyseal elements on the lateral sacral borders, with similar nodules on the corresponding iliac joint surface, points to this area as the major site of growth. Depending on whether growth is primarily at the sacral or iliac margin, the shape of the sacrum may be altered. Consequently, a female sacrum (usually coupled with an unusually wide iliac blade) may be narrower and have a smaller index than many males. Depending on how growth is distributed, the sacrum may vary from a fairly regular pentagon or triangle to one with wasp-waist indentations. The number of segments articulating with the ilium can vary from two to three, with occasional accessory articulations in the postauricular area. The segment number does not seem to vary by sex or race.

The variable pattern of sacroiliac growth presents one set of problems in assessing sacral widening. Other problems arise from variable sacral structure. Generally, maximum breadth of sacrum is used as an indicator of differentiating growth. But the "first" sacral segment may actually be a lumbar vertebra that became sacralized. Does one then measure sacral width at the next segment? What can be used for a body size indicator? Width of an upper sacral body that has not undergone widening?

Measuring sacral length presents even greater problems. If there are four or six segments, which should be measured? Sacral curvature is variable. The sacral promontory may be at the top vertebra or between the first and second bodies. Curvature varies from deep to nearly flat. One must choose between a length taken with a tape or a chord measured with a caliper. It is no wonder that Derry (1912), Trotter (1926), Fawcett (1937), and others find wide variability in sacral indices.

The sacral auricular surface is wide and flat in males, but has a narrow groove corresponding to the ridged iliac surface. The shape of these mortised joint surfaces in males suggests that the narrow elevated female joint is more mobile. Supporting this is the ankylosis of the upper surface that occurs in about 50% of older men (Brooke, 1924), but almost never in women. Women, on the other hand, tend to have arthritic or inflammatory changes in these surfaces. The number and position of sacral segments articulating with the ilium varies in humans. Analogous variation varies by genus in pongids. It would be reasonable to expect sex or race variations in humans, but these have not been shown.

UPPER EXTREMITIES

Dwight (1894) described the male clavicle as strong, long, and boldly curved, and the female clavicle as slight, short, and straight. He felt that size and strength were more reliable sex characteristics than curvature. Terry (1932) and Woo (1938) have also reviewed race and sex differences.

In the United States, football injuries probably account for the majority of old fractures in clavicles, so these might serve as sex indicators. Since the 1940s, when shoulder-strap purses became popular, weights on the left shoulder may have modified clavicle shape. Males are now starting to carry these purses as a fashion item, though mailmen, newsboys, caddies, and others have habitually carried loads in this way.

Bainbridge and Genovés (1956) have reported sex differences in the scapula. Vallois (1928, 1946), concluding a series of studies on the scapula, felt that the eight types he found could be referred to races. The scapular vertebral border, the glenoid fossa, and the spine are the portions most likely to survive. The blade is usually paper-thin, and the axillary and upper borders are equally fragile. Dwight (1894) reported that the glenoid surface area is a useful sex indicator, because it is correlated with humeral head size. Differences in marginal sharpness, shape of the articular surface, or other characters are not dismissed.

Women's shoulders are usually narrower than their hips, with this ratio reversed in men. Shoulder:hip breadth indices in the living (Table 4) tend to confirm this. Tradition opines that the "carrying angle"—the angle of the forearm with the humerus—should be greater in women, so that their forearms could clear their wider hips. As described by Dwight (1894), "It is generally thought that the female humerus is more slanting . . . [and] makes a smaller lateral angle with the extended and supinated forearm; but Berteaux's measurement makes the difference too slight to be worth much." Later studies, as Dwight predicted, show such overlap in both sexes as to make this indicator valueless for sex identification.

Measurements of the humeral condylo-diaphyseal angle by Bodel (1939) and Snow (1940) show a range of about 71–94° in males, 73–95° in females, with a difference between the means (about 1°) so slight as to be useless.

Before birth and in infancy, the humeral shaft twists so as to bring the humeral head, elbow, forearm, and wrist into an alignment compatible with upright posture. (The femur and leg bones undergo an analogous adjustment.) With a mean of 117° in the orang and a range of 140–178° in humans, torsion seemed for a while to be a promising race indicator. Studies failed to produce the desired distribution for evolutionary racial ranking (Matthews, 1887). More recently, Krahl and Evans (1945) and Krahl (1976), measuring torsion and allowing for rotation, found strong side differences. The wide variation and overlapping distributions showed, as usual, less relation to sex or race than to function.

Themido (1926) recorded head, shaft, and condyle dimensions in humeri of known and unknown sex. Except for head diameter and circumference, most dimensions showed the usual overlap. The dividing head diameter for the sexes was about 44 mm for both femur and humerus. Dorsey (1897) gives similar figures and notes that femur and humerus head dimensions are about the same size and that the humeral head may or may not be larger than the femoral, with neither correlation nor regularity. His major difference with other authors is that he asserts that sex differences are greater in Europeans than in "the lower races."

Septal apertures in the lower end of the humerus vary widely by race, side, and sex. These perforations in the olecranon fossa occur a few millimeters proximal to the lower epiphyseal plate and usually appear after adolescence. Hrdlička (1932) noted that they were much more common in women than in men and more frequent in the left humerus. Similar apertures occur in pongids and in other mammals. Human frequencies range from under 5% to nearly 60%. Most authors report highest frequencies in women, on the left side, and in less well-nourished individuals or groups. Akabori (1934), Trotter (1934), and, more recently, Glanville (1967) all comment that the predominant common characteristic seems to be the strength of the bone. These foramina seem related primarily to occupational or nutritional stresses; association with sex or race is cultural rather than genetic.

Humerus: radius indices traditionally reflect shorter forearms in whites and in women; but again, there are no consistent sex or race differences (cf. Table 5) (Trotter and Gleser, 1952, 1958, 1977).

LOWER EXTREMITIES

Every leg joint interested nineteenth-century anthropologists. These might indicate the stage at which humans attained truly upright posture and thus help to distinguish the "lower races" from those more advanced. Accordingly, the acetabulum, knee, ankle, and foot joints were examined meticulously. The lower back is also involved in squatting. "Squatting facets" are one of a complex of traits that may occur in many combinations. This evidence needs careful interpretation, for Hewes (1955) sketches numerous ways of squatting, involving different degrees of flexing one or both legs. "Squatting facets" on the lower anterior tibial margin of Punjabis, both infant and adult, were examined by Charles (1894a,b). Were they a hereditary preadaptation or acquired after birth? Although this part of the epiphysis is still cartilaginous in early childhood, traces of facets seemed to be present. Their occurrence in nonsquatting populations is frequent enough to make them, alone, of dubious value for diagnosing race, nationality, or sitting habits.

In extreme hyperflexion, femur–acetabulum contact may produce facets on the anterior neck of the femur as well as a "notch" in the upper margin of the acetabulum. Muscular tension may lead to femoral bowing and development of crista aspera on the posterior femoral surface. Stresses may also contribute to femoral and tibial flattening (Hepburn, 1897).

At the knee, pressure on the posterior margin of the femoral condyles may result in posterior (and upward or lateral) extension of the joint surfaces and retroversion of the tibial head. Tension on the ligaments may remodel both the intracondylar space of the femur and the tibial spines (Charles, 1894a). Arthritic changes may also occur at the knee, with eroded areas on the posterior condylar surfaces of both tibia and femur (rather than more anteriorly or centrally placed, as in standing). These stresses may also affect the patella by altering the frequency and size of vastus notches or patches of patellar erosion.

At the ankle, pressure on the anterior tibial surface should produce "squatting facets" and remodeling of the astragalus (Cameron, 1923). In the foot, hyperflexion of the toes during kneeling or squatting may produce patterns such as those described by Ubelaker (1979) in prehistoric Ecuadoreans.

In the lower trunk, habitual squatting may alter the apparent lumbar curve (Snow, 1948) by compressing anterior vertebral body heights. Indices of anterior:posterior body height have also been interpreted as evidence for a stooped "Neanderthal" posture and cave man shuffle. Indeed, it is quite possible that changes in the curvature of the cervical spine, skull base, and shoulders may also accompany habitual postures of the lower trunk.

In searching for good examples of "squatting facets," the clearest examples were usually found in female skeletons. Obviously these prehistoric women were not sitting idly around campfires. Instead, they were working: processing skins, grinding grain, or doing other hard, strenuous jobs that could best be done by kneeling, squatting, or being in some similar posture for long periods of time.

Taken in the context of other cultural evidence, scars of occupation may provide indirect evidence for race (i.e., sitting on the ground rather than on chairs). Activities are probably better evidence for sex than for race and may even suggest chronology; these may provide indirect evidence as to race or sex.

Alternative explanations have been advanced for flattened long bone shafts. Platymeria has been associated with nutrient conservation (Gillman, 1874; Hoyme and Bass, 1962), but also with stress (Buxton, 1938). Obviously, interpretation in any particular case must depend on what other factors are present and their degree of development.

Widened hips in women ought to produce an "imbalance" in femoral weight bearing, with femoral heads farther from the midline than in males. Dwight (1894) comments, "The angle [the femoral neck] makes with the shaft . . . is nearer a right angle in shorter femurs, and if a short femur joins a broad pelvis, as in woman, by so much more is the angle decreased. . . . This . . . I long taught with perfect good faith. . . ." Dwight found the average about the same (125°) in both males and females, with a range of 110° to 144°. He further comments that the shortest female femora have angles below the average for males or larger femora.

The predicted more oblique femur shaft in women should also have a more acute bicondylar angle, to articulate with a properly placed tibial head. Again, as with its humeral analogue, expected conditions are not found.

Stewart (1962), Walensky (1965), and Gilbert (1976) studied racial differences in the place and degree of anterior femoral curvature. U.S. black femora were somewhat straighter than those of U.S. whites, with the point of maximum curvature between the trochanter and midshaft. White femora showed maximum curvature nearer midshaft. Amerindian and Eskimo femora were most strongly curved, with strong linea aspera (Hrdlička, 1939). Except for fetal bones, there were too few subadult femora available to allow Walensky to estimate the age at which these curvature patterns first appeared. It is therefore uncertain whether place and degree of curvature are racial or are associated primarily with racial differences in lifestyle. Following White (1799) who had dissected one black cadaver, Hrdlička (1939) also mentioned straightness of bones as a black trait. The basis for this statement is not evident.

Dwight (1894) and Dorsey (1897) reported some evidence for larger articular surfaces in most male long bones. For Pearson and Bell (1917/19), a femoral head diameter of 44 mm divided males from females. Hrdlička (1944, 1945) reported similar proportions in Alaska natives and other populations. Again, whether this difference is a function of body size or is a real, hormonally mediated sex difference is uncertain. In the case of the Alaska natives, sex differences in the degree of strenuous activity would not seem to be causal, though activity might be a factor in other populations.

Patek (1926) reported a sex difference in angulation of the foot during walking. Age differences within American women suggested that this is due more to social conventions regarding ladylike gait than to anatomical structure. The skeleton is not likely to reflect this habit.

Deformed feet are a reliable indicator of sex and class status in Chinese women in the geographical areas and during the time periods that the practice of foot binding was customary. The custom had already reached western China about A.D. 1000, but was then primarily used for young girls "intended for the gay life" (Gernet, 1962). It later became an upper-class status symbol. Absence of deformity has no significance.

Popular legend periodically attributes the high frequency of champion black athletes to anatomical peculiarities. Body build, i.e., relatively long limbs—especially distal segments—as reported by Todd and Lindala (1928), Todd (1929), and Trotter and Gleser (1952, 1958), may offer some mechanical advantage in some sports.

During the 1930s, popular notions concerning leg structure were invoked to explain the success of black runners and jumpers. According to theory, Negroes had a long tibia, short calf muscles, and a somewhat longer calcaneus. Cobb (1934, 1936, 1942) demonstrated that these stereotypes were both groundless and inconsequential. A long heel bone would improve jumping leverage only if the foot had a high arch, but equally popular legend held that blacks had low arches and flat feet. The long calcaneus is also imaginary, being the result of a subcutaneous fat pad. With the cooperation of Jesse Owens, 1936 Olympic champion, Cobb demonstrated Owens' lack of most of the anatomical characters needed for athletic success. More important, Cobb also demonstrated the wide overlap in racial distributions for most of these characters. Aside from the usual sex differences in size, Steele (1976) saw no great race differences.

Separation of the big toe from the rest of the foot leaves no known osteological evidence unless in facets on the metatarsal bones. The La-Ferrassie Neanderthal is said by Boule and Vallois (1957) to have this apelike feature. Unfortunately, this illustration of the foot bones in matrix does not show this expected primative feature. This characteristic was of considerable interest during World War II, as a possible way of distinguishing between the Japanese, who wore thonged sandals, and the Chinese, who did not. It was found to be of limited practical value because most soldiers wore shoes in combat.

THE DISCRIMINANT FUNCTION APPROACH

The primary purpose of discriminant function analysis is to reduce subjective judgment, and the need for trained expertise. A second claimed advantage is that all bones will be evaluated on "the same evidence." If the clearest evidence for sex is a large parturition scar in one pelvis and a wide sciatic notch in another, it would seem ill-advised to insist on using only ischium:pubis index and femur head diameter as sex criteria. Unless the formulas include horizontal pelvic measurements, their major component is body size, and the populations' degree of sexual dimorphism will influence their effectiveness. They may be useful for identifying bones from peoples of similar body size and build, especially at range extremes, where help is least needed. To be usable, all needed parts must be present. If race, and therefore the correct formula, is unknown, determinations on bones of intermediate size may not be trustworthy.

Since the development of the discriminant function statistic by Fischer (1940), physical anthropologists have found it to be an effective quantitative approach to sex and race determination. The justification for this application is that morphological variation may be better assessed if the skeleton and its parts are considered as a system and analyzed in terms of the factors that are collectively postulated to explain it (Novotny, 1986). The first studies using this premise were published by Thieme and Schull (1957), Hanihara (1959), Giles and Elliot (1962a), and Howells (1965).

Sex determination is amenable to discriminant function analysis based on the assumption that the two sexes will produce a bimodal curve (Thieme and Schull, 1957). Hanihara (1959) was able to obtain an accuracy rate of 90% from a Japanese sample using only three dimensions from the skull. Giles (1970) demonstrated that a similar approach can be successfully applied to Caucasoid and Negroid populations as well. It was also noted that the degree of sexual dimorphism is about the same in all major race groups, although the contribution of a particular variable to a function differs from one population to the next. Therefore, one would expect the variables used in each assessment to have population-specific weights. Table 8 lists sex determination accuracies for blacks (B), whites (W), Mongoloids (M), and American Indian (I) populations.

Discriminant function studies have proliferated and produced techniques that can be used on every major bone as well as fragmentary skeletal remains. Because the pelvis exhibits the most obvious sexual dimorphism of any skeletal component, studies have concentrated in this area. Within the pelvic girdle, the acetabulum and sciatic region have received the most attention (e.g., Jovanović and Živanović, 1965; Kelley, 1979b; Schulter-Ellis et al., 1983, 1985). The use of pubic and ischial lengths alone yields an accuracy of 94% to 97% in major race groups, including the Japanese and American blacks and whites. The figure is even higher (98%) when acetabular size is also included in the formula (Schulter-Ellis et al., 1985).

Lower extremity bones, however, should not be ignored because, as also noted in Table 8, certain measurements from the femur and tibia can provide nearly 87% discrimination between the sexes. These findings are especially important when one considers that such a high percentage can be obtained from even a fragment of a bone. In recent years, research has been extended to the ribs (İşcan, 1985), humerus, radius, and ulna (Steel, 1972; Černý and Komenda, 1980; Allen et al., 1987), sacrum (Stradalova, 1975; Kimura, 1982a), femur (DiBennardo and Taylor, 1982; İşcan and Miller-Shaivitz, 1984a), tibia (Pettener et al., 1980; İşcan and Miller-Shaivitz, 1984b), talus, and calcaneus (Steele, 1976). Krogman and İşcan (1986) list several formulas from these and other bones from several populations.

A number of problems associated with this procedure have been discovered and detailed accordingly (Defrise-Gussenhoven, 1966; Howells, 1969; Giles, 1970; Van Vark, 1985; DiBennardo, 1986). Important considerations include sample size and the rationale for variable selection (Van Vark, 1985). Furthermore, it has been demonstrated that discriminant function sexing formulas should be population specific to account for race-linked differences in sexual dimorphism (Kajanoja, 1966; Boulinier, 1968; Henke, 1971).

Discriminant function statistical analyses were also utilized as a quantitative method to distinguish one race group from another. As expected, the cranium has been the focus of this assessment (Giles and Elliot, 1962a; Crichton, 1966; Rightmire, 1970; Gill et al., 1988). Despite the general success of this methodology, some concerns have been raised. With few exceptions (e.g., Giles and Elliot, 1962b), these functions have been designed to discriminate between only two populations at one time. Another problem is the existence of intrapopulational variation (Birkby, 1966; Snow et al., 1979). Therefore, the formulas from one population should not be applied to another population (Birkby, 1966).

Postcranial differences between races have also been examined. Earlier studies have shown that statistically significant racial differentials existed in many dimensions of, for ex-

TABLE 8. Accuracy Rate of Sex Determination in Various Bones Using the Discriminant Function Formulas in Different Racial Groups

Bone or structure	No. of variables	Race[a]	Percent accuracy	Source
Face and neurocranium	4	N	85	Giles (1970)
	4	C	86	Giles (1970)
	4	M	90	Hanihara (1959)
Mandible	3	N	85	Giles (1970)
Ribs	4	C	83	İşcan (1985)
Innominate	2	N	97	
	2	C	98	Schulter-Ellis et al. (1983, 1985)
Ischium and pubis	2	N	96	Kimura (1982a)
	2	C	94	Kimura (1982a)
	2	M	97	Kimura (1982a)
Sacrum	2	N	83	Kimura (1982b)
	2	C	80	Kimura (1982b)
	2	M	75	Kimura (1982b)
Femur				
Head	1	N	90	
	1	C	90	İşcan and Miller-Shaivitz (1984a)
Midshaft circ	1	N	73	
	1	C	84	İşcan and Miller-Shaivitz (1984a)
	1	I	85	Black (1978)
Tibia				
Prox epiphy br	1	N	86	
	1	C	87	İşcan and Miller-Shaivitz (1984b,c)
Nutr fora circ	1	N	80	
	1	C	77	İşcan and Miller-Shaivitz (1984b,c)
Calcaneus	2	C	79	Steele (1976)
Talus	2	C	83	Steele (1976)

[a] M, Mongoloid; N, Negroid; C, Caucasoid; I, American Indian.

ample, the scapula (Flower, 1879), ribs (Lanier, 1944; Loth and İşcan, 1987), long bones (Schultz, 1937; Modi, 1957), and pelvis (Howells and Hotelling, 1936; Letterman, 1941). Recent studies concentrate primarily on the pelvic girdle (Flander, 1978; İşcan, 1983), its associated structures like the sciatic notch and acetabulum (Schulter-Ellis and Hayek, 1984), and techniques combining dimensions of several bones (DiBennardo and Taylor, 1983).

Table 9 presents race determination accuracies for Caucasoid, Negroid, and Mongoloid populations. Clearly, the cranium is the most reliable part of the skeleton for determining race. Interestingly, yet not unexpectedly, the pelvis is the second most racially diagnostic region, particularly in one dimension—the transverse breadth of the inlet. Prediction rates at this site range from 75% to 88%. Adding measurements from a long bone (e.g., the femur) to pelvic formulas increased classification accuracy to over 90%. Many of these functions can be found in Krogman and İşcan (1986).

MAKING DECISIONS

The available evidence for deciding race and sex for any specimen is usually both metric and morphological. The first step in making a decision is to list all of the evidence on each point and evaluate it. Some items, such as size of the brow ridge, might reflect both race and sex. Others, such as pelvic morphology, might relate primarily to sex. Parturition scars might in themselves be decisive, while size might be equivocal. Although a decision as to race or sex is the objective, a record of the evidence used and how it was evaluated could prove to be of great value if it were necessary 1) to defend the conclusions or 2) to change an opinion in the light of new evidence. Whether race or sex is

TABLE 9. Accuracy Rate of Race Determination in Various Bones Using the Discriminant Function Formulas

Bone or structure	No. of variables	Race[a]	Percent accuracy	Source
Face	1	C I	M = 80–95 F = 91–95	Gill et al. (1988)
Face and neurocranium	7	N C I	M = 80–95 F = 88–93	Giles and Elliot (1962b)
Pelvic inlet	1	N C	M = 75–77 F = 79–88	İşcan (1983)
Innominate and femur	15	N C	M = 94–97 F = 88–92	DiBennardo and Taylor (1983)
Innominate and femur	3	N C	M = 82 F = 78 M = 84 F = 77	Schulter-Ellis and Hayek (1984)
Pelvis, femur, and tibia	10	N C	M = 95 F = 91	Krogman and İşcan (1986)
Femur	4 4	N C	M = 77 F = 67	Krogman and İşcan (1986)
Tibia	4 4	N C	M = 83 F = 71	Krogman and İşcan (1986)

[a] N, Negroid; C, Caucasoid; I, American Indian.

decided first is, in most cases, a matter of personal preference, for each should be reviewed in the light of the other and also by considering additional factors such as culture.

DECISIONS AS TO SEX

An orderly procedure is to list evidence for sex/race by skeletal component, assigning some coding for significance. In deciding sex, pelvic parts are usually more significant than the skull. The skull, in turn, is probably more significant than long bones. We should be aware of our subconscious assumption that this skeleton is that of a normal person, average in most respects. We should remember also that although most adults are clearly male or female, most experts agree that identification of sex is rarely possible in more than 80–90% of skeletons, so we should include M?, ?, and F? in our opinions. Absence of clearly evident sex characters may have been one of that person's physical features in life.

Within the pelvis, the presence of parturition scars is highly significant, for it is hard to think of any activity that could mimic them in males. Their absence, however, does not necessarily mean male sex. According to Census figures (U.S. Bureau of the Census, 1988), the percentage of American women who have not borne children by age 20 (well over 50%) decreases to about 10% by age 50. Not all pregnant women have deliveries that leave scars. In our mothers and in many Third World women, it matters little whether a particular pit or groove is evidence of pregnancy or of childbirth; but in an increasing number of modern urban women, pregnancy is not always terminated in the traditional manner. For the future, it may become useful to distinguish between scars of pregnancy and scars of parturition.

We assume that if the skeleton is a female, she underwent the usual kind and degree of anterior pelvic enlargement at adolescence, and that, if a male, he did not. We may be able to estimate, from statistics on the percentage of women with "android" pelves or of difficult deliveries due to pelvic inadequacies, that some unknown, probably small, percentage of women may lack some of the usual morphological clues as to sex. The question to be asked is, Is there evidence of anterior pelvic growth at adolescence? The evidence may lie in the shape of the subpubic arch, the ischium:pubis index, the shape of the symphysis, the presence or absence of Phenice's (1969) triangle, or some other feature. These are not independent phenomena; they are simply expressions of one single process: anterior pelvic growth. Accordingly, they count as a *single* point of evidence, not a list of independent features. The number and/or clarity of the evidence might lead to a relatively high weighting for "yes." Yet Hanna and Washburn (1953), using ischium : pubis index, were unable to determine the sex of about 10% of their Eskimo pelves. Discriminant functions, and even the experienced eye, are unable to determine sex in 10% of pelves. The fault lies not with the method, but with the pelvis.

Growth at the sacroiliac joint can produce a complex set of characters; a wide iliac blade, a wide sacrum, a wide preauricular sulcus, and a wide, shallow sciatic notch are clear indicators of female sex. But "narrow" for any one of these does not necessarily mean male. Sacrum and ilium should always be articulated, when present, to evaluate enlarging growth in the posterior pelvis. If both ilium and sacrum are narrow, it would appear that posterior widening did not take place. This usually means male. The iliac and sacral indices, wherever they are measured, will vary accordingly, as will the sciatic notch. To some extent a wide preauricular sulcus may reflect this growth, although part of its form may reflect pregnancy. Postauricular shape and morphology may also suggest the presence or extent of remodeling. Because sacrum, ilium, and (to some extent) ischium are involved in the remodeling of the posterior pelvis, evidence may not be as clear for remodeling around the pubic symphysis, and this may lead to lower weightings for this group of factors.

Arthritic changes in sacroiliac and symphyseal surfaces suggest mobility; when this is a consequence of pregnancy stresses, it is highly significant (Putschar, 1976). On the other hand, it may simply reflect the sacroiliac joint form, which seems less stable in women than in men. Either way, evidence of mobility suggests female sex. Ankylosis of the sacroiliac joint, at least unilateral, seems to be found almost exclusively in men (Brooke, 1924). If present, arthritis or ankylosis would be highly significant and should have a fairly high weighting; if absent, these would be of little significance and would rate a low score or an "x," as unobservable.

Only in the pelvis is there direct evidence as to sex; that is, bony modifications relating to childbearing, or preparation for it. Strictly speaking, this too is indirect evidence, for not all women bear children.

The evidence for sex elsewhere in the skeleton is indirect: size and robusticity, which show a tremendous range of variation with much overlap; cultural phenomena; and a few physical characters, of unknown etiology, associated with sex.

Whether expressed as cranial capacity, long bone length, or some other dimension, size is a single characteristic. It might be helpful to assess odds for male/female sex for several bones, in terms of distance from means. This might produce pattern inconsistencies that might suggest differences in body proportions associated with race or sex. Whether robusticity is another aspect of size or reflects primarily a person's degree of activity, and thus his occupation, has yet to be decided. Studies of sex differences in bony muscle markings in nonhumans, both primate and nonprimate, would help to decide whether they reflected hormone levels or simply level of activity. Such studies would help in assessing their value as sex characters in humans.

When an activity is more or less restricted to one sex and is widespread in a group, its presence is likely to offer reliable evidence as to sex. This, however, presupposes that the anthropologist has fairly extensive and accurate cultural information. Arthritis at the atlanto-occipital joint in a young woman might suggest that she habitually carried loads on her head. Chipped incisors might suggest opening bobby pins. But habits change: they can be adopted by one part of a society but abandoned by another, or discarded altogether. The weight to be assigned varies from time to time as the custom prevails. If present, cultural signs may be highly significant; if absent, they may be of no diagnostic value either way.

Once the various evidence is assembled, it needs to be ranked, weighted, and combined. We are not concerned here with the probability with which a particular combination of characters may be found together. The probability of several events is the product of the probability of each. Is a person with this cranial capacity, height, and bi-iliac width more likely to be male or female? The answer may be found by weighting and summing the probabilities for each factor and estimating their joint probability. Sometimes we may also have to consider conditional probability, i.e., if the probability of a second event depends on a prior associated event. This is akin to procedures used in arriving at business decisions when several alternative actions are possible and a variety of factors must be considered (Schlaifer, 1959).

How does one calculate and use weighting factors? For metric characters we might adapt z-scores. Thus we might average the z-scores for all long bone lengths or other size characters.

DECISIONS AS TO RACE

Although bones are biological specimens, it is most practical to make both initial and final determinations in terms of bureaucratic race. If a person has been employed, enrolled in school, or engaged in any activity that is monitored by U.S. federal agencies, that person is likely to have been listed as one of the officially recognized groups: "white," "black," "American Indian or Alaskan native," "Asian or Pacific Islander," or "Hispanic." The disappearance and description of that person are likely to have been reported in one of these categories. It is in these lists that the authorities will probably look first for a preliminary identification. The second most likely alternative, if the person was a recent immigrant, would be in terms of nationality. The third probability would be in terms of community recognition and cultural identification. Biological matters, such as mixed ancestry and the strains involved, which are what the anthropologist sees, to the police are simply matters of further descriptive detail to confirm identification.

Most of the racial evidence is found in the face and lower jaw. Except for evidence for cultural practices, which may be seen in the skull vault or joints, deciding race on the basis of long bones or other postcranial parts is exceedingly risky. Again, even in the face, racial traits are difficult to assess clearly until after adolescence. Even after adolescence, experts err. Unless there is some absolutely trustworthy point of evidence, only "undecided" or "possibly . . ." is justified.

Bureaucratic white and black probably reflect social race reasonably closely, for they emphasize how the person is accepted by the community. However there are many persons whose ancestry is almost totally white but who prefer to be known as black, and vice versa.

Amerindian and Asiatic Mongoloid biological features are best combined by the anthropologist in reaching a preliminary identification. Unless there is clear evidence for a national origin, it is wisest not to try to distinguish Amerindians from other Mongoloids. Coon (1958), Hrdlička (1942), and many experienced anthropologists have remarked on the striking resemblance of Amerindians to some of the Mongoloid peoples of Asia, citing this as additional evidence for the Asiatic origin of the American Indian. If resemblances in the living are so strong, one can expect difficulty in separating skeletal remains. Without some cultural clues, such as dental work, cranial deformity, or the like, one should proceed cautiously. Yet, it may be possible to recognize some regional populations of Amerindians (Neumann, 1952) or Europeans (Coon, 1939).

Similar cautions apply to other major groups. Many Hispanics have obvious Amerindian ancestry, but this varies with their country of origin. Peruvians, Puerto Ricans, Mexicans, and Chileans are all Hispanics, but biological components vary greatly, even within these groups. When does one add "possibly Hispanic" to the report on a skeleton diagnosed as white, black, or Amerindian? This is a decision that can wait until late in the process of identification and is best based on knowledge of the community.

Having decided upon the major group to which a skeleton most likely belongs, go no further. It is hard enough to tell a living Korean from a living Chinese or Japanese. With only a skeleton, this should not be attempted. It might be possible to eliminate a Hispanic of primarily Amerindian ancestry because there is no evidence for other expected strains. "Unlikely" is safer than "impossible" when queried about this.

FUTURE DEVELOPMENTS IN FORENSIC ANTHROPOLOGY

Race and sex characters appear to fall into two general groups. The metric characters, including the indices derived from them, usually show great variability and wide zones of overlap. These are easily described to students and to law enforcement personnel. Numerical probabilities for race and/or sex can be assigned, but their distributions make it difficult to assign an identification with more than paired probabilities. However, with most of the anthropologist's criteria coming from standard U.S. whites, blacks, and Amerindians, the chances for accuracy with these groups are pretty high.

The range of morphological variability, which the anthropologist sees during 20–40 years' experience handling bones, may be analyzed and organized so as to somewhat reduce the students' learning time. Hrdlička's *Practical Anthropometry* (1939) reflects over 40 years' experience, mostly with bone. When Stewart (1952) prepared the fourth edition of this work, he added an additional 30 years. The person who has read about skeletal identification is just as much in need of practice and experience as the new medical graduate. There is an additional handicap, though, because few of the traditional race and sex indicators have been properly studied, so that there is little data on how these traits actually vary.

Few data, either metric or morphological, are available for members of the "new" populations that are even now coming into laboratories for identification. The anthropologist's odds for success are best when dealing with standard U.S. blacks, whites, and Amerindians. It must be recognized that standards based on these populations, or inferred from unidentified archaeological materials or even older studies of the living, may not always be applicable to skeletal materials from other peoples. The material currently being brought in for study is often from younger individuals and is frequently from parts of the world where even the living are inadequately known.

The anthropologist is faced also with several new sources of change that may affect his data. A major source of physical change is socioeconomic and nutritional. Studies from many areas indicate that the younger people (Meredith, 1976), both sedentes and migrants, are both taller and heavier. Body proportions, such as relative sitting height and relative limb segment lengths, have been altered by changes in growth patterns. Changes in body build in children of recent Southeast Asian immigrants are evident when compared with the parental generation, although they have not yet been documented and quantified. In a few cases we note that means for size by age have increased. But we do not know yet whether the means have increased because the whole range has shifted or because the lower end of the range has been eliminated or both.

Changes produced by altered diet and living conditions may be more basic than we suspect. Many features that we have regarded as genetic may be cultural or ecologic. Studies on child-care practices have suggested that the head shape of some Middle Eastern people is primarily cultural (Ewing, 1950), a conclusion anticipated by Boas (1912). The "typical" female pelvic shape observed by Topinard (1878) in Paris dissecting room women has turned out to represent inadequate nutrition (Angel and Olney, 1981) rather than normal femininity. We should not be surprised by other changes in our traditional beliefs. The flattened skull base and rounded "black" forehead also may be socioeconomic and disappear from both populations and race trait lists. If some of our sex and race stereotypes regarding the skeleton are less than real, we should discover this as soon as possible, rather than pass on misinformation to our students and to those who consult us.

Certain studies are urgently needed as follows:

1. Updates of our anthropometric knowledge of major recent immigrant groups.
2. Updates of our knowledge of how changed environments and diets affect body size and form.
3. New data on people of mixed racial heritage and their growth patterns.
4. Expanded knowledge of the ages at which skeletal changes related to sex and race appear in the juvenile skeleton.
5. Examination of previously unexplored parts of the skeleton for characters associated with sex and race; we cannot say there are no differences until we have looked.
6. Monitoring of young girls to see whether premature pregnancy and early use of the birth control pill alters bone growth, body proportions, and final height.

7. Studies of skeletal development of teen age athletes treated with steroids to improve performance.

Data on other populations now in the United States are urgently needed. There may be skeletal collections available for study overseas. With present political conditions, it is unrealistic to hope that overseas collections will be accessible for study, even to professionals in those countries. The alternatives are studies on living persons from those countries and a concerted effort to make maximum use of the bodies and/or bones that become available.

In some medical and dental schools, gross anatomy is considered passé, a necessary evil that must be taught to freshmen. Medical school anatomists should be alerted to the unique research potential embodied in cadavers of New Americans and the value of establishing skeletal collections comparable to those founded by Cobb, Terry, Hamann-Todd, and others (İşcan, 1988). It may become advisable to transfer existing skeletal collections to anthropology departments where they can be maintained, expanded, and used. Skeletal remains that become available should be deposited in one or two central study collections, possibly on long-term loan.

Law enforcement personnel and medical examiners should be asked to cooperate in helping to assemble such bony remains, or at least to make them available for study before their final disposition. In some states, organ donor forms are routinely presented to applicants for driver's licenses. Perhaps these consent forms could be expanded to include skeletal research. Assembling a skeletal collection, documented as fully as possible, of modern peoples of Africa, Asia, East and West Indies, and the Americas—of *all* ages and racial backgrounds—will be a slow and expensive undertaking. As much information as possible should be gathered: handedness, health, ancestry, etc. (İşcan, 1988). The records of the Terry collection, which include death masks, measurements before dissection, hair samples, and other data, are an invaluable starting place.

Anthropologists, who understand the practical value of such collections, will have to educate physicians, clergy, law enforcement personnel, politicians, grief counselors, and others to the potential benefits of these collections. When cemeteries must be moved, perhaps an adaptation of the British solution might be developed. At St. Bride's, London, skeletons of nineteenth-century (and earlier) parishioners are stored in boxes in the church basement. In compliance with religious beliefs, they are in consecrated ground, but they are at the same time accessible for study. Research proposals are submitted to a committee consisting of representatives of the church with appropriate scientific advisors. Perhaps other families might find a similar concept acceptable. One Washington, D.C., area cemetery has long suggested that people distressed at the prospect of inhumation should consider above-ground burial in ventilated vaults that are "clean, dry."

Many profitable studies of skeletal material already on hand are possible. These should begin with simple morphological observations. Subtle differences that can be detected only with computer assistance are not likely to be useful to the anthropologist trying to reconstruct a living human being, nor are they likely to add materially to our understanding of human variation.

New studies of old bones should be supplemented with studies of the living. When Hrdlička came to Washington, D.C., in 1903, he was already advocating periodic physical surveys of the U.S. population. These are still needed, now more than ever. A few anthropometric studies of children, adolescents, and Armed Forces personnel are better than nothing. To be truly useful, the series must be divided for analysis into rational biological and geographical subgroups and should include many more measurements. This will mean reeducating granting agencies and the public to allay fears that the data may be used to the subjects' disadvantage.

Cooperation and support may be increased by the expectation that practical applications of the data gained could be profitable for everyone. For example, the makers of school buses might be persuaded that sponsoring growth studies, which include leg lengths of 6-year-olds, would not only make for safer and more comfortable buses, but would also be a legitimate tax deduction. The number of industries needing current anthropometric data is legion. Perhaps one day anthropologists can work, wearing shirts that fit, sitting at desks of the proper height, while their children climb onto school buses with steps and seats they can reach. The potential cost:benefit ratio is high and positive.

For the anthropologist reconstructing life, such data could provide guidance in applying currently available data and planning research to fill in the most urgent gaps in our knowledge.

REFERENCES

Akabori E (1934) Septal apertures in the humerus in the Japanese, Ainu, and Koreans. Am J Phys Anthropol 18: 395–400.

Allbrook DB (1955) The east African vertebral column. Am J Phys Anthropol 13:489–513.

Allen JC, Bruce MF, and MacLaughlin SM (1987) Sex determination from the radius in humans. Hum Evol 2:373–378.

Allen JP, and Turner EJ (1988) We the People: An Atlas of American Ethnic Diversity. New York: Macmillan.

Angel JL (1969) The bases of paleodemography. Am J Phys Anthropol 30:425–438.

Angel JL, and Kelley JO (1986) Posterior ramus edge inversion: A new racial trait. Am J Phys Anthropol 69:172 (abstract).

Angel JL, and Olney LM (1981) Skull base height and pelvic inlet depth from prehistoric to modern times. Am J Phys Anthropol 54:197 (abstract).

Appleton VB (1927) Growth of Chinese children in Hawaii and in China. Am J Phys Anthropol 10:237–252.

Bailit H, and Hunt EE (1964) The sexing of children's skeletons, from teeth alone and its genetic implications. Am J Phys Anthropol 22:171–173.

Bainbridge D, and Genovés ST (1956) A study of sex differences in the scapula. J R Anthropol Inst 86(2):109–134.

Bayer LM, and Gray H (1934) Anthropometric standards for working women. Hum Biol 6:472–489.

Beddoe J (1870) On the Stature and Bulk of Man in the British Isles. London: Asher.

Beddoe J (1885) The Races of Britain: A Contribution to the Anthropology of Western Europe. Bristol: Arrowsmith.

Berry B (1963) Almost White. New York: Macmillan.

Birkby WH (1966) An evaluation of race and sex identification from cranial measurements. Am J Phys Anthropol 24:21–27.

Black T III (1978) A new method for assessing the sex of fragmentary skeletal remains: Femoral shaft circumference. Am J Phys Anthropol 48:227–231.

Boas F (1912) Changes in the bodily form of descendants of immigrants. Am Anthropol 14:530–562.

Bodel JK (1939) Determination of the condylo-diaphysial angle of the humerus. Am J Phys Anthropol 25:333–339.

Bolk L (1917) On metopism. Am J Anat 22:27–47.

Boule M, and Vallois HV (1957) Fossil Man. New York: Dryden Press.

Boulinier G (1968) La détermination du sexe des crânes humains â l'aide des fonctions discriminantes. Bull Mem Soc Anthropol Paris 3:301–316.

Bowles GT (1977) The People of Asia. New York: Scribner.

Boyd WC (1950) Genetics and the Races of Man. Boston: Little Brown.

Brooke R (1924) The sacroiliac joint. J Anat 58(4):299–305.

Burkitt AN (1924) The physical characters of the Australian aboriginal. Proceedings of the Pan-Pacific Scientific Congress, pp 248–251.

Buxton LHD (1925) The Peoples of Asia. New York: Knopf.

Buxton LHD (1938) Platymeria and platycnemia. J Anat 73:31–36.

Cameron J (1920) The naso-orbito-alveolar index: A new craniometric method, including a description of a specially designed indexometer for estimating it. Am J Phys Anthropol 3:63–76.

Cameron J (1923) Osteology of Western and Central Eskimo. Report of the Canadian Arctic Expedition 1913–'18. Vol. 12, Part C, Ottawa.

Cave AJE (1937) The anatomical and obstetrical significance of the sacro-iliac notch. J Anat 72:140–142 (abstract).

Černy M, and Komenda S (1980) Sexual diagnosis by the measurements of humerus and femur. Sb Pr Pedogog Fak Univ Palack Olomouc Biol 2:147–167.

Černy M, and Komenda S (1982) Reconstruction of body height based on humerus and femur lengths (material from Czech lands). IInd Anthropology Congress of Aleš Hrdlička, Universitas Carolina Pragensis, pp 475–479.

Charles RH (1894a) The influence of function as exemplified in the morphology of the lower extremity of the Panjabi. J Anat Physiol 28:1–18.

Charles RH (1894b) Morphological peculiarities in the Panjabi and their bearing on the question of acquired characters. J Anat Physiol 28:271–280.

Cobb WM (1934) The physical constitution of the American Negro. J Negro Educ 3:340–388.

Cobb WM (1936) Race and runners. J Health Phys Educ 7: 1–8.

Cobb WM (1942) The physical anthropology of the American Negro. Am J Phys Anthropol 29:113–223.

Connolly CJ (1926) The location of nasion in the living. Am J Phys Anthropol 9:349–353.

Coon CS (1939) The Races of Europe. New York: Macmillan.

Coon CS (1958) An anthropogeographic excursion around the world. Hum Biol 30:29–42.

Coon CS (1981) Adventures and Discoveries: The Autobiography of Carleton S. Coon. Englewood Cliffs, NJ: Prentice-Hall.

Coon CS, Garn SM, and Birdsell JB (1950) Races: A Study of Race Formation in Man. Springfield, IL: Charles C Thomas.

Coon CS, and Hunt EE Jr (1965) The Living Races of Man. New York: Knopf.

Crichton JM (1966) A multiple discriminant analysis of Egyptian and African Negro crania. Papers of the Harvard University Peabody Museum 57:47–67.

Damon A (1965) Stature increase among Italian-Americans: Environmental, genetic, or both? Am J Phys Anthropol 23:401–408.

Damon A, and Crichton JM (1965) Body disproportions and occupational success in bus and truck drivers. Am J Phys Anthropol 23:63–68.

Damon A, and McFarland RA (1955) The physique of bus and truck drivers: With a review of occupational anthropology. Am J Phys Anthropol 13:711–742.

Davenport CB, and Steggerda M (1929) Race Crossing in Jamaica. Washington, DC: Carnegie Institute.

Defrise-Gussenhoven E (1966) A masculinity-femininity scale based on a discriminant function. Acta Genet 16: 198–208.

Deniker J (1900) The Races of Man: An Outline of Anthropology. New York: Scribner.

Deniker J (1926) Les Races et les Peuples de la Terre. Paris: Masson.

Derry DE (1909) Note on the innominate bone as a factor in the determination of sex: With special reference to the sulcus preauricularis. J Anat Physiol 43:266–276.

Derry DE (1912) The influence of sex on the position and composition of the human sacrum. J Anat Physiol 46: 184–192.

Derry DE (1923) On the sexual and racial characters of the human ilium. J Anat 58:71–83.

DiBennardo R (1986) The use and interpretation of common computer implementation of discriminant function analysis. In KJ Reichs (ed): Forensic Osteology. Springfield, IL: Charles C. Thomas, pp 218–228.

DiBennardo R, and Taylor JV (1982) Classification and misclassification in sexing the black femur by discriminant function analysis. Am J Phys Anthropol 58:145–151.

DiBennardo R, and Taylor JV (1983) Multiple discriminant function analysis of sex and race in the postcranial skeleton. Am J Phys Anthropol 61:305–314.

Dorsey GA (1897) A sexual study of the articular surfaces of the long bones in aboriginal American skeletons. Boston Med Surg J 137(4):80–82.

Dureau A (1873) Des caractères sexuels du crane humaine. Rev Anthropol 2:475–487.

Dwight T (1881) The sternum as an index of sex and age. J Anat Physiol 15:327–330.

Dwight T (1890) The sternum as an index of sex, height and age. J Anat 24:527–535.

Dwight T (1894) The range and significance of variations in the human skeleton. Boston Med Surg J 131(4):73–76, 97–101.

Dwight T (1904/05) The size of the articular surfaces of the long bones as characteristic of sex: An anthropological study. J Anat 4:19–32.

y'Edynak G (1976) Long bone growth in western Eskimo and Aleut skeletons. Am J Phys Anthropol 45:569–574.

Eiben O (1981) Physique of female athletes: Anthropological and proportional analysis. In J Borms, M Hebbelinck, and A Venerando (eds): The Female Athlete: A Socio-Psychological and Kinanthropometric Approach. Basel: Karger.

Eickstedt EF von (1934) Rassenkunde und Rassengeschichte der Menschheit. Stuttgart: Enke.

Ericksen MF (1978) Aging in the lumbar spine: III. L5. Am J Phys Anthropol 48:247–250.

Ericksen MF (1982) Aging changes in thickness of the proximal femoral cortex. Am J Phys Anthropol 59:121–130.

Ewing JF (1950) Hyperbrachycephaly as influenced by cultural conditioning. Papers of the Peabody Museum of American Archaeology and Ethnology, Vol. 23, No. 2. Cambridge: Harvard University.

Fawcett E (1937) The sexing of the human sacrum. J Anat 72:633.

Fischer E (1913) Die Rehobother Bastards und das Bastardierungsproblem beim Menschen. Jena: Fischer.

Fischer RA (1940) The precision of discriminant function. Ann Eugen 10:422–429.

Flander LB (1978) Univariate and multivariate methods for sexing the sacrum. Am J Phys Anthropol 49:103–110.

Flower WH (1879) On the scapular index as a race character in man. J Anat 14:13–17.

Folkmar D (1911) Dictionary of Races or Peoples. U.S. Immigration Commission No. 662. Washington, DC: U.S. Government Printing Office.

Garn SM, Nagy JM, and Sandusky ST (1972) Differential sexual dimorphism in bone diameters of subjects of European and African ancestry. Am J Phys Anthropol 37:127–129.

Genovés S (1967) Proportionality of the long bones and their relation to stature among Mesoamericans. Am J Phys Anthropol 26:67–77.

Gernet J (1962) Daily Life in China on the Eve of the Mongol Invasion, 1250–1276. Stanford: Stanford University Press.

Gilbert BM (1976) Anterior femoral curvature: Its probable cause and utility as a criterion of racial assessment. Am J Phys Anthropol 45:601–604.

Giles E (1970) Discriminant function sexing of the human skeleton. In TD Steward (ed): Personal Identification in Mass Disaster. Washington, DC: National Museum of Natural History, pp 99–107.

Giles E, and Elliot O (1962a) Negro-white identification from the skull. VIe Congres Int Sci Anthropol Ethnol Paris 1:179–184.

Giles E, and Elliot O (1962b) Race identification from cranial measurements. J Forensic Sci 7:147–157.

Gill GW, Hughes SS, Bennett SM, and Gilbert BM (1988) Racial identification from the midfacial skeleton with special reference to American Indians and whites. J Forensic Sci 33:92–99.

Gillman H (1874) The Moundbuilders and platycnemism in Michigan. Smithsonian Annual Report, 1873, pp 364–390.

Glanville EV (1967) Perforation of the coronoid-olecranon septum: Humero-ulnar relationships in Netherlands and African populations. Am J Phys Anthropol 26:85–92.

Goldstein MS (1939) The development of the bridge of the nose. Am J Phys Anthropol 25:101–117.

Goldstein MS (1943) Demographic and Bodily Changes in Descendants of Mexican Immigrants: With Comparable Data on Parents and Children in Mexico. Austin: University of Texas, Institute of Latin-American Studies.

Greulich WW (1976) Some secular changes in the growth of American-born and native Japanese children. Am J Phys Anthropol 45:553–568.

Greulich WW, and Pyle SI (1950) Radiographic Atlas of Skeletal Development of the Hand and Wrist. Stanford: Stanford University Press.

Greulich WW, and Thoms H (1939) An x-ray study of the male pelvis. Anat Rec 75:289–299.

Hamilton M (1975) Sexual dimorphism: Secular trend of adaptation. Am J Phys Anthropol 42:305 (abstract).

Hanihara K (1959) Sex diagnosis of Japanese skulls and scapulae by means of discriminant functions. J Anthropol Soc Nippon 67:21–27.

Hanna RE, and Washburn SL (1953) The determination of the sex of skeletons, as illustrated by a study of the Eskimo pelvis. Hum Biol 25:21–27.

Hartle JA (1962) A study of the Mongoloid face. Unpublished Ph.D. thesis, Columbia University, New York.

Henke W (1971) Methodisches zur Geschlechtsbestimmung und zum morphometrischen Vergleich von menschlichen Skelettserien. Ph.D. dissertation, Kiel.

Hepburn D (1897) The platymeric, pilasteric and popliteal indices of the race collections of femora in the Anatomical Museum of the University of Edinburgh. J Anat Physiol 31:116–156.

Hewes GW (1955) World distribution of certain postural habits. Am Anthropol 57:231–244.

Hiernaux J (1975) The People of Africa. New York: Scribner.

Hoffman M (1936) Heads and Tales. New York: Charles Scribner and Sons.

Hooton EA (1918) On certain Eskimoid traits in Icelandic skulls. Am J Phys Anthropol 1:53–76.

Hooton EA (1930) The Indians of Pecos Pueblo: A Study of Their Skeletal Remains. New Haven: Yale University Press.

Houghton P (1974) The relationship of the pre-auricular groove of the ilium to pregnancy. Am J Phys Anthropol 41:381–389.

Houghton P (1975) The bony imprint of pregnancy. NY Acad Med Bull 51:655–661.
Houghton P (1977) Rocker jaws. Am J Phys Anthropol 47: 365–369.
Howells WW (1943) Physical anthropology as a technique. Am J Phys Anthropol 1:355–361.
Howells WW (1965) Determination du sexe du bassin par fonction Discriminante: Etude du material du Doctor Gaillard. Bull Mem Soc Anthropol Paris, XI serie, 7:95–105.
Howells WW (1969) The use of multivariate techniques in the study of skeletal populations. Am J Phys Anthropol 31:311–314.
Howells WW, and Hotelling H (1936) Measurements and correlations on pelves of Indians of the southwest. Am J Phys Anthropol 21:91–106.
Hoyme LE (1957) The earliest use of indices for sexing pelves. Am J Phys Anthropol 15:537–546.
Hoyme LE (1963a) Sex differentiation in the human pelvis: Its bearing on problems of identification. D. Phil. thesis, Oxford University.
Hoyme LE (1963b) The relation of age and sex ratios to health, longevity, and culture in aboriginal skeletal populations. Am J Phys Anthropol 21:402 (abstract).
Hoyme LE, and Bass WM (1962) Human skeletal remains from the Tollifero (Ha6) and Clarksville (Mc14) sites, John H. Kerr Reservoir basin, Virginia. Bureau Am Ethnol Bull 182:329–400.
Hoyte DAN, and Enlow DH (1966) Wolff's law and the problem of muscle attachment on resorptive surfaces of bone. Am J Phys Anthropol 24:205–213.
Hrdlička A (1919a) Anthropometry. Am J Phys Anthropol 2:43–67.
Hrdlička A (1919b) Anthropometry: B. Introduction to anthropometry. Am J Phys Anthropol 2:175–194.
Hrdlička A (1919c) Anthropometry: C. Anthropometry on the living: Instruments. Am J Phys Anthropol 2:283–319.
Hrdlička A (1919d) Anthropometry: D. Skeletal parts: The skull. Am J Phys Anthropol 2:401–428.
Hrdlička A (1920) Shovel-shaped teeth. Am J Phys Anthropol 3:429–465.
Hrdlička A (1932) The humerus: Septal aperture. Anthropology (Prague) 10:31–96.
Hrdlička A (1939) Practical Anthropometry. Philadelphia: Wistar Institute Press.
Hrdlička A (1942) Peoples of the Soviet Union. Washington, DC: Smithsonian War Background Series, No. 3.
Hrdlička A (1944) The Anthropology of Kodiak Island. Philadelphia: Wistar Institute Press.
Hrdlička A (1945) The Aleutian and Commander Islands and Their Inhabitants. Philadelphia: Wistar Institute Press.
Hunt EE, and Gleiser I (1955) The estimation of age and sex of preadolescent children from bones and teeth. Am J Phys Anthropol 13:479–487.
Imbelloni J, and Dembo A (1938) Deformaciones Intencionales del Cuerpo Humano de Caracter Etnico. Buenos Aires: J. Anesi.
İşcan MY (1983) Assessment of race from the pelvis. Am J Phys Anthropol 62:205–208.
İşcan MY (1985) Osteometric analysis of sexual dimorphism in the sternal end of the rib. J Forensic Sci 30: 1090–1099.
İşcan MY (1988) Rise of forensic anthropology. Yrbk Phys Anthropol 31:203–230.
İşcan MY, and Derrick K (1984) Determination of sex from the sacroiliac: A visual assessment technique. Fla Sci 47: 94–98.
İşcan MY, and Miller-Shaivitz P (1984a) Determination of sex from the femur in blacks and whites. Collegium Antropol 8:169–177.
İşcan MY, and Miller-Shaivitz P (1984b) Determination of sex from the tibia. Am J Phys Anthropol 64:53–58.
İşcan MY, and Miller-Shaivitz P (1984c) Discriminant function sexing of the tibia. J Forensic Sci 29:1087–1093.
Ivaniček F (ca. 1952) Unpublished study of skull thickness. U.S. National Museum.
Jit I, Jhingan V, and Kulkarni M (1980) Sexing the human sternum. Am J Phys Anthropol 53:217–224.
Johnston FE, and Snow CE (1961) The reassessment of the age and sex of the Indian Knoll skeletal population: Demographic and methodological aspects. Am J Phys Anthropol 19:237–244.
Jovanović S, and Živanović S (1965) The establishment of the sex by the greater sciatic notch. Acta Anat 61:101–107.
Kajanoja P (1966) Sex determination of Finnish crania by discriminant function analysis. Am J Phys Anthropol 24: 29–34.
Keith A (1919) The differentiation of mankind into racial types. Smithsonian Annual Report, 1919, pp 443–453.
Keith A (1948) A New Theory of Human Evolution. London: Watts.
Kelley MA (1979a) Parturition and pelvic changes. Am J Phys Anthropol 51:541–545.
Kelley MA (1979b) Sex determination with fragmented skeletal remains. J Forensic Sci 24:154–158.
Kimura K (1976) On the skeletal maturation of Japanese-American white hybrids. Am J Phys Anthropol 44:83–89.
Kimura K (1982a) A base-wing index for sexing the sacrum. J Anthropol Soc Nippon 90 (Suppl):153–162.
Kimura K (1982b) Sex differences of the hip bone among several populations. Okajimas Folia Anat Jpn 58:266–273.
Krahl V (1976) The phylogeny and ontogeny of humeral torsion. Am J Phys Anthropol 45:595–599.
Krahl VF, and Evans FG (1945) Humeral torsion in man. Am J Phys Anthropol 3:229–253.
Krogman WM, and İşcan MY (1986) The Human Skeleton in Forensic Medicine. Springfield, IL: Charles C Thomas.
Lanier RR Jr (1944) Length of the first, twelfth, and accessory ribs in American whites and Negroes: Their relationship to certain vertebral variations. Am J Phys Anthropol 2:137–146.
Letterman GS (1941) The greater sciatic notch in American whites and Negroes. Am J Phys Anthropol 28:99–116.
Loth SR, and İşcan MY (1987) The effect of racial variation on sex determination from the sternal rib. Am J Phys Anthropol 72(2):227 (abstract).
Lundy JK (1983) Regression equations for estimating living stature from long limb bones in South African Negro. S Afr J Sci 79:337–338.
Marett JRH (1936) Race, Sex and Environment: A Study of Mineral Deficiency in Humans. London: Hutchinson.
Marett RR (1935) Head, Heart and Hands in Human Evolution. New York: Holt.
Martin R (1928) Lehrbuch der Antropologie. Jena: Fischer.
Matthews W (1887) An apparatus for determining the angle of torsion of the humerus. J Anat Physiol 21:536–538.
McKern TW, and Stewart TW (1957) Skeletal age changes in young American males. Analysed from the standpoint of age identification. Environmental Protection Research Division (Quartermaster Research and Development Center, U.S. Army, Natick, MA), Technical Report No. EP-45.
Meier A (1949) A study of the racial ancestry of the Mississippi college Negro. Am J Phys Anthropol 7:227–239.
Meredith HV (1976) Findings from Asia, Australia, Europe and North America on secular changes in mean height of children, youths, and young adults. Am J Phys Anthropol 44:315–326.

Mo S (1983) Estimation of stature by long bones of Chinese male adults in South China. Acta Anthropol Sin 2:80–85 [in Chinese].

Modi JP (1957) Medical Jurisprudence and Toxicology. Bombay: Tripathi private.

Mourant AE (1959) Blood Groups: Genetical Variation in Human Populations. Oxford: Pergamon.

Neumann GK (1952) Archeology and race in the American Indian. In JB Griffin (ed): Archaeology of Eastern United States. Chicago: University of Chicago Press.

Novotny V (1986) Sex determination of the pelvic bone: A systems approach. Anthropologie 24:197–206.

Ohyama S, Hisanaga A, Inamasu T, Yamamoto A, Hirata M, and Ishinishi N (1987) Some secular changes in body height and proportion of Japanese medical students. Am J Phys Anthropol 73:179–183.

Ortner DJ (1966) A recent occurrence of an African type tooth mutilation in Florida. Am J Phys Anthropol 25: 177–180.

Oschinsky L (1954) The Racial Affinities of the Bagandas and the Bantu Tribes of British East Africa. Cambridge: W. Heffer.

Oschinsky L (1962) Facial flatness and cheekbone morphology in Arctic Mongoloids: A case for morphological taxonomy. Anthropologica 4:349–377.

Oschinsky L (1964) The Most Ancient Eskimos: The Affinities of Dorset Culture Skeletal Remains. Ottawa: Canadian Research Centre for Anthropology, University of Ottawa.

Oschinsky L, and East DA (1964/65) The cranial morphology of Arctic Mongoloids: A Statistical Study. Ottawa: National Museum of Canada.

Patek S (1926) The angle of gait in women. Am J Phys Anthropol 9:273–291.

Pearson K, and Bell J (1917/19) A study of the long bones of the English skeleton. I. The femur. Ch. 1–4 in Draper's Co. Research Mem University of London. Biom. Series X.

Peng S, and Zhu F (1983) Estimation of stature from skull, clavicle, scapula and os coxa of male adults of southern China. Acta Anthropol Sin 2:253–259 [in Chinese].

Pettener D, Gualandi PB, and Cavicchi S (1980) La determinazione del sesso mediante analisi multivariata di caratteri metrici del tibia. Antropol Contemp 3:363–372.

Phenice TW (1969) A newly developed visual method of sexing the os pubis. Am J Phys Anthropol 30:297–301.

Putschar WGJ (1976) The structure of the human symphysis pubis with special consideration of parturition and its sequelae. Am J Phys Anthropol 45:589–594.

Reynolds EL (1947) The bony pelvis in prepuberal childhood. Am J Phys Anthropol 5:165–200.

Riesenfeld A (1956) Shovel-shaped incisors and a few other dental features among the native peoples of the Pacific. Am J Phys Anthropol 14:505–521.

Rightmire GP (1970) Bushman, Hottentot and South African Negro crania studied by distance and discrimination. Am J Phys Anthropol 33:169–196.

Roberts DF, and Bainbridge DR (1963) Nilotic physique. Am J Phys Anthropol 21:341–370.

St. Hoyme LE (1982) A simple statistical method for estimating sex distribution and dimensions in dissociated long bone series. Ossa 7:119–127.

St. Hoyme LE (1984) Sex differences in the posterior pelvis. Collegium Antropol 8:139–154.

St. Hoyme LE, and Gindhart PS (1978) Evaluation of 2-D anthropomorphic template ("Oscar") and 3-D anthropomorphic device (H-point machine) in relation to heights and body proportions of American drivers. Department of Transportation HS-803-77B.

Saksena SS (1974) A quantitative method of morphological assessment of hybridization in the U.S. Negro-white crania. Am J Phys Anthropol 41:269–278.

Sauter MR, and Privat F (1954) Sur un nouveau procede metrique de determination sexuelle du bassin osseux. Bull Soc Suisse Anthropol Ethnol 31:60–84.

Schlaifer R (1959) Probability and Statistics for Business Decisions. An Introduction to Managerial Economics Under Uncertainty. New York: McGraw Hill.

Schulter-Ellis FP, and Hayek LC (1984) Predicting race and sex with an acetabulum-pubis index. Collegium Antropol 8:155–162.

Schulter-Ellis FP, Hayek LA, and Schmidt OJ (1985) Determination of sex with a discriminant analysis of new pelvic bone measurements. Pt. II. J Forensic Sci 30:178–185.

Schulter-Ellis FP, Schmidt OJ, Hayek L-A, and Craig J (1983) Determination of sex with a discriminant analysis of new pelvic bone measurements. Pt. I. J Forensic Sci 28:169–180.

Schultz AH (1930) The skeleton of the trunk and limbs of higher primates. Hum Biol 1:303–438.

Schultz AH (1937) Proportions, variability and asymmetries of the long bones of the limbs and the clavicles in man and apes. Hum Biol 9:281–328.

Sheldon WH, Dupertuis CW, and McDermott E (1954) Atlas of Men. New York: Harper.

Snow CC, Hartman S, Giles E, and Young FA (1979) Sex and race determination of crania by calipers and computers: A test of the Giles and Elliot discriminant functions in 52 forensic science cases. J Forensic Sci 24:448–460.

Snow CE (1940) Condylo-diaphysial angles of Indian humeri from North Alabama. Alabama Museum of Natural History Paper 6, Geological Survey of Alabama, Birmingham.

Snow CE (1948) Indian Knoll skeletons of site OH 2, Ohio County, Kentucky. Univ Kentucky Rep Anthropol 4(3, part 2):381–554.

Snow CE (1974) Early Hawaiians. Lexington: University of Kentucky Press.

Sonder E, and Knussmann R (1985) Zur Korperhohenbestimmung mannlicher Individuen aur Femur-, Tibia-, und Humerus-Fragmenten. Morphol Anthropol 75:131–153.

Stafford EW, and Counter SA (1988) Descendants of the [1904 Peary] expeditions. National Geographic 174:414–429.

Steel FLD (1972) The sexing of the long bones, with reference to the St. Bride Series of identified skeletons. J R Anthropol Inst Great Britain Ireland 92:212–222.

Steele DG (1976) The estimation of sex on the basis of the talus and calcaneus. Am J Phys Anthropol 45:581–588.

Steele DG, and McKern TW (1969) A method for assessment of maximum long bone length and living stature from fragmentary long bones. Am J Phys Anthropol 31: 215–227.

Stevenson PH (1924) Age order of epiphyseal union in man. Am J Phys Anthropol 7:53–93.

Stewart TD (1934) Sequence of epiphyseal union, 3rd molar eruption and suture closure in Eskimos and American Indians. Am J Phys Anthropol 19:433–452.

Stewart TD (1943) Relative variability of Indian and white cranial series. Am J Phys Anthropol 1:261–270.

Stewart TD (ed) (1952) Practical Anthropometry. Philadelphia: Wistar Institute Press.

Stewart TD (1957) Distortion of the pubic symphyseal surface in females and its effect on age determination. Am J Phys Anthropol 15:9–18.

Stewart TD (1962) Anterior femoral curvature: Its utility for race identification. Hum Biol 34:49–62.

Stewart TD (ed) (1970) Personal Identification in Mass Disasters. Washington, DC: Smithsonian Institution.

Stradalova V (1975) Sex differences and sex determination on the sacrum. Anthropologie 13:237–244.
Straus WL Jr (1927) The human ilium: Sex and stock. Am J Phys Anthropol 11:1–28.
Tanner JM (1962) Growth at Adolescence: With a General Consideration of the Effects of Hereditary and Environmental Factors Upon Growth and Maturation from Birth to Maturity. Oxford: Blackwell.
Terry RJ (1932) The clavicle of the American Negro. Am J Phys Anthropol 16:351–379.
Themido AA (1926) Contribuções para o estudo da antropologia Portuguesa: VII Sobre algunos caracteres sexuais dos humeros Portugueses. Rev Univ Coimbra 10:103–173.
Thieme FP, and Schull WJ (1957) Sex determination from the skeleton. Hum Biol 29:242–273.
Thompson DW (1917) On Growth and Form. London: Cambridge University Press.
Todd TW (1929) Entrenched Negro physical features. Hum Biol 1:57–69.
Todd TW, and Lindala A (1928) Dimensions of the body: Whites and American Negroes of both sexes. Am J Phys Anthropol 12:35–119.
Todd TW, and Tracy B (1930) Racial features in the American Negro cranium. Am J Phys Anthropol 15:53–110.
Topinard P (1878) Anthropology. London: Chapman and Hall.
Torgersen J (1951) The developmental genetics and evolutionary meaning of the metopic suture. Am J Phys Anthropol 9:193–210.
Trotter M (1926) The sacrum and sex. Am J Phys Anthropol 9:445–450.
Trotter M (1934) Septal apertures in the humerus of American whites and Negroes. Am J Phys Anthropol 19:213–227.
Trotter M, and Gleser GC (1951) Trends in stature of American whites and Negroes born between 1840 and 1924. Am J Phys Anthropol 9:427–440.
Trotter M, and Gleser GC (1952) Estimation of stature from long bones of American whites and Negroes. Am J Phys Anthropol 10:463–514.
Trotter M, and Gleser GC (1958) A re-evaluation of estimation of stature based on measurements of stature taken during life and of long bones after death. Am J Phys Anthropol 16:79–123.
Trotter M, and Gleser GC (1977) Corrigenda to "Estimation of stature from long limb bones of American whites and Negroes. American Journal of Physical Anthropology (1952)." Am J Phys Anthropol 47:355–356.
Ubelaker DH (1979) Skeletal evidence for kneeling in prehistoric Ecuador. Am J Phys Anthropol 51:679–685.
UNESCO (1952) Statement on Race. Geneva: UNESCO.
U.S. Bureau of the Census (1988) Statistical Abstract of the United States, 108th edition. Washington, DC: U.S. Government Printing Office.
Vallois HV (1928) L'omoplate humaine, étude anatomique et anthropologique. Bull Mem Soc Anthropol Paris 9: 129–168.
Vallois HV (1946) L'omoplate humaine, étude anatomique et anthropologique. Bull Mem Soc Anthropol Paris 7:16–100.
Vallois HV (1957) Le poids comme caractère sexuel des os longs. L'Anthropologie 61:45–69.
Van Vark GN (1985) Multivariate analysis in physical anthropology. In PR Krishnaiah (ed): Multivariate Analysis—IV. Amsterdam: Elsevier, pp 599–611.
Verneau R (1875) Le Bassin dans les Sexes et dans les Races. Paris, (Thesis).
Vogt KC (1865) Lecons sur L'homme, sa Place dans la Terre. Paris: Reinwald.
Walensky N (1965) A study of anterior femoral curvature in man. Anat Rec 151:559–570.
Wallman KK and Hodgdon J (1977) Race and Ethnic Standards for Federal Statistics and Administrative Reporting. Statistical Reporter 77-10:450–454.
Washburn SL (1948) Sex differences in the pubic bone. Am J Phys Anthropol 6:199–207.
Washburn SL (1949) Sex differences in the pubic bone of Bantu and bushman. Am J Phys Anthropol 7:425–432.
Weiner JS (1954) Nose shape and climate. Am J Phys Anthropol 12:615–618.
Weiss KM (1972) On the systematic bias in skeletal sexing. Am J Phys Anthropol 37:239–250.
Weslager CA (1943) Delaware's Forgotten Folk: The Story of the Moors and Nanticokes. Philadelphia: University of Pennsylvania Press.
White C (1799) An Account of the Regular Gradations in Man and in Different Animals and Vegetables and from the Former to the Latter. London: C. Dilly.
Wolpoff MH (1968) Climatic influence on the skeletal nasal aperture. Am J Phys Anthropol 29:405–424.
Woo J-K (1949) Racial and sexual differences in the frontal curvature and its relation to metopism. Am J Phys Anthropol 7:215–226.
Woo J-K (1950) *Torus palatinus.* Am J Phys Anthropol 8: 81–111.
Woo TL (1937) A biometric study of the human malar bone. Biometrika 29:113–123.
Woo TL (1938) An anthropometric study of the Chinese clavicle. Acad Sin Anthropol J 1:1–565.
Woo TY, and Morant GM (1934) A biometric study of the flatness of the facial skeleton. Biometrika 26:196–250.
Zaaijer T (1893) Der sulcus preauricularis ossis ilei. Verh K Akad Series 2, Vol. 1, Amsterdam: Wetensch.

Reconstruction of Life From the Skeleton
© 1989 Alan R. Liss, Inc., pages 95–108

Chapter 6

Nonmetric Skeletal Variation

Shelley R. Saunders
Department of Anthropology, McMaster University, Hamilton, Ontario L8S 4L9, Canada

INTRODUCTION

Nonmetric skeletal variants are features that are usually recorded as being present or absent. Over 200 variants have been described for the skull (Ossenberg, 1976) and an almost equal number for the infracranial skeleton (Le Double, 1912; Saunders, 1978; Winder, 1981). Though they are not to be confused with general morphological features such as chin form or nasal aperture shape, the dichotomous nature of nonmetric traits often wavers when, upon closer examination, one can recognize more than two states of trait manifestation. Many different names have been used to describe these traits (Table 1). The term "nonmetric" simply signifies that these features are difficult to measure on an interval scale, thus it has become the term of common usage. A major contribution to our understanding of the nature and formation of these variants is Ossenberg's (1969) classification of cranial traits into several categories based on arrested or excessive bone formation, soft tissue relationships, and/or regional factors (Table 2). These categories are not always mutually exclusive, but they provide a set of workable criteria by which analyses can proceed. Particularly interesting are variants (such as third trochanter of the femur or atlas bridging over the vertebral artery) that resemble atavisms or "throwbacks" and that are often constant skeletal features in other animals.

In the last 20 years a voluminous literature has accumulated that is dedicated to assessing the value of nonmetric traits for making inferences about prehistoric population relationships. The theoretical approach of these studies follows a biological population model, which assumes that these traits are primarily under genetic control. In large unselective lists of traits it is always possible to identify some that are obviously pathogenic or mechanically induced and do not qualify under the model, but in most instances such distinctions are not precise.

HISTORICAL BACKGROUND

Nonmetric traits were observed and recorded as curiosities by ancient Greeks and early European anatomists (Ossenberg, 1969), but investigations into the biological nature of skeletal variants first burgeoned in the early nineteenth century. These traits served as supporting evidence for several early theories of form. The idealistic morphologists of the German *Naturphilosophen,* who were searching for a universal morphological theory in a preevolutionary period, concluded that the structures of all organisms represented a unity of plan or a limited number of archetypes (Russell, 1916). The "vertebral" theory represents one aspect of this grander theory in which the skull was said to be composed of fused vertebrae, an idea that is embryologically correct in principle (Huxley, 1864). Skeletal variants at the cranio-

TABLE 1. Names Given to Skeletal Morphological Variants

Emphasizing discontinuity
- Discrete traits
- Discreta
- Discontinuous traits
- Anomalies
- Atavisms
- Nonmetrical characters
- Minor variants
- All-or-none attributes

Emphasizing underlying continuity
- Quasi-continuous traits
- Epigenetic polymorphisms
- Threshold characters

vertebral border supposedly represented remnants of the elemental vertebrae.

The extremist recapitulation theory professed by Ernst Haeckel (Haeckel, 1879) saw the growth and development of form in the individual as a direct model for the evolution of life. Many human skeletal variants that resembled constant features in the lower mammals were seen as vestiges of the evolutionary stages through which the developing organism had passed (Saunders, 1978).

The polygenist theory, which hierarchically ranked the living races of man, marshaled observations of the presence of skeletal variants (which appeared to be reversions to ancestral conditions) in certain of the "lowest" races, as evidence for racial primitiveness (Morton, 1839; Scott, 1893). It is these early racial studies that generated the idea that trait frequencies might be used for "population" comparisons.

More extensive anatomical and anthropological monographs, which dealt with one or a number of traits; appeared in the early part of this century. Most were descriptive (Le Double, 1903, 1906, 1912) and did much to synthesize data on all known traits, with considerable attention being paid to the relationships between bone and soft tissue structures and observations of trait presence in early development. But there was a lack of consistency in reporting, and little attention was paid to side of the body, sex, age, or geographic group differences in trait incidence.

A model for the genetic control of minor skeletal variants was first proposed by Grüneberg (1952). He observed that single gene mutations in mice could induce the formation of a number of minor skeletal variants as part of their syndromic effects. However, these variants could also reach high frequencies in normal mice of certain inbred strains. Over 50 variants were subsequently identified in the mouse skeleton (Grüneberg, 1963). It was found that there were no strict correlations be-

TABLE 2. Classes of Traits[a]

Hyperostotic[b]
- Characterized by an excess of ossification into structures that are normally composed of cartilage, ligaments, or dura
- Trochlear spur
- Pterygospinous bridge
- Clinoclinoid and caroticoclinoid bridging
- Atlas bridging (posterior and lateral)
- Supratrochlear spur of the humerus

Hypostotic[c]
- Characterized by incomplete ossification or by arrested development reflecting the retention of an immature or embryonic stage
- Tympanic dehiscence
- Trace of os japonicum
- Infraorbital suture
- Septal aperture of the humerus
- Sternal aperture

Foramina, canals, and grooves for blood vessels and nerves
- Supraorbital notch or foramen
- Frontal grooves
- Accessory optic canal[b]
- Zygomaticofacial foramen (absent or number present)
- Supraclavicular nerves pierce clavicle

Supernumerary vault sutures (most are intercorrelated)
- Lambdoid wormian bones
- Pterionic ossicle
- Parietal notch ossicle
- Asterionic ossicle

Craniobasal
- Divided hypoglossal canal[b]
- Ossified apical ligament[b]
- Jugular canal bridging[b]

Spinal
- Cervical transverse foramen double[b]
- Number of presacral vertebrae
- Lumbosacral spina bifida (occulta)[c]

Prominent bony processes
- Third trochanter of the femur[b]
- Peroneal trochlea of the calcaneus[b]

Facet variations
- Double condylar facet
- Anterior-middle facet variations of the calcaneus

[a] This is an exemplary list; traits selected are those that have been well defined, produce relatively low intraobserver error, and in most cases are apparently resistant to environmental stress. An important class of variations not included here because they are so difficult to identify in archaeological samples are accessory bones of the carpus and tarsus.

[b,c] Traits that could also be placed into hyper/hypostotic pattern of trait variation.

tween parents and offspring for the presence of variants within a strain, indicating that traits did not follow a simple Mendelian pattern of inheritance. Thus, in an inbred strain, individuals with or without a trait are genetically alike. The presence of a trait or discontinuity in the phenotype is determined by a physiological threshold. Individuals who surpass the threshold will manifest the trait; for those who do not, the trait is absent.

The most intensively studied variant in mice was absence of the third molars (Grüneberg, 1952). It was found that the absence of the tooth is a discontinuous character arising from an underlying continuous distribution, the size of the tooth rudiment. The size of the tooth germ is determined by the genetic constitution of the individual and influenced by the genetic constitution of the mother, the maternal environment, and prenatal and postnatal environmental factors (Fig. 1). The genes involved are multiple genes with small, additive effects. Absence occurs if tooth germ size falls below a critical level, about five days after birth in the case of mice (Grewal, 1962). Thus, the expressions of size variations are affected by generalized and localized factors; whatever influences size will indirectly affect the presence of third molars. The underlying continuous variable was not specifically identified for all other traits, but was generally assumed to exist. Grüneberg called these traits "quasi-continuous" characters to emphasize their similarity to metric characters. As with metric characters, the multiple genes controlling for quasi-continuous characters are remote from their phenotypic effects.

Other investigators examined the causes of trait variation in inbred lines (Searle, 1954a,b; Deol and Truslove, 1957; Howe and Parsons, 1967). A variety of factors, including sex, litter size, maternal age, asymmetry, parity, and gestation length, all had some effect on trait variability, particularly the first four listed. However, residual, intangible nongenetic factors accounted for over 80% of the variance in three-quarters of the 20 traits examined by Searle (1954a). Studies of the influence of diet on trait variation in inbred lines found that a change in diet causes changes in body size, usually mediated through maternal physiology, so that the frequencies of skeletal variants are altered (Searle, 1954b). This could be accomplished by altering the position of the physiological threshold or by shifting the mean or changing the variance of the continuous distribution. Consequently, any factor that affects size during development might alter trait presence. Should sex differences in skeletal size arise, then the variant would manifest itself more in one sex than the other. If sides should be differentially affected by size factors, then trait presence would be asymmetrical.

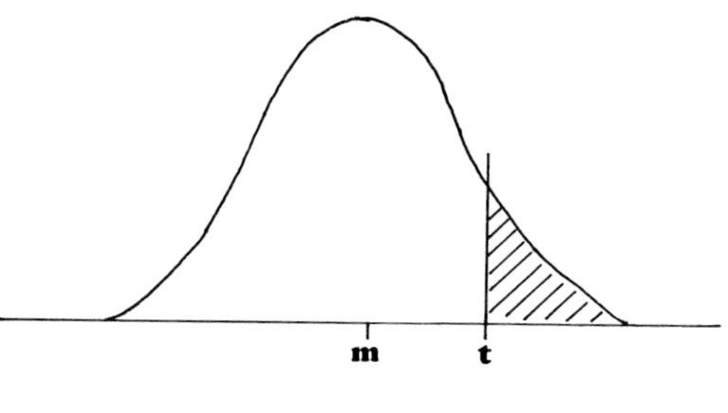

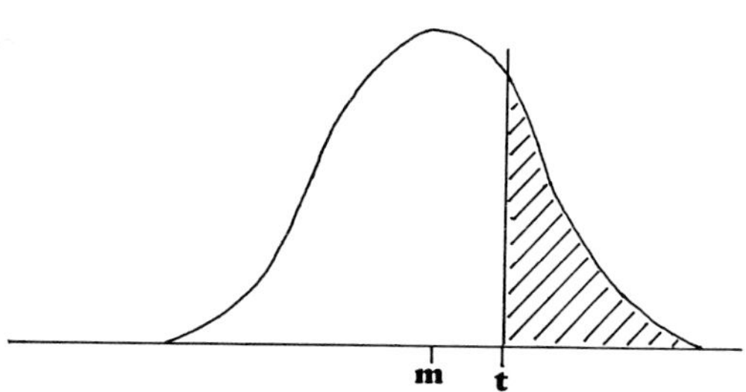

Fig. 1. The quasi-continuous model proposes that a trait or character has an underlying continuity (termed *liability* in the context of human diseases). A threshold (t) imposes a discontinuity on visible expression so that those below the threshold are "unaffected" and those above it are "affected." The continuous variation of liability is both genetically and environmentally influenced and can be thought of as a physiological process such as the development of a skeletal element. Two populations with different incidences (hatched areas) for one nonmetric trait are illustrated. The variance of liability is the same in the two groups but the means (m) differ.

Minor skeletal variants were subsequently found to occur in wild populations of mice, other rodents, and other vertebrates (Deol, 1958; Berry and Searle, 1963; Rees, 1969; Sjøvold, 1977). In a study of nonmetric trait frequencies in wild mouse populations, Berry (1963) attributed intersample variability to geographical factors, minimizing any effects of diet, although he admitted that such effects could be masked by sample bias. Calculating mean measures of divergence for British and worldwide mouse samples using a multivariate statistic that combined individual trait frequencies, he concluded that nonmetric variants can be used to genetically characterize natural or random-bred populations even though his calculated measures of divergence produced no recognizable patterns in the measures of separation. There were contradictory results in several instances.

A later paper by Berry and Berry (1967) is usually taken to be the stimulus for human population studies using nonmetric skeletal traits. Although this idea already existed in the anthropological literature and had been put into practice by several workers (Laughlin and Jorgenson, 1956; Brothwell, 1959), Berry and Berry's major contributions were a lengthy list of cranial traits and the application of the multivariate Smith-Grewal statistic, which allowed for the calculation of the average distances between sample populations.

The tenor of Berry and Berry's article was to treat nonmetric traits as superior to metric variables of the skeleton in population studies. Any effects of sex, age, side, and intertrait correlations on trait frequencies, as well as the possibility of major environmental effects, were seen as minimal in human skeletal samples and could be discounted. This claim and the fact that nonmetric traits could be scored on fragmentary bones were seen as the major advantages of these characters in dealing with small archaeological samples. According to Berry and Berry (1967), simple trait frequencies in skeletal samples could act as "genetic markers" to assess biological variability in ancient populations.

A plethora of studies subsequently applied nonmetrics to population comparisons following the Berry and Berry trait list and statistical method (Jantz, 1970; Finnegan, 1972; Birkby, 1973; McWilliams, 1974). Opinions coalesced into two factions: those who thought nonmetric traits could not satisfactorily distinguish skeletal populations compared to metric traits and those who thought they were good discriminators.

As a result of this debate, criticisms of nonmetric traits have focused on methodological problems and, secondarily, on theoretical considerations. It is important to resolve whether the effects of developmental and environmental factors on trait expression in human skeletal samples are minimal enough to allow lumping of samples and still produce meaningful sample comparisons. The appropriateness and robusticity of the statistical methods of comparison have also received considerable attention (Sjøvold, 1973; Green and Suchey, 1976; Finnegan and Cooprider, 1978).

On another level is the fundamental question of the validity of the biological population model. Are nonmetric traits (and metric variables) valid morphological discriminators of skeletal samples? If so, are they also valid biological discriminators? Direct tests of genetic and environmental hypotheses are needed, as are critical evaluations of certain assumptions made in using the model.

METHODOLOGICAL PROBLEMS

Symmetry and Asymmetry of Trait Incidence

Most nonmetric traits occur on either side of the body. After the publication of Berry and Berry's work, a long debate developed over how to record and treat bilateral traits in sample comparisons. Although there are a number of options (Green et al., 1979; Wijsman and Neves, 1986), there are two favored methods. The first calculates trait incidence by individual (number of individuals exhibiting the trait on either or both sides/total number of individuals). The second records trait incidence by the proportion of sides (number of sides with trait present/total number of sides). Those choosing the individual method have argued that the use of sides assumes that the expression of traits is independent between sides. Yet tests of side interdependence are strongly positive for the great majority of cranial and infracranial traits (Korey, 1970; Buikstra, 1972; Saunders, 1978; Molto, 1983). On the other hand, proponents of the side method argue that scoring by individual leads to an underestimation of the true population frequency in cases of poorly preserved skeletal material.

Bilaterally scored variants are not side independent, nor are they perfectly correlated. The ratios of unilaterality to bilaterality of trait expression are high for many traits (Trinkaus, 1978; Molto, 1983) and can produce disparate trait incidences between individual and side count methods, thus altering measures of sample divergence (Zegura, 1975; Sjøvold, 1977). Although statistical adjustments have been proposed that use side frequencies simultaneously but separately (Green et al., 1979; Wijsman and Neves, 1986), they are difficult to use with poorly preserved samples. Besides, these corrections do not address the basic question of the biological meaning of bilateral trait expression.

Ossenberg (1981) has proposed that unilateral expression is due to genetic influences. As genetic liability for a trait increases so does the probability of bilateral occurrence. However, McGrath et al. (1984) point out that this hypothesis is inconsistent with the concept of liability as applied to quasi-continuous traits. If liability is the underlying graded attribute of trait expression that is assumed to be normally distributed and influenced by both genetic and environmental factors, then there is no apparent physical or mechanical process that would explain the progression from unilateral to bilateral expression. In fact, Korey (1970, 1980) and others (Saunders, 1978; Winder, 1981) observed that bilateral trait incidence increases with developmental age for cranial and infracranial traits. Thus, unilateral occurrence appears to be a developmental transitional phase within individuals. Asymmetry is attributed to random environmental disruptions occurring during development.

Genetic influence was tested (McGrath et al., 1984) by calculating estimates of the heritability of asymmetry for a series of 13 nonmetric traits in rhesus macaque skeletons with known genetic relationships. The estimates were found to be low, arguing against any genetic influence on asymmetrical expression. Genetic correlations between sides for trait presence were found to be generally high, indicating that the genetic basis of the two sides of an individual is the same. While cautioning that genetic correlations and heritability estimates are population specific and results from nonhuman samples cannot necessarily be generalized to human remains, McGrath and coauthors argue that scoring of nonmetric trait frequencies should be by individual. It is contended that nonmetric trait asymmetry is due to "fluctuating asymmetry" produced by random nongenetic disruptions in development that reflect the organism's level of developmental homeostasis or ability to develop symmetrically. If this model is correct, there is no reason why reporting trait frequency by either side cannot obtain an estimate of the true population frequency, because fluctuating asymmetry is randomly expressed on either side.

McGrath et al. (1984) argue that the levels and heritabilities of fluctuating asymmetry for nonmetric traits should be assessed because they will estimate the population's ability to canalize development. But nonmetric traits can also be influenced by directional asymmetry wherein there is a greater development of a character on one side of the body or the other. Ossenberg (1969) and Molto (1983) report a higher frequency of hyperostotic cranial traits on the left side of the skull and a slight tendency for hypostotic traits to favor the right side. It was suggested this is due to slight retardation of ossification and richer innervation on that side associated with cerebral dominance. Saunders (1978) and Winder (1981) found some infracranial traits to be consistent with hyper/hypostotic expectations. In this case, significantly asymmetric hyperostotic traits are right side dominant owing to the slight effects of cerebral dominance on limb bone asymmetry. Although directional asymmetry is minimal enough as to have little effect on sample distance calculations, its existence cannot be ignored in trait etiology.

Effects of Sex and Age

According to the quasi-continuous inheritance model, size differences manifested through sexual dimorphism should affect trait frequencies (Grüneberg, 1952). These effects have been claimed to be minimal in human population studies (Berry and Berry, 1967). But a number of nonmetric distance studies have found statistically significant intersex variation both for individual traits and for the multivariate distances calculated from archaeological samples (Jantz, 1970; Finnegan, 1972; Corruccini, 1974a; Saunders, 1978). Solutions to the problem of sex-dependent traits have variously involved omitting such traits from an analysis, omitting one sex from the distance calculations for sex-associated traits, or keeping the proportions of sexes approximately equal. None of these solutions is quite satisfactory since all run the risk of removing or diluting potentially valuable intrapopulation heterogeneity and thereby diminishing interpopulation discrimination (Corruccini, 1974a; Harris, 1977; Finnegan, 1978).

Studies of human skeletal samples of documented sex have all found that the number of traits significantly affected by sex exceeds those expected by chance (Corruccini, 1974a; Berry, 1975; Finnegan, 1978; Cosseddu et al., 1979). However, the researchers reach different conclusions with regard to their results mainly because their statistical methods and trait lists are not comparable. The range of opinions can be summarized as follows:

1. Any sex differences in trait frequencies that exist are random and can be disregarded.

2. Slight differences due to sexual dimorphism can be expected, but they usually don't affect distance studies of small archaeological populations.

3. Sex differences exist for many traits and might contribute significant information to distance studies.

There is evidence that in certain trait categories size influence is mediated through sexual dimorphism. Several workers have detected an association between hyperostotic traits and higher male incidence, whereas females displayed more hypostotic traits, which could be attributed to reduced size and bone robusticity in females or a reduction of the developmental program resulting in small size and the retention of immature features (Ossenberg, 1969; Saunders, 1978; Molto, 1983). There appear to be no consistent sex-related patterns for foraminal traits, but Ossenberg (1969) reports a higher female incidence for several craniobasal traits.

It would seem logical to assume that populations with less sexual dimorphism might exhibit fewer significantly sex-associated traits than populations with greater degrees of sexual dimorphism. The few tests of this hypothesis have not supported it (Sjøvold, 1977; Winder, 1981). Sex differences in trait incidences do not appear to be explained merely by differences in body size. More recently, it has been suggested that males and females respond differently to alterations in skeletal growth such that trait presence may be associated with small bone size in one sex and large bone size in the other (Dahinten and Pucciarelli, 1983; Richtsmeier et al., 1984). Clearly, further examinations of sex differences in skeletal development can only improve our understanding of how nonmetric traits are formed.

Age variability is an important causative component of a quasi-continuous trait because these variants are the end points of genetically controlled and environmentally mediated developmental processes. Age variability in nonmetric trait incidence has been documented in mice (Self and Leamy, 1978) and also in humans (Ossenberg, 1969; Korey, 1970; Buikstra, 1972; Saunders, 1978; Winder, 1981; Molto, 1983), although the main effect occurs in the active growth period. Most workers agree that subadults must be excluded from samples in order to remove the age effect. On the other hand, there is still considerable debate over the effect of adult age changes on trait frequency. Studies of skeletal samples of docu-

TABLE 3. Age Stability of Certain Nonmetric Traits[a]

Age stable over the entire age span
Cranial
Jugular canal bridging
Divided hypoglossal canal
Paracondylar process
Squamoparietal synostosis
Frontal grooves
Pterygospinous bridge (foramen of Civinini)
Infracranial
Supratrochlear spur of the humerus
Bipartite patella
Number of presacral vertebrae
Age stable in Postadolescents
Cranial
Metopism
Pterygobasal bridging
Accessory optic canal
Ossified apical ligament
Wormian bones
Parietal process of temporal squama
Clinoid bridging
Infracranial
Spina bifida occulta
Atlas bridging
Ossified apical ligament (of atlas)
Sternal aperture
Double condylar facet
Anterior/middle facets of the calcaneus separated

[a] This is a very conservative list; it is not intended to be exhaustive. Traits were chosen if they were shown to be age independent based on several studies. Some traits have been excluded because of difficulties with scoring. Demonstrating age dependence depends on adequate sample sizes of accurately documented age at death. Sources include Ossenberg (1969), Corruccini (1974a), Berry (1975), Finnegan (1978), Saunders (1978), Dodo (1980, 1986), Winder (1981), and Molto (1983).

mented age have come to conflicting conclusions, generally because of the use of different statistical methods, variations in sample sizes, and different trait lists (Corruccini, 1974a; Berry, 1975; Finnegan, 1978).

When age effects are examined by trait category, a general trend of age progressiveness is found for hyperostotic traits and age regressiveness for hypostotic traits (Ossenberg, 1969; Saunders, 1978; Winder, 1981; Molto, 1983). This suggests that continued periosteal bone growth in the adult period contributes to the formation of "excess bone" traits and the obliteration of "lack of bone" traits. Nevertheless, studies of fetal and infant bones have identified certain specific traits as being age stable (Table 3) (Ossenberg, 1969; Saunders, 1978; Dodo, 1980, 1986).

Researchers conducting population studies must assess the magnitude of sex and age effects within samples before conducting intersample comparisons. Careful examinations of the soft tissue relationships of trait formation can help to identify those traits that are predominantly manifestations of the sex hormones or the aging process (Saunders, 1978). Although there may be a remote genetic predisposition to develop a bony process or an accessory articular facet, environmental factors predominate, and skeletal samples demographically different in age and sex structure cannot be compared.

Intertrait Correlations

Mouse genetic studies demonstrated that major genes can have an effect on the concurrent incidence of several minor skeletal variants via manifold or pleiotropic effects. Pleiotropism is a developmental phenomenon that arises as a result of coordinated gene action in different parts of the body or by a cascade of secondary and tertiary effects produced by the gene product (Grüneberg, 1963). If minor skeletal variants are controlled by an underlying normally distributed liability for trait expression that is composed of a large number of genetic and nongenetic factors, then correlations between traits should be low (Truslove, 1961).

However, the mouse researchers recognized interactions between traits for certain obvious biological reasons. These include 1) traits associated because they are alternate expressions of the same underlying variable and 2) traits associated because of a common developmental manifestation due to either regional (topographical) effects during growth or a common developmental phenomenon such as arrested growth.

Experiments with diet (Searle, 1954b; Dahinten and Pucciarelli, 1983) have also demonstrated that common environmental factors can similarly affect certain traits.

Tests of intertrait correlations in human samples have usually shown them to be low and random (Berry and Berry, 1967; Kellock and Parsons, 1970; McWilliams, 1974; Suchey, 1975). However, Sjøvold (1977) demonstrated that discovering significant correlations between traits is largely a function of sample size. As samples increase into the hundreds, genetic and/or environmental correlations may be discovered. In addition, detecting correlations for dichotomous variables depends on an appropriate statistic, in this case the phi coefficient, which most closely approximates the chi-square distribution (Benfer, 1970; Sjøvold, 1977; Saunders, 1978; Molto, 1983). Sjøvold (1977) concluded that, in general, nonmetric traits can be assumed to be correlated for both genetic and environmental reasons. However, he stated that for the small sample sizes available to researchers of human populations, intercorrelations will not affect the distance studies to any greater extent than would random fluctuations of independent variables. Yet, detecting intertrait associations reveals meaningful information about trait etiologies. In the case of humans, such detections may clarify genetic and environmental sources of variability within and between populations.

Several investigators have identified traits that are parts of a common variable (Ossenberg, 1976; Saunders, 1978; Molto, 1983). Others have recognized apparently common developmental pathways such as the associations found between hypostotic traits and accessory sutural bones (Ossenberg, 1969). There also seems to be a common pattern of expression for craniobasal variations (Ossenberg, 1969) and spinal variants (Saunders, 1978) that reflect regional patterns of development.

Nonmetric traits may be correlated with one another if they follow common developmental pathways or are influenced by similar phenomena. Comparisons of nonmetric and metric variables are revealing in this regard. When the incidences of nonmetric traits have been compared to general body size, the correlations are low (Corruccini, 1974b; Sjøvold, 1977). On the other hand, comparisons of trait presence and specific skeletal measurements have been positive both for single-trait (Bennett, 1965; Lozanoff et al., 1985) and multitrait studies (Corruccini, 1976; Saunders, 1978; Cheverud et al., 1979; Winder, 1981; Richtsmeier et al., 1984). Some have observed a general tendency for hyperostotic traits to be associated with large dimensions and hypostotic traits with small dimensions, which would reflect the common influence of a general size factor. Another interpretation is that both metric and nonmetric traits are determined by the growth and development of the soft tissues and functional spaces of the skeleton that act both locally and on a broader scale (Cheverud et al., 1979; Richtsmeier et al., 1984). Clarification of common trait etiologies will only come from more detailed studies of their development during the early growth period.

Inter- and Intraobserver Error

Until recent years, there was little formal testing of the precision and reliability with which nonmetric traits could be scored both between and within observers. On the other hand, although the charge can be made that many nonmetric researchers have been uncritical and unimaginative in copying lists of traits from secondary sources, it is true that a number of workers have eliminated traits of dubious value from their trait batteries, including those that show obvious evidence of pathogenic, dietary, or functional influence or ambiguity in expression (Korey, 1970; Buikstra, 1972; Suchey, 1975; Ossenberg, 1976; Molto, 1983).

Direct checks of interobserver error have reported very high deviations for at least several traits, usually those that could have been predicted to be problematic. For example, De Stefano et al. (1984) report substantial interobserver differences in recording foraminal traits such as ethmoid foramen position and mastoid foramen position. Error was somewhat less for the complete expression of hypoglossal canal bridging than for the partial formation state of this trait. In fact, intraobserver error tests bear out the following general conclusions:

1. Partial trait manifestations are presently totally uncomparable between observers and are subject to considerable error even by one observer (Saunders, 1978; Molto, 1983). The situation is somewhat better for dental traits because of the availability of standard casts illustrating trait expression (Nichol and Turner, 1986).

2. For the cranium, identification of accessory foramina and traits that reflect tendinous or ligamentous attachments are most problematic (Buikstra, 1972; Ossenberg, 1974; Suchey, 1975; Molto, 1979; De Stefano et al., 1984).

3. For the infracranial skeleton, greatest error occurs with the identification of articular facet extensions and certain tori and tubercles (Saunders, 1978). However, the biological meaning of a number of these traits is questionable.

As things stand at present, data of different observers are not directly comparable (Thoma, 1981; Rösing, 1984), yet neither are those for craniometrics (Utermohle and Zegura, 1982). The acceptable level of intraobserver scoring consistency is conventionally set at 95% (Korey, 1970; Molto, 1983), although one study of dental morphological traits accepts up to 10% discrepancies at the two or more grade level of multistate traits (Nichol and Turner, 1986). Assessment of intraobserver error should be standard procedure in any study, particularly if the samples are scored at widely spaced intervals (Zegura, 1975; Molto, 1979).

Careful trait descriptions do exist in the early literature (Lillie, 1917) and have recently received much deserved attention (Ossenberg, 1976; Dodo, 1980, 1986; Hauser and De Stefano, 1985). Past neglect of the issue of scoring error and trait characterization unfortunately casts doubt on the results of earlier past studies. A warning given two decades ago is still relevant today, "the success of future work in this field is dependent on the precision used in recording data" (Anderson, 1968:142).

THEORETICAL CONSIDERATIONS: GENETIC HYPOTHESES AND THE BIOLOGICAL POPULATION MODEL

Early investigators of human skeletal samples recognized that nonmetric traits might be inherited. Often the inferred evidence of a genetic basis came from the fact that a trait made its appearance before birth (Adams, 1934; Keyes, 1935). Obviously this kind of observa-

TABLE 4. Criteria for Assessing Quasi Continuity

1. On close investigation, the existence of more than two stable levels of a character, reflecting an underlying continuity
2. Sensitive to developmental influences—laterality and sex
3. Sensitive to environmental influences—maternal age and parity, both of which may produce increasing proportions of fluctuating asymmetry among the offspring
4. Positive association between the degree of trait expressivity in probands and increasing incidence of affected relatives when more than two grades of trait expressivity are observed
5. Positive association between the first sib's trait condition and that of a subsequent sib
6. Positive association between trait population frequency (total trait incidence) and expressivity on an intergroup basis

tion does not negate the influence of environment since trait presence could be influenced by maternal physiology or the prenatal environment. Nor does age dependence deny a genetic basis since inherited features may be delayed in ontogeny. Nevertheless, equivalent trait frequencies in the fetuses and adults of several populations would suggest predominantly genetic control.

Early studies of relatives either simply reported the familial tendencies for certain traits or, if pedigrees were analyzed, the common conclusion was that the traits fit a simple Mendelian pattern of inheritance. Because trait frequencies detected in relatives of affected individuals did not usually match with expected Mendelian ratios, the provisos of "reduced penetrance" and "variable expressivity" were used as escape clauses (Edwards, 1960).

The quasi-continuous model of inheritance was a significant contribution to explaining many skeletal variants, but pedigree data from relatives could often fit either the quasi-continuous or Mendelian models (Reich et al., 1972). In fact, quasi-continuous traits often simulate single-locus models when the trait is common in the population and the correlation between relatives is high (Edwards, 1960). Grüneberg's (1952) criteria for recognizing quasi-continuous traits are helpful in this regard, as are others based on pedigree data (Table 4) (Sofaer, 1969; Stern, 1973; Falconer, 1981). These criteria have been used to test the goodness of fit of dental traits (Sofaer, 1969; Scott, 1973; Harris, 1977) and some skeletal traits (Saunders and Popovich, 1978) to the quasi-continuous model. However, in most cases a fit is inferred simply because traits appear as minor variants of the skeleton.

Determination of the proportion of variation in nonmetric trait expression that is due to genetic variation has not been realized for human populations. No one has yet compiled large human pedigree samples, either living or dead, in which nonmetric traits can be identified and recorded. If variants are continuous or quasi-continuous, the relative importance of heredity can be determined by calculating the heritability, which is the proportion of total phenotypic variance that is due to additive genetic variance (V_A/V_P) or the actions of multiple genes, each having small effects. It is important to note that the remainder of the phenotypic variance includes dominant gene effects, any effects of the interaction between genotype and environment, and the effects of environmental factors alone. Estimates of the additive variance can be calculated from the degree of resemblance between relatives. Falconer (1981) provides a statistical method for quasi-continuous traits in which the only information required is the percentage incidence of the trait in the general population and the incidence in relatives of affected individuals. Falconer's method assumes that there are no effects from dominance or masking effects of major genes and that liability for trait expression is normally distributed or can be transformed for mathematical analysis.

Only a very few researchers have studied heritability of nonmetric skeletal traits. Self and Leamy's (1978) study of random-bred house mice found heritabilities to be generally low for a series of 11 cranial traits. They attributed this to a relatively recent emergence of the sample population from its inbred strain. The only other studies of the heritability of skeletal nonmetric traits are Cheverud and Buikstra's (1981a,b) investigations of 14 cranial traits in rhesus macaque skulls from Cayo Santiago. Falconer's method for threshold traits was used with 135 mother-offspring pairs and calculated separately by side. Resulting heritabilities for the right side range from −0.22 to 1.12, but none are significantly greater than one or less than zero. These results are seen as generally moderate, because over one-half of the heritabilities are greater than 0.5, which is interpreted as a considerable amount of genetic variation. Cheverud and Buikstra found heritabilities for hyper/hypostotic traits to be significantly higher than for foraminal traits, a result they attributed to trait etiology. Hyper/hypostotic traits were said to be produced by less variable ossifications of connective tissue, while foraminal traits would have several developmental sources. The variation in composite foraminal traits could be lower than the variation in the parts that compose them, thereby producing lower genetic variation estimates. However, heritabilities calculated from left-side trait incidences did not support this argument (McGrath et al., 1984).

There are a number of problems and constraints inherent in heritability studies of threshold traits. The assumption of normality of the underlying liability can be wrong if there are single genes with large effects or major environmental factors acting on liability. Estimates of heritability are subject to greater error because of the loss of information when working with dichotomized variables. Large standard errors in the estimates, found by Cheverud and Buikstra (1981a,b), diminish the strength of the conclusions. In addition, it is not possible to partition out the variance due to common environment shared by relatives unless one can test the consistency of heritability estimates in different sorts of relatives. Richtsmeier and McGrath (1986) tested for this in a cross-fostering study of random-bred mice and found only four of 35 traits to have statistically significant heritability values. Finally, and most important, heritability measures are specific to populations and cannot be generalized beyond them. A change in environmental variability or genetic variability can alter the heritability without altering the mean incidence of a trait in the population. More complex segregation analyses of different sorts of relatives would be useful for detecting the effects of major genes or environmental interactions on nonmetric traits.

The biological population model for nonmetric traits assumes that distances based on these traits are directly proportional to distances based on gene frequencies (Berry and Berry, 1967) and that it can be used for testing evolutionary hypotheses about genetic change in human populations, such as inferring gene flow, genetic admixture, or constructing evolutionary trees. Success with this model has been variable. Nonmetric traits do sometimes discriminate satisfactorily among populations of different racial origin (Ossenberg, 1976). Distance statistics generated by nonmetric traits sometimes do correlate with metric, linguistic, geographic (Ossenberg, 1977; Sjøvold, 1977), chronologic (Rothammer et al., 1982), and even genetic data (Brewer-Carias et al., 1976; Lane, 1978; Szathmary and Ossenberg, 1978), but there are exceptions (Jantz, 1970; Rightmire, 1972; El-Najjar, 1974; Carpenter, 1976; Thoma, 1981).

Unfortunately, the biological validity of distance studies of prehistoric samples is difficult to verify. The observation that two populations are distinguishable by nonmetric trait incidence does not prove genetic dissimilarity because it is a phenotypic observation; rather, environmental differences in time and space might have caused the differentiation. Absence of distinction between two populations does not necessarily imply genetic homogeneity because dominance or environmental effects could be obscuring any genetic differences. Finally, although morphological data (metrics and nonmetrics) may be compared to geographic, linguistic, or cultural data, this does not imply genetic comparisons are being made since genetic populations may migrate, become more culturally homogeneous by diffusion, or assimilate other cultural groups.

One way of testing the biological population model is to compare trait frequency data to gene frequency data for tests of genetic admixture in parental and hybrid populations. The distance between the hybrid population and two parental populations should be linear, and the hybrid should fall between the parental frequencies. Corruccini et al. (1982) compared cranial/dental nonmetric and odontometric distances calculated for an early slave population and twentieth-century blacks and whites to estimates of genetic admixture expected for such populations. The results from both classes of data are discordant with expected genetic distance, particularly for nonmetric traits. Yet, there are some difficulties with interpreting these results because the sample populations may not be representative of the gene frequency data that was gathered from the literature.

A further test of the genetic hypothesis compared nonmetric trait frequencies to gene frequency data collected from populations of Brazilian blacks, whites, and mulattos from the same region (Wijsman and Neves, 1986). Estimates of admixture obtained from the gene frequency data fit expectations, with the mulatto population falling between the other two. On the other hand, distances calculated from the nonmetric trait frequencies are nonlinear; the mulattos do not fall between the two parental populations. Several criticisms might be leveled at this study. The mulatto skeletal sample is small and the trait battery includes many traits that are correlated, subject to intraobserver error or inherently difficult to score. However, as the authors point out, if these traits produce more "noise" than "signal" then the parental populations would not differ significantly in trait frequency, which they do. The authors' further examination of individual traits show that only a small proportion of traits place mulattos intermediate between blacks and whites. Explanations for the discordant results could be dominance, threshold, or environmental effects.

Major gene effects have not been convincingly demonstrated for any specific human nonmetric trait. However, we should expect that genetic syndromes that alter bone ossification can induce the expression of certain variants, since they do so in experimental animals (Grüneberg, 1963). Significant environmental effects have been demonstrated for some individual traits, implicating factors such as trauma (Ossenberg, 1970) or mechanical stress (Mayhall, 1970; Ossenberg, 1981; Axelsson and Hedegaard, 1985; Lozanoff et al. 1985). Experimental studies of the effects of poor nutrition on trait incidence in other animals show that some but not all traits are significantly altered by nutritional deficiencies, which cause disturbances in ossification (Dahinten and Pucciarelli, 1981, 1983). If some traits can be shown to have a specific nutritional component, then in fact they can be used to study populations in nutritionally deficient environments.

The great weight of population-directed research has shown that nonmetric traits should not necessarily be better than metric traits at morphological discrimination for both theoretical and methodological reasons (Corruccini, 1974a; Cheverud et al., 1979); but they should not be any worse (Ossenberg, 1976). The quasi-continuous etiological model includes the expectation that traits will be affected by developmental and environmental factors. If these characters "are but the by-products of continuous variables" (Grüneberg, 1952:112), then there is no inherent reason why they should fare any better than metric traits in population studies. In fact, many nonmetric skeletal variants can arise from *either* a predominantly genetic or environmental source, as evidenced by the existence of phenocopies. These are nonspecific environmental perturbations that mimic or copy genetic perturbations. As an example, the formation of wormian bones or accessory bones of the rat cranium can be induced by experimental deformation (Pucciarelli, 1974), though we know that these traits are concentrated in certain inbred mouse lines and human pedigrees (Torgersen, 1951; Deol and Truslove, 1957). It is obvious that genetic influences and environmental stimuli have the same causal status during skeletal development. Both play the role of evocators rather than complete causes; in both cases, the relevant trigger calls forth one of a limited, preexisting set of developmental pathways. I would suggest here that a focus of investigations on atavistic-like nonmetric traits may be revealing and useful. Work with other animals has shown that skeletal variation is bounded; there is a tendency toward the appearance of atavistic forms (Alberch, 1983). This boundedness suggests that the developmental program is constrained and that the apportionment of morphological variation is nonrandom; the implications are evolutionary as well as physiological.

It is my contention that the poor performance of nonmetric traits in discriminating skeletal populations in many instances is attributable to the particular lists of traits used and to the considerable difficulties involved with trait description and scoring precision. Painstaking studies have demonstrated how few traits may be regarded as reliable indicators of morphological divergence based on different kinds of tests.

An important limitation of skeletal population studies is the nature of the skeletal samples themselves. The silent assumption that interpopulation variability detected by osteological variables is necessarily biological in origin is a major methodological hurdle because skeletal samples are temporal populations, varying in time and in composition (Cadien et al., 1974; Lane, 1978). Their approximation to true breeding populations is decidedly remote.

CONCLUSIONS

What directions should research on human nonmetric traits take? Further tests of genetic hypotheses should be conducted. Investigating trait variation in cases of human population admixture and examining the parents and offspring of marriages between individuals of different ancestry are two ways of evaluating whether additive gene effects are predominant for nonmetric traits. Further heritability studies of different traits would be bolstered by comparisons of different sorts of relatives to test for environmental covariation and data from a variety of populations to see if heritability estimates are generally comparable across populations. If the appropriate samples could be gathered, complex segregation analyses could search for both major gene effects and environmental covariance between relatives at the same time. This approach would most likely require data from living individuals.

Studies that use nonmetric traits to assess morphological relationships are still important, but genetically based conclusions must be approached with caution. Those studies that do not make inferences about specific genetic relationships but simply test for familial correlations still provide data for anthropological interpretations. For example, demonstrations of nonrandom trait patterns in cemeteries may indicate family clusters. Such differences can be due to both common genes and common environmental effects. But as long as the investigator simply wishes to test for nonrandomness in mortuary patterns and not propose complex genetic explanations, then the bounds of allowable theoretical assumptions are not exceeded. The same situation would apply to attempts to assign individual skeletons to a family, archaeological sample, or larger group, as in forensic cases or cases of isolated skeletal finds. Such classifications are simply based on assumptions of morphological relatedness. When surveying skeletal samples, investigators should be on the lookout for individual cases of genetic syndromes or pathological conditions that induce skeletal variants as phenocopies of minor variants.

Finally, and most important, it is quite clear from the variability of results produced by multitrait studies, no matter what hypotheses are being tested, that the most profitable direction of research is to examine traits on an individual basis when testing modes of inheritance, determining environmental effects, or exploring trait development through fetal dissection or functional analyses. We also need more detailed assessments of ranked schemes of trait expression such as those developed for dental morphological traits. If scoring error can be minimized, closer approximations to the continuous variables underlying trait expression allow more detailed testing of genetic and environmental hypotheses, provide ways of relating morphology to developmental processes, and permit the use of more powerful statistical methods for sample comparisons.

REFERENCES

Adams JL (1934) The supracondyloid variation in the human embryo. Anat Rec 59:315–333.

Alberch P (1983) Morphological variation in the neotropical salamander genus *Bolitoglossa*. Evolution 37:906–919.

Anderson J (1968) Skeletal "anomalies" as genetic indicators. In DR Brothwell (ed): The Skeletal Biology of Earlier Human Populations. Oxford: Pergamon Press, pp 135–148.

Axelsson G, and Hedegaard B (1985) Torus palatinus in Icelandic schoolchildren. Am J Phys Anthropol 67:105–112.

Benfer RA (1970) Associations among cranial traits: Brief communication. Am J Phys Anthropol 32:463.

Bennett KA (1965) The etiology and genetics of wormian bones. Am J Phys Anthropol 23:255–260.

Berry AC (1975) Factors affecting the incidence of non-metrical skeletal variants. J Anat 120:519–535.

Berry RJ (1963) Epigenetic polymorphism in wild populations of *Mus musculus*. Genet Res 4:193–220.

Berry RJ, and Berry AC (1967) Epigenetic variation in the human cranium. J Anat 101:361–379.

Berry RJ, and Searle AG (1963) Epigenetic polymorphism of the rodent skeleton. Proc Zool Soc Lond 140:577–615.

Birkby WH (1973) Discontinuous morphological traits of the skull as population markers in the prehistoric Southwest. Ph.D. dissertation, University of Arizona.

Brewer-Carias CA, le Blanc S, and Neel JV (1976) Genetic structure of a tribal population, the Yanomamo Indians: XIII. Dental microdifferentiation. Am J Phys Anthropol 44:5–14.

Brothwell D (1959) The use of non-metrical characters in the skull in differentiating populations. Ber 6 Tag Dtsch Ges Anthropol Kel 103:103–109.

Buikstra JE (1972) Hopewell in the Lower Illinois River Valley. Ph.D. dissertation, University of Chicago.

Cadien JE, Harris EF, Jones WP, and Mandarino LJ (1974) Biological lineages, skeletal populations and microevolution. Yrbk Phys Anthropol 18:194–201.

Carpenter JC (1976) A comparative study of metric and non-metric traits in a series of modern crania. Am J Phys Anthropol 45:337–344.

Cheverud JM, and Buikstra JE (1981a) Quantitative genetics of skeletal nonmetric traits in the rhesus macaques on Cayo Santiago. I. Single trait heritabilities. Am J Phys Anthropol 49:43–49.

Cheverud JM, and Buikstra JE (1981b) Quantitative genetics of skeletal nonmetric traits in the rhesus macaques on Cayo Santiago. II. Phenotypic, genetic and environmental correlations between traits. Am J Phys Anthropol 54: 51–58.

Cheverud JM, Buikstra JE, and Twichell E (1979) Relationships between non-metric skeletal traits and cranial size and shape. Am J Phys Anthropol 50:191–198.

Corruccini RS (1974a) An examination of the meaning of cranial discrete traits for human skeletal biological studies. Am J Phys Anthropol 40:425–446.

Corruccini RS (1974b) The relation between ponderal index and discrete traits and measurements of the skull. Hum Biol 46:219–231.

Corruccini RS (1976) The interaction between nonmetric and metric cranial variation. Am J Phys Anthropol 44: 285–294.

Corruccini RS, Handler JS, Mutaw RJ, and Lange FW (1982) Osteology of a slave burial population from Barbados, West Indies. Am J Phys Anthropol 59:443–460.

Cosseddu GG, Floris G, and Vona G (1979) Sex and side differences in the minor nonmetrical cranial variants. J Hum Evol 8:685–692.

Dahinten SL, and Pucciarelli HM (1981) Effect of sex, age and nutrition on discontinuous traits from rat skull. Acta Anat 110:159–163.

Dahinten SL, and Pucciarelli HM (1983) Effects of protein-calorie malnutrition during suckling and post-weaning periods on discontinuous cranial traits in rats. Am J Phys Anthropol 60:425–430.

Deol MS (1958) Genetical studies on the skeleton of the mouse: XXIV. Further data on skeletal variation in wild populations. J Embryol Exp Morphol 6:569–574.

Deol MS, and Truslove GM (1957) Genetical studies on the skeleton of the mouse: XX. Maternal physiology and variation in the skeleton of C57BL mice. J Genet 55:288–312.

De Stefano GF, Hauser G, Guidotti A, Rossi S, Gualdi Russo E, and Brasili Gualandi P (1984) Reflections on interobserver differences in scoring nonmetric cranial traits (with practical examples). J Hum Evol 13:349–355.

Dodo Y (1980) Appearance of bony bridging of the hypoglossal canal during the fetal period. J Anthropol Soc Nippon 88:229–238.

Dodo Y (1986) Observations on the bony bridging of the jugular foramen in man. J Anat 144:153–165.

Edwards JH (1960) The simulation of Mendelism. Acta Genet 10:63–70.

El-Najjar MY (1974) People of Canyon de Chelly: A study of their biology and culture. Ph.D. dissertation, University of Arizona.

Falconer DS (1981) Introduction to Quantitative Genetics. London: Longman.

Finnegan M (1972) Population definition on the Northwest Coast by analysis of discrete character variation. Ph.D. dissertation, University of Colorado.

Finnegan M (1978) Non-metric variation of the infracranial skeleton. J Anat 125:23–37.

Finnegan M, and Cooprider K (1978) Empirical comparisons of distance equations using discrete traits. Am J Phys Anthropol 49:39–46.

Green RF, and Suchey JM (1976) The use of inverse sine transformations in the analysis of non-metric cranial data. Am J Phys Anthropol 45:61–68.

Green RF, Suchey JM, and Gokhale DV (1979) The statistical treatment of correlated bilateral traits in the analysis of cranial material. Am J Phys Anthropol 50:629–634.

Grewal MS (1962) The development of an inherited tooth defect on the mouse. J Embryol Exp Morphol 10:202–211.

Grüneberg H (1952) Genetical studies on the skeleton of the mouse IV. Quasi-continuous variations. J Genet 51: 95–114.

Grüneberg H (1963) The Pathology of Development. Oxford: Blackwell.

Haeckel E (1879) The Evolution of Man: A Popular Exposition of the Principal Points of Human Ontogeny and Phylogeny, 3rd Ed. New York: Appleton.

Harris E (1977) Anthropologic and genetic aspects of the dental morphology of Solomon Islanders, Melanesia. Ph.D. dissertation, Arizona State University.

Hauser G, and De Stefano GF (1985) Variations in form of the hypoglossal canal. Am J Phys Anthropol 67:7–11.

Howe WL, and Parsons PA (1967) Genotype and environment in the determination of minor skeletal variants and body weight in mice. J Embryol Exp Morphol 17:283–292.

Huxley TH (1864) Lectures on the Elements of Comparative Anatomy. London: J Churchill.

Jantz RL (1970) Change and variation in skeletal populations of Arikara Indians. Ph.D. dissertation, University of Kansas, Lawrence.

Kellock WL, and Parsons PA (1970) A comparison of the incidence of minor non-metrical cranial variants in Australian aborigines with those of Melanesia and Polynesia. Am J Phys Anthropol 33:235–240.

Keyes JEL (1935) Observations on 4000 optic foramina in human skulls of known origin. Arch Ophthalmol 13:538–568.

Korey KA (1970) Characteristics of the distributions of non-metric variants of the skull. MA thesis, University of Chicago.

Korey KA (1980) The incidence of bilateral nonmetric skeletal traits: A reanalysis of sampling procedures. Am J Phys Anthropol 53:19–23.

Lane RA (1978) The Allegany Seneca: A test of the genetic reliability of nonmetric osteological traits for intrapopulation analysis. Ph.D. dissertation, University of Texas, Austin.

Laughlin WS, and Jorgenson JB (1956) Isolate variation in Greenlandic Eskimo crania. Acta Genet 6:3–12.

Le Double AF (1903) Traite des Variations des Os du Crane et leur Signification au Point de vue de l'Anthropologie. Paris: Vigot Freres.

Le Double AF (1906) Traite des Variations des Os de la Face de l'Homme. Paris: Vigot Freres.

Le Double AF (1912) Traite des Variations de la Colonne Vertebrale de l'Homme. Paris: Vigot Freres.

Lillie RD (1917) Variations of the canalis hypoglossis. Anat Rec 13:131–144.

Lozanoff S, Sciulli PW, and Schneider KN (1985) Third trochanter incidence and metric trait covariation in the human femur. J Anat 143:149–159.

Mayhall JT (1970) The effect of culture change upon the Eskimo dentition. Arctic Anthropol 7:117–121.

McGrath JW, Cheverud JM, and Buikstra JE (1984) Genetic correlations between sides and heritability of asymmetry for nonmetric traits in rhesus macaques on Cayo Santiago. Am J Phys Anthropol 64:401–411.

McWilliams KR (1974) Gran Quivira Pueblo and biological distance in the U.S. Southwest. Ph.D. dissertation, Arizona State University.

Molto JE (1979) The assessment and meaning of intraobserver error in population studies based on discontinuous cranial traits. Am J Phys Anthropol 51:333–344.

Molto JE (1983) Biological Relationships of Southern Ontario Woodland Peoples: The Evidence of Discontinuous Cranial Morphology. Ottawa: National Museums of Canada, Archaeological Survey of Canada, Paper No. 117.

Morton SG (1839) Crania American or, a comparative view of the skulls of various aboriginal nations of North and South America. Philadelphia: John Pennington.

Nichol CR, and Turner CG (1986) Intra- and interobserver concordance in classifying dental morphology. Am J Phys Anthropol 69:299–315.

Ossenberg NS (1969) Discontinuous morphological variation in the human cranium. Ph.D. dissertation, University of Toronto.

Ossenberg NS (1970) The influence of artificial cranial deformation on discontinuous morphological traits. Am J Phys Anthropol 38:357–371.

Ossenberg NS (1974) Origins and relationships of Woodland peoples: The evidence of cranial morphology. In E Johnston (ed): Aspects of Upper Great Lakes Anthropology; Papers in Honour of Lloyd A Wilford. St. Paul: Minnesota Historical Society, pp 15–339.

Ossenberg NS (1976) Within and between race distances in population studies based on discrete traits of the human skull. Am J Phys Anthropol 45:701–716.

Ossenberg NS (1977) Congruence of distance matrices based on cranial discrete traits, cranial measurements, and linguistic-geographic criteria in five Alaskan populations. Am J Phys Anthropol 47:93–98.

Ossenberg NS (1981) An argument for the use of total side frequencies of bilateral nonmetric skeletal traits in population distance analysis: The regression of symmetry on incidence. Am J Phys Anthropol 54:471–479.

Pucciarelli HM (1974) The influence of experimental deformation on neurocranial wormian bones in rats. Am J Phys Anthropol 41:29–37.

Rees JW (1969) Morphological variation in the cranium and mandible of the white tailed deer (*Odocoileus virginianus*): A comparative study of geographical and four biological distances. J Morphol 128:95–112.

Reich T, James JW, and Morris CA (1972) The use of multiple thresholds in determining the mode of transmission of semicontinuous traits. Ann Hum Genet 36:163–184.

Richtsmeier JT, Cheverud JM, and Buikstra JE (1984) The relationship between cranial metric and nonmetric traits in the rhesus macaques from Cayo Santiago. Am J Phys Anthropol 64:213–222.

Richtsmeier JT, and McGrath JW (1986) Quantitative genetics of cranial nonmetric traits in randombred mice: Heritability and etiology. Am J Phys Anthropol 69:51–58.

Rightmire GP (1972) Cranial measurements and discrete traits compared in distance studies of African Negro skulls. Hum Biol 44:263–275.

Rösing FW (1984) Discreta of the human skeleton: A critical review. J Hum Evol 13:319–323.

Rothammer F, Quevedo S, Cocilovo JA, and Llop E (1984) Microevolution in prehistoric Andean populations: Chronologic nonmetric variation in northern Chile. Am J Phys Anthropol 65:157–162.

Russell ES (1916) Form and Function. A Contribution to the History of Animal Morphology. London: John Murray.

Saunders SR (1978) The Development and Distribution of Discontinuous Morphological Variation of the Human Infracranial Skeleton. Ottawa: National Museums of Canada, Archaeological Survey of Canada, Paper No. 81.

Saunders SR, and Popovich F (1978) A family study of two skeletal variants: Atlas bridging and clinoid bridging. Am J Phys Anthropol 49:193–204.

Scott GR (1973) Dental morphology: A genetic study of American white families and variation in living Southwest Indians. Ph.D. dissertation, Arizona State University.

Scott JH (1893) Osteology of the Maori and Moriori. Royal Society of New Zealand Transactions and Proceedings 26:1–64.

Searle AG (1954a) Genetical studies on the skeleton of the mouse: IX. Causes of variation within pure lines. J Genet 52:68–102.

Searle AG (1954b) Genetical studies on the skeleton of the mouse: XI. The influence of diet on variation within pure lines. J Genet 52:413–424.

Self SG, and Leamy L (1978) Heritability of quasi-continuous skeletal traits in a randombred population of house mice. Genetics 88:109–120.

Sjøvold T (1973) The occurrence of minor, non-metrical variants in the skeleton and their quantitative treatment for population comparisons. Homo 24:204–233.

Sjøvold T (1977) Non-metrical divergence between skeletal populations. Ossa 4 (Suppl 1):1–133.

Sofaer JA (1969) The genetics and expression of a dental morphological variant in the mouse. Arch Oral Biol 14: 1213–1223.

Stern C (1973) Principles of Human Genetics. San Francisco: W.H. Freeman.

Suchey JM (1975) Biological distance of prehistoric central California. Populations derived from non-metrical traits of the cranium. Ph.D. dissertation, University of California.

Szathmary E, and Ossenberg NS (1978) Are the biological differences between North American Indians and Eskimos truly profound? Curr Anthropol 19:673–701.

Thoma A (1981) The pattern of quasi-continuous variation in *Homo sapiens*. J Hum Evol 10:303–310.

Torgersen J (1951) Hereditary factors in the sutural pattern of the skull. Acta Radiol 36:374–382.

Trinkaus E (1978) Bilateral asymmetry of human skeletal non-metric traits. Am J Phys Anthropol 49:315–318.

Truslove GM (1961) Genetical studies on the skeleton of the mouse: XXX. A search for correlations between some minor variants. Genet Res 2:431–438.

Utermohle CJ, and Zegura SL (1982) Intra and inter-observer error in craniometry: A cautionary tale. Am J Phys Anthropol 57:303–310.

Wijsman EM, and Neves WA (1986) The use of nonmetric variation in estimating human population admixture: A test case with Brazilian blacks, whites, and mulattos. Am J Phys Anthropol 70:395–405.

Winder S (1981) Infracranial nonmetric variation: An assessment of its value for biological distance analysis. Ph.D. dissertation, Indiana University.

Zegura SL (1975) Taxonomic congruence in Eskimoid populations. Am J Phys Anthropol 43:271–284.

Reconstruction of Life From the Skeleton
© 1989 Alan R. Liss, Inc., pages 109–127

Chapter 7

Congenital Abnormalities in Skeletal Populations

Spencer Jay Turkel
School of Natural Sciences, New York Institute of Technology, Old Westbury, New York 11568

INTRODUCTION

The purpose of this chapter is to demonstrate the importance of congenital malformations in the study of paleopathology. The chapter begins with a discussion of the nature of malformations in modern populations; this is followed by a presentation of some examples from ancient populations.

A major handicap in such studies is the problem of clearly defining what is meant by the phrase "congenital malformation." A variety of terms are used synonymously. "Congenital" is derived from the Latin and means "born together"; it is often replaced by "birth," a word derived from Old English. Both indicate that something is present at or before parturition. Whether or not an observable characteristic, per se, must be present at birth is questionable; perhaps only the etiological factor must be present. "Malformation," derived from the Latin *malus* meaning "evil" combined with *formatio* meaning "formation," has a pejorative sense. Thus, the characteristic is thought of as an evil thing. The words "abnormality," from the Latin *ab* meaning "away from" and *norma* meaning "rule," or "anomaly," from the Greek for the same meanings, connote that the characteristic is somehow against nature's laws. Similarly, "defect," from the Latin *deficere* meaning "to fail," suggests that the individual is not formed successfully.

The latter term indicates that a characteristic is either unusual or clinically significant. The focus on their clinical aspects distinguishes congenital malformations from mere anatomical variants or variations. Nevertheless, both anomaly and abnormality refer to structures that are not standard. Perhaps the underlying distinction is that congenital malformation refers to physiological variants that decrease survivability or reproductive success, whereas anatomical variations are neutral morphological deviations from the mean. It is difficult to support such a dichotomy, however. Thus, from Heinonen and associates:

> There is no general agreement about what constitutes a malformation. In this study, children were considered to be malformed when they had structural defects at or soon after birth, including tumors and syndromes that tend to be prominently associated with structural defects. (Heinonen et al., 1977: 31)

> Major malformations were defined as those which were potentially life-threatening or which were major cosmetic defects. (Heinonen et al., 1977:65)

This definition is obviously clinically oriented, but nevertheless does not provide criteria for deciding what constitutes "a life-threatening structural or a major cosmetic defect."

Not all investigators have placed the emphasis on the "defective" nature of congenital malformations; some have taken a statistical approach. Thus, according to the World Health Organization:

> . . . "malformation" does not necessarily connote only structural maldevelopment, but may also include functional and biochemical entities. For the present purpose teratology is considered to concern developmental deviations of a structural, functional or biochemical nature that are initiated pre-natally. The functional category includes behavioral parameters and the biochemical category metabolic parameters. "Embryopathy" is synonymous with "developmental deviation." (WHO, 1967:7)
>
> There is a continuum of variations from the hypothetical norm to the extreme deviant, and there is no logical place at which to draw the line of separation. The distinction between minor variation and frank malformation, therefore, is an arbitrary one and each investigator must establish his own criteria and apply them to spontaneous and induced malformations alike. (WHO, 1967;13)

McIntosh (1959) expressed the problem of definition quite clearly:

> Concerning the grotesque and unusual there is no debate . . . [On the other hand we find the] fuzzy nature of the boundary lines of the items to be scored, requiring arbitrary and usually unsatisfactory drawing of cut-off lines separating, on an *ad hoc* basis, what is to be regarded as abnormal and unexpected from the normal or expected . . . The problem must be viewed as a whole, not subdivided according to the rarity, or the lethality, or the supposed clinical significance of individual lesions. (McIntosh, 1959:139–140)

The issue, then, is whether congenital malformations represent an arbitrarily defined set within the tails of a normal distribution or are "real" and separable entities (McKusick, 1969), producing a polymodal distribution of normal and congenitally malformed individuals. Resolution of the problem is not yet possible, because hard data on variations within both normal and malformed populations are not available for most characteristics.

ANTHROPOMETRY

The present inability to view congenital malformations within the context of a variable population can be blamed on the obvious lack of anthropometry in the majority of studies. Gorlin et al. (1976) were highly critical of the qualitative, nonmetrical descriptions of congenital malformations, citing especially the example of "hyper-" and "hypotelorism":

> Distance between the eyes may appear to be abnormal depending upon the width of the face, the form of the glabellar area, the presence of epicanthic folds, the shape and width of the nose. Furthermore, one must accurately define what one means by ocular hypertelorism. Does one refer to boney interorbital distance, interpupillary distance, or inter-inner-canthal distance? How accurate are these measurements in an active, uncooperative patient? (Gorlin et al., 1976:xiv)

Farkas (1981) collected a good data base on cephalic anthropometrics, primarily directed toward clinical problems of some Canadian populations. Merlob et al. (1984) took 37 measurements on 198 Israeli newborns. Measurements were arrayed in respect to gestational age. Normal values were considered to lie within two standard deviations of the average. The authors then listed congenital malformations associated with extreme values.

Difficulties in the general application of these and similar studies lay in the specificity of the ethnic/racial composition of the populations measured and the necessarily limited range of measures made. Perhaps more importantly, all measurements were taken from "normal" subjects. Whereas it was proposed that extreme values may suggest the presence of a congenital malformation, the statistical relationship of the specific measure and a congenital malformation remains to be demonstrated. Nevertheless, it is encouraging that physicians are beginning to recognize the importance of anthropometry.

One area of clinical interest where anthropometric studies have made considerable contributions is in the evaluation of normal vs. abnormal growth in stature. The stature of a patient can be compared to standardized tables of the subject's appropriate age, sex, and race, even taking into consideration the height of the parents (e.g., Tanner, 1976). Evaluation of children can include predictions of their adult height (e.g., Tanner et al., 1983).

In addition to evaluating stature, it may be important to evaluate proportions of body parts with respect to overall stature. Among patients who have "abnormally" short stature, is this factor due to a proportionate reduction in both the limbs and the trunk or to a disproportionate shortening in either the limbs or the trunk? At one time, patients with disproportionately short limbs were lumped together as "achondroplastic dwarfs," and those with disproportionately short trunks had "Morquio's disease" (Rimoin, 1979). Anthropometrical analysis has split these disorders into numerous conditions. For example, shortening of the limbs can affect primarily the proximal segments (i.e., thigh and arm) or the middle segment (i.e., leg and forearm), conditions known as rhizomelia and mesomelia, respectively. Attention to greater detail in these disorders has led to a better understanding of variability for specific conditions as well as a clearer differentiation of related conditions (Rimoin and Horton, 1978; Rimoin, 1979).

TABLE 1. International Nomenclature of Constitutional Diseases of Bones

A. Osteochondrodysplasias ("abnormalities of cartilage and/or bone growth and development")
   1. Defects of growth of tubular bones and/or spine
      a. Identifiable at birth (25 subtypes)
      b. Identifiable in later life (23 subtypes)
   2. Disorganized development of cartilage and fibrous components of skeleton (11 subtypes)
   3. Abnormalities of density of cortical diaphyseal structure and/or metaphyseal modeling (24 subtypes)

B. Dysostoses ("malformation of individual bones, singly or in combination")
   1. Dysostoses with cranial and facial involvement (7 subtypes)
   2. Dysostoses with predominant axial involvement (7 subtypes)
   3. Dysostoses with predominant involvement of the extremities (26 subtypes)

C. Idioipathic osteolyses (3 subtypes)

D. Miscellaneous disorders with osseous involvement (11 subtypes)

E. Chromosome aberrations ("primary metabolic abnormalities")
   1. Calcium and/or phosphorus (6 subtypes)
   2. Complex carbohydrates (15 subtypes)
   3. Lipids (3 subtypes)
   4. Nucleic acids (1 type)
   5. Amino acids (1 type)
   6. Metals (1 type)

Modified from Maroteaux (1986).

ETIOLOGY AND PATHOGENESIS

A major stumbling block has been a lack of understanding of both the etiology and the pathogenesis of the major congenital malformations, thereby placing a heavy reliance on the classification of phenotypes. The International Nomenclature of Constitutional Diseases of Bone (Maroteaux, 1986) has an hierarchical system in which five major classes of disorders are further subdivided. It is necessarily a hodgepodge of taxa defined either etiologically, pathogenetically, or phenetically (Table 1).

The absence of a consistent etiological classification has led to doubt concerning the relationships of various diseases and has raised problems in the identification of individuals as members of these groups (Feingold, 1977). Discussions within the medical community are reminiscent of the splitter/lumper controversies in paleoanthropology (McKusick, 1969). This analogy is quite apt, since much of the early work has been essentially typological, focusing on particular congenital malformations as though each were a specific "disease."

A good example of congenital malformation used in an approach to disease has been the study of craniostenosis. Many investigators looked myopically at the sutures without noting concomitant features (e.g., Bolk, 1915). Cohen (1979), however, showed that premature sutural obliteration occurred as a primary feature in 11 chromosomal syndromes, 26 monogenetic syndromes, two chemically induced syndromes, and 17 syndromes of unknown etiology. In addition, craniosynostosis was a secondary feature of 22 other conditions, including hemolytic anemias, hyperthyroidism, rickets, and rubella syndrome.

Many of these typological difficulties have resulted from the specialized interests of the investigator. Thus, Warkany has pointed out that "if there are no eye defects, the syndrome does not exist in ophthalmology" (Warkany, 1974:3).

Attempts to extricate the study of congenital malformations from typology have recently been undertaken. A growing number of investigators are turning to numerical taxonomy (e.g., Evans, 1982; Ward and Meaney, 1984). Computer-assisted methods for analyzing data are also proving useful (e.g., Estabrook, 1977; Lowry et al., 1977).

More common, however, are published works attempting to "clarify" the problems of taxonomy by offering alternate nomenclatures for classes of congenital malformations. These nomenclatures often focus on differing pathogenetic processes (e.g., Hermann and Opitz, 1974; McKusick, 1974; Smith, 1975). A consensus regarding nomenclature was attempted in 1975 (Christiansen et al., 1975), with little compliance, and again in 1982 (Spranger et al., 1982).

In the system proposed by Spranger et al. (1982), the focus was on "errors of morphogenesis." This assumed some morphogenetic sequence, which was termed "normal development." Various deviations from normal development were envisioned:

Malformation: a morphologic defect of an organ, part of an organ, or larger region of the body resulting from an intrinsically abnormal developmental process.

Disruption: a morphologic defect of an organ, part of an organ, or larger region of the body resulting from an extrinsic breakdown of, or an interference with, an originally normal developmental process.

Deformation: an abnormal form, shape, or position of a part of the body caused by mechanical forces.

Dysplasia: an abnormal organization of cells into tissues and its morphologic results (i.e., dyshistogenesis).

These pathogenetic processes can result in the phenotypic expression of single or multiple defects, depending upon the degree of damage done to the embryo. However, to understand how deviations from normal development occur, it is first necessary to make assumptions concerning normal developmental patterns. There are two basic models used for explaining the morphogenesis of the embryo: the developmental field and the epigenetic landscape models.

In the former model, areas of primitive totipotential tissues are determined to become specific tissue types by the induction of neighboring environments (Lehtonen and Saxen, 1986). The latter model describes the channeling of relatively undifferentiated tissues into narrower options of development (Waddington, 1962).

Although multiple defects arise from disturbances affecting numerous morphogenetic fields, a disturbance within a single morphogenetic field may also produce multiple defects if that field is responsible for the development of a series of structures, and, especially, if it is affected early. According to Spranger et al. (1982), the former situation gives rise to a "syndrome," whereas the latter gives rise to a "sequence."

Both syndromes and sequences are caused by a single pathogenetic agent. It is also possible that multiple but causally independent agents may occur simultaneously, thereby affecting more than one developmental field. This situation produces an "association."

Because little is known of the actual pathomorphogenesis of congenital malformations, attention is more often focused on the frequency of phenotypes within populations or, more commonly, among families. The term "expression" refers to the degree of malformation present in an individual, whereas the term "penetrance" refers to the percentage of individuals in the population who express to any degree the phenotype when the appropriate etiological factors are present (Skinner, 1983).

Difficulties in interpreting variable degrees of expression result from the recognition of variation in the underlying etiologic processes. For example, similar phenotypes (often referred to as "phenocopies") may be caused by different genotypes, i.e., heterogeneity, and dissimilar phenotypes may be caused by the same genotype, i.e., pleiotropy. This raises an important question: When one finds variability in the severity of expression among individuals does it represent heterogeneity or pleitropy?

Interpreting variability is even more complicated when the disorder is not the result of unifactorial inheritance. Differences in the severity of expression within a population may represent the cumulative effect of multiple loci, i.e., polygenesis (Carter, 1977), the synergistic interaction of multiple loci, i.e., epistasis, or the interaction of a genetic predisposition with environmental impacts, i.e., multifactorial inheritance. An additional factor is whether the interaction between phenotype and genotype produces a continuous distribution in variability or is a threshold effect.

The relationship of etiological factors to pathogenetic processes is brought about by the vulnerability of tissues and organs during "critical periods" of development. The critical periods are classically determined by moments when cells are differentiating, proliferating, and/or migrating. These are thought to be the moments of most rapid organization (Scott, 1986). This concept of the discrete critical period, essentially limited to prenatal development, was challenged by Marker (1977), who pointed out that the genesis of the limb skeleton could better be divided into six major phases spanning the complete prenatal and postnatal growth of the individual: 1) preimplantation, 2) implantation, 3) preblastemal, 4) classical critical period, 5) period of synthesis, and 6) period of mineralization.

In the course of each phase, the developing individual is prone to different etiological agents. More importantly, the consequences of exposure to the etiological agent also differs at each stage. During the preimplantation phase, etiological agents tend to be genetically determined and lead to "faulty" cell lines. These "faulty" cells either produce abnormal enzymes, produce normal enzymes in abnormal amounts or at incorrect times, or do not normally respond to normal stimuli. Disturbances occurring during the implantation or preblastemal phases usually result in such severe malformation that spontaneous abortion follows.

During the classical critical period, which spans the embryonic and fetal developmental stages, pathogenetic factors usually result in the loss of cell mass in proliferating limb buds. Agents that attack nuclei result in hypoplasias or aplasia, as well as polydactylies. Agents that attack germ layers result in bizarre distal malformations. Agents that interfere with timing or induction interactions lead to aplasia, hypoplasia, or polydactylies.

During the period of synthesis there is secretion and maturation of the mesenchymal intercellular substance. Disturbances will lead to dysostoses of individual bones. The period of mineralization will also include the proper maintenance and remodeling of adult bone.

Hence the International Nomenclature of Constitutional Diseases of Bone (Maroteaux, 1986) includes congenital malformations that are apparent at birth, such as achondroplasia, as well as congenital malformations that do not develop until later, such as metaphyseal chondrodysplasia (variety of subtypes).

Merker's (1977) expansion of the concept of the critical period helps to explain the increase in mortality with age from congenital abnormalities, as described below.

In addition to the different periods at which a congenital malformation may actually appear, increased rates of mortality and/or morbidity with age may result from increasing severity with age. More importantly, difficulties in diagnosis cause incidence rates based on observations of newborns to underestimate actual rates. McKeown and Record (1960) found that rates observed at birth were significantly lower than observations made five years later in the same sample population. Neel (1958) had made similar observations on a Japanese sample in which congenital malformations noted at birth were compared to congenital malformations noted nine months after birth. The rates that changed the most were those that were difficult to diagnose immediately, such as cardiac malformations and congenital hip displacement, whereas less subtle congenital malformations, such as anencephaly, spina bifida aperta, and cleft lip with or without cleft palate changed only slightly. Thus, a prospective study by McIntosh et al. (1954) noted that:

> Only 43% of the malformations presented signs, symptoms or [radiographic] abnormalities which were observable at birth . . . Less than one-fifth (18.1%) of all malformations were unrecognized until the follow-up examination at one year. (McIntosh et al., 1954:512)
>
> Except for the central nervous system, every organ system group had a markedly higher incidence of malformation among neonatal deaths than among stillbirths. Among stillbirths and neonatal deaths combined, the incidence was about the same (from 13–18%) for all organ groups except for respiratory system and skin. In live-born infants, the pattern was quite different. The musculo-skeletal system was affected in the highest proportion of infants (2.8%), followed by skin with 1.6%. This

> may be, in part, a reflection of the greater ease of diagnosis of minor external defects than of minor internal defects. (McIntosh et al., 1954:517)

GENERAL EPIDEMIOLOGY

Congenital malformations represent a major cause of mortality in human populations. In the United States at the present time, congenital malformations are the fifteenth leading cause of death in all ages, representing 5.5 deaths/100,000 population (National Center for Health Statistics, 1986). In relation to age-specific, proportionate mortality rates among the 15 leading causes of death, congenital malformations are even more important in the younger age groups. Under 1 year of age congenital malformations are in second place (236/100,000), following "certain conditions originating in the perinatal period." Between 1 and 14 years, they fall slightly to third place (2.6/100,000), following accidents and malignant neoplasms, which are first and second, respectively. Their position falls considerably between 15 and 24 years to sixth place (1.1/100,000), following accidents, suicide, homicide, malignant neoplasms, and diseases of the heart, in that order. In the ensuing age categories, congenital malformations represent only a small proportion of deaths in relation to the other leading causes. Nevertheless, this proportionate standing in the older groups is somewhat misleading because of the relatively larger increases in the mortality rates of other diseases with age. The age-specific mortality rates of congenital malformations actually increase steadily after 34 years of age, from 1.1/100,000 in the 15–34 age group to 6.6/100,000 in the age 85 and older group, a 600% increase!

Congenital malformations may also result in varying degrees of nonlethal dysfunction, thereby contributing to morbidity. Emery and Rimoin (1983) estimated the overall genetic contributions to mortality and morbidity in the United States; it was thought to be quite high. A chromosomal abnormality was found in 60% of abortuses, 7% of perinatal deaths, and one in every 200 newborns. One in every 50 newborns had a major congenital abnormality, and one in every 100 newborns had a unifactorial genetic disorder. The rates for unifactorial disorders per 1,000 population were autosomal Dominant, 7.0; autosomal Recessive, 2.5; and X-linked, 0.5.

Emery and Rimoin (1983) further calculated that 10% to 25% of all children had a disorder that was at least in part genetic, with 5% entirely genetic. One percent of adults had either unifactorial or chromosomal disorders.

McKusick (1986) enumerated 1,906 disorders in which a unifactorial genetic etiology was demonstrated and an additional 2,001 in which a unifactorial genetic etiology was highly suspected.

In a prospective study of 5,964 pregnancies, McIntosh et al. (1954) found the overall rate of congenital malformations to be 7.5%. The percentage was lowest in the live-birth group. In the non-live-birth groups, the rates of congenital malformations increased from 13% in abortuses to 23% in intrapartum deaths to 29% in neonatal deaths.

> The differences among antepartum, intrapartum and neonatal rates may indicate that many malformations which are compatible with intrauterine life impose a fatal hazard at parturition, while others are incompatible with extrauterine life. (McIntosh et al., 1954:509)

CROSS-CULTURAL EPIDEMIOLOGY

It is difficult to make accurate comparisons of the incidence rates of congenital malformations among populations for a variety of reasons:

1. The higher priority of interest in infectious and nutritional diseases in poor populations.
2. Variable proportions of births outside a professional health system.
3. Underdeveloped systems of reporting health statistics.
4. Variations in the methods of observation, definition, and diagnosis.

Whereas congenital malformations are common as a group, the individual types are generally rare. The most common types, such as spina bifida aperta, are found in 1–2/1,000 in the population (Table 2). Some syndromes have been described only in a few families or in single individuals (Table 3).

TABLE 2. Relatively Common Syndromes (Rates Within Populations)[a]

Osteogenesis imperfecta congenita	1/40,000
Osteogenesis imperfecta tarda	1/25,000
Achondroplasia	1/25,000
Mucopolysaccharidosis type I (Hunter)	1/100,000
Mucopolysaccharidosis type II (Hurler)	1/50,000
Mucopolysaccharidosis type III (San Filippo)	1/50,000
Mucopolysaccharidosis type IV (Morquio)	1/100,000

[a] Frequencies are derived from Wiedemann et al. (1985).

Stevenson et al. (1966) attempted to compare worldwide rates of congenital malformations at birth from 24 health centers (Table 4). They defined 14 categories of malformation, most of which were further subdivided. The rates of total congenital malformations averaged 13/1,000 births, but there was great variation among the centers.

Variations in rates were also seen within the different types of congenital malformations defined by Stevenson et al. (1966). Neural tube defects were relatively low in Chile, Colombia, Malaysia, and the Philippines and were high in Egypt and, especially, Ireland. This is in general keeping with other studies that have shown spina bifida to be most common in the northern latitudes (Leck, 1984).

The categories of harelip with cleft palate, harelip without cleft palate, and cleft palate are generally grouped into two, with the first two merged. The rationale is that clefts of the maxillary portion of the palate are not generally found without harelip (Fig. 1). It is believed that the process of fusion begins in the posterior maxilla and continues anteriorly. On the other hand, the palatine portion of the palate fuses separately and later. Therefore, posterior

TABLE 3. Relatively Rare Syndromes (Total Number of Individuals Diagnosed)[a]

Achondrogenesis	85
Mesomelic dysplasia (Nievergelt)	15
Craniosynostosis (Crouzon)	100
Craniosynostosis (Apert)	150
Chondrodysplasia punctata (rhizomelic form)	36
Diastrophic dysplasia	70

[a] Frequencies are derived from Wiedemann et al. (1985).

TABLE 4. Worldwide Rates of Congenital Malformations (Per 1,000 Population)

Above average (>14/1,000)	
South Africa (white)	22
Panama	21
Ireland	20
Australia (white)	18
Czechoslovakia	17
Yugoslavia	16
Brazil	16
Average (12–14/1,000)	
Colombia	14
Spain	13
South Africa (Bantu)	13
Mexico	13
Egypt	12
Hong Kong	12
Below average (<12/1,000)	
Malaysia	10
Philippines	9
South Africa ("colored")	9
Chile	9
India	6

Modified from Stevenson et al. (1966).

clefts are somewhat independent of anterior clefts. Highest frequencies of cleft lip with or without cleft palate were found in the Asian populations of Malaysia and Hong Kong and also among South African whites and Chileans. Low rates were found among South African Bantu and "coloreds"and Yugoslavs.

The incidence of "talipes" was found to be relatively low in Egypt, India, Hong Kong, Ireland, the Philippines, and South African Bantu and "coloreds," whereas it was high in Panama, South African whites, and Yugoslavs. Unfortunately, this category was difficult to define, because many observers give the designation of "talipes" to any number of unrelated foot anomalies.

In this series, Stevenson and coworkers noted high frequencies of congenital hip displacement in Colombia and Yugoslavia. North American Indian groups were not included in this survey, however, and it is generally known that they have considerably higher frequencies of congenital hip displacement than whites.

Polydactyly was most common in South African Bantu, which is in keeping with the well-known high incidences among blacks. It was also high in Colombia, Brazil, and Panama, which are all populations that may have large black intermixture.

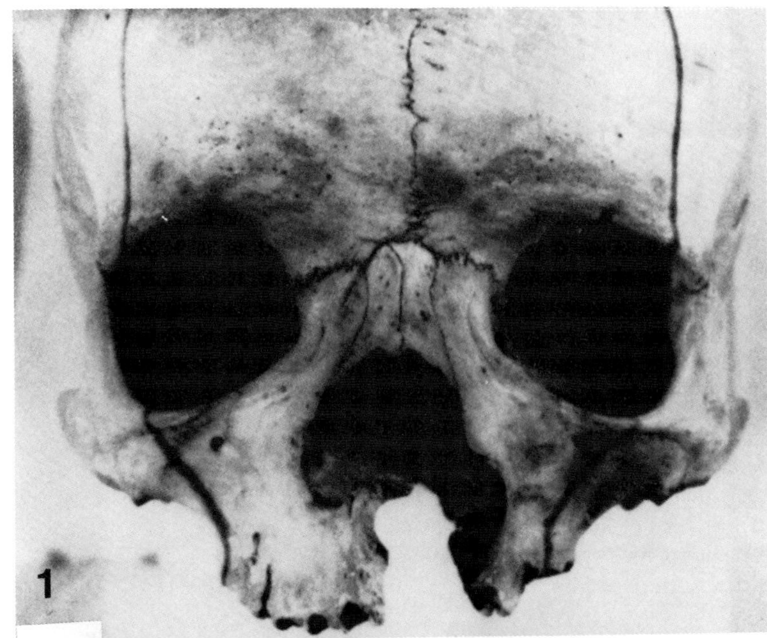

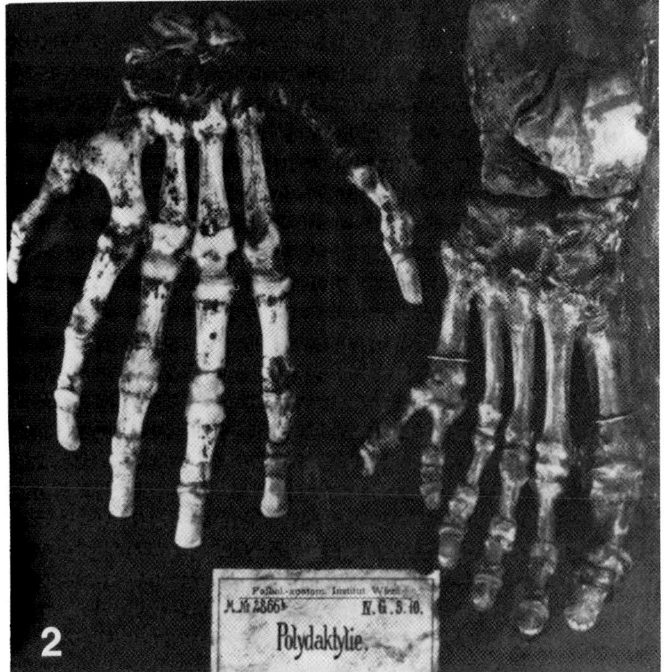

Fig. 1. Cleft lip and cleft palate in a Pacific Islander. (Reproduced from Ortner and Putschar, 1981, with permission of Smithsonian Contributions to Anthropology.)

Fig. 2. Polydactyly of the right hand and the right foot. (Reproduced from Ortner and Putschar, 1981, with permission of Smithsonian Contributions to Anthropology.)

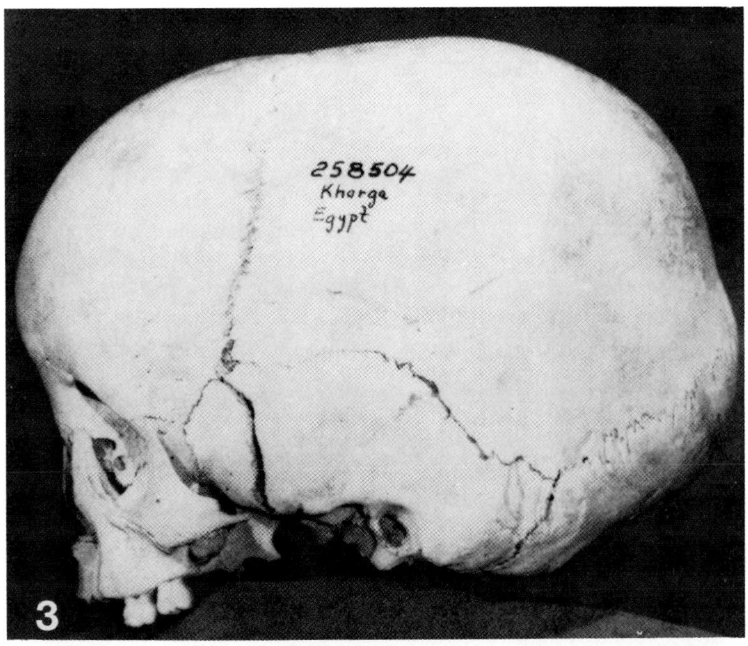

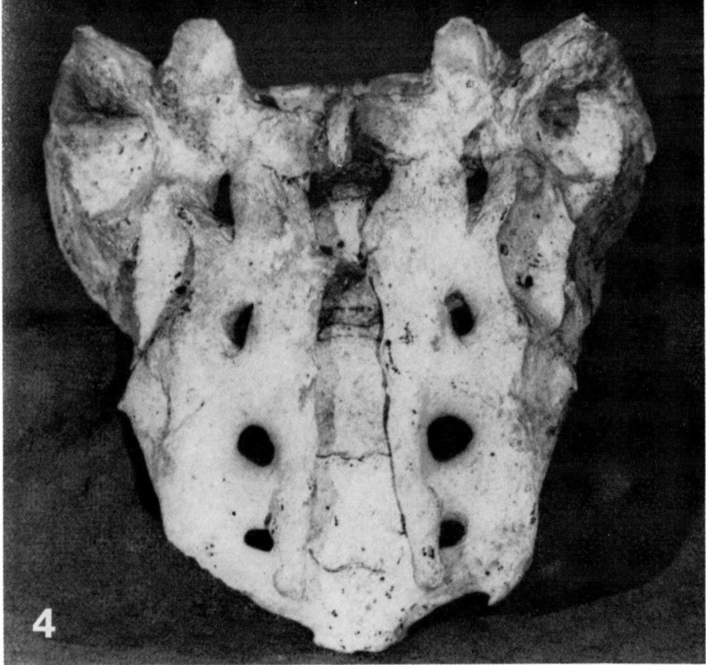

Fig. 3. Scaphocephaly in a young child from ancient Egypt. (Reproduced from Ortner and Putschar, 1981, with permission of Smithsonian Contributions to Anthropology.)

Fig. 4. Spina bifida in the sacrum of a young adult from the Bronze Age of Jordan. (Reproduced from Ortner and Putschar, 1981, with permission of Smithsonian Contributions to Anthropology.)

TABLE 5. Differences in Rates of Congenital Malformations in the United States (Per 1,000 Population)

	Major	Minor
Whites	46.03	32.79
Blacks	45.65	22.93
Puerto Ricans	37.78	27.32

Reproduced from Heinonen et al., 1977, with permission of Publishing Science Group, Inc.

South African Bantu and Yugoslavs were relatively high in general skeletal malformations, whereas Malaysians were relatively low. These categories appear too broad, which is perhaps why little discrimination between populations could be made.

Heinonen et al. (1977) surveyed congenital malformations found in 12 U.S. medical centers. Ethnic/racial differences were compared among whites, blacks, and "Puerto Ricans." Overall rates (per 1,000 population) were basically similar (Table 5). When "major" congenital malformations were separated from "minor," whites (32.79) were somewhat higher than blacks (22.93), with Puerto Ricans intermediate (27.32). Blacks were lowest overall in congenital malformations of the central nervous system (4.54), Puerto Ricans were highest (7.56), and whites were intermediate (5.75), although blacks were highest in microcephaly.

In relation to congenital malformations of the musculoskeletal system, blacks appear to have the highest rate (17.39), with Puerto Ricans the lowest (9.01) and whites intermediate (11.75). However, a closer look points out that most of the black rate is due to an extraordinarily high rate of polydactyly (Fig. 2), nearly nine times that of the white and Puerto Rican rates. Except for their intermediate rates of hypoplasia of a limb or a limb part, blacks are lowest for all other musculoskeletal malformations. Similarly, blacks have the lowest rates for syndromes excluding trisomy-21 (1.9), whereas whites have the highest rates (2.7), with Puerto Ricans intermediate (2.3).

One major difficulty in comparative studies is the inability of precisely defining the populations ethnically and racially and of accurately identifying individuals. This is a problem in most of the published studies. For example, many British studies compare rates of congenital malformations in whites and blacks with "Asians." The Asian population in these studies are generally from India or Pakistan and are therefore racially Caucasoid rather than Mongoloid. Similarly, the term "Puerto Rican," as used colloquially by non-Hispanics in New York City, often refers to any Spanish speaker. Thus it hardly conforms to the notion of an ethnic group, let alone a racial group. This vitiates many comparative analyses. In the prospective study of McIntosh et al. (1954), the mothers were classed as white and nonwhite (but no attempt was made to classify the fathers).

> A large part of the population is Puerto Rican and the color distinction was based on the mother's statement as to race. It is probable that the nonwhite group is more homogeneous racially than is the white, since most Puerto Ricans claim white parentage regardless of pigment considerations. (McIntosh et al., 1954;508)

The effect of race on the expression and/or diagnosis of congenital malformations may be significant. Stewart (1972) cautioned that scaphocephaly (Fig. 3), caused by premature closure of the sagittal suture, can be overlooked in blacks because of a different pattern of skull form. In whites and Mongoloids, scaphocephaly produces a characteristic keel-shaped elevation of the skull along the suture. In blacks, however, the bulbous frontal and projecting occiput are separated by a depression along the sagittal suture.

Emanuel et al. (1968) studied the physical features of Taiwanese children, comparing those with cytologically diagnosed trisomy-21 with controls. They found that "there is no single sign which is pathognomonic" for Down's syndrome. There was great individual variation in expression of the classic signs, such as speckled iris, as well as superimposition of sexual (e.g., palate height) and racial (e.g., "Mongoloid fold") features, which confused the subjectively determined stigmata.

Cultural variability in mating patterns may also affect rates of genetic disorders. Young (1987) found that in Great Britain, the South Asian Muslim immigrants, who practiced first cousin consanguinity, had higher rates of recessive lethal malformations than whites. Similarly, Terry et al. (1983) found that although

Muslim Pakistanis had a lower overall rate of genetic disorders than Hindu Indians, the former had significantly higher rates of chromosomal defects and multiple abnormalities. The Muslim groups tended to marry at a later age than the Hindus. In addition, the Hindus had a very low frequency of first cousin marriage, whereas the Muslims had a high rate.

These caveats notwithstanding, there are a number of congenital malformations that appear to have a differential prevalence among living ethnic/racial groups. The high prevalence of polydactyly in blacks has been cited above. It is well known that American Indian populations differ from American whites in having higher incidences of congenital hip displacement, especially among the Navaho and Manitoba (Woolf et al., 1968). Spondylolisthesis appears among the Eskimo (Stewart, 1931) and cleft lip/palate among the Sioux and Navaho. Unfortunately the variation among the different American Indian groups is not well documented. In addition, other ethnic groups are known to have a relatively higher incidence of specific musculoskeletal congenital malformations, such as increased talipes equinovarus among the Maori (Howie and Phillips, 1970). Of course, it has been known for some time that congenitally abnormal hemoglobins, which also show an uneven ethnic distribution, can produce skeletal deformations.

ANTHROPOLOGICAL STUDIES

Anthropologists can be helpful to clinicians in the study of congenital malformations in a number of areas, one of which is anthropometry. Physical anthropologists are generally well trained in anthropometry and are not only familiar with many of the technical and practical problems in the taking of these measurements but are also sensitive to the questions of statistical representativeness of samples. More importantly, the relationship of linear measurements to concepts of body form is also a longstanding concern among anthropologists. Naturally, these problems must be adequately solved before a meaningful taxonomy can be established (Ward and Meaney, 1984). In addition, anthropologists are familiar with the methods of pedigree analysis and the problems associated with defining ethnic and/or racial groups. Solving these problems is crucial for any epidemiological study.

A further area in which the anthropologist can aid the clinician is in the analyses of skeletal populations. Such analyses may corroborate findings from other sources. This is particularly apparent in studies of vertebral anomalies. Spina bifida refers to a midline fusion defect in the vertebral arch (Fig. 4). The standard literature rates the prevalence of spina bifida in S1 as quite high, approaching 25% of the population (e.g., Schmorl and Junghanns, 1971). Brothwell and Powers (1968) compiled prevalence rates for skeletal populations of the British Isles and found approximately 17% of some degree of opening of the S1 spinous tubercle. However, some studies have indicated that the vertebral arch may not fuse dorsally until considerably later than is generally accepted in the literature (Sutow and Pryde, 1956; Turkel and Taylor, 1986). These studies suggest that the actual prevalence of spina bifida of S1 in adults is significantly lower than 25%. Brothwell and Powers (1968) did not consider age in his series.

Merbs and Wilson (1960) studied spinal anomalies among the Sadlermiut Eskimo. They observed spina bifida occulta in a number of skeletons and derived the following age-specific distribution: <14, 4/4 (100%); 14–18, 2/7 (29%); >18 (males), 7/28 (25%); >18 (females), 1/33 (3%).

Although the sample size is quite small, we do see a steady decrease in the frequency of spina bifida with age, especially among the females who drop to only 3%. On the other hand, it appears that the males retain a relatively large prevalence at 25%. Is this difference in prevalence between males and females due to a sex-linked genetic predisposition or to differing culturally induced environmental traumas between the sexes?

Actually, it may also be possible to interpret the male/female differences on the basis of age, especially given the recognized faster rates of skeletal maturation in females (e.g., Krogman and İşcan, 1986). Sutow and Pryde (1956) found 52% spina bifida in S1 of 18-year-old Japanese males compared to 30% in 18-year-old Japanese females. Turkel and Taylor (1986) found that the prevalence of spina bifida of S1 did not stabilize until age 35. Hence, it is possible that the male sample of Merbs and

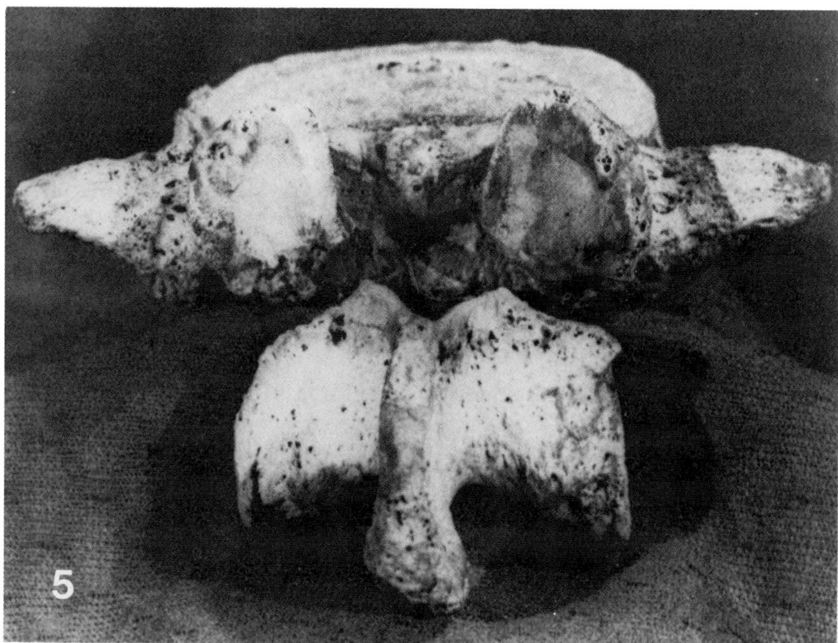

Fig. 5. Spondylolysis in a lumbar vertebra of a young adult male from the Bronze Age of Jordan. (Reproduced from Ortner and Putschar, 1981, with permission of Smithsonian Contributions to Anthropology.)

Wilson (1960) is younger than their female sample. Unfortunately, Merbs and Wilson (1960) give us only an overall age distribution for their adult sample. Although the average ages of the males (34.3) and females (35.5) are comparable, we find that 44% of the males were younger than 31 years, whereas only 36% of the females were younger than 31.

A more classic example is Stewart's (1931, 1953) study of lumbar spondylolysis at the pars interarticularis among Alaskan natives (Fig. 5). His findings, along with others (e.g., Merbs and Wilson, 1960; Lester and Shapiro, 1968), have put the frequency of spondylolysis among the Eskimo at 20–40%, as compared to less than 10% among white Americans (Wiltse et al., 1976). Stewart (1953) further demonstrated that the prevalence of defective vertebrae increased with age. This led him to reject his earlier hypothesis that the high population prevalence was due to inheritance. He suggested instead that hyperflexion of the lumbar spine while the knees were extended caused repeated small trauma resulting in fatigue fractures.

Clinical studies on American whites are in complete agreement with Stewart's observations concerning age distribution (Wiltse et al., 1976). On the other hand, pedigree studies do indicate that there is a strong genetic component to spondylolysis (e.g., Shahriaree et al., 1979). Clinical histories of white American patients with spondylolysis fail to discover traumas or unusual postures antecedent to the diagnosis (Taillard, 1976). It is possible that spondylolisthesis is a defect resulting from a disturbance in Merker's critical phase 6 (i.e., the period of mineralization, see above).

Bennett (1967) studied craniosynostotic skulls found among Southwest American Indian archaeological populations. Although he was unable to develop overall prevalence rates, he did compare the relative rates in which specific sutures were prematurely closed in skulls showing some form of craniosynostosis. His findings were in accord with clinical studies on modern populations (e.g., David et al., 1982).

ANTHROPOLOGICAL INTERPRETATIONS OF HERITABLE ANOMALIES

The majority of anthropological works concerned with congenital malformations in skeletal populations has been directed toward documenting the presence of specific defects in these ancient populations (e.g., Brothwell, 1967; Brothwell and Powers, 1968). This has not been quite so simple, however, because of conditions of preservation, as well as difficulties in diagnosis (e.g., Steinbock, 1976; Ortner and Putschar, 1981; Zimmerman and Kelley, 1982). These difficulties, inherent within the study of paleopathology, should not condemn us to the limited task of finding and tabulating the prevalence of congenital malformations. Certainly there is some larger anthropological meaning to be extracted. Some interesting attempts have been made to use the presence of congenital malformations in archaeological populations as evidence in support of other issues.

Since most congenital malformations are found in such low frequencies within a population, increased prevalence should carry some significant implications. One possibility is consanguinity among individuals with the defect. Thus, Ferembach (1963) suggested that approximately 180 burials from Taforalt, Morocco, represented an endogamous group because of their relatively high frequency of spina bifida and other vertebral anomalies. Similarly, Bennett (1973) suggested that a relatively high frequency of an unusual vertebral anomaly (i.e., partial sacralization of L6, with spina bifida) found among protohistoric Medoc American Indians indicated a small, stable, inbred population.

Smith (1973) found individuals buried at the Natufian site of Hayonim to have a relatively high frequency of congenital absence of M3. She suggested that this represented a more or less permanently settled family who buried their dead in the same cave over numerous generations. This was then related to changes in subsistence patterns.

Angel (1964) examined family burials in Bronze Age Mediterranean cities. He found evidence of thalassemia with a "scattered occurrence in families, perhaps among siblings." He related this to the increased risk of malaria following agricultural expansion (see also Livingstone, 1958).

ANTHROPOLOGICAL INTERPRETATIONS OF NONHERITABLE ANOMALIES

Although the overwhelming number of congenital malformations appear to have a primarily genetic basis, there are some defects caused by in utero environmental traumas. When present, these anomalies can help to evaluate the degree of environmental stress on a population.

Infectious diseases were the first documented environmental teratogens. Mead (n.d., quoted by Watson, 1749) noticed that infants born to mothers exposed to smallpox could contract the disease in utero. Hutchinson (1909) described stigmata of congenital syphilis. Gregg (1941) demonstrated the teratogenic effects of rubella.

Noninfectious environmental teratogens may also produce congenital malformations. Murphy (1929) demonstrated the hazards of ionizing radiation. Thalidomide was the first chemical proved to be teratogenic in humans (McBride, 1961). Although there are presently many suspected chemical teratogens, few have been found that actually do affect humans (Persaud et al., 1985).

One possibly significant prenatal stressor, however, is malnutrition. Warkany and Nelson (1940) experimentally produced skeletal abnormalities in the offspring of rats reared on a deficient diet. Venkata (1962) reported statistically significant lower birth weights and higher mortality rates among infants born to malnourished mothers than those born to well-nourished mothers in India. Apte and Iyengar (1972) determined that fetal weight was closely related to body fat and protein composition. Krishnamachari and Iyengar (1975) found greater bone density among newborns of well-nourished mothers compared with those malnourished in India.

It is also of interest that relative nourishment of the mother has differential effects according to race. For example, Bissenden et al. (1981a) found that South Asian women needed to show signs of better nutrition in their second trimester than whites in order to have "normal weight" babies. This meant that the South Asian women had greater skin-fold thickness and weight gain during pregnancy. In addition, and more importantly, the well-nourished South Asian women who gave birth to "normal weight" babies showed a biochemical difference in urine analysis as compared to well-nourished whites. Furthermore, Bissenden et al. (1981b) found that low birth weight in South

Asian babies was more often the result in poor prenatal nutrition, whereas low birth weight in whites was more often the result of complications in the pregnancy of well-nourished mothers. They were able to lower the rates of low birth weight in South Asian babies by giving protein supplements to the mothers. Rush et al. (1980) attempted to increase the birth weights of black American babies through protein supplements to the mothers in the second trimester. Not only were they unable to increase the birth weights, but they increased the incidence of preterm births and associated neonatal deaths. There was also significant growth retardation up to 37 weeks of gestation. These studies indicate that prenatal nutrition is superimposed on racial factors during development. Polednak (1986) suggested that developmental processes differ according to race.

Cook and Buikstra (1979) compared nutritional stress between Middle Woodland and Late Woodland populations of the Lower Illinois Valley. They noted circular dental caries secondary to hypoplasia in both the deciduous and permanent teeth, thereby referring developmental stress to specific pre- and postnatal developmental periods. They discovered that children with enamel defects showed relatively higher rates of anemia, infectious disease, and weanling age mortality. Cook and Buikstra did not find significant differences between the two Woodland populations with respect to the timing of developmental stress. However, they reported that the Late Woodland population had a statistically significant higher frequency of circular caries. They concluded that the nutritional environment for the Late Woodland children was more stressful than that for the Middle Woodland children.

CULTURE AND CONGENITAL MALFORMATION

Another anthropological concern in regard to congenital malformations is the reaction of the population to the appearance of malformed births. One way of gauging this is through differential burial. A well-known case is that of an anencephalic individual (Fig. 6) from the catacombs of Hermopolis (Warkany, 1959). It was buried with sacred animals, perhaps indicating the less-than-human regard in which it was held or, alternately, its sacredness.

Dawson (1927) enumerated nine achondroplastic individuals (Fig. 7) from elite burials of ancient Egypt. The context of their entombments, as well as numerous artistic and written records, indicated that some achondroplastics maintained great wealth and attained high social status. Of course, the exhumation of Egyptian mummies has been biased toward the elite classes; therefore, the existence and fortunes of nonelite achondroplastics was not reported. Dawson (1927) also pointed out that figurines and amulets representing dwarfs were thought to have magical significance, especially in regard to childbirth (Fig. 8).

Ballantyne (1894) listed 62 birth defects from ancient Assyrian written records. Tablets enumerated individual defects with concomitant prognostications with regard to the fortunes of the country and/or household in which the births occurred. Not all of the predictions were for calamity (e.g., a deformed tongue [#18] could presage world peace!). Ballantyne was impressed by the nearly scientific objectivity of the various descriptions: "In this tablet at least none of the recorded anomalies can be regarded as impossible, and therefore mythical" (Ballantyne, 1894:137). Cicero (Falconer, 1908) noted that the term "monstrum," i.e., to show (hence our word monster) was used in reference to events or objects that had divining properties.

On the other hand, Aristotle (Peck, 1942) proposed that congenital malformations were examples of incomplete development of the human form and therefore expressed varying degrees of animal form. This was echoed later by Harvey (1651). Warkany (1959) related instances during the seventeenth century in which people were executed because the birth of malformed children, or even animals, was thought to have been the result of bestiality.

Representations of congenital malformations in art may also indicate a significant relationship of the malformed individual with the culture. Dawson's (1927) discussion of the magical status dwarfs held in ancient Egypt was noted above. He also pointed out that some mythological creatures appeared to be based on achrondroplastics. Schatz (1901, quoted by Barrow, 1970) believed that "many mythological monsters may have arisen from observations of developmental abnormalities." Brooks

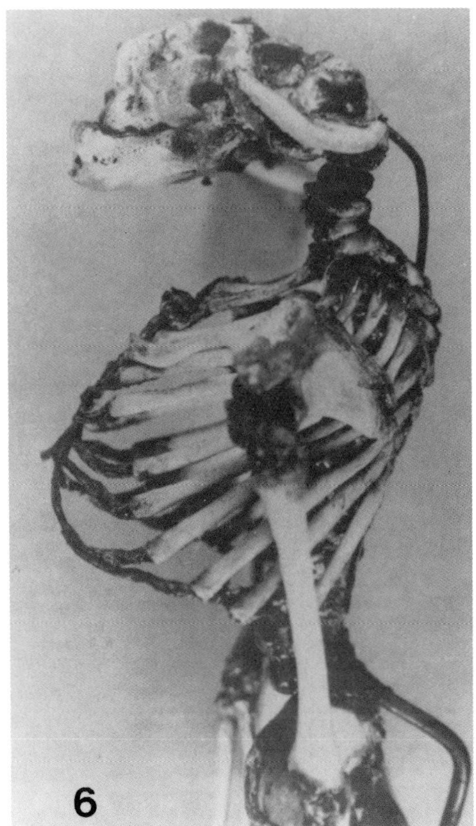

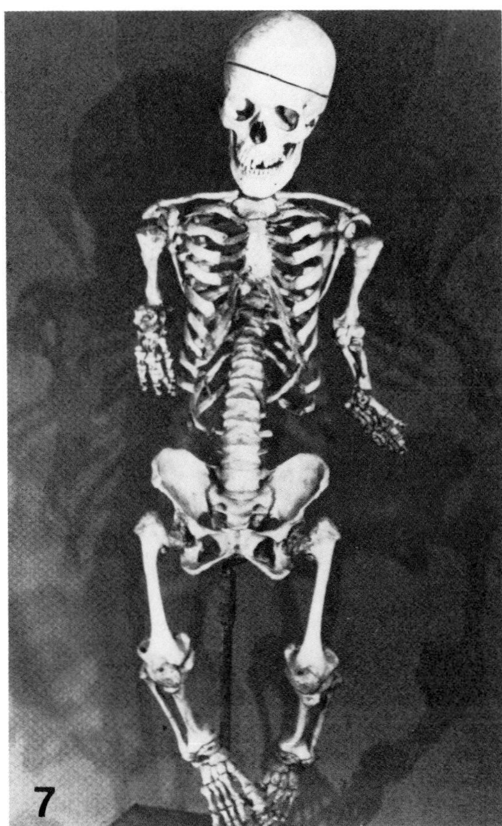

Fig. 6. An anencephalic skeleton of a neonate. (Reproduced from Zimmerman and Kelley, 1982, with permission of Praeger Publishers.)

Fig. 7. An achondroplastic neonate. (Reproduced from Ortner and Putschar, 1981, with permission of Smithsonian Contributions to Anthropology.)

and Hohenthal (1963) refer to pottery depicting "hare-lip" in pre-Columbian California; it was noted above that cleft lip, with or without cleft palate, is relatively high among American Indians. Brodsky (1943) made a case for the diagnosis of congenital malformations in Oceanic art and legend.

Murdy (1981) interpreted the Olmec were-jaguar motif in relation to congenital malformations. He points to similarities in the grotesque form of the mythologic being with possible malformations in humans resulting from spina bifida:

> The fact that the head is disproportionately large even for a baby . . . could be due to hydrocephalus; the limply hanging legs may be the result of the paraplegia or even death . . . , usually associated with myelomeningocele. The accentuated facial feature of the child may represent pain, perhaps due to the urethral failure and subsequent infection often associated with myelomeningocele . . . This pained expression may have reminded the Olmec of the jaguar's snarl, which, coupled with the cleft forehead, was sufficient to complete the analogy and fusion of the two representations. (Murdy, 1981:865)

Murdy goes on to suggest that this defect may have been more common among the ruling class, because of endogamy, with the were-jaguar motif becoming "a religious symbol of their distinct position in society." This is further used as evidence by Murdy that the Olmec had reached the level of a chiefdom.

Murdy's scenario becomes even more plausible if the diagnosis of the congenital malformation is changed to Merkel's syndrome. In this syndrome there is usually microcephaly with sloping forehead, cranial rachischisis with exencephalocele, and cleft palate, along with other anomalies of the face, limbs, and viscera (Opitz and Howe, 1969). All of these malformations are consistent with the peculiarities of the were-jaguar head and face. Furthermore, Young and Clarke (1985) found a high incidence of Merkel's syndrome among immigrants to Great Britain from Gurjat, Pakistan, where first cousin consanguineous marriage is common. On the other hand, no skeletons have been diagnosed with this syndrome from American archaeological sites; however, this may be due to missed diagnosis. Stewart (1975) cautions that exencephalocele may be mistaken for attempted trephination (Fig. 9).

CONCLUSIONS

Worldwide surveys, as well as comparisons of groups within populations, demonstrate that congenital malformations have differential rates according to ethnic/racial background. The significance of such variance, however, often remains unexplored. The majority of congenital malformations in the "industrial" countries are genetic disorders, and genetic disorders have also been described for all other communities studied.

Differential rates in genetically controlled traits can be understood from the standpoint of population genetics. First, mutation rates will vary among populations. Second, initial differences in mutation rates will be maintained if barriers to gene flow between populations exist. Third, in small populations genetic drift may cause further increases or decreases in the rates. Fourth, magnification of rates, especially in recessive traits, will occur if consanguineous matings are practiced. In addition, delayed childbearing will increase rates of chromosomal anomalies. Fifth, natural selection will modify rates. Sixth, cultural attitudes may also influence rates through sexual selection or infanticide.

The presence of a heritable congenital malformation within a population, therefore, may give us information concerning mating practices both within the population and between neighboring populations. It may also give us information concerning cultural and ecological changes that cause a shift in selective pressures.

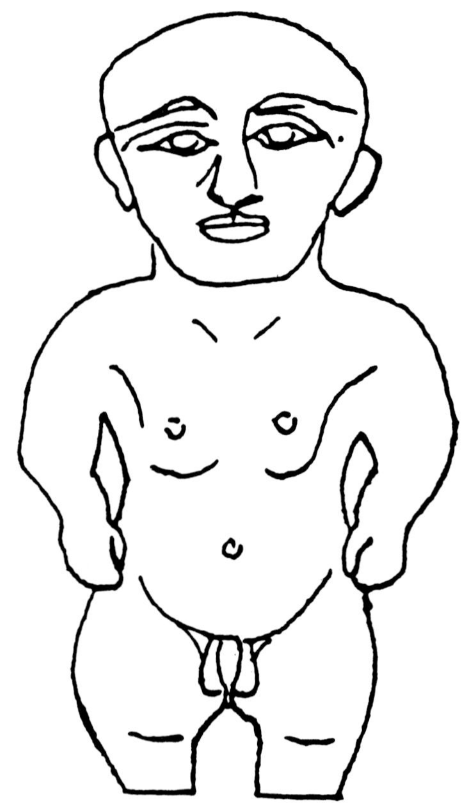

Fig. 8. A drawing of an amulet representing an achondroplastic individual. (Reproduced from Dawson, 1927, with permission of Annals of Medical History.)

Differential rates in nonheritable congenital malformations also provide considerable information. These disorders result from environmental prenatal insults. Most commonly, these stressors are due to nutritional deficiencies in or infection of the mother during pregnancy. Exposure of the mother to environmental toxins and medications is also traumatic. Because these factors are ecological, they are highly influenced by cultural practices. Such cultural activities as, for example, population control, subsistence and settlement patterns, differential treatment of women, prenatal food taboos, and control of communicable disease and sanitation will have an impact on the rates. Culture

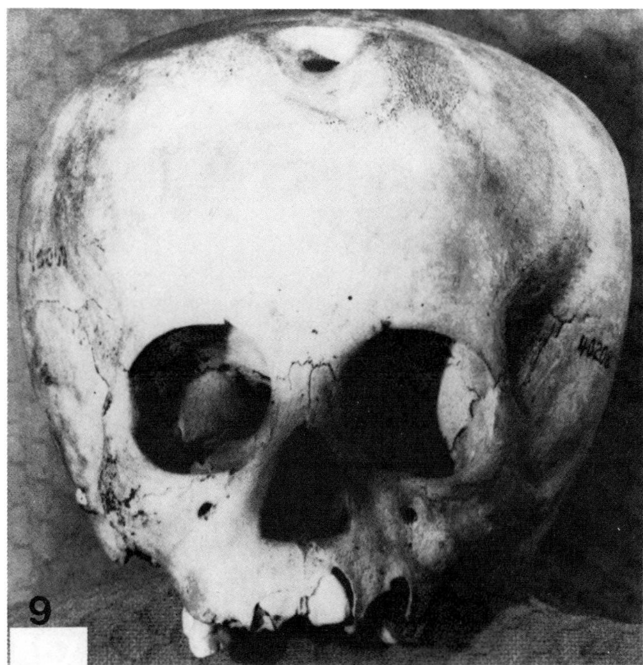

Fig. 9. An exencephalocele in the frontal bone of an ancient Peruvian. (Reproduced from Ortner and Putschar, 1981, with permission of Smithsonian Contributions to Anthropology.)

contact with other populations, either in the form of warfare or trade, may bring new diseases or increase nutritional stress. In addition, drought, flood, temperature change, and other environmental catastrophes will have severe consequences.

The reactions of the community to the appearance of a congenital malformation is of importance anthropologically. Prevalence rates and age at death reflect both biological fitness and cultural fitness. Infanticide and ostracism obviously decrease fitness. On the other hand, rates will be relatively higher if the individuals are fully accepted or even supported by the community. The attitudes of the community, in turn, are influenced by their beliefs concerning the etiology of congenital malformations and their feelings concerning their responsibilities toward the disadvantaged. In a stratified society, the fate of handicapped individuals depends on the class into which they are born.

In order to properly interpret this information, however, it is imperative to develop prevalence or incidence rates. There are a number of difficulties in developing these rates. First are the problems in diagnosis. Although physical anthropologists easily recognize deviations from the normal pattern of development, recognition of a specific, usually rare, syndrome is often a different matter. General paleopathology texts focus on the more common disorders, especially those already described from skeletal populations. Medical texts, on the other hand, usually focus on gross descriptions of facial form, limb development, and soft tissue defects, providing less information of use for the analysis of the skeleton than for the analysis of the living patient. Skeletons collected for study from individuals with rare syndromes are more rare than the syndromes. Postmortem damage, deterioration, and deformation of skeletal material impose further obstacles.

The reportage of individual skeletons that demonstrate a specific congenital malformation is helpful. It provides a means of opening a dialogue, especially insofar as developing a correct procedure for diagnosis. It also allows some knowledge of the spatial and temporal extents of birth defects. For interpretation and comparison, however, only rates will be sufficient. Therefore, it is necessary that estimates of the population size and the number of afflicted individuals be provided whenever possible.

REFERENCES

Angel JL (1964) Osteoporosis: Thalassemia? Am J Phys Anthropol 22:369–374.

Apte IV, and Iyengar L (1972) Composition of the human foetus. Br J Nutr 27:305–312.

Ballantyne JW (1894) The teratological records of Chaldea. Teratologia 1:127–142.

Barrow MV (1970) A brief history of teratology to the 20th century. Teratology 4:119–130.

Bennett KA (1967) Craniostenosis: A review of the etiology and a report of new cases. Am J Phys Anthropol 27:1–10.

Bennett KA (1973) Lumbo-sacral malformations and spina bifida occulta in a group of proto-historic Modoc Indians. Am J Phys Anthropol 36:435–440.

Bissenden JG, Scott PH, Hallum J, Mansfield HN, Scott P, and Wharton BA (1981a) Anthropometric and biochemical changes during pregnancy in Asian and European mothers having well grown babies. Br J Obstet Gynaecol 88:992–998.

Bissenden JG, Scott PH, King J, Hallum J, Mansfield HN, and Wharton BA (1981b) Anthropometric and biochemical changes during pregnancy in Asian and European mothers having light for gestational age babies. Br J Obstet Gynaecol 88:999–1008.

Bolk L (1915) On the premature obliteration of sutures in the human skull. Am J Anat 17:495–523.

Brodsky I (1943) Congenital abnormalities, teratology and embryology: Some evidence of primitive man's knowledge as expressed in art and lore in Oceania. Med J Aust 1:417–420.

Brooks ST, and Hohenthal WD (1963) Archaeological defective palate crania from California. Am J Phys Anthropol 21:25–32.

Brothwell DR (1967) Major congenital anomalies of the skeleton: Evidence from earlier populations. In DR Brothwell and AT Sandison (eds): Diseases in Antiquity. Springfield, IL: Charles C Thomas, pp 423–446.

Brothwell DR, and Powers R (1968) Congenital malformations of the skeleton in earlier man. In DR Brothwell (ed): The Skeletal Biology of Earlier Human Populations. London: Pergamon Press, pp 173–203.

Carter CO (1977) Principles of polygenic inheritance. Birth Defects 13(3a):67–74.

Christiansen RL (1975) Proposed guidelines for the classification, nomenclature, and naming of morphologic defects. Syndrome Ident 3:1–8.

Cohen MM Jr (1979) Craniosynostosis and syndromes with craniosynostosis. Birth Defects 15(5b):13–65.

Cook DC, and Buikstra JE (1979) Health and differential survival in prehistoric populations: Prenatal dental defects. Am J Phys Anthropol 51:649–664.

David DJ, Poswillo D, and Simpson D (1982) The Craniosynostoses: Causes, Natural History, and Management. Berlin: Springer-Verlag.

Dawson WR (1927) Pygmies, dwarfs and hunchbacks in ancient Egypt. Ann Med Hist 9:315–326.

Emanuel I, Shuang S, and Yeh E (1968) Physical features of Chinese children with Down's syndrome. Am J Dis Child 115:461–468.

Emery AEH, and Rimoin DL (1983) The nature and incidence of genetic disease. In AEH Emery and DL Rimoin (eds): Principles and Practice of Medical Genetics. New York: Churchill Livingstone, pp 1–3.

Estabrook GF (1977) Objective methods for classification and the study of birth defects. Birth Defects 13(3a):5–11.

Evans JA (1982) Numerical taxonomy in the study of birth defects. In TVN Persaud (ed): Genetic Disorders, Syndromology and Prenatal Diagnosis. New York: Alan R. Liss, pp 139–160.

Falconer WA (1908) Cicero: De Senectute, De Amicitia, De Divinatione. Boston: Harvard University Press.

Farkas LG (1981) Anthropometry of the Head and Face in Medicine. New York: Elsevier.

Feingold M (1977) Introduction. Birth Defects 13(3a):1–3.

Ferembach D (1963) Frequency of spina bifida occulta in prehistoric human skeletons. Nature 199:100–101.

Gorlin RJ, Pindborg JJ, and Cohen MM Jr (1976) Syndromes of the Head and Neck. New York: McGraw-Hill.

Gregg NM (1941) Congenital cataract following German measles in the mother. Trans Ophthalmol Soc Aust 3:35–46.

Harvey W (1651) Disputations Touching the Generation of Animals (trans. G Whitteridge). Boston: Blackwell.

Heinonen OP, Slone D, and Shapiro S (1977) Birth Defects and Drugs in Pregnancy. Littleton, MA: Publishing Science Group.

Hermann J, and Opitz JM (1974) Naming and nomenclature of syndromes. Birth Defects 10(7):69–86.

Howie RN, and Phillips LI (1970) Congenital malformations in the newborn. NZ Med J 71:65–71.

Hutchinson J (1909) Syphilis, 2nd Ed. London: Cosell.

Krishnamachari KAVR, and Iyengar L (1975) Effect of maternal malnutrition on the bone density of neonates. Am J Clin Nutr 28:482–486.

Krogman WM, and İşcan MY (1986) The Human Skeleton in Forensic Medicine. Springfield, IL: Charles C Thomas.

Leck I (1984) The geographical distribution of neural tube defects and oral clefts. Br Med J 40:390–395.

Lehtonen E, and Saxen L (1986) Control of differentiation. In F Falkner and JM Tanner (eds): Human Growth, A Comprehensive Treatise, Vol. 1, 2nd Ed. New York: Plenum Press, pp 27–51.

Lester CW, and Shapiro HL (1968) Vertebral arch defects in the lumbar vertebrae of prehistoric American Eskimos. Am J Phys Anthropol 28:43–47.

Livingstone FB (1958) Anthropological implications of the sickle-cell gene distribution in West Africa. Am Anthropol 60:553–562.

Lowry RB, Rocheleau J, and Kellor L (1977) Comparison of existing classifications for coding congenital malformations and genetic syndromes. Birth Defects 13(3a):53–59.

Maroteaux P (1986) International nomenclature of constitutional diseases of bones. Birth Defects 22(4).

McBride WG (1961) Thalidomide and congenital abnormalities. Lancet 2:1358.

McIntosh R (1959) The problem of congenital malformations. J Chronic Dis 10:139–151.

McIntosh R, Merritt KK, Richards MR, Samuels MH, and Bellows MT (1954) The incidence of congenital malformations: A study of 5,964 pregnancies. Pediatrics 14: 505–522.

McKeown T, and Record RG (1960) Malformations in a population observed for five years after birth. In GEW

Wolstenhome and CM O'Connor (eds): Ciba Foundation Symposium on Congenital Malformations. Boston: Little Brown, pp 2–21.

McKusick VA (1969) On lumpers and splitters, or the nosology of genetic disease. Birth Defects 5(1):23–32.

McKusick VA (1974) Nomenclature of syndromes. Birth Defects 10(7):61–63.

McKusick VA (1986) Mendelian Inheritance in Man, 7th Ed. Baltimore: Johns Hopkins University Press.

Merbs CG, and Wilson WH (1960) Anomalies and pathologies of the Sadlermiut Eskimo vertebral column. Bull Natl Mus Can 180:154–179.

Merker H (1977) Considerations on the problems of the critical period during development of the limb skeleton. Birth Defects 13(1):179–202.

Merlob P, Yakov S, and Reisner SH (1984) Anthropometric measurements of the newborn infant. Birth Defects 20(7):1–52.

Murdy C (1981) Congenital deformities and the Olmec were-jaguar motif. Am Antiq 46:861–871.

Murphy DP (1929) Ovarian irradiation and the health of the subsequent children. Surg Gynecol Obstet 48:766–779.

National Center for Health Statistics (1986) Annual summary of births, marriages, divorces, and deaths: United States, 1985. Monthly Vital Stat Rep 34 (13 September).

Neel JV (1958) A study of major congenital defects in Japanese infants. Am J Hum Genet 10:398–445.

Opitz JM, and Howe JJ (1969) The Merkel syndrome. Birth Defects 5(2):167–179.

Ortner DJ, and Putschar WGJ (1981) Identification of pathological conditions in human skeletal remains. Smithsonian Contrib Anthropol 28.

Peck AL (1942) Aristotle: Generation of Animals. Boston: Harvard University Press.

Persaud TVN, Chudley AE, and Skalko RG (1985) Basic Concepts in Teratology, New York: Alan R. Liss.

Polednak AP (1986) Birth defects in blacks and whites in relation to prenatal development. Hum Biol 58:317–335.

Rimoin DL (1979) Variable Expressivity in the Skeletal Dysplasias. Birth Defects 15(5b):91–112.

Rimoin DL, and Horton WA (1978) Short stature. Part I. J Pediatr 92:523–528.

Rush D, Stein Z, and Susser MA (1980) A randomized controlled trial of prenatal nutritional supplementation in New York City. Pediatrics 65:685–697.

Schmorl G, and Junghanns H (1971) The Human Spine In Disease and Health, 2nd Ed. (trans. EF Besemann). New York: Grune and Stratton.

Scott JP (1986) Critical periods in organizational processes. In F Falkner and JM Tanner (eds): Human Growth, A Comprehensive Treatise, Vol. 1, 2nd Ed. New York: Plenum Press, pp 181–196.

Shahriaree H, Sajadi K, and Rooholamini SA (1979) A family with spondylolisthesis. J Bone Joint Surg [Am] 61: 1256–1258.

Skinner R (1983) Unifactorial inheritance. In AEH Emery and DL Rimoin (eds): Principles and Practice of Medical Genetics, Vol. 1. New York: Churchill Livingstone, pp 65–74.

Smith DW (1975) Classification, nomenclature, and naming of morphologic defects. J Pediatr 87:162.

Smith P (1973) Family burials at Hayonim. Paleorient 1: 69–71.

Spranger J, Benirschke K, Hall JG, Lenz W, Lowry RB, Opitz JM, Pinsky L, Schwarzacher HG, and Smith DW (1982) Errors of morphogenesis: Concepts and terms. J Pediatr 100:160–165.

Steinbock RT (1976) Paleopathological Diagnosis and Interpretation. Springfield, IL: Charles C Thomas.

Stevenson AC, Johnston HA, Stewart MIP, and Golding DR (1966) Congenital malformations. Bull WHO (Suppl 34).

Stewart TD (1931) Incidence of separate neural arch in the lumbar vertebrae of Eskimos. Am J Phys Anthropol 16: 51–62.

Stewart TD (1953) The age incidence of neural-arch defects in Alaskan natives considered from the standpoint of etiology. J Bone Joint Surg [Am] 35:937–950.

Stewart TD (1972) Racial differences in the manifestation of scaphocephaly. Am J Phys Anthropol 37:451.

Stewart TD (1975) Cranial dysraphism mistaken for trephination. Am J Phys Anthropol 42:435–438.

Sutow WW, and Pryde AW (1956) Incidence of spina bifida occulta in relation to age. Am J Dis Child 91:211–217.

Taillard WF (1976) Etiology of spondylolisthesis. Clin Orthop 117:30–39.

Tanner JM (1976) Charts for the diagnosis of short stature and low growth velocity, allowance for height of parents and prediction of adult height. Birth Defects 12(6):1–13.

Tanner JM, Whitehouse RH, Cameron N, Marshall WA, Healy MJR, and Goldstein H (1983) Assessment of Skeletal Maturity and Prediction of Adult Height (TW2 Method), 2nd Ed. New York: Academic Press.

Terry PB, Condie RG, Mathew PM, and Bissenden JG (1983) Ethnic differences in the distribution of congenital malformations. Postgrad Med J 59:657–658.

Turkel SJ, and Taylor JV (1986) Classification of spina bifida occulta in the sacrum and its application to the identification of skeletal remains. Paper presented at the 39th Annual Meeting of the American Academy of Forensic Sciences, New Orleans, February 1986.

Venkata CPS (1962) Maternal nutritional status and its effect on the newborn. Bull WHO 26:193–201.

Waddington CH (1962) New Patterns in Genetics and Development. New York: Columbia University Press.

Ward RE, and Meaney FJ (1984) Anthropometry and numerical taxonomy in clinical genetics. Am J Phys Anthropol 64:147–154.

Warkany J (1959) Congenital malformations in the past. J Chronic Dis 10:84–96.

Warkany J (1974) Overview of malformation syndromes. Birth Defects 10(7):1–5.

Warkany J, and Nelson RC (1940) Appearance of skeletal abnormalities in the offspring of rats reared on a deficient diet. Science 92:383–384.

Watson W (1749) Some accounts of the fetus in utero being differently affected by the smallpox. Phil Trans R Soc Lond 46:235–239.

Wiedemann H-R, Gorsse K-R, and Dibbern H (1985) An Atlas of Characteristic Syndromes, 2nd Ed. (trans. MF Passarge). Chicago: Year Book Medical Publishers.

Wiltse LL, Newman PH, and Machab I (1976) Classification of spondylolisis and spondylolisthesis. Clin Orthop 117:23–29.

Woolf CM, Koehn JH, and Coleman SS (1968) Congenital hip disease in Utah. Am J Hum Genet 20:430–439.

World Health Organization (1967) Principles for the testing of drugs for teratogenicity. WHO Tech Rep Ser 364:1–18.

Young ID (1987) Malformations in different ethnic groups. Arch Dis Child 62:109–111.

Young ID, and Clarke M (1985) Lethal malformations and perinatal mortality: A 10 year review with comparison of ethnic differences. Br Med J 295:89–91.

Zimmerman MR, and Kelley MA (1982) Atlas of Human Paleopathology. New York: Praeger.

Reconstruction of Life From the Skeleton
© 1989 Alan R. Liss, Inc., pages 129–160

Chapter 8

Skeletal Markers of Occupational Stress

Kenneth A. R. Kennedy
Section of Ecology and Systematics, Division of Biological Sciences, Cornell University, Ithaca, New York 14853

INTRODUCTION

In Lewis Carroll's classic, *Alice's Adventures in Wonderland,* when Alice came upon the blue caterpillar seated on a mushroom smoking his hookah she was in a diminutive condition, a stress response from eating some cake. Confused by the crisis of her identity, Alice was unable to respond to the caterpillar's question, "Who are you?" The caterpillar, taking a sensibly Lockean view that personal identity is based upon continuity and consistency of memories, sought to assist Alice by asking her to recite a familiar poem. Normally, Alice would have had no difficulty in reciting "Father William," but in her altered state she offers her own version:

"You are old," said the youth, "and your jaws are too weak
For anything tougher than suet;
Yet you finished the goose, with the bones and the beak—
Pray, how did you manage to do it?"

"In my youth," said his father, "I took to the law,
And argued each case with my wife;
And the muscular strength, which it gave to my jaw,
Has lasted the rest of my life."

In Alice's parody of Robert Southey's didactic poem about how to live long and well, Lewis Carroll does not suggest that Father William inherited his remarkable masticatory properties; rather, these were acquired in the course of the old man's occupation in legal debate. Although these verses are more appropriate to Wonderland than to the pragmatic realm of skeletal biology, they accentuate the fact that irregularities of osseous and dental tissues may develop under conditions of prolonged and continued stress imposed by some habitual, or occupational, activity. Popular concepts of this interrelationship of morphological structure and behavioral function embrace bowlegged cowboys and thirsty long-fanged vampires, but markers of occupational stress have scientific importance when applied to clinical problems of industrial and athletic medicine and to efforts to reconstruct lifeways from the human skeleton by paleontologists, paleodemographers, and forensic anthropologists.

This chapter describes some 140 markers of occupational stress that are reported in published medical and anthropological sources and that have come to the attention of the author in the course of field research in southern Asia and in forensic anthropology cases brought to the Human Biology Laboratory at Cornell University.

HISTORICAL BACKGROUND

Interest in markers of occupational stress has its origin in the medical literature of trade and military diseases that emerged in the mid-sixteenth century in Europe. Georgius Agricola (1494–1555) wrote a 12-volume work, published in 1556, about mining, which includes an account of diseases and accidents suffered by miners in Bohemia and Silesia. The Faustian alchemist and surgeon Paracelsus (1493–1541) published theories about respiratory diseases of miners, which he made to fit his notion of the sunless abyss of Tartarus where Zeus punished the Titans (Paracelsus, 1567). The first systematic exposition of industrial medicine, however, appeared in 1700 with the publication of *De Morbis Artificum Diatriba* by Bernardino Ramazzini (1633–1714), professor of medicine at the University of Modena and, after 1700, at the University of Padua. The English translation of Ramazzini's opus appeared in 1705 with the title *A Treatise on the Diseases of Tradesmen* and earned the Italian professor the title of "father of industrial medicine." His perception of the relationships between certain metals and symptoms of metallic poisoning among artisans and painters led to formulation of remedial procedures as well as recognition that an individual's occupation was the source for understanding problems of health. Ramazzini's motto—*Medici munus plebeios curantis est interrogare quas artes exerceant*—is appropriate as well to the anthropological investigator of markers of occupational stress in human skeletal material.

One of Ramazzini's admirers was Charles Turner Thackrah (1795–1833), apothecary, general practitioner, and poor-law physician to the textile workers at Bean Ing, a factory in Leeds. In the course of his medical training under Astley Cooper at Guy's Hospital, London, the young Thackrah read the English translation of Ramazzini's treatise. In 1831 he published his own comprehensive study of industrial medicine in England, *The Effects of the Principal Arts, Trades, and Professions, and of Civic States and Habits of Living, on Health and Longevity* (Meiklejohn, 1957). Among the trade diseases with which Thackrah was familiar were skeletal conditions of pelvic deformation and vertebral scoliosis characteristic of weavers who sat for long periods of time at their looms. He recognized that these malformations were exacerbated by the harsh conditions of labor and malnutrition prevalent in the early days of England's industrial revolution. The chronic inflammatory condition of ischial bursitis, which can produce bilateral osteitic ischial tuberosities and is known as "weaver's bottom," was appreciated by the Elizabethans as well, as demonstrated in Shakespeare's selection of the name "Bottom" for his weaver in *A Midsummer Night's Dream.*

By the latter part of the nineteenth century, a number of anatomists and surgeons became aware that the skeleton may reveal a broad spectrum of morphological and size irregularities that could be related to life habits. Among them was William Arbuthnot Lane (1856–1943), demonstrator of anatomy at Guy's Hospital and famous for his operations for fractures and cleft palates. In 1887 Lane observed:

> When we find a condition of the skeleton differing from the normal and obviously not the result of disease, I think we are justified in concluding that the variation must have resulted from the performance of some purpose or function in addition to those normally performed during the life of that individual alone. (Lane 1887b:586)

Lane's practice brought him face-to-face with working-class people whose bodies had been shaped by years of heavy physical labor; many of his patients exhibited modifications of the sternum and clavicle, which he attributed to carrying heavy loads. In his description of the skeleton of a dissection room cadaver whose trade was known to be that of a shoemaker, Lane defined an occupation as follows:

> One, which, when the person engaged in it is in very indigent circumstances [and] is carried on without variation during the whole adult lifetime of the individual, and is not, as in many kinds of labour, relinquished of necessity as old age approaches for others which are less laborious. (Lane 1888:593)

Lane used the phrase "pressure changes" to refer to the anatomical markers developed in response to habitual activities in order to distinguish them from markers of trauma and bone modifications associated with advancing age. Although "very indigent circumstances" are not a necessary component of conditions contributing to the development of markers of occupational stress, Lane's awareness of the habitual and prolonged factors involved in marker formation is consistent with what we know today about these anatomical features.

During the five decades separating the appearance of Thackrah's treatise on trade diseases and the publication of Lane's dissection room and clinical studies, a small body of scholars emerged, many of whom were trained in medicine, who were preoccupied with questions about the anatomical and evolutionary distinctions between apes, the "civilized and savage races," and prehistoric hominids whose bones were excavated from archaeological sites. Among these early physical anthropologists were Paul Broca (1824–1880), who in 1868 described platycnemia in his study of fossil hominid remains from the Dordogne Valley, and Leonce Pierre Manouvrier (1850–1927), who attributed this feature to the hyperactivity of the tibialis posticus muscle among inhabitants of mountainous countries with rough terrains that had to be traversed during hunting activities (Manouvrier, 1888). Diminution in frequency of platycnemia in Europeans was ascribed to the habits of civilization, and Manouvrier was certain as to the primitive nature of the trait, since he had encountered it in the tibiae of apes. Platycnemia was reported in skeletal material from prehistoric sites in France (Pruner-Bey, 1868), Germany (Schaaffhausen, 1882), Switzerland (Studer, 1886), and Pomerania (Virchow, 1886), in megalithic graves in Stolzenberg (Jahn, 1886), in nineteenth-century men from Denbighshire in England (Busk, 1871; Dawkins and Busk, 1870), among South Sea Islanders (Virchow, 1880b), and in various human populations extant today (Kuhff, 1881; Topinard, 1885; Virchow, 1880a; Wyman, 1871).

Another frequently observed anatomical variable was faceting on portions of the tibia and talus, which was attributed to squatting posture. The history of observations and interpretations of squatting facets is reviewed by Trinkaus (1975), who cites Arthur Thomson (1858–1935), lecturer on human anatomy at the University of Oxford, as recognizing that the skeletal morphology of the tibia and foot bones can be altered by habitual squatting. It was a professor of anatomy at the Medical College at Lahore (now in Pakistan), R. Havelock Charles (1858–1934), who suggested that Neanderthals squatted, a conclusion he reached through his familiarity with the studies of the Cannstadt and Spy fossils by Fraipont (1888) and Lohest (Fraipont and Lohest, 1887) and his own observations of the sitting postures of Punjabis (Charles, 1893–1894). Discussion of squatting facets by Marcellin Boule (1861–1942), in his treatise on the La Chapelle-aux-Saints Neanderthals (1911–1913), assured the place of this morphological feature in subsequent studies of fossil hominids (McCown and Keith, 1939; Taylor, 1968), although controversies have arisen over this marker of occupational stress (Regnault, 1898). The effects of habitual squatting on other bones of the lower extremities and pelvis were examined by British anatomists (Barnett, 1954; Buxton, 1938; Charles, 1893–1894; Martin, 1932; Thomson, 1890; Turner, 1887).

The synthesis of industrial medicine and physical anthropology with respect to markers of occupational stress was achieved by the British anatomist, William Turner (1832–1916), professor of anatomy at the University of Edinburgh from 1867 to 1903. In his lecture to the Royal Medical Society of Edinburgh on 5 November 1886, Turner asked if specialization of skeletal structures, form, and proportions had taken place in each human race to such an extent as to stamp the races with definitive anatomical characters, even if the normal range of morphological variation of traits for populations and the species is considered. He concluded that:

> Within certain limits the forms of the bones are without question influenced by the muscular apparatus which is attached to them. . . . If then the habits of life of one race call into play some special group of muscles, which are not, through a difference in habit, so constantly employed in another race, then I have no doubt that the form of the bone, not merely as regards the prominence of the processes to which the muscles are attached, but the relative area of the surfaces of attachment, would undergo a corresponding modification. . . . I believe, therefore, that we may in some degree ascribe the differences in the configuration of the skeleton in various races of men to the influence of habit operating through muscular action and pressure upon the bones, when in a comparatively plastic condition, and in the course of years of moulding them into the form which they present in the adult man.

. . . Descent and habits are therefore two great factors to be considered in the study of the variations which one meets with in the skeletons of the different races of men" (Turner 1887:486, 489, 492).

In nineteenth-century America there were a number of medically trained writers who contributed to some branch of anthropology, but they were as indifferent to markers of pathological stress as they were to the signs of occupational habits. John Collins Warren (1778–1856), Samuel G. Morton (1779–1851), Josiah Clark Nott (1804–1873), and Joseph Leidy (1823–1891) were pathologists who were aware of a variety of stresses in their patients, but they did not extend their knowledge of skeletal deformation and irregularities to their descriptions of prehistoric human skeletal remains. The earliest notable American study of prehistoric human skeletons from the viewpoint of pathology was carried out by one of Leidy's students, Joseph Jones (1833–1896), who excavated skeletons in the southeastern United States and considered that some of them bore signs of syphilis. Within the decade following the publication of Jones's treatise in 1876, paleopathology was well established at the Peabody Museum at Harvard University under Jeffries Wyman (1814–1874) and Frederic W. Putnam (1839–1915), but the emphasis was on trauma, anomalies, and clinically diagnosed pathological conditions. It was not until the era of Aleš Hrdlička (1869–1943) at the Smithsonian Institution in Washington, D.C., that serious attention was given to markers of occupational stress and disease (Jarcho 1966:3–8).

INDUSTRIAL AND ATHLETIC MEDICINE

During the full century that separates us from the time of Turner's address to the Royal Society of Edinburgh and the appearance of Jones's treatise on pre-Columbian treponemal lesions, medical practitioners and dissection room anatomists have continued to note markers of occupational stress in the course of clinical practice, while anthropologists have done the same in the context of research into the skeletal biology of living and ancient populations. These efforts have been undertaken, for the most part, independently of one another, with the result that neither medical clinicians nor physical anthropologists are very aware of the published sources about markers of occupational stress generated by each other's profession. Synthetic studies of the subject, which combine research data of industrial medicine and anthropological skeletal biology, do not exist, and a historical survey of the literature in both fields reveals that sources appear sporadically and are written according to a wide range of scientific standards of observation and publication. Most of the references to markers of occupational stress in the clinical literature are included in larger works, as in Lewin's (1959) text on disabilities of the foot and ankle.

Much of the published literature about industrial medicine concentrates on studies of stigmata of manual laborers. A classic study in this field was undertaken by Francesco Ronchese (1945, 1948) of the Department of Dermatology, Boston University School of Medicine. Although directed to stress modifications of the skin, Ronchese's work, *Occupational Marks and Other Physical Signs: A Guide to Personal Identification,* includes cases of dental modification resulting from chronic stress along with descriptions of "equestrian's buttocks," "stenographer's spread," "housemaid's knee," "stone-cutter's ring," "florist's fingertips," and "lover's elbow bursitis." Ronchese recognized that "occupational marks or marks due to habits . . . are of considerable scientific value to personal identification" (Ronchese 1948:54), an insight seldom shared by his medical colleagues, who limited the search for individual characteristics to abnormalities related to congenital and infectious diseases, sporadic anomalies, inherited or familiar peculiarities, effects of prenatal trauma, and similar events of a medical history (Dutra, 1944; Smith, 1939). Ronchese included these variables, but emphasized the value of documenting markers reflecting behavioral habits and life-styles.

As industrial medicine became a highly specialized field by the middle of the present century (Hunter, 1962, 1969), it found itself allied with orthopedics and athletic or sports medicine. A 1981 census of medical practitioners in the United States revealed that 600 surgeons were members of the American Orthopaedic Society, while 5,000 physicians were affiliated with the American College of Sports Medicine (Clark et al., 1981). Most recently emergent is the specialty of arts medicine, the solace for dancers, painters, musicians, and other artists (Rowes, 1986)—even breakdancers whose repertoire of stresses includes "jumper's knee" and "manhole syndrome" (the fate of joggers and breakdancers who suffer crushed bones and egos by falling into open manholes). Knee strain from improper use of exercise equipment in health clubs has added "machinery knee" to this list of new stressors (Nagle, 1984).

While great riches are to be found in the clinical literature by the anthropologist sufficiently adventurous to explore its depths and broad distribution, a limiting factor is that the emphasis is on soft tissue modifications that may not be represented in dried bone. Radiographic analysis serves to bring some observations of the industrial and sports physician into the purview of the anthropologist, but the fact remains that dried bone is seldom encountered by the clinician in the course of practice, and medical interpretations of bony lesions lack the sophistication of observation offered by the trained paleopathologist in human skeletal biology (Bugyi and Kausz, 1970). Given these circumstances, as well as the differences in scientific orientation of medicine and anthropology, it is not surprising that research on markers of occupational stress has developed quite independently.

ANTHROPOLOGICAL RESEARCH

The anthropological literature of markers of occupational stress is found in sources associated with the closely allied research areas of paleontology, paleodemography, and forensic anthropology. Practitioners of these fields share methodological backgrounds in human skeletal biology, osteology, and dental anthropology along with theoretical orientations to human evolution and biological diversity of living and ancient populations. Examples of the paleontological context include studies of squatting facets among Neanderthals (Trinkaus, 1975) and observations of supinator crest hypertrophy in the ulnae of Mesolithic Gangetic hominids that are related to spear-throwing activity (Kennedy, 1983). J. Lawrence Angel (1946) correlated skeletal changes of the pelvis and lower extremities of ancient Greeks from Neolithic to medieval Byzantine times to locomotor stress in rough terrain and discussed disease factors in ancient Aegeans (Angel, 1959, 1960, 1964, 1971, 1982), prehistoric Californians (Angel, 1966), and in freed black populations buried in Philadelphia (Angel et al., 1985b, 1987; Kelley and Angel, 1987). Leigh's (1925) study of dental pathology of native Americans in the context of nutrition and the natural environment was a significant contribution to dental anthropology, but it was Steven Molnar's (1972) survey of dental functions among various prehistoric populations that served as the impetus for recent studies of dental markers of occupational stress and culture (Goodman et al., 1984; Larsen, 1985; Schulz, 1977).

Paleodemographic studies of prehistoric populations undergoing transition of socioeconomic adaptations from hunting-foraging to agricultural-pastoral practices have been compiled in a volume edited by Mark Cohen and George J. Armelagos (1984). Several contributors to the work—*Paleopathology at the Origins of Agriculture*—refer to specific markers of occupational stress within the broader framework of populational reactions to growth and development, disease, rates of mortality, and other demographic factors. The study of activity-induced pathological conditions in the Sadlermiut population of Arctic Canada by Charles Merbs (1983) is an important study of disease responses to occupational stressors. This is an exception in the paleodemographic literature where life-styles from skeletal material are limited to discussions of mortality and disease (Edynak, 1976; Fedeli and Masali, 1978; Rose, 1985; Zarek, 1966). Larsen (1987) provides a useful synthesis of recent advances made in bioarchaeology, an emerging discipline that emphasizes the study of human skeletal and dental tissues in relation to analysis of diet, nutrition, disease, and behavior.

Forensic anthropologists, who have the most to gain from a familiarity with markers of occupational stress in their medical-legal pursuits toward personal identification, have produced few published accounts of their case studies and laboratory observations. The *Bibliography of References on Forensic Anthropology*, edited by William G. Eckert (1974), does not include markers of occupational stress within the classification of 14 topical headings, nor does Clyde Snow mention these variables in his introduction to the bibliography or in his summary of the state of the art of forensic anthropology published in *Annual Review of Anthropology* in 1982. This omission is perpetuated in recent textbooks on forensic anthropology (Stewart, 1979), human osteology (Bass, 1969, 1979, 1987), and pathology of human skeletal remains (Ortner and Putschar, 1981). Although Wilton Krogman (1935) does not discuss markers of occupational stress in his earlier works, the second edition of *The Human Skeleton in Forensic Medicine* mentions several published sources (Krogman and İşcan 1986:401–412). Studies of nonmetric variations of the human skeleton include mention of specific markers (Berry and Berry, 1967; Finnegan, 1978, 1983; Finnegan and Faust, 1974; Saunders, 1978). More often, however, markers are discussed in the context of anatomical descriptions of given populations (e.g., Angel, 1966, 1979; Angel et al., 1985b; Cameron, 1934; Grimm, 1959; Merbs, 1983; Tainter, 1980; Trotter, 1937, 1964, 1967); descriptions of specific markers are few (e.g., Angel et al., 1985a; Kelley, 1982; Kennedy, 1983; Levy, 1968; Scher, 1978).

The anthropologist who has contributed most significantly to the study of markers of occupational stress is the late J. Lawrence Angel (1915–1986), curator in the physical anthropology section of the National Museum of Natural History, Smithsonian Institution. For 40 years he collected data on the skeletal biology of the ancient peoples of the Mediterranean basin, and his knowledge of markers of occupational stress contributed to his success as a forensic anthropologist in the identification of human remains (Kernan, 1977). A posthumous contribution to forensic anthropology that incorporates data about markers of occupational stress is in the process of preparation and final editing by Margaret C. Caldwell. Among other important contributors to this topic are Donald J. Ortner of the Smithsonian Institution, Charles F. Merbs of Arizona State University, and Stephen Molnar of Washington University. Citations of the contributions of these anthropologists, along with those of the late Calvin Wells (1908–1978) of Castle Museum, Norwich, are contained in Table 1.

RESPONSES OF BONE TO STRESS

In 1892, Julius Wolff (1836–1902), a German anatomist, stated that "the form of the bone being given, the bone elements place or displace themselves in the direction of the functional pressure and increase or decrease their mass to reflect the amount of functional pressure." Wolff's Law of Transformation describes responses of bone to mechanical forces whereby remodeling takes place in well-vascularized subchondral areas in order to resist stress. Lipping, spurring, and exostoses of various kinds occur in order to expand the bony framework so that the load may be dissipated and lowered per unit area. The gross deformity that results from severe and prolonged stress forms the marker of occupational stress that can be observed macroscopically (Radin et al., 1972).

Another kind of response involves muscles that directly influence the morphology of bone at loci other than joint surfaces. Thus compression, while stimulating bone growth, may also lead to resorption if exceeding limits of response or affecting blood supply. Here the primary factor responsible for elevated tubercles, crests, and tuberosities is muscle pull upon these structures to which muscle is attached. Tension increases osteogenesis and the mass of bone beneath a muscle, the result being an elevated area of insertion formed by Sharpey's fibers, which extend from the connective tissue mass of muscle directly into the cortical bone. These fibers become covered over by deposits of new bone (Hoyte and Enlow, 1966).

Wolff's law was one approach toward understanding phenotypic changes in bone, but it is understood today that direct muscle pull can also be related to cortical recession (endosteal growth) where tension is acting in a manner associated with resorption rather than deposition. Earlier anatomists assumed that muscle and tendon markings constituting the superstructures of tubular bones were related only to the external bone table; recent research has established that external compacta are often shifted from an endosteal position, that resorptive areas may underlie muscles, and that alternating sequences of resorption and deposition for both bony surfaces may occur irrespective of the muscular attachments. In short, the inner table of bone changes in direct harmony with changes in the outer table, and tuberosities may have an outer surface that is resorptive.

The manufacture and maintenance of bone is performed by mesenchymal cells, which have the primary function of making new cells by mitotic division when a stimulus reaches them, and metabolically specialized cells, which do not divide but have the capacity to make new bone, govern ion exchange between blood and bone, and do metabolic work of bone resorption and formation. The differentiated metabolically specialized cells begin as osteoclasts resorbing bone and later become bone-making osteoblasts. In the third and final stage of their life, these cells become surrounded by products of their own manufacture. The division of labor by cells allows for continued replenishment of material for remodeling, growth, and lesion repair (Frost, 1966). Bone turnover is highest under conditions of pathological stress, and the limits of bone plasticity may be exceeded by agents of certain abnormalities of biochemistry, metabolism, hormonal and enzymatic activity, and vascular and neuronal changes. However, nonpathological conversion occurs during early bone growth and during later life as haversian remodeling takes place. As whole bone changes, various parts and areas of bone become relocated; hence remodeling involves a combination of resorptive and depositional functions over periosteal and endosteal surfaces. Haversian conversion involves replacement of existing cortical bone by secondary osteons (Enlow, 1976).

Although the term "stress" is applied to discussion of occupational markers, the term has a more specific meaning in biomechanics. Evans (1957:4–5) defines stress as "intermolecular resistance within an object to the action of an outside force which is applied to it" and gives the example of internal resistance within leg bones as a result of compressional force applied to them by body weight when standing erect. Stress may be conceived, as well, as mutual force or action between contiguous surfaces of bodies caused by external force (Thieme, 1950:18). Stress lines produced by compressive loading of a model made of rubber or plastic resemble trabecular structures of natural bone formed during growth.

"Strain" refers to deformation or distortion of an object whereby linear dimensions are changed when force is applied. The force may be tensile, which tends to pull or lengthen an object, or compressive, which pulls it together and shortens it. An example of strain is alteration in body size after stretching.

"Shear" results from applied forces that tend to cause two contiguous parts of a body to slide relatively to each other in a direction parallel to their plane of contact, as takes place in dislocation of certain bones or in normal joint action of articular facets of vertebrae; "torsion" involves twisting.

These responses to the push and pull of force are involved in the formation of markers of occupational stress, becoming manifested macroscopically if an area of bone is affected by a force or load that exceeds the bone's elastic limit so that the area of stress does not return to its original form. Pressure tolerance varies for different bones and for portions of the same bone, but excessive stress and strain can lead to bone destruction and necrosis. If the limits of elasticity are not exceeded, new bone formation is stimulated, a critical factor in healing.

When a tubular bone surface becomes less concave as an external force is applied, the net loss of bone appears at the surface as a result of osteoclastic activity. Greater concavity of a bone surface when an external force is applied leads to a net increase in bone at that surface as a result of osteoblastic activity. This correlation may be caused by an electrical voltage generated at the surface of bones that are deformed by bending (Epker and Frost, 1965).

Classic sources on osteogenesis and physiology of bone tissue (McLean and Urist, 1955; Murray, 1985), mechanical adaptations of bones and joints (Currey, 1984; Evans, 1957, 1966; Johnson, 1966; Townsley, 1948), muscle growth and function in relation to skeletal morphology (Hoyte and Enlow, 1966; Scott, 1957), and skeletal plasticity (Hughes, 1968) contribute toward an understanding of marker formation, but these offer very few cases of specific markers of occupational stress. The clinical milieu of these and other anatomical studies means that most cases of stress are associated with pathological conditions rather than with the lifeways of individuals and the cultures of non-Western populations.

CLASSIFICATION OF MARKERS

The great diversity of markers of occupational stress reported in medical and anthropological literature may be classified according to types of stressors.

Attrition

Enamel, dentine, and related dental structures may undergo varying degrees of wear caused by ingestion of abrasive particles, by grinding of teeth in normal occlusion of the jaws, and by objects held or moved about in the mouth when the dentition functions as a tool or accessory hand. Severe dental attrition may involve lesions penetrating the pulp cavity. There is some regeneration of dentine under the stress of attrition, but if the rate of attrition is too severe and persistent, production of new dentine will not keep pace with wear. Tooth realignment or evulsion, often accompanied by caries and abscess formation, may follow. Abrasion of osseous tissue is involved when bones are in direct contact at joint surfaces because of deterioration of intervening structures under severe osteoarthritic conditions. The result is eburnation of the bones at points of articulation.

Enthesopathic Lesions

Enthesopathic lesions at loci of muscular insertions caused by hypertrophy of relevant muscles form rough patches, irregularities, and osteophytes on bone. These may be induced by mechanical strain from forces external to the body, as with carrying heavy burdens on the head, which can result in fractures of the spinous processes of cervical vertebrae (Levy, 1968). They may be induced in other cases from internal forces, as with hypertrophy of the supinator crest on the proximal ulna as a result of supination and hyperextension of the arm in spear throwing, slinging, and pitching (Kennedy, 1983). The habitual squatting posture of many ancient and modern peoples also causes enthesopathic changes from internal forces within the skeletomuscular system (Trinkaus, 1975). Marked lines of attachment for flexor ligaments on palmar surfaces of the phalanges of the right hand of a first millennium B.C. mummy from Thebes have been attributed to flexion of the fingers in a firm grasp, as in holding a stylus (Kennedy et al., 1986). The mummy in question is identified from historical sources as Penpi, a scribe, and bones of the macerated skeleton suggest that he was right-handed. Postcranial bones provide markers of occupational stress indicative of the cross-legged seated posture of Egyptian scribes.

Trauma

Lesions due to sudden or gradually imposed stress may result in bone fractures. Osteogenesis arises from periosteum and endosteum at some distance from the fracture line, and repair moves toward the gap, enveloping and replacing fibrocartilaginous callus. New bone arises from cells with osteogenetic potency, and as it advances into the callus, prevascular connective tissue cells are drawn into the osteogenetic process and are transformed into osteoblasts. Thus cartilaginous callus of bone is replaced by new bone (McLean and Urist, 1955). Trauma of the dentition occurs with tooth chipping, displacement, and evulsion (Molnar, 1972).

Bone Degeneration

Bone degeneration takes the form of atrophic loss of substance or volume of bone, as in osteoporosis, or reorientation of trabeculae, as occurs when subchondral bone is subjected to repeated loading. As microfractures heal, bone becomes rigid and initiates a sequence of changes: impulse loading, trabecular microfracture, bone remodeling, resultant stiffening of bone, increased stress on articular cartilage, cartilage breakdown, joint degeneration (Radin et al., 1972). Joint degeneration and osteoporosis are accelerated under conditions of heavy physical labor, obesity, and various stressors of life-style (Chalmers and Ho, 1970; Mashkara, 1971).

Nutrition

As a component of nutrient resource availability, food quality, social status, environment, and life-style, nutrition is the basis of the individual's capacity to attain full ontogenetic development. In the context of skeletal maturity, body size, and stature, nutrition is a marker of occupational stress. Nutritional deficiency has been cited as the cause of platymeria, platycnemia, and platybrachia (Buxton, 1938), although nonnutritional factors may be involved as well. Diaphyseal bowing is diagnostic of a number of pathological stressors, including treponemal diseases and rickets.

Sexual Dimorphism

The harder physical labor in which men engage imposes greater skeletomuscular robusticity upon bones, the sizes of which may be under the control of genetic and hormonal factors. Since greater force is placed upon areas of muscle insertion than on areas of muscle origin, those portions of tubular bones bearing insertions are characteristically more robust. Occupational effects have been considered in determination of sex from skeletons. The humerus has been selected for this type of analysis, and it reveals differences between males and females (France, 1985) with results that are similar to those found in discriminant function sexing of the tibia (İşcan and Miller-Shaivitz, 1984). Spondylosis and spondylolithesis are twice as frequent in males than in females, again reflecting the heavier physical labor performed by men (Thieme, 1950). A combined skeletal sample of 134 hunter-gatherers and agriculturalists from northwestern Alabama showed that no relationship was discovered between arthritis at the knee and any femoral measurement or strength estimate, although arthritis at the hip was significantly greater in individuals with larger femora. When the sexes and cultural groups were separated, only agricultural males exhibited a significant association between arthritis at the knee and dimensions and cortical area of the femur. These same agricultural males had larger and stronger femoral diaphyses than any other part of the sample, a situation that leads Bridges (1989) to conclude that degenerative joint disease may occur in response to factors other than those imposed by habitual activities or traumatic injuries. Bridges (1987) notes that not all degenerative bone changes of the elbow and shoulder should be attributed to weapon use, especially in cases where less dramatic, more mundane activities may prevail among members of both sexes.

Racial Differences

Ecological conditions rather than racial factors are more important in cases involving stress reactions of bones and teeth. Therefore, it is interesting to observe that people of Asiatic descent have a high incidence of arthritic knees and low incidence of pelvic arthritis, whereas in Eurasians the knees and hips are equally involved (Radin et al., 1972). Students of Asiatic martial arts note that Orientals have greater freedom of movement in the medial aspect of the knee joint than do Caucasians (Klein, 1977). Habitual sitting postures and walking patterns may be related to these so-called racial differences (Amako, 1960).

Age Differences

Age characteristics of lower limb skeletal changes in persons engaged in physical labor have been studied in factories in the U.S.S.R. (Mashkara, 1971).

The markers of occupational stress listed in Table 1 are seldom the consequence of a single stress factor. Sex, age, social status, nutritional quality and quantity, life-style, and general health profile are critical components in the genesis of a specific marker. Criteria employed in the selection of the markers in this study have been 1) reports of irregularities of bones and teeth that are attributed to occupational activity by medical and anthropological investigators and 2) data that are available in published sources. Descriptions of anatomical structures, stress factors, and occupational activities are taken from the published works cited in the reference column of Table 1 (Fig. 1, 2). Evaluation of each entry is not included in the present study as this is best reserved for a subsequent analysis. In human beings, these markers are not tested experimentally. When animals are used in experiments involving relationships of muscle to bone (Avis, 1959; Horowitz and Shapiro, 1955; Washburn, 1947), parallels with markers of occupational stress in humans are not obvious. Therefore, occupational activities must be inferred from clinical records in industrial and athletic medicine, ethnographic accounts, and the archaeological and historical records. Human skeletal collections with which some hospital and occupational data are associated, as with the Terry and Todd collections in the United States, are invaluable sources for assessing the significance of certain markers of occupational

TABLE 1. Markers of Occupational Stress

Skeletal component	Anatomical structure	Stress factor	Occupational activity	Reference
Mandible	Sharp tubercles on medial and lateral aspects of anterior-superior surfaces of mandibular condyles	Forward projection of the mandible and extension of pterygoid muscles	Clarinet playing	Angel and Caldwell (1984)
Tympanic portion and acoustic meatus of temporal bone	Auditory exostoses (auditory tori)	Exposure of the ear canal to cold water	Habitual diving for exploitation of aquatic food resources by Upper Paleolithic and Mesolithic Europeans, native Californians, Tasmanians	Frayer (1988)
Temporomandibular joint	Osteoarthritis, especially of left temporomandibular joint	Masticatory pressure	Softening skins and boots by chewing. Objects held in the left hand by Sadlermiut women	Merbs (1983)
Vertebral column	Lower lumbar spondylolisthesis, with compression of lumbar disks and other osteophytic development	Flexion of the spine with immobility of the pelvis and lower extremities	Lifting heavy objects combined with sitting many hours in a kayak by Sadlermiut men	Merbs (1983)
	"Snowmobiler's back." Compression of vertebrae	Vertical compressive force	Sledding and tobogganing over rough terrain by Sadlermiuts	Merbs (1983)
			Snowmobile riding	Roberts et al. (1971)
			Cart riding by medieval Germans	Grimm (1959)
	Reduction of lumbar curvature. Defects in neural arches	Sharp, sudden torsion movements; lumbar flexion	Bending the waist while keeping the legs extended at the knee when sitting in a kayak	Stewart (1956)
	Predominant kyphosis with slight scoliosis and little compensatory lordosis	Flexion and lateral bending	Long periods of sitting. Identification of a tailor from eighteenth–early nineteenth-century cemetery in Norwich, England	Wells (1967)
	Robusticity of superior articular processes of L-5; robusticity of joint of L-5 and first sacral vertebra; irregular margins of lumbar bodies and markers of lumbar stress; irregular margins of sacroiliac joint	Extension and free rotation of thorax and flexion of the pelvis against the leg; excessive loading of left acetabular margins	Shoveling and throwing heavy materials. Ship trimmer brought to Guy's Hospital, London, in 1886. (Ship trimming involves arranging coal so that the ship's equilibrium is stable. Coal shoveled and thrown great distances)	Lane (1887a)

Scoliosis with convexity of curvature toward the side of the body that supports the burden	Flexion and lateral bending	Carrying heavy burdens on the shoulder by nineteenth-century English laborers	Lane (1885)
	Flexion and lateral bending	Stone mining by Tuscan alabaster miners near Volterra and Pisa	Hunter (1962)
Scoliosis and pelvic deformation	Flexion and lateral bending	Long periods of sitting at a weaving loom combined with nutritional deficiency. Nineteenth-century English weavers	Thackrah (1831)
"Porter's neck." Fractures of vertebral arches; forward dislocation of vertebrae with sheering of the pedicles; herniation of the disks. Most injuries affect region of C-1 to C-4	Compression of vertebral disks and fractures from force pressing downward on the head and cervical column	Carrying heavy loads (90 kg or more) on the top of the head. Grain porters from Salisbury, Rhodesia (Zambia)	Levy (1968)
"Milker's neck." Compressive fracture of the cervical spine with subluxation and compressive fracture of the lower cervical bodies. Most injuries affect region of C-6 to C-7	Hyperflexion of the cervical bodies	Milking a cow when the milker's head is pushed against the animal's flank and the animal shifts position, thereby loading the milker's neck	Olin et al. (1982)
Thoracic osteoarthritis with spondylosis; enlargement of the articular processes of the thoracic vertebrae; scoliosis; vertebral body expansion	Flexion and lateral bending of the thoracic region	Strenuous physical activity in lifting and hauling (cannon?) by sailors of King Henry VIII flagship *Mary Rose* (sank 1545 off Isle of Wight)	Stirland (1985b)
Schmorl's disk hernation. Crescent-shaped lesions in the lower thoracic and lumbar vertebral bodies; intervertebral osteochondrosis; continued stress may result in destruction of the vertebral plate and spondylitis deformans	Flexion and lateral bending	Generalized physical stress among prehistoric hunter-forager and urban populations	Kelley (1982)

Continued

TABLE 1. Markers of Occupational Stress—Continued

Skeletal component	Anatomical structure	Stress factor	Occupational activity	Reference
Vertebral column *continued*	Gross osteoarthrosis of the cervical spine and spinal cord injury; most injuries affect region of C-1 to C-4; acute kyphotic angulation localized in one disk space; cervical lordosis	Flexion and lateral bending	Carrying heavy loads on top of the head by Cape Province black laborers; wood carrying and water carrying by black females; grain sack carrying by black males	Scher (1978)
	Fracture of cervical spines; severe osteoarthritis of spines	Sudden impact of force on the top of the head	Acapulco divers who break the impact of the water in daily dives of over 100 feet with the tops of their heads rather than with their hands held in front of their heads	Radin et al. (1972)
	Spondylolisthesis, spondylolisthesis, and herniation of vertebral disks	Stress resulting from erect posture when lumbar curvature involves a shearing component of vertical compressive force	Ecological factors of intensive physical labor by ancient and historic males from northern latitude populations of Eskimos and Lapps	Thieme (1950)
Sternum	Absence (destruction) of the manubrioglandiolar (clavicular) articulation	Force applied in a downward direction to the lateral end of the clavicle and rib 2 and to the manubrium	Heavy load carrying upon the back by nineteenth-century English laborers	Lane (1887b)
	Manubriogladiolar joint infused and assuming the character of a hinge joint	Movement of joint around a transverse axis and extreme flexion under pressure	Placement of the last of a boot against the chest by nineteenth-century English shoemakers. Autopsy subject at Guy's Hospital, London	Lane (1888)
Ribs	Osteoarthritis of costovertebral joints, especially in thoracic area of T-4 through T-9	Elevation	Elevation of ribs when carrying heavy objects by Sadlermiut women carrying children on their backs	Merbs (1983)
	Flattening of ribs 6 through 8 with incurved lower sternum and fused angle of Lewis	Bracing of ribs with the pelvis and immobility of the thoracic cage	Stays with straight supports in corsets. Worn by American Colonial women	Angel et al. (1985a)

	Ridged lateral reaction and anterior twisting of ribs 9 through 12, flattening of vertebral spines T-11 through T-13	Bracing of ribs with the pelvis and immobility of the thoracic cage	Corsets with sharply concave sides plus straight steel stays. Worn by American nineteenth-century women (Terry Collection 1846–1896 births)	Angel et al. (1985a)
	Flattening of spines T-5 through L-5 with "healed fracture" wave	Bracing of ribs with the pelvis and immobility of the thoracic cage	Modern back braces	Angel et al. (1985a)
Clavicle	Robusticity of lateral end of clavicle which occurs also on rib 2	Force applied in a downward direction to the lateral end of the clavicle and rib 2	Carrying heavy loads in both hands with arms extended along the sides of the body by milkman carrying pails for long distances	Lane (1887b)
	Robusticity of sternoclavicular joint surfaces with minute particles of bone scattered through a dense fibrous wedge of osseous tissue and replacing the fibro-cartilage attachment	Force applied to lateral end of the clavicle in a backward and downward direction	Hand sewing by a shoemaker. Autopsy subject at Guy's Hospital, London	Lane (1888)
	Prominent attachment of origin of pectoralis major	Circumduction of the arms	Slinging with both arms elevated above the head by prehistoric Minorcan men	Cameron (1934)
Scapula	Bilateral osteoarthritis of acromioclavicular joints	Elevation of the arms	Kayak paddling and harpoon throwing. Harpoon thrown from seated position in a kayak by Sadlermiut men	Merbs (1983)
	Osteoarthritis of left glenoid cavity	Extension of the arms	Use of the bow held in the left hand by Sadlermiut men	Merbs (1983)
	Bilateral osteoarthritis of the glenoid cavity		Skin scraping by Sadlermiut women	Merbs (1983)
	Os acromiale or bipartite acromion. Nonfusion of the acromion process	Tearing of the rotator cuff due to continued and heaving loading of the right or left arm	Protracted and continued use of the English longbow by archers of King Henry VIII flagship *Mary Rose* (sank 1545 off Isle of Wight)	Stirland (1985a)

Continued

TABLE 1. Markers of Occupational Stress—Continued

Skeletal component	Anatomical structure	Stress factor	Occupational activity	Reference
Humerus	Bilateral bowing of diaphyses; convexity of bow directed laterally; deep groove for musculospiral (radial) nerves; prominent posterior portion of deltoid tuberosity; encroachment of articular surface of humeral head on to the superior aspect of the anatomical neck	Circumduction and abduction of the arm	Slinging with both arms elevated above the head by prehistoric Minorcan men	Cameron (1934)
	Platybrachia	Nutritional deficiency	Deficiency of bone in relation to surfaces required for normal muscular attachments	Buxton (1938)
	Exostosis of the medial epicondyle from its lower edge into a vertically descending osteophyte	Hyperactivity of pronator teres, flexor carpi radialis, palmaris longus, flexor digitorum superficialis, and flexor carpi ulnaris	Javelin throwing among Neolithic Saharans of Niger; modern golf players	Dutour (1986)
Radius	Bilateral stress fracture of mixed sclerotic and periosteal types	Supination of the arm with a heavy load	Field-gun running. Muzzle of a heavy gun is caught and carried across the forearms in competitive military sport activity	Farquharson-Roberts and Fulford (1980)
			Carrying heavy loads with the elbows bent among masons and bakers	Gentry (1972)
	Unilateral right-side lesions, spicules, and osteophytes on the radial tuberosity at the site of insertion of biceps brachii; small lesion on the distal face of the olecranon fossa of the ulna at point of contact with the olecranon process at full elbow extension; bilateral asymmetry of humeri	Flexion of the right elbow against a strong external force with an external rotation of the shoulder while the left arm is extended to a compressive force	Archery among Neolithic Saharans of Niger and Mali	Dutour (1986)

Ulna	Hypertrophy of supinator crest and fossa	Supination and hypertension of arm	Spear throwing, use of sling and atlatl, pitching missiles by modern athletes and Mesolithic Gangetic populations	Kennedy (1983, 1985)
	Exostoses on medial surface of ulnar notch; bone chipping	Supination and hyperextension of arm	Baseball pitching	King (1969)
	Anconeus ridge elevation	Extension at humeroulnar joint	Carrying heavy objects by cradling them in both arms. Eskimo populations	Plummer (1984)
	Subcutaneous cellulites at the elbow	Extension and flexion at glenohumeral joint combined with humeroulnar extension and flexion	Pounding action when an individual stands over a vessel and pounds a pestle equal to his own stature, as in earlier industrial method of crushing lead silicate glaze	Hunter (1969)
	Hypertrophy of supinator crest and depressed fossa	Pronation and supination of the forearm with humeroulnar extension	Manipulation of iron with a long reach with elbows extended by black slaves at Catoctin furnace, Maryland	Kelley and Angel (1983)
			Heavy physical labor by blacks, slave and free, buried in Baptist cemetery between 1823 and 1843 in Philadelphia	Angel et al. (1985b)
	Large, flattened, and slightly curved exostoses on the posterior superior surfaces of the right and left olecranon processes, especially of the right side	Stress on the insertion of the triceps brachii tendon in extension of the elbow	Net casting, woodcutting, and blacksmithing among Neolithic Saharans of Niger and Mali; modern baseball players	Dutour (1986)
	Hypertrophy of the proximal one-half of ulna of right or left arm. Chronic circumferential periostitis secondary to trauma	Hammering action of forearm against pelvis and chaps	Professional rodeo-cowboy bareback bronco riders in Nebraska. Only one arm is allowed to come in contact with rigging cinched to the horse	Claussen (1982)
Joint surfaces				
Shoulder	Lipping, porosity, and eburnation of joint surfaces of acromial facet of clavicle, glenoid fossa, and humerus head	Elevation, depression, circumduction at glenohumeral joint	General stress response of lower-status individuals of Middle Woodland Illinois Valley populations	Tainter (1980)

Continued

TABLE 1. Markers of Occupational Stress—Continued

Skeletal component	Anatomical structure	Stress factor	Occupational activity	Reference
Joint surfaces *continued*				
Elbow	Lipping, porosity, and eburnation of capitulum, radial head, and radial notch of ulna	Pronation and supination	General stress response of lower-status individuals of Middle Woodland Illinois Valley populations	Tainter (1980)
	Lipping, porosity, and eburnation of medial and lateral borders of trochlea, coronoid, radial and olecranon fossae, and olecranon process of ulna	Flexion and extension	General stress response of lower-status individuals of Middle Woodland Illinois Valley populations	Tainter (1980)
Knee	Lipping, porosity, and eburnation of lateral and medial condyles of tibia, lateral and medial condyles of femur, and lateral and medial surfaces of patella	Flexion and extension	General stress response of lower-status individuals of Middle Woodland Illinois Valley Populations	Tainter (1980)
Upper extremities	Significant increase in diaphyseal dimensions in all arm bones; increase in bowing and torsional strengths of middle to distal area of humeral diaphysis, decrease in bilateral asymmetry	Vigorous flexion and extension at humeroradial and radiocarpal joints	Grinding corn with a long wooden pestle and hollowed log mortar by southeastern U.S. Indian women	Bridges (1985)
Elbow	"Atlatl elbow." Lipping and eburnation of capitulum from frictional removal of cartilage over this surface of the humerus	Flexion and extension of the elbow. Pronation and supination of the hand and forearm.	Spear throwing and use of the atlatl by Early Horizon California men; seed grinding of Early Horizon California women	Angel (1966)
	"Atlatl elbow." Porosity, eburnation, and destruction remodeling of the capitulum	Pronation and supination; flexion	Intensity of elbow use by Eskimos	Ortner (1968)
	"Atlatl elbow." Degenerative joint disease	Rotation of the elbow	Varieties of repetitive activities by males and females of Archaic hunter-gatherers and Mississippian agriculturalists from northwestern Alabama	Bridges (1987)

	Osteoarthritis of the humeroradial joint	Pronation and supination	Kayak paddling by Sadlermiut men	Merbs (1983)
	Osteoarthritis of the humeroulnar joint	Flexion and extension	Kayak paddling by Sadlermiut men	Merbs (1983)
	"Dog-walker's elbow." Lateral epicondylitis of the joint	Sudden tugging and traction on extended and pronated arm	Walking a dog on a short leash when the animal is not trained to heel	Davis (1981) Mebane (1981)
	"Hooker's elbow." Lateral epicondylitis of the joint	Frequent elevation and depression of the partially flexed	Ice fishing when the fisherman sits over a hole in the ice and repeatedly jerks his arm upward on a fishing line attached to a stick	Dahl et al. (1981) Davis (1981)
Elbow and shoulder	Join degeneration and osteoarthritic changes	Repetitious impact loading	Use of pneumatic drills. Fingers and wrists are not affected	Radin et al. (1972)
Wrist	Osteoarthritis of ulnarcarpal joints, especially of the left hand	Ulnar flexion	Kayak paddling when left hand is used as a pivot for the double-bladed paddle by Sadlermiut men	Merbs (1983)
	Osteoarthritis of ulnarcarpal joints and radioulnar joints, especially of the left hand	Ulnar flexion	Cutting skins using the left hand. Skins are held in the right hand by Sadlermiut women	Merbs (1983)
Hand				
Pollex	"Cowboy thumb." Fracture along transverse or longitudinal planes of diaphysis	Fracture	Gripping the saddle horn while flying off the saddle in rodeo riding or while riding mechanical barroom bulls	Davis (1981)
Phalanges	Marked lines of attachment for flexor ligaments on palmer surfaces of first phylangeal row of the right hand	Flexion in firm grasp	Grasping a stylus by an Egyptian scribe from Thebes, Third Intermediate period	Kennedy et al. (1986)
Intermetacarpal joints	"Seamstress's fingers." Osteoarthritis and marked attachments for ligaments of intermetacarpal joints of the right hand	Flexion; forceful opposition of thumb and index finger	Driving bone needles through tough skins in sewing by Sadlermiut women	Merbs (1983)

Continued

TABLE 1. Markers of Occupational Stress—Continued

Skeletal component	Anatomical structure	Stress factor	Occupational activity	Reference
Pelvis	Senile osteoporosis		Consequences of lighter work pattern and reduced physical stress of technologically more advanced populations (Sweden, United Kingdom) compared to poorer populations (China, African Bantu speakers)	Chalmers and Ho (1970)
Acetabulum	Large size of ischial portion of facies lunata combined with prominent rim and deep groove for obturator externus	Abduction and flexion	Squatting and sartorial postures by Punjabis	Charles (1893–1894)
Sacroiliac joint	Accessory sacroiliac facets at level of the second posterior sacral foramina and adjacent to the posterior superior iliac spines	Weight bearing; vertebral loading in flexion; axial compression of vertebral column	Carrying infants or other loads on the back over the lumbar-sacral region. East African women	Trotter (1937, 1964, 1967)
Innominate	"Weaver's bottom." Bilateral osteitic craggy appearance of the ischial tuberosities	Chronic inflammatory condition of tissues and ischial bursitis	Long periods of sitting by weavers, coachmen, bargees, tailors (but not shoemakers)	Wells (1967)
	Bilateral osteitis, craggy appearance of the ischial tuberosities combined with lateral bowing of the fibulae	Ischial periostitis. Curvature of fibulae due to pressure from the feet resting under the legs in a crossed-legged sitting position; inversion at subtalar joint	Long periods of sitting. Identification of a tailor from eighteenth–early nineteenth-century cemetery in Norwich, England	Wells (1967)
Femur	Articular anterior-superior border of the femoral neck is prominently curved and forms a well-marked convexity	Hyperflexion of hip and knee with hyperdorsiflexion of ankle and subtalar joints	Squatting posture by Punjabis	Charles (1893–1894)
	Prolongation of the internal condylar articular surface superior to the origin of gastrocnemius, hence the superior surface of the internal condyle is articular	Hyperflexion of hip and knee with hyperdorsiflexion of ankle and subtalar joints	Squatting posture by Punjabis	Charles (1893–1894)

"Mountaineer's gait." Erosion of the reaction area of the femoral neck	Tightening of the ligaments of the hip joint during extension	Active walking and running in hilly terrain by ancient Greeks	Angel (1960, 1964)
"Poirier's facet." Facet produced by the extension of the articular surface of the head on the anterior surface of the neck	Flexion of the knee and extension of the hip joint	Sitting posture with knees flexed and buttocks on a low seat (6 inches above the ground). Yoruba of western Nigeria, prehistoric Greeks	Angel (1960, 1964) Kostick (1963) Odgers (1931) Poirier and Charpy (1911) Sauser (1936)
"Cervical eminence." Smooth mound or ridge extending from the femoral tubercle (superior cervical tubercle) along the anterior-superior aspect of the neck to the head	Flexion of the knee and extension of the hip joint	Squatting posture and prolonged standing or walking	Kostick (1963)
"Peritrochlear groove." Gutterlike groove formed by the medial trochlear margin which may become converted into a tunnel in periarticular osteoarthritis. It extends to a notch that demarcates the trochlea from the condylar surface	Flexion of the knee and extension of the hip joint	Squatting posture and prolonged standing or walking	Kostick (1963)
"Posterior cervical (acetabular) imprint." Facet on the posterior aspect of the neck that is limited laterally by tubercle bordering the medial margin of the groove for the obturator externus tendon	Flexion of the knee and extension of the hip joint	Squatting posture and prolonged standing or walking	Kostick (1963)
"Charles's facet." Facet behind and above medial epicondyle and extending to the adductor tubercle. It is a part of the gastrocnemius bursa	Flexion of the knee and extension of the hip joint	Squatting posture by Neander 1 and Spy 2 Neanderthal specimens	Charles (1893–1894) Klaatsch (1900) Kostick (1963)
"Tibial imprint." Impression on the posterior aspect of the distal end of the femoral diaphysis, marked above by the medial condyle	Flexion of the knee and extension of the hip joint	Squatting posture	Kostick (1963)

Continued

TABLE 1. Markers of Occupational Stress—Continued

Skeletal component	Anatomical structure	Stress factor	Occupational activity	Reference
Femur *continued*	"Osteochondritic imprint." A hole or plaquelike bony excrescence on the upper posterior portion of the lateral condyle	Flexion of the knee and extension of the hip joint	Squatting posture	Kostick (1963)
	"Martin's facet." Crescentic facet formed by extension of the trochlear surface onto the lateral aspect of the lateral condyle	Flexion of the knee and extension of the hip joint	Squatting posture by Australian aborigines	Kostick (1963) Martin (1932)
	"Supratrochlear facet and imprint." Facet produced by the extension of the superior margin of the lateral trochlear surface on to the neighboring diaphysis	Flexion of the knee and extension of the hip joint	Squatting posture	Kostick (1963)
	Facets or osteochondritic imprints on the posterior-superior femoral condyles	Hyperflexion of hip and knee with hyperdorsiflexion of ankle and subtalar joints	Squatting posture by Neanderthals and modern *Homo sapiens*	Trinkaus (1975)
	Groove on the femoral intercondylar line from the posterior cruciate ligament	Hyperflexion of hip and knee with hyperdorsiflexion of ankle and subtalar joints	Squatting posture by Neanderthals and modern *Homo sapiens*	Trinkaus (1975)
	Intercondylar line is crossed by a distinct groove for the posterior cruciate ligament. The line is more convex upward	Hyperflexion of hip and knees with hyperdorsiflexion of ankle and subtalar joints	Squatting posture	Martin (1932)
	"Anterior cervical imprint" or "fossa of Allen" or "imprint of Berteaux." Impression on the anterior and inferior aspects of the medial part of the neck, adjacent to the head	Hyperflexion of hip and knees with hyperdorsiflexion of ankle and subtalar joints	Rapid descent of a steep slope; rough-country gait by prehistoric Greeks	Angel (1959, 1960, 1964) Kostick (1963) Meyer (1924) Odgers (1931)
	Platymeria	Nutritional deficiency	Nutritional deficiency of "primitive peoples" causes deficiency of bone in relation to the area needed for muscular attachments	Buxton (1938)

		Tension of gluteus maximus pulling upon femoral surface of its insertion thereby drawing outward the proximal third of the diaphysis	Squatting posture by Maori of New Zealand	Turner (1887)
	Pilasterism	Upright posture	Activities connected with sea and fishing habits. Native Americans from coast of Georgia	Oetteking (1930)
Tibia	Rounding of the posterior margin of the lateral tibial condyle, especially of its medial portion. The posterior margin of the medial tibial condyle has a distinct angulated edge	Hyperflexion of the knee	Squatting posture	Charles (1893–1894) Huard and Montagne (1950, 1953) Klaatsch (1900) Thomson (1889) Virchow (1900)
	Retroversion of tibial head	Hyperflexion of the knee	Squatting posture by Punjabis	Aitken (1905) Cameron (1934) Charles (1893–1894) Huard and Montagne (1950, 1953) Klaatsch (1900) Morganthaler (1955)
		Hyperflexion of the knee	Active running in rough terrain. Early Horizon California populations	Angel (1966)
	"Quadricipital groove." Proximal end of tibia has a distinct groove produced by tendon of the ligamentum patellae; retroversion of the tibial head; lateral lipping of the quadricipital groove	Flexion of knee	Squatting posture by central Indian populations	Kate and Robert (1965)
	"Squatting facets." Flexion facets at the anterior surface of the distal end of the tibia at the ankle	Flexion of knee	Squatting posture by Punjabis	Charles (1893–1894)
	"Squatting facets." Flexion facets at the anterior surface of the distal end of the tibia at the ankle	Flexion of knee	Squatting posture. Various populations of India	Singh (1959)

Continued

TABLE 1. Markers of Occupational Stress—Continued

Skeletal component	Anatomical structure	Stress factor	Occupational activity	Reference
Tibia *continued*	"Lateral squatting facet." Facet continuous with the trochlear surface making a sharp angle with the line of curvature	Dorsiflexion of tibiotalar joint	Squatting posture by Punjabis. Rare in European adults but occurs in fetuses of both Indians and Europeons	Barnett (1954)
			Squatting posture. Neanderthals and modern *Homo sapiens*	Trinkaus (1975)
	Platycnemia	Stress from soleus and deep plantar-flexors of the feet	Active running in rough terrain by Early Horizon California populations	Angel (1966)
		Nutritonal deficiency	Nutritional deficiencies of "primitive people" causes deficiency of bone in relation to the area needed for muscular attachments	Buxton (1938)
		Flexion. Undue prominence of the origin of tibialis posticus	Squatting posture by British Neolithic populations	Cameron (1934)
		Flexion. Undue prominence of the origin of tibialis posticus	Climbing and hunting by "those races, the members of which dwell in rough countries"	Thomson (1889)
Fibula	Bilateral fracture of proximal one-third of diaphysis	Flexion of the knee and dorsiflexion of the ankle	Jumping from a squatting position during military gymnastics in Athens, Greece	Symeonides (1980)
Knee	"Miner's knee." Osteoarthritis with lesions of the menisci	Flexion	Stooping or squatting while hewing a low seam of coal. Knees kept flexed. European miners.	Bürkle-de la Camp (1937)
		Excessive external rotation or internal femur rotation when foot is dorsiflexed and knee is flexed	Movements executed in martial arts where Caucasians are more severely affected than Asians	Klein (1977)
	"Musher's knee." Iliotibial band irritation, usually of one leg, leading to osteoarthritic modifications of the joint	Rapid hyperextension	Sharp backward kicking of the leg executed by a team driver at the rear of a dogsled to spur team to greater speed over snowy and icy ground by Arctic natives and sportsmen	Dahl et al. (1981) Davis (1981)

Foot				
Talus	Prolongation of the external side of the trochlear articular surface that encroaches on the superior surface of the neck	Dorsiflexion of tibiotalar joint	Squatting posture by Punjabis	Charles (1893–1894)
		Dorsiflexion of tibiotalar joint	Squatting posture. Various populations of India	Das (1959) Singh (1959)
	"Medial squatting facet." Facet on superior lateral surface of the neck of the talus articulating with facet on the anterior surface of the distal end of the tibia	Dorsiflexion of tibiotalar joint	Squatting posture found "almost invariably in savage races." Due to climbing in apes	Thomson (1889, 1890)
	Facies externa accessoria corporis tali	Dorsiflexion, medial rotation, and eversion of the subtalar joint	Squatting posture by Japanese	Morimoto (1959)
Calcaneum	Unilateral or bilateral vertically oriented exostosis at the locus of insertion of the Achilles tendon and adductor hallucis; bony spur extends to the posterior-inferior tuberosity	Plantar enthesopathy involving stress on adductor hallucis muscle	Long-distance running among Neolithic Saharans of Niger; modern joggers running on hard surfaces; spontaneous lesion in aged and obese individuals (most comon among females)	Dutour (1986)
	"Rider's bone." Exostoses and fractures	Repeated forceful impact of the heel on the ground	Riding and dismounting in a horse where stress is placed on the heel by farmers and cowboys in the United States	Angel (1982)
	"Policeman's heel." Bursitis and formation of a calcaneal bony spur at any of several loci; early stages are "floor-walker's foot," "World's Fair heels," and "exposition heels"	Pull on the attachment of the plantar fascia	Walking on hard pavements	Lewin (1959)

Continued

TABLE 1. Markers of Occupational Stress—Continued

Skeletal component	Anatomical structure	Stress factor	Occupational activity	Reference
Foot *continued*				
Metatarsals and first proximal phalanx	"Executive foot." Metatarsals display facets and/or small bony extensions on the superior surface of the first proximal phalanx, which extends distally from the proximal articular surface, elevated 2 to 4 mm above the normal surface of the bone	Extension of the metatarsophalangeal joints	Kneeling, resting, or work posture with body weight producing considerable joint reaction force at metatarsophalangeal joints by populations of late Integration period in south coast of Equador	Ubelaker (1978, 1979)
	Metatarsophalangeal osteochondritis	Extension of the metatarsophalangeal joints	"Executives" sitting at desks with their heels off the floor and weight on their toes	Lewin (1959)
Hallux	"Golfer's big toe." Exostoses and a rim of bone encircling the head of the first metatarsal. Extreme arthritis	Plantar flexion of the tibiotalar joint and eversion of the subtalar joint while weight is on the great toe	Pivoting movement of the golfer when using a club	Lewin (1941)
Dentition	Grooves on occlusal surfaces of anterior teeth	Wear	Use of the dentition as a tool in preparation of materials for production as utilitarian objects. Use of plant materials for this purpose by Indians of the Great Basin	Larsen (1985)
	Anterior tooth loss	Wear/trauma	Use of the teeth for power grasping in holding sled reins or fish lines. Trauma from wrestling and fighting by Sadlermiut men	Merbs (1983)
			Softening skins with the teeth. Sadlermiut women	Merbs (1983)
	Grooves on occlusal and approximal surfaces of anterior teeth	Wear	Cordage manufacture by prehistoric California Indians at Stone Lake site	Schulz (1977)

Fracture of occlusal edges of anterior teeth	Trauma	Opening bobby-pins with the teeth	Ronchese (1948)
Serrated occlusal surfaces of anterior teeth	Wear	Holding and cutting thread. Seamstress and tailor	Ronchese (1948)
Deep denting of occlusal surfaces of central incisors	Wear	Holding tacks and nails in the mouth by upholsterers	Ronchese (1948)
Ellipsoid aperture formed by occlusing upper and lower central incisors	Wear	Pipe smokers holding a pipe in the mouth	Dechaume (1938)
Greater abrasion of lower incisors than of upper incisors in the same dentition	Wear	Stripping bark from tree branches warmed in a fire and retaining ash and gritty substances by natives of Northern Territory of Australia	Barrett (1977)
Attrition of canine and premolar teeth	Wear	Sharpening a spear or digging stick and pressure flaking a stone tool by natives of Northern Territory of Australia	Barrett (1977)
Chipped dental enamel from lingual marginal ridges of lower teeth and buccal marginal ridges of upper teeth	Trauma	Holding a spear shaft between the teeth for straightening by natives of Northern Territory of Australia	Barrett (1977)
Attrition of premolar and molar teeth, often most severe on one side of the mouth, with rounding of buccal margins in the region where a masticatory quid is "parked" when not being chewed	Wear	Chewing tobacco	Barrett (1977)
Heavier wear on incisors and canines than on posterior dentition	Wear	Shanidar I Neanderthal who held objects in his teeth to compensate for loss of his right hand; La Ferrassie I Neanderthal teeth are similarly worn, and he had a damaged right arm	Coon (1966)

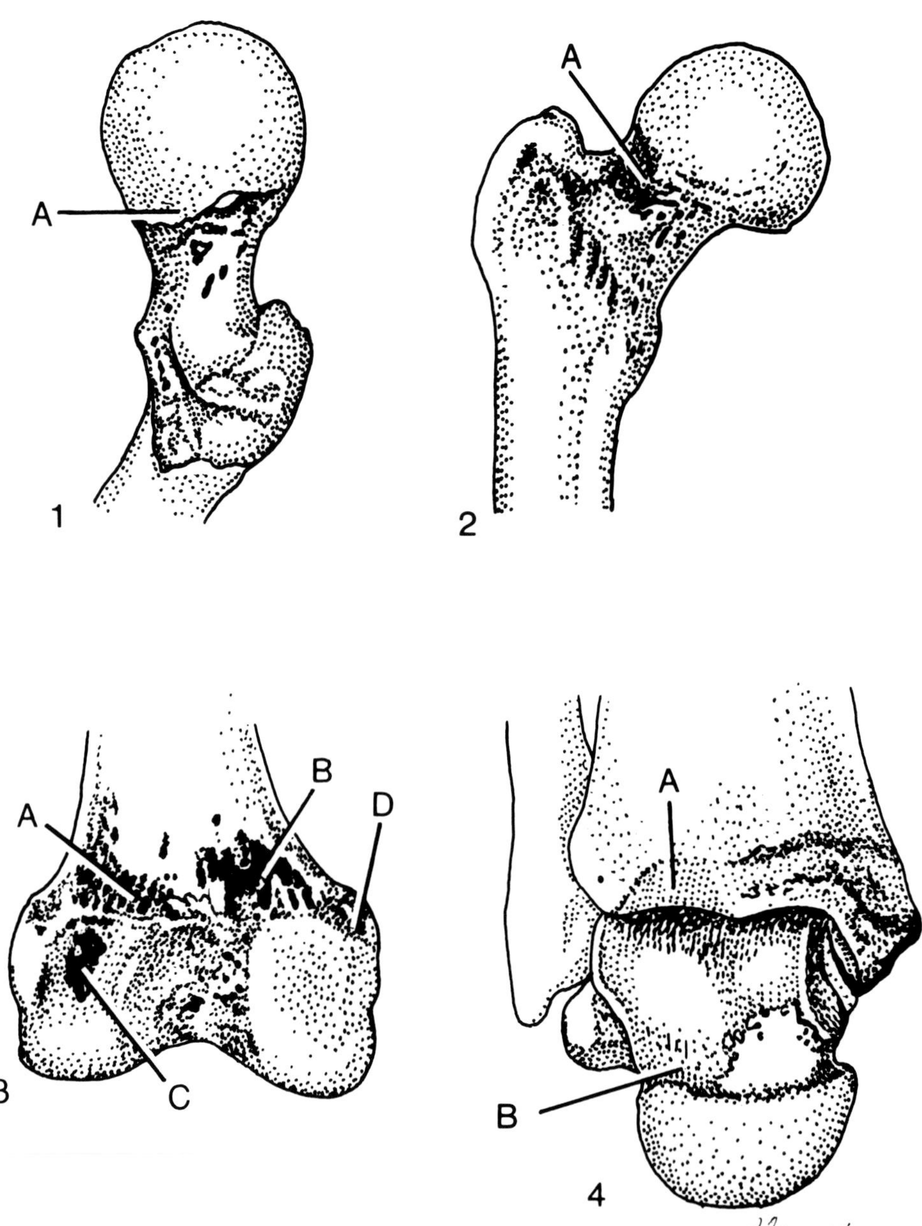

Fig. 1. **1:** A, Convexity of the anterior-superior border of the femoral neck. **2:** A, Poirier's facet. **3:** A, Lateral tibial imprint; B, medial tibial imprint; C, osteochondritic imprint; D, Charles's facet. **4:** A, Flexion facet on tibia; B, flexion facet on talus (not drawn to scale).

stress, but conclusions reached from the study of such series are still outside the arena of laboratory experimentation. In short, anthropological understanding of the causes of markers and their correct identification await further investigation by skeletal biologists familiar with the sources summarized in this survey.

DISCUSSION AND CONCLUSIONS

Markers of occupational stress are one expression of bone plasticity under pressure of

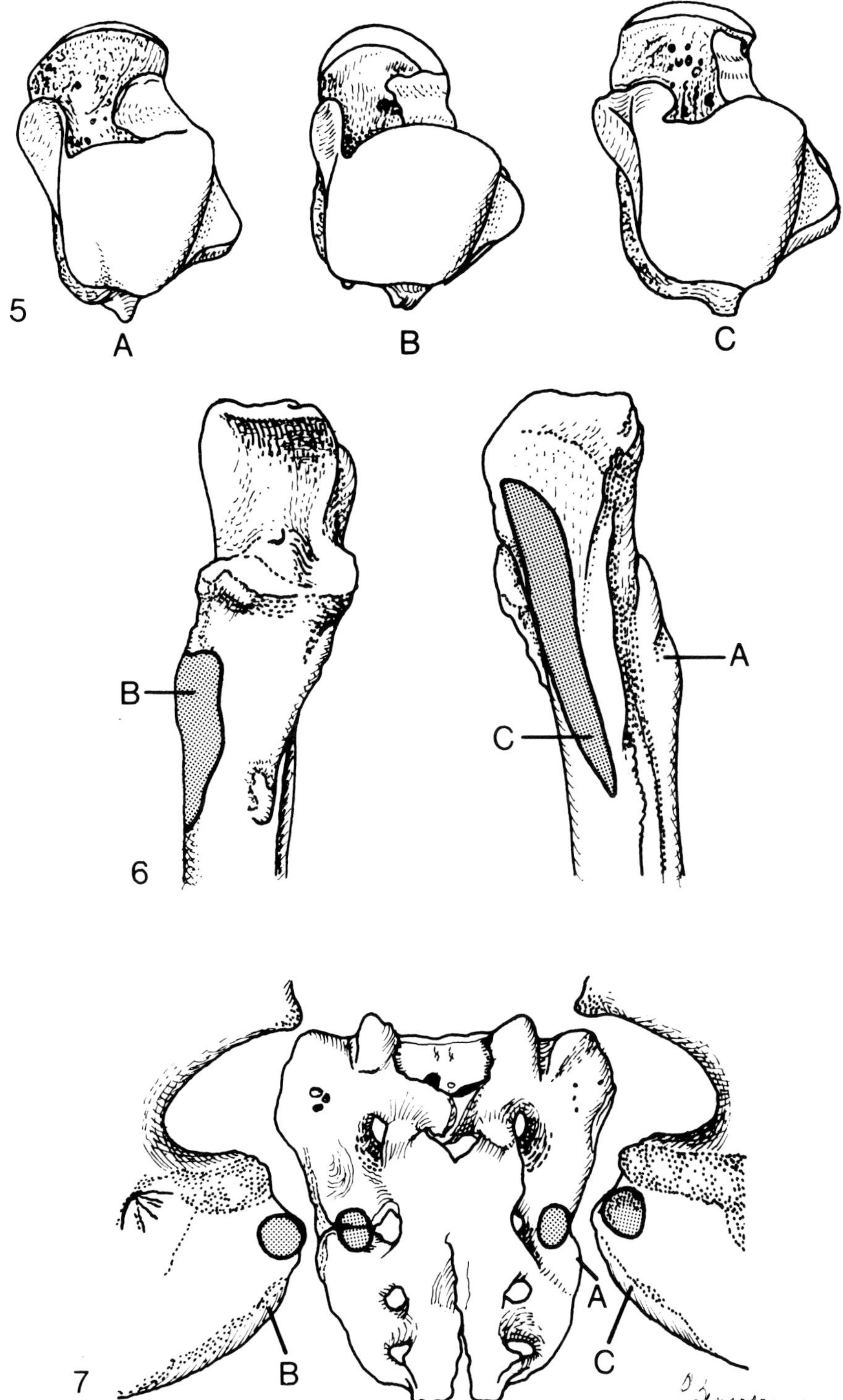

Fig. 2. **5:** A, Lateral flexion facet on talus; B, lateral flexion facet on talus with lateral extension on the trochlear surface; C, lateral flexion facet on talus with medial and lateral extensions on the trochlear surface. **6:** A, Supinator crest on the ulna; B, attachment of supinator muscle; C, attachment of anconeus muscle. **7:** A, Accessory sacroiliac facets on the sacrum; B and C, accessory sacroiliac facets on left and right innominates (not drawn to scale).

extracorporeal and internal forces that are *not* attributable to disorders of disease, metabolism, biochemistry, hormonal and enzymatic imbalances, or neuronal and vascular disorders. Irregularities of skeletal morphology have been observed by medical and anthropological researchers for over a century, but in human beings these markers are not tested experimentally. Occupational activities must be inferred from clinical records, ethnographic accounts, and archaeological and historical sources.

Interpretations vary a great deal as to a specific activity involved in the formation of a given bony or dental irregularity. Pilasterism has been attributed to walking and running across hilly terrain as well as to nutritional deficiency by different investigators, while others have explained the feature entirely on the basis of the assumption of squatting postures.

There has been a tendency to isolate a single occupational activity as the cause of a given enthesopathic lesion, as is seen in the literature about spear throwing, slinging, baseball pitching, and related behaviors. At the other end of the speculative spectrum are statements that an entire suite of morphological traits may be the consequence of a single pattern of behavior, i.e., squatting posture or running over rough terrain.

There has not been any systematic organization of data about markers of occupational stress, and much of the present lore is anecdotal and seldom finds its way into published reports. This is the challenge implicit in this survey of the subject, all of which returns us to Alice, who not only had to endure the eccentric behavior of the Mad Hatter at the tea party (whose occupation of felting cloth for hat making affected his brain through mercury poisoning), but who also learned from the Mock Turtle that the stresses of an education in French, music, and washing could modify a real turtle into the sentimental creature that led her in the lobster quadrille.

ACKNOWLEDGMENTS

I owe to the late Dr. J. Lawrence Angel my awakening of interest in markers of occupational stress when, late on a bleak November afternoon in 1977, we examined together the skeleton of an unknown individual in his office at the Smithsonian Institution. The robust muscular attachments on the clavicles led Larry to consider the possibility that these were the remains of a man who had played a trumpet or trombone, an observation that later contributed to the correct identification of this individual as a deceased musician. In pursuing this interest in my own practice and teaching of forensic anthropology, I have benefited from the generosity of Miss Margaret C. Caldwell, M.A., who provided me with a list of some published sources on the subject of markers of occupational stress. To Dr. Deedra McClearn of the Section of Ecology and Systematics, Cornell University, I am indebted for valuable suggestions relevant to the table that appears in this chapter. Miss Laura Linke of Ithaca, New York, has been an extremely able and venturesome archivist in our search for relevant literature.

REFERENCES

Agricola G (1556) De Re Metallica. Basel: J. Froben and N. Bishoff.

Aitken DM (1905) A note on the variation of the tibia and astragalus. J Anat Physiol 39:489–491.

Amako T (1960) On the injuries of the menisci in the knee joint of Japanese. J Jpn Orthop Surg Soc 33(12):1289–1322.

Angel JL (1946) Skeletal change in ancient Greece. Am J Phys Anthropol 4(1):69–97.

Angel JL (1959) Femoral neck markings and human gait. Anat Rec 133(2):244.

Angel JL (1960) Human gait, hip joint and evolution. Am J Phys Anthropol 18(4):361.

Angel JL (1964) The reaction area of the femoral neck. Clin Orthop 32:130–142.

Angel JL (1966) Early skeletons from Tranquillity, California. Smithsonian Contrib Anthropol 2(1).

Angel JL (1971) The People of Lerna. Washington, DC: Smithsonian Institution Press. (Published simultaneously by the American School of Classical Studies at Athens.)

Angel JL (1979) Osteoarthritis in prehistoric Turkey and medieval Byzantium. In E Cockburn, H Duncan, and JM Riddle (eds): Arthritis: Modern Concepts and Ancient Medicine. Proc Henry Ford Hosp Med J 27(1):38–43.

Angel JL (1982) Osteoarthritis and occupation (ancient and modern). In VV Novotny (ed): IInd Anthropological Congress of Aleš Hrdlička. Pragensis: Universitas Carolina, pp 443–446.

Angel JL, and Caldwell PC (1984) Death by strangulation: A forensic anthropological case from Wilmington, Delaware. In TA Rathbun and JE Buikstra (eds): Human Identification: Case Studies in Forensic Anthropology. Springfield, IL: Charles C Thomas, pp 168–175.

Angel JL, Kelley JO, and Schneider G (1985a) Bony effects of vanity on spinal pain: 18th century stays versus later corsets. Paper presented at the Physical Anthropology Section of the 37th Annual Meeting of the American Anthropological Association, Washington, DC.

Angel JL, Kelley JO, Parrington M, and Pinter S (1985b) Stresses of first freedom: 19th century Philadelphia. Abstracts of papers presented at the 54th Annual Meeting of the American Association of Physical Anthropologists, Knoxville, TN.

Angel JL, Kelly JO, Parrington M, and Pinter S (1987) Life stresses of the free black community as represented by the First African Baptist Church, Philadelphia, 1823–1841. Am J Phys Anthropol 74:213–229.

Avis V (1959) The relation of the temporal muscle to the form of the coronoid process. Am J Phys Anthropol 17(2):99–104.

Barnett CH (1954) Squatting facets on the European talus. J Anat 88:509–513.

Barrett MJ (1977) Masticatory and non-masticatory uses of teeth. In RVS Wright (ed): Stone Tools as Markers. Canberra: Australian Institute of Aboriginal Studies, pp 18–23.

Bass WM (1969) Recent developments in the identification of human skeletal material. Am J Phys Anthropol 30(3): 459–461.

Bass WM (1979) Developments in the identification of human skeletal material (1968–1978). Am J Phys Anthropol 51(4):555–562.

Bass WM (1987) Human Osteology: A Laboratory and Field Manual, 3rd Ed. Columbia: Missouri Archaeological Society.

Berry AC, and Berry RJ (1967) Epigenetic variation in the human cranium. J Anat 101(2):361–379.

Boule M (1911–1913) L'Homme fossile de la Chapelle-aux-Saints. Ann Paleontol 6:111–172; 7:21–56, 85–192; 8:1–70.

Bridges PS (1985) Structural changes of the arms associated with habitual grinding of corn. Abstract of paper presented at the Bioarchaeology Symposium, 54th Annual Meeting of the American Association of Physical Anthropologists, Knoxville, TN.

Bridges PS (1987) Osteological correlates of weapon use. Paper presented at the 86th Annual Meeting of the American Anthropological Association, Chicago.

Bridges PS (1989) Osteoarthritis, diaphyseal dimensions and strength of the femur in the prehistoric Southeastern United States. Abstract of paper presented at the 58th Annual Meeting of the American Association of Physical Anthropologists, San Diego.

Broca P (1868) Sur les cranes et ossements des Eyzies. Bull Soc Anthropol Paris, Serie 2 3:350–392, 432–446.

Bugyi B, and Kausz J (1970) Radiographic determination of the skeletal age of the young swimmers. J Sports Med Phys Fitness 10:269–270.

Bürkle-de la Camp H (1937) Uber Meniscusschaden. Arch Orthop Unfallchir 37:354–368.

Busk G (1871) On the discovery of platycnemic men in Denbighshire. J Ethnol Soc Lond 2(4):450–468.

Buxton LHD (1938) Platymeria and platycnemia. J Anat 73:31–36.

Cameron J (1934) The Skeleton of British Neolithic Man. London: Williams and Norgate.

Chalmers J, and Ho KC (1970) Geographical variations in senile osteoporosis: The association with physical activity. J Bone Joint Surg [Br] 52:667–675.

Charles RH (1893–1894) The influence of function, as exemplified in the morphology of the lower extremity of the Panjabi. J Anat Physiol 28:1–18.

Clark M, Shapiro D, Coppolo V, Friendly DI, and Sandza R (1981) The sports surgeons. Newsweek, 28 September: 70–71.

Claussen BF (1982) Chronic hypertrophy of the ulna in the professional rodeo-cowboy. Clin Orthop 164:45–47.

Cohen MN, and Armelagos GJ (eds) (1984) Paleopathology at the Origins of Agriculture. New York: Academic Press.

Coon CS (1966) The Origin of Races. New York: Alfred A. Knopf.

Currey J (1984) The Mechanical Adaptations of Bones. Princeton: Princeton University Press.

Dahl W, Matthews K, Midthun J, and Sapin P (1981) "Musher's knee" and "hooker's elbow" in the Arctic. N Engl J Med 304(12):737.

Das AC (1959) Squatting facets on the talus in U.P. (Uttar Pradesh) subjects. J Anat Soc India 8(2):90–92.

Davis M (1981) Odd ailments: A random sampling of strange disorders, as reported in American and British medical journals. Discover 2:48–50.

Dawkins WB, and Busk G (1870) On the discovery of platycnemic men in Denbighshire. Br Assoc Rep 40:148.

Dechaume M (1938) Lesions buccales, dentaires et maxillaires dans les maladies professionnelles. Arch Mal Prof Hyg Toxicol Ind 1:200–220.

Dutour O (1986) Enthesopathies (lesions of muscular insertions) as indicators of the activities of Neolithic Saharan populations. Am J Phys Anthropol 71(2):221–224.

Dutra FR (1944) Identification of person and determination of cause of death from skeletal remains. Arch Pathol 38: 339–349.

Eckert WG (1974) The Bibliography of References on Forensic Anthropology. Wichita: Inform (International Reference Organization in Forensic Medicine and Sciences).

Edynak GJ (1976) Life-styles from skeletal material: A medieval Yugoslav example. In E Giles and JS Friedlaender (eds): The Measures of Man: Methodologies in Biological Anthropology. Cambridge, MA: Peabody Museum Press, pp 408–432.

Enlow DH (1976) The remodeling of bone. Yrbk Phys Anthropol 20:19–34.

Epker BN, and Frost HM (1965) Correlation of bone resorption and formation with the physical behavior of loaded bone. J Dent Res 44:33–41.

Evans FG (1957) Stress and Strain in Bones; Their Relation to Fractures and Osteogenesis. Springfield, IL: Charles C Thomas.

Evans FG (ed) (1966) Studies on the Anatomy and Function of Bone and Joints. New York: Springer-Verlag.

Farquharson-Roberts MA, and Fulford PC (1980) Stress fracture of the radius. J Bone Joint Surg [Br] 62(2):194–195.

Fedeli M, and Masali M (1978) Osteopathology caused by work activity in early Egyptians. Paper presented at the 2nd European Meeting of the Palaeopathology Association, 1978, Turin, Italy.

Finnegan M (1978) Non-metric variation of the infracranial skeleton. J Anat 125(1):23–37.

Finnegan M (1983) Supplement to "Bibliography of human and nonhuman non-metric variation." Unpublished manuscript, Osteology Laboratory, Kansas State University.

Finnegan M, and Faust MA (1974) Bibliography of human and nonhuman non-metric variation. Research Reports of the Department of Anthropology 14, University of Massachusetts.

Fraipont J (1888) Le tibia dans la race de Neanderthal; etude comparative de l'incurvation de la tete du tibia, dans ses rapports avec la station verticale chez l'homme et les anthropoides. Rev Anthropol, Serie 3 3:145–158.

Fraipont J, and Lohest M (1887) La race humaine de Neanderthal ou de Canstadt en Belgique: Recherches ethnographiques sur des ossements humains, decouvertes dans les depots quaternaires d'une grotte a Spy et determination de leur age geologique. Arch Biol 7:587–757.

France DL (1985) Occupational effects on the determination of sex in the humerus. Abstract of paper presented at the Physical Anthropology Section, 37th Annual Meeting, American Academy of Forensic Sciences, Las Vegas.

Frayer DW (1988) Auditory exostoses and evidence for fishing at Vlasac. Curr Anthropol 29(2):346–349.

Frost HM (1966) Morphometry of bone in palaeopathology. In S Jarcho (ed): Human Palaeopathology. New Haven: Yale University Press, pp 131–150.

Gentry J (1972) La maladie des insertions des tendons. Cah Med Lyon 48:4685–4690.

Goodman AH, Martin DL, Armelagos GJ, and Clark G (1984) Indications of stress from bone and teeth. In MN Cohen and GJ Armelagos (eds): Palaeopathology at the Origins of Agriculture. New York: Academic Press, pp 13–49.

Grimm H (1959) Vorgeschichtliches, fruhgeschichtliches und mittelalterliches Fundmaterial zur Pathologie der Wirbelsaule. Nova Acta Leopold 21:5–44.

Horowitz SL, and Shapiro HL (1955) Modification of the skull and jaw architecture following removal of the masseter muscle in the rat. Am J Phys Anthropol 13(2):301–308.

Hoyte DAN, and Enlow DH (1966) Wolff's law and the problem of muscle attachment on resorptive surfaces of bone. Am J Phys Anthropol 24(2):205–214.

Huard P, and Montagne M (1950) Le squelette humain et l'attitude accroupie. Bull Soc Etudes Indochin 25:401–426.

Huard P, and Montagne M (1953) Le squelette humain et la station en flexion. Presse Med 61:1305–1307.

Hughes DR (1968) Skeletal plasticity and its relevance in the study of earlier populations. In DR Brothwell (ed): Skeletal Biology of Earlier Human Populations. London: Pergamon Press, pp 31–55.

Hunter D (1962) The Diseases of Occupation, 3rd Ed. London: English Universities Press.

Hunter D (1969) The Diseases of Occupation, 4th Ed. Boston: Little, Brown.

İşcan MY, and Miller-Shaivitz P (1984) Discriminant function sexing of the tibia. J Forensic Sci 29(4):1087–1093.

Jahn U (1886) Platyknemische Tibien aus dem megalithischen Grabe von Stolzenburg. Z Ethnol 18:607.

Jarcho S (1966) The development of the present condition of human palaeopathology in the United States. In S Jarcho (ed): Human Palaeopathology. New Haven: Yale University Press, pp 3–42.

Johnson LC (1966) The principles of structural analysis. In S Jarcho (ed): Human Palaeopathology. New Haven: Yale University Press, pp 68–81.

Jones J (1876) Explorations of the aboriginal remains of Tennessee. Smithsonian Contrib Knowl 22:259:1–158.

Kate BR, and Robert SL (1965) Some observations on the upper end of the tibia in squatters. J Anat 99:137–141.

Kelley JO, and Angel JL (1983) The workers of Cotoctin furnace. Md Archaeol 19(1):2–17.

Kelley JO, and Angel JL (1987) Life stresses of slavery. Am J Phys Anthropol 74:199–211.

Kelley MA (1982) Intervertebral osteochondrosis in ancient and modern populations. Am J Phys Anthropol 59(3):271–279.

Kennedy KAR (1983) Morphological variations in ulnar supinator crests and fossae, as identifying markers of occupational stress. J Forensic Sci 28(4):871–876.

Kennedy KAR (1985) Importance of markers of occupational stress on bones and teeth in personal identification case studies. Abstract of paper presented at the Physical Anthropology Section, 37th Annual Meeting of the American Academy of Forensic Sciences, Las Vegas.

Kennedy KAR, Plummer J, and Chiment J (1986) Identification of the eminent dead: Penpi, a scribe of ancient Egypt. In K Reichs (ed): Forensic Osteology: The Recovery and Analysis of Unknown Skeletal Remains. Springfield, IL: Charles C Thomas, pp 290–307.

Kernan M (1977) Breathing life into dry bones. Smithsonian 7(11):116–123.

King JW (1969) Analysis of the pitching arm of the professional baseball player. Clin Orthop 67:116–123.

Klaatsch H (1900) Die wichtigsten Variationen am Skelet der freien unteren Extremitat des Menschen und ihre Bedeutung fur das Abstammungsproblem. Ergeb Anat Entwickl 10:599–719.

Klein KK (1977) Why Caucasian martial artists have greater knee problems. Black Belt 15:46–48.

Kostick EL (1963) Facets and imprints on the upper and lower extremities of femora from a western Nigerian population. J Anat 97:393–402.

Krogman WM (1935) Life histories recorded in skeletons. Am Anthropol 37:92–103.

Krogman WM, and İşcan MY (1986) The Human Skeleton in Forensic Medicine, 2nd Ed. Springfield, IL: Charles C Thomas.

Kuhff GA (1881) De la platycnemie dans les races humaines. Rev Anthropol, Serie 2 4:256–259.

Lane WA (1885) Changes produced by pressure in the bony skeleton of the trunk and shoulder girdle. Guy's Hosp Rep 43:321–434.

Lane WA (1887a) A remarkable example of the manner in which pressure-changes in the skeleton may reveal the labour-history of the individual. J Anat Physiol 21(3):385–406.

Lane WA (1887b) The causation of several variations and congenital abnormalities in the human skeleton. J Anat Physiol 21(4):586–610.

Lane WA (1888) The anatomy and physiology of the shoemaker. J Anat Physiol 22(4):593–628.

Larsen CS (1985) Dental modifications and tool-use in the western Great Basin. Am J Phys Anthropol 67(4):393–402.

Larsen CS (1987) Bioarchaeological interpretations of subsistence economy and behavior from human skeletal remains. Adv Archaeol Method Theor 10:339–445.

Leigh RW (1925) Dental pathology of Indian tribes of varied environmental and food conditions. Am J Phys Anthropol 8(2):179–199.

Levy LF (1968) Porter's neck. Br Med J 2:16–19.

Lewin P (1941) The Foot and Ankle: Their Injuries, Diseases, Deformities and Disabilities. Philadelphia: Lea and Febiger.

Lewin P (1959) The Foot and Ankle: Their Injuries, Diseases, Deformities and Disabilities, 4th Ed. Philadelphia: Lea and Febiger.

Manouvrier LP (1888) Memoire sur la platycnemie chez l'homme et chez les anthropoides. Mem Soc Anthropol Paris, Serie 2 3:469–548.

Martin CP (1932) Some variations in the lower end of the femur which are especially prevalent in the bones of primitive people. J Anat 66:371–383.

Mashkara KI (1971) Age characteristics of lower limb skeletal changes in persons engaged in physical labor. Arkh Anat Gistol Embriol 61:88–94 [in Russian with English abstract].

McCown TD, and Keith A (1939) The Stone of Mount Carmel II: The Fossil Human Remains from the Levalloiso-Mousterian. Oxford: Clarendon Press.

McLean FC, and Urist MR (1955) Bone: An Introduction to the Physiology of Skeletal Tissue. Chicago: University of Chicago Press.

Mebane WN (1981) Dog-walker's elbow. N Engl J Med 304(10):613–614.

Meiklejohn A (1957) The Life, Work and Times of Charles Turner Thackrah, Surgeon and Apothecary of Leeds (1795–1833). Edinburgh and London: E. and S. Livingston.

Merbs CF (1983) Patterns of activity-induced pathology in a Canadian Inuit population. National Museum of Man Mercury Series, Archaeological Survey of Canada No. 119.

Meyer AW (1924) The "cervical fossa" of Allen. Am J Phys Anthropol 7(2):257–269.

Molnar S (1972) Tooth wear and culture: A survey of tooth functions among some prehistoric populations. Curr Anthropol 13:511–526.

Morganthaler PW (1955) Quelques remarques au sujet de l'inclinaison et de la retroversion du tibia. Bull Schweiz Ges Anthropol Ethnol 31:45–59.

Morimoto I (1959) The influence of squatting posture on the talus of the Japanese. Med J Shinshu Univ 4(3):417–432.

Murray PDF (1985) Bones: A Study of the Development and Structure of the Vertebrate Skeleton. With an introduction by BK Hall. Cambridge: Cambridge University Press.

Nagle M (1984) Breakdancing fans find new ways to break bodies. USA Today, 9 July 1984, D-1.

Odgers PNB (1931) Two details about the neck of the femur. 1. The eminentia; 2. The empreinte. J Anat 65:352–362.

Oetteking B (1930) Pilasterism and platycnemism. Indian Notes 7:164–174.

Olin MS, Young HA, Seligson D, and Schmidek HH (1982) An unusual cervical injury occurring during cow milking. Spine 7(5):514–515.

Ortner DJ (1968) Description and classification of degenerative bone changes in the distal joint surfaces of the humerus. Am J Phys Anthropol 28(2):139–156.

Ortner DJ, and Putschar WGJ (1981) Identification of pathological conditions in human skeletal remains. Smithsonian Contrib Anthropol 28.

Paracelsus (1567) Von der Bergsucht oder Bergkrancheiten drey Bucher, inn dryzehn Tractat verfast und beschriben worden. . . . Dilingen: Sebaldum Meyer.

Plummer J (1984) Supinatur crest development in Alaskan Eskimos. Honors thesis in Ecology, Systematics and Evolution, Cornell University.

Poirier P, and Charpy A (1911) Traite d'Anatomie, 2d Ed. Paris: Masson et Cie Editeurs.

Pruner-Bey F (1868) Discussion sur les ossements humains des Eyzies. Bull Soc Anthropol Paris, Serie 2 3:416–432.

Radin EL, Paul IL, and Rose RM (1972) Role of mechanical factors in pathogenesis of primary osteoarthritis. Lancet 1(7749):519–522.

Ramazzini B (1700) De Morbis Artificum Diatriba. Modena: A. Capponi.

Ramazzini B (1705) A Treatise on the Diseases of Tradesmen. London: Andrew Bell, Ralph Smith, Daniel Midwinter, and others.

Regnault F (1898) Forme des surfaces articulaires du membre inferieur. Bull Soc Anthropol Paris, Serie 4 9:535–544.

Roberts VL, Noyes FR, Hubbard RP, and McCabe J (1971) Biomechanics of snowmobile injuries. J Biomech 4:569–577.

Ronchese F (1945) Calluses, cicatrices and other stigmas as an aid to personal identification. JAMA 128(13):925–932.

Ronchese F (1948) Occupational Marks and Other Physical Signs: A Guide to Personal Identification. New York: Grune and Stratton.

Rose JC (ed) (1985) Gone to a better land: A biohistory of a rural black cemetery in the post-reconstruction South. Arkansas Archaeological Survey Research Series No. 25.

Rowes B (1986) Body: To deal with their special needs, painters and performers can turn to a new speciality: Arts medicine. People Weekly 26(21):101–103.

Saunders SR (1978) The development and distribution of discontinuous morphological variation of the human infracranial skeleton. National Museum of Man Mercury Series, Archaeological Survey of Canada No. 81.

Sauser G (1936) Eminentia colli femoris dorsalis (Ein neuer osteologischer Befund am menschlichen Schenkhals). Z Rassenk 3:286–291.

Schaaffhausen HJ (1882) Neue vorgeschichtliche Denkmale und Funde im Rheinthal: Platyknemie. Dtsch Ges Anthropol Korresp-Blatt 10:167–171.

Scher AT (1978) Injuries to the cervical spine sustained while carrying loads on the head. Paraplegia 16:94–101.

Schulz PD (1977) Task activity and anterior tooth grooving in prehistoric California Indians. Am J Phys Anthropol 46(1):87–92.

Scott JH (1957) Muscle growth and function in relation to skeletal morphology. Am J Phys Anthropol 15(2):197–234.

Singh I (1959) Squatting facets on the talus and tibia in Indians. J Anat 93:540–550.

Smith S (1939) Studies in identification. No. 3: The importance of physical deformities. Police J Lond 12(3):274–285.

Snow CC (1982) Forensic anthropology. Annu Rev Anthropol 11:97–131.

Stewart TD (1956) Examination of the possibility that certain skeletal characters predispose to defects in the neural arches. Clin Orthop 8:44–60.

Stewart TD (1979) Essentials of Forensic Anthropology. Springfield, IL: Charles C Thomas.

Stirland A (1985a) Possible correlation between acromiale and occupation in the burials from the *Mary Rose.* Paper presented at the 5th European Meeting of the Palaeopathology Association, Siena, Italy.

Stirland A (1985b) The *Mary Rose* burials: Pathology, with special reference to some lesions possibly related to occupational activity. Paper presented at the 12th Annual Meeting of the Palaeopathology Association, Knoxville, TN.

Studer T (1886) Bericht uber menschlicher Skeletknochen bei Sutz am Bieler See. Z Ethnol 18:714–717.

Symeonides PP (1980) High stress fractures of the fibula. J Bone Joint Surg [Br] 62(2):192–193.

Tainter JA (1980) Behavior and status in a Middle Woodland mortuary population from the Illinois valley. Am Antiq 45(2):308–313.

Taylor JV (1968) The Neanderthal tibia. Ph.D. thesis, Columbia University.

Thackrah CT (1831) The Effects of the Principal Arts, Trades, and Professions, and of Civic States and Habits of Living, on Health and Longevity; with a Particular Reference to the Trades and Manufactures of Leeds; and Suggestions for the Removal of Many of the Agents, Which Produce Disease, and Shorten the Duration of Life. London: Longman, Rees, Orme, Brown, and Green. (2nd Ed. greatly enlarged with slight change of title, 1832.)

Thieme FP (1950) Lumbar breakdown caused by erect posture in man with an emphasis on spondylolisthesis and herniated intervertebral discs. Anthropological Papers of the Museum of Anthropology, University of Michigan No. 4.

Thomson A (1889) The influence of posture on the form of the articular surfaces of the tibia and astragalus in the different races of man and in the higher apes. J Anat Physiol 23:616–639.

Thomson A (1890) Additional note on the influence of posture on the form of the articular surfaces of the tibia and astragalus in the different races of man and the higher apes. J Anat Physiol 24:210–217.

Topinard P (1885) Elements d'Anthropologie Generale. Paris: A. Delahaye et E. Lecrosnier.

Townsley W (1948) The influence of mechanical factors on the development and structure of bone. Am J Phys Anthropol 6(1):25–45.

Trinkaus E (1975) Squatting among the Neanderthals: A problem in the behavioral interpretation of skeletal morphology. J Archaeol Sci 2:327–351.

Trotter M (1937) Accessory sacro-iliac articulations. Am J Phys Anthropol 22(2):247–255.

Trotter M (1964) Accessory sacroiliac articulations in East African skeletons. Am J Phys Anthropol 22(2):137–142.

Trotter M (1967) Variation of the sacroiliac union. Med Biol Illus 17:50–53.

Turner W (1887) On variability in human structure, as displayed in different races of men, with special reference to the skeleton. J Anat Physiol 21(3):473–495.

Ubelaker DH (1978) Human Skeletal Remains: Excavation, Analysis, Interpretation. Chicago: Aldine.

Ubelaker DH (1979) Skeletal evidence for kneeling in prehistoric Ecuador. Am J Phys Anthropol 51(4):679–686.

Virchow R (1880a) Bericht uber internationalen prahistorischen Congress in Lissabon. Z Ethnol 12:333–355.

Virchow R (1880b) Schadel-und Tibiaformen von Sudsee-Insulanern. Z Ethnol 12:112–120.

Virchow R (1886) Bericht uber Prahistorische-anthropologische verhaltnisse in Pommern. Z Ethnol 18:598–639.

Virchow R (1900) Das Knie japanischer Hocker. Verh Berl Ges Anthropol Ethnol Urgesch 32:385–396.

Washburn SL (1947) The relation of the temporal muscle to the form of the skull. Anat Rec 99:239.

Wells C (1967) Weaver, tailor or shoemaker? An osteological detective story. Med Biol Illus 17:39–47.

Wolff J (1892) Das Gesetz der Transformation der Knochen. Berlin: A. Hirschwald.

Wyman J (1871) Flattening of the tibia. Fourth Annual Report of the Trustees of the Peabody Museum of American Archaeology and Ethnology 1871:21.

Zarek JM (1966) Dynamic considerations in load bearing bones with special reference to osteosynthesis and articular cartilage. In FG Evans (ed): Studies on the Anatomy and Function of Bones and Joints. New York: Springer-Verlag, pp 40–51.

Reconstruction of Life From the Skeleton
© 1989 Alan R. Liss, Inc., pages 161–189

Chapter 9

Trauma

Charles F. Merbs
Department of Anthropology, Arizona State University, Tempe, Arizona 85287

INTRODUCTION

Damage to the skeleton from trauma has a venerable antiquity, going back to the origin of bone itself. Trauma occurs as a result of violent encounters with environmental hazards, inter- and intraspecies conflicts, and, in rare instances, self-mutilation and suicide. Humans are able to use their superior hands and brains to create their own trauma-producing instruments, ranging from crude crushing and cutting weapons to the sophisticated ultradestructive weaponry of modern warfare. Conversely, humans utilize trauma, primarily in the form of surgery, as a medical procedure.

Steinbock (1976) divided the subject of trauma into five major categories: 1) fractures, 2) crushing injuries, 3) bone wounds caused by sharp instruments (including arrow and spear wounds, scalping, trephination, sincipital T scarring, and amputation), 4) dislocations, and 5) transverse (growth-arrest) lines. Ortner and Putschar (1981) made use of eight categories under the heading of trauma: 1) fracture, 2) dislocation, 3) deformation, 4) scalping, 5) mutilation, 6) trephination, 7) traumatic problems arising from pregnancy, and 8) sincipital T mutilation. With the qualifier "acute" included in his chapter heading, Knowles (1983) included seven subjects under trauma: 1) fractures, 2) dislocations (acetabular flange lesions and arthrosis), 3) exostoses, 4) Schmorl's nodes, 5) osteochondritis dissecans, 6) surgery (trephination and amputation), and 7) evidence of wounds and weapons. It is clear from these examples that there is much more agreement than disagreement as to what should be included under the heading "trauma." This author will follow the pattern set by his predecessors, using all of their categories with the exception of growth-arrest lines, a topic that can be handled more effectively in the context of growth and development. Conversely, fatigue (stress) fractures, although not the result of acute trauma, fit more comfortably into this section than a category dealing specifically with the effects of stress and microtraumata on the skeleton. Pathological fractures may also be included here, even though the "trauma" that produces them may be nothing more than normal movement. Tooth loss, particularly if intentional or a result of accident, is also appropriately dealt with under the heading of trauma, especially because the healing of the alveolus closely resembles the healing of bone fractures in other parts of the skeleton. Furthermore, it is useful to look at trauma in the broader context of human behavior, such as circumstances that produce trauma, the effects on individuals and populations, and medical efforts to heal the results of traumatic stress.

FRACTURES

Types

Some obvious ways to describe a fracture include noting the bone affected, the location of

TABLE 1. Terms Commonly Used in Reference to Fractures

articular—involving the articular (joint) surface of a bone
avulsion—fragment of bone pulled off by a muscle at the site of its insertion
Barton's—fracture of the distal end of the radius
Bennett's—longitudinal fracture of the first metacarpal running into the carpometacarpal joint and complicated by subluxation
boxer's—fracture of the proximal or distal extremity of a metacarpal bone (frequently seen in boxers)
buttonhole—fracture in which the bone is perforated by a missile
capillary—hairlike fracture
chauffeur's—fracture of the radial styloid process produced by a twisting or snapping injury (frequently seen in chauffeurs and truck drivers)
closed—fracture that does not communicate with the external environment
Colles'—fracture toward the distal end of the radius in which the distal fragment is displaced posteriorly
comminuted—fracture in which a bone is divided into more than two parts
complete—fracture that divides a bone into separate parts
compound—fracture in which disruption of soft tissue results in communication with the external environment
compression—fracture in which a bone is crushed by compressive forces (most frequently involving the anterior portion of a vertebral body)
concertina—compression fracture in which the entire vertebral body is compressed about equally
depressed—fracture in which a part of the bone has been depressed below its surface
direct—fracture occurring at the specific point of injury and due to the injury itself
displaced—fracture in which the broken ends have moved some distance from each other
Duverney's—fracture of the ilium just below the anterior superior spine
epiphyseal—disruption of a bone between its epiphysis and diaphysis
fatigue—fracture caused by unusual bone stress or repeated microtrauma
green-stick—fracture in which one side of the bone is broken while the other side is bent (seen most often in children)
grenade-thrower's—fracture of the humerus caused by muscular contraction (associated with throwing heavy objects)
hangman's—fracture of cervical vertebrae with anterior dislocation of the axis
impacted—fracture in which one fragment is driven into another
incomplete—fracture that does not divide the bone into separate parts
indirect—fracture occurring at a site other than that of direct injury
intercondylar—fracture occurring between the condyles of a bone
intrauterine—fracture of a fetal bone in utero
Jefferson's—bursting fracture of the atlas
lead-pipe—fracture in which the cortex of the bone is slightly compressed and bulged on one side with a slight crack on the opposite side
linear—fracture that extends parallel to the long axis of a bone
lip—fracture of the posterior edge (lip) of the acetabulum (may be associated with dislocation of the hip)
longitudinal—see linear fracture
march—stress fracture, usually involving a metatarsal (associated with marching, hiking, etc.)
midnight—oblique fracture of the proximal phalanx of the fifth toe
Monteggia's—fracture of the shaft of an ulna with dislocation of the head of the radius (associated with parrying a blow with the forearm)
multiple—two or more separate fractures in the same bone
oblique—fracture in which the break extends oblique to the long axis of the bone
open—see compound fracture
parry—see Monteggia's fracture
pathologic—fracture of a bone previously weakened by other pathology
Pauwel's—fracture of the proximal neck of the femur with varying degrees of angulation
perforating—see buttonhole fracture
pertrochanteric—fracture of the femur passing through the greater trochanter
pond—depressed fracture of the skull in which a fissure circumscribes the affected area giving it a circular form
Pott's—fracture of the distal tibia with associated ligamentous damage or injury to the medial malleolus of the tibia
simple—see closed fracture
Smith's—fracture toward the distal end of the radius in which the distal fragment is displaced anteriorly (also known as a reverse Colles' fracture)
spiral—fracture produced by torsion in which the break spirals around the bone
spondylolysis—fracture in the neural arch of a vertebra, usually between the superior and inferior articular processes

TABLE 1. Terms Commonly Used in Reference to Fractures—Continued

spontaneous—see pathologic fracture
sprinter's—fracture of the anterior superior or anterior inferior iliac spine, a fragment of bone being pulled off by muscular violence (as at the start of a sprint)
stellate—fracture having a central point from which fissures radiate
Stieda's—fracture of the internal condyle of the femur
stress—see fatigue fracture
supracondylar—fracture through the distal shaft of the humerus
torsion—see spiral fracture
transcervical—fracture through the neck of the femur
transverse—fracture with the break at a right angle to the long axis of the bone
ununited—fracture in which the separated parts remain ununited after healing
Wagstaffe's—separation at the medial malleolus of the tibia
wedge—anterior compression fracture of a vertebral body

Definitions are primarily from Hilt and Cogburn (1980).

the fracture on the bone, and the shape of the fracture. Commonly occurring fractures have been given special designations (Table 1). Some bear the names of the people who first described them (Barton, Colles, Monteggia, Stieda, etc.); some were named for their appearance (buttonhole, concertina, green-stick, lead-pipe, etc.); some were named to reflect the forces that produced them (compression, depression, stress, torsion, etc.); some were named for activities with which they are associciated (boxing, grenade throwing, marching, sprinting, etc.); and some were named according to their anatomical location (articular, epiphyseal, pertrochanteric, transcervical, etc.).

Fractures may also be described as incomplete, when the affected bone is not divided into separate parts, or complete, when it is so divided. A comminuted fracture is a complete fracture in which the affected bone is divided into more than two parts. The shape of the fracture, whether transverse, oblique, or spiral, is also considered. Other commonly used categories include green-stick, depression, compression, impacted, stress (fatigue), intra-articular, avulsion, and epiphyseal separation. Fractures may also be designated as simple (closed), or compound (open), the latter indicating a fracture that communicates with the external environment. This designation is significant because a compound fracture would allow organisms to gain direct access to the bone with resultant infection. Another important category is that of pathological (or spontaneous) fracture, where the bone involved has already been weakened by other pathology. This weakening may be localized, as in the case of lytic lesions produced by a metastatic carcinoma or tuberculosis, or generalized, as seen in the collagen-deficient bones of individuals with osteogenesis imperfecta.

Healing

A bone fracture usually causes a rupture of blood vessels in the bone marrow and the periosteum, and sometimes in adjacent muscles, with subsequent development of a large hematoma around the fracture (Weinmann and Sicher, 1955:314–315). The normal process of healing involves six overlapping stages: 1) the blood of the hematoma coagulates, usually six to eight hours after the accident; 2) the blood clot becomes organized with young connective tissue (granulation tissue) and 3) is gradually transformed into fibrous (temporary) callus; 4) the fibrous callus is replaced by primary bony callus, which in turn 5) is replaced by secondary bone callus; and, finally, 6) the affected bone undergoes functional reconstruction (Weinmann and Sicher, 1955:315–328). The callus mass usually increases in size from four to six weeks after the injury and then diminishes gradually. It is interesting to note that although primary bony callus is readily identifiable histologically, it does not show up in radiographs and is very poorly preserved in archaeological contexts. However, the age of the individual is an important factor. In young children, union usually occurs quite rapidly, callus often becoming visible radiologically within two weeks with the bone being consolidated in four to six weeks. Union occurs more slowly in adults, consolidation usually taking about three months and even extending to four or five

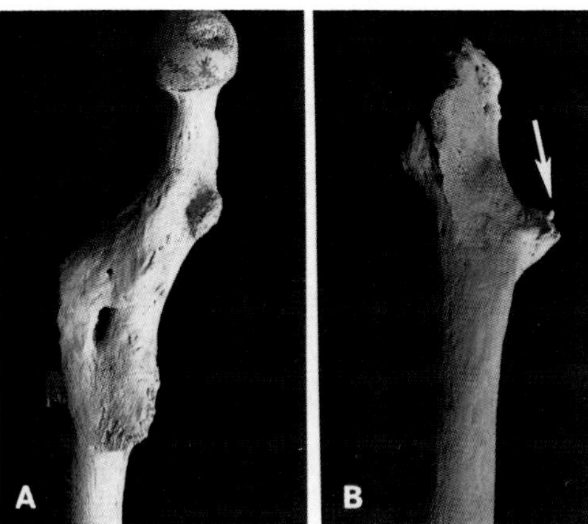

Fig. 1. **A:** Compound fracture of femoral shaft with large draining sinus. Right femur (SDMM 1915-2-344); Chavina, Peru. **B:** Healed but ununited fracture through femoral neck (arrow); head not recovered. Right femur (SDMM 1915-2-342); Chavina, Peru. (Photos courtesy of SDMM.) Specimen codes used here and in the following figure legends: ASU, Arizona State University, Tempe; CMC, Canadian Museum of Civilization, Ottawa; SDMM, San Diego Museum of Man; UW, University of Wisconsin, Madison.

months in the case of a large bone like the femur.

The healing of a compound fracture will proceed in normal fashion if it has not become infected. Infected fractures show considerable disturbance in the healing process, including the development of periostitis and osteomyelitis. In such cases the resorption of necrotic bone and the development of new bone are retarded or may not occur at all. The final outcome of a compound fracture will depend on the duration of the infection and on the amount of bone lost at the site of fracture. Callus development generally begins when the acute infection becomes chronic. Infections of long duration or involving excessive amounts of bone loss may prevent bony union. An example of a comminuted compound fracture involving the proximal half of the shaft of a right femur was found at Chavina, Peru (Fig. 1A). A large sinus with a drainage opening indicates that infection was present at the time of death.

Healing may be complete at the time of death, even to the point that extensive remodeling had occurred or was in process. In either case the osteological changes make it quite obvious that the fracture occurred while the individual was still alive. When the fracture occurs near or at the time of death, however, the absence of any signs of healing can make it difficult, if not impossible, to distinguish from postmortem damage.

Ununited Fractures

The healing process may also result in nonunion, with or without the development of a movable joint (arthrosis). In an example from the Libben site in Ohio (Lovejoy and Heiple, 1981:533), healed fractures of a left radius and ulna resulted in a functional pseudoarthrosis between the two bones in the vicinity of the fractures. Nonunion results from failure to effect complete immobilization of the separated parts, thus making it impossible for the developing bone callus to consolidate. Some degree of immobilization, often adequate in itself to allow union, will occur voluntarily in the sufferer because of the extreme pain experienced when the fractured limb is moved. Inadequate splinting may also allow sufficient movement to prevent union.

In many cases a fracture may go undetected with no attempt to immobilize the bone. An example of such nonunion is a right ulna from Matucana, Peru, where a fracture through the trochlear notch, probably never detected as a fracture and thus never immobilized, remained ununited (Fig. 2A). Fracture of the neck of a right femur from Chavina, Peru, resulted in a permanent separation of the head from the shaft (Fig. 1B). The extremely light weight of the femur suggests that it had undergone extensive mineral loss through disuse. Also, failure to recover the head portion of this bone suggests that it may have been resorbed. Resorption of a broken ununited part can occur if its blood supply is disrupted. The occasional resorption of one portion of an ununited scaphoid in the wrist occurs because the fracture separates the resorbing bone part from its normal blood supply.

Resorption of a distal fragment, or simply a failure to recover it, may result in confusing nonunion with amputation. The fracture through the olecranon fossa of the right humerus of Shanidar I has been interpreted as an ununited fracture (failing recovery of the distal portion of the bone and the remainder of the

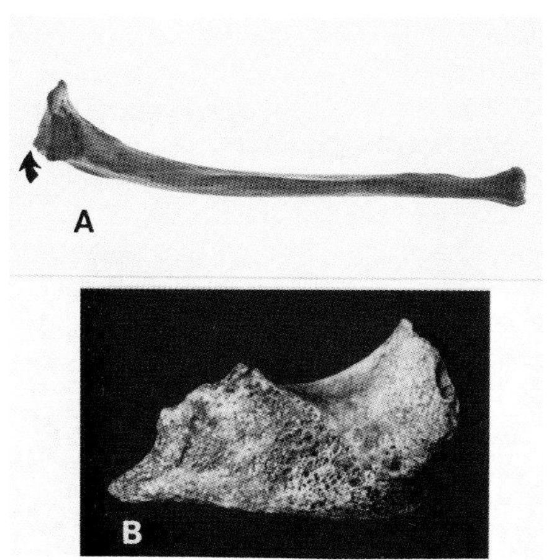

Fig. 2. **A:** Healed but ununited fracture through trochlear notch (arrow); olecranon not recovered. Right ulna (SDMM 1915-2-669); Matucana, Peru. **B:** Healed but ununited fracture or amputation through trochlear notch (shaft not recovered). Left ulna (ASU Ch77-115B/65); Nuvakwewtaqa, Arizona. (Photos courtesy of ASU.)

arm) or an amputation (Trinkaus and Zimmerman, 1982:66). The fact that careful examination of the burial area failed to produce the missing parts favors the amputation hypothesis. An ununited fracture through the trochlear notch of an ulna recovered from Nuvakwewtaqa (Chavez Pass), Arizona (Fig. 2B), a situation almost identical to that already described for an ulna from Matucana, Peru, also resulted in nonrecovery of the distal part. Because of the fact that the original context of this burial had been totally destroyed by looters prior to excavation, the nonrecovery in this instance could not be taken as support for an amputation hypothesis.

Another fairly common ununited fracture that is usually not recognized as such is spondylolysis, a fracture occurring between the superior and inferior articular processes of a vertebra. Rare cases of spontaneous union in spondylolysis have been reported, and union has occasionally been achieved through the application of elaborate devices to immobilize the affected region (Wiltse et al., 1975). In the great majority of cases the parts remain ununited.

Poorly United Fractures

Problems such as failure to reduce the fracture, incorrect apposition of the separated parts, or incomplete immobilization of the affected area, may result in a shortening, angulation, or rotation of the affected bone. If any of these results is extensive, it may lead to deformity, degenerative pathology, and functional disability. The original Neandertal specimen, recovered in Germany in 1856, had suffered a fractured proximal ulna that healed with marked deformity (Schaefer, 1957). A healed comminuted fracture of the distal femur from the site of Nuvakwewtaqa, Arizona, resulted in severely limited flexion while allowing considerable hyperextension of the knee (Fig. 3). This fracture obviously made walking very difficult, particularly over the rough terrain of this site.

The healing process may, in some instances, provide information on medical intervention. It seems quite clear from the occasional recov-

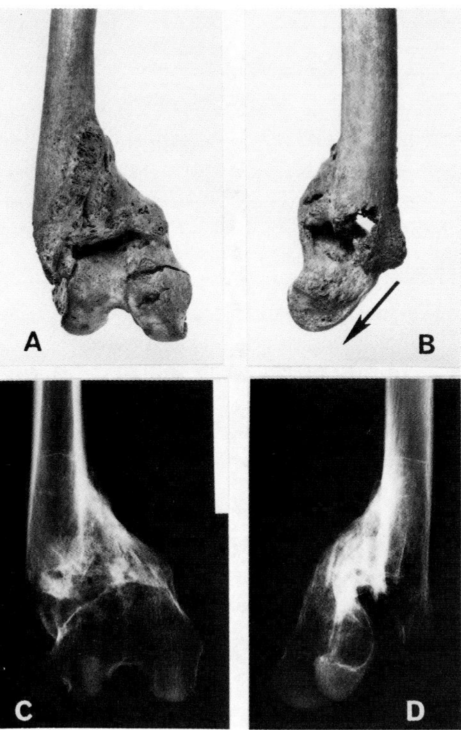

Fig. 3. Poorly healed fracture of distal femur. Right femur (ASU Ch80-77.5N/196.5E); Nuvakwewtaqa, Arizona. **A:** Anterior view. **B:** Lateral view (arrow indicates orientation of condyles). **C:** Radiograph, anteroposterior view. **D:** Radiograph, mediolateral view. (Photos courtesy of ASU.)

ery of ancient splints (Majno, 1975:75) and the survival of traditional medical practitioners called "bonesetters" among present-day Indian groups, such as the Hopi, that the art of reducing a fracture and immobilizing the affected bone was well known in antiquity. However, while it may be safe to assume that a badly healed fracture received no medical treatment or inadequate treatment, it may not be the case that a well-healed fracture received treatment. One only has to look at some of the well-healed fractures found in wild gibbons (Schultz, 1939) to be impressed with what nature can accomplish without human intervention.

Secondary Changes

Fractures, even those that are apparently well healed, can cause other changes in the skeleton. This has already been noted in the case where a fractured femoral neck appears to have produced osteoporosis in the bone. The previously mentioned right humerus from Shanidar I is another such case. The fractures suffered by this bone (or associated nerve damage) severely affected the right clavicle and scapula as well as the humerus (Trinkaus and Zimmerman, 1982:64). Compared with the normal left arm, the size of the clavicular shaft has been reduced by 10 to 15%, the height of the scapular spine by about 35%, and the size of the humeral shaft by about 45%. This size reduction is due to hypotrophy, if it occurred during growth, or atrophy, if it occurred during adulthood. Fractures may also lead to the disruption of joint mechanics resulting in osteoarthritis (degenerative joint disease). A fracture in the distal shaft of a left fibula belonging to a Sadlermiut Eskimo from the Canadian Arctic caused extensive arthritic disruption of the adjacent tibiotalar articulation (Merbs, 1983:94).

Even apparently well-healed fractures may have effects, sometimes quite subtle, on related aspects of the skeleton. In two examples from the Sundown site in Arizona, multiple but reasonably well-healed fractures in the upper part of the skeleton had clearly changed some aspects of the biomechanics of the upper limbs resulting in noticeable anatomical changes (Merbs and Vestergaard, 1985). A fracture of the right clavicle and fractures of the spinous processes of at least the first three thoracic vertebrae (all well healed) resulted in marked asymmetry of the humeri. The right humerus is 10 mm longer than the left, and the angle its head forms with the shaft is 17° greater. The right humerus also shows some degree of lateral rotation and contains a prominent osteophyte lateral to the radial fossa. The second individual has healed fractures of the right scapular blade and left ulna, and again the two humeri show considerable asymmetry. The right humerus is 8 mm shorter than the left and has a deep groove between its trochlea and medial epicondyle.

Depression and Compression Fractures

Strictly speaking, a depression fracture is produced by a force applied to just one side of a bone, whereas a compression fracture requires forces from two sides. The distinction is difficult to make, however, when one considers that the second force operating to produce a compression fracture is most often merely the resistance to the initial force. In the case of a "depression" fracture involving the cranial vault, the outer cortex of the bone is clearly depressed inward while the underlying diploe is "compressed." If the inner cortex is also involved, it and the compressed diploe will also be "depressed." Referring to such fractures as "depressed" rather than "compressed" often becomes a matter of convention rather than accurate description.

Depression fractures have been observed on crania of *Homo erectus* (Weidenreich, 1943) and may even go back to the time of *Australopithecus* (Dart, 1949). Trinkaus and Zimmerman (1982:68–69) report a "crushing" fracture involving the lateral orbital region on the left side of a Neandertal skull, Shanidar I. Large depression fractures involving the cranium frequently result in death, as in the case of the "pond" fracture sustained by an individual from Nuvakwewtaqa, Arizona (Fig. 4A). The sharp margins of the fracture lines indicate that no healing had occurred before death. Humans are remarkably resilient, however, and the severity of cranial depression fractures that can sometimes be survived is truly amazing. An example is a cranium from Cinco Cerros, Peru, in which a large area on the right side of the skull has been depressed so deeply as to severely affect the inner table (Fig. 4B). Two fracture lines extend outward from the depression, one

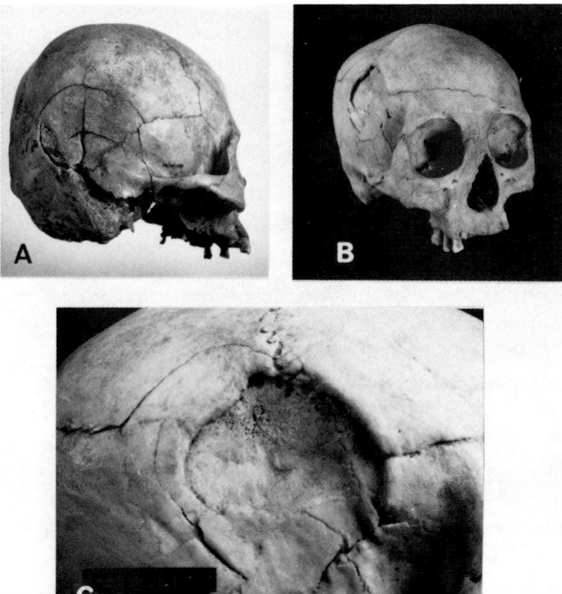

Fig. 4. **A:** Unhealed depression (pond) fracture. This cranium also contains cut marks (not visible on photo) that encircle the vault. Cranium (ASU 6104-1); Nuvakwewtaqa, Arizona. (Photo courtesy of ASU.) **B:** Healed depression (pond) fracture. Cranium (SDMM 1915-2-348); Cinco Cerros, Peru. **C:** Close-up of B. (Photos courtesy of SDMM.)

completely crossing the frontal bone to pterion on the opposite side, and the other extending downward across the temporomandibular articulation. The smooth nature of the edges of the fracture lines and the filling in with new bone where parts were separated indicate that healing had been well along or complete by the time the individual died.

In an interesting study that focused on the North Channel Islands and adjacent mainland of southern California, Walker (1981) found a high frequency (22.4%) of well-healed depressed cranial fractures among the island dwellers and a much lower frequency (3.3%) among the mainlanders. The similar size and shape of the depressions suggested to Walker that they were produced by a blunt weapon, and he attributes the higher frequency of lesions among the islanders to intense competition for limited resources. Walker also noted a dramatic decline in such injuries when comparing earlier and later island series, a change he associates with the introduction of new weaponry, particularly the bow and arrow.

Depression fracturing may also affect other parts of the skeleton, particularly the ends of long bones where the cortex is thin and the underlying cancellous bone somewhat compressible. Merbs (1985) describes a fracture of this type involving the lateral condyle of the left tibia of an Anasazi Pueblo woman buried at the bottom of the Grand Canyon. The fracture, clearly outlined by three break lines, covers about two-thirds of the condylar surface and produced a depression 7 mm deep. The likely cause of this fracture was a fall that occurred while the affected leg was fully extended. In this position the femoral condyle would have acted like a hammer to produce the depressed fracture in the tibia. It is interesting to note that the femoral condyle in this case shows no evidence of fracturing.

When subjected to strong vertical forces, the vertebral body is particularly vulnerable to crushing. Generally it is the anterior portion of the vertebra that is affected, the body thus assuming a wedge-shaped appearance. Another type of fracture affecting the vertebral body is the so-called "concertina" fracture, in which the entire body is uniformly compressed. This type of fracture is more likely to occur in old adults and is associated with general skeletal breakdown. Similar to the concertina fracture is the so-called "fish vertebra" condition. Associated with osteoporosis, this condition results when the intervertebral disk presses in upon a weakened vertebral body, producing depressions in the center of the body that extend to the periphery. The concave body surfaces thus resemble those seen in fish vertebrae.

Another condition of traumatic origin that results in depressed body surfaces is herniation of the vertebral disk, better known to radiologists as Schmorl's node. This condition is generally confined to central areas of the body, the periphery retaining its normal flat surface (Merbs, 1983:119). Disk herniation lesions are generally irregular in appearance, the depressed area often showing a very roughened surface. Disk herniations are frequently seen in the same vertebrae as compression fractures, suggesting that they were produced by the same traumatic event.

Disk herniation may sometimes be confused with other conditions, such as "cupping," that have nothing to do with mechanical forces. Associated with sickle-cell anemia, the cupping is caused by circulatory stasis and ischemia, and the depression produced is generally smooth and quite regular. Other nontrauma pathological conditions that destroy portions of the disk surface may also be confused with disk herniation, most notably tuberculosis and coccidioidomycosis. It is also important to note that the vertebral body may be subjected to fracturing other than simple compression (see Merbs, 1983:115).

Vertebral compression fracturing is most often associated with falls, and it was a common occurrence in the early days of parachute jumping before landing procedures were improved. (This author suffered such a fracture [first lumbar] in a fall from a ladder while trimming a palm tree.) Some measurable expression of vertebral compression was found in 36 of 80 adult Sadlermiut Eskimos (Merbs, 1983:110). The high incidence of vertebral compression fracturing in this population is attributed primarily to riding on a komatik, a simple platform sled lacking any form of shock absorber. As the vehicle moves rapidly over ice roughened by pressure ridges or rocks hidden by snow, vertical forces, sometimes quite violent, are transmitted directly to the vertebral column of the rider. The Eskimo condition is thus similar to one known in orthopedics as "snowmobiler's back," also characterized by vertebral compression fractures, which is occasionally observed in people who ride snowmobiles over rough terrain (Roberts et al., 1971). Sadlermiut males were affected with a slightly higher frequency than females (47 to 43%), but of greater interest is the difference in distribution of affected vertebrae in the two sexes, with females showing greatest involvement in the midthoracic region (T5–T9) and males in the lower thoracic–upper lumbar region (T11–L2) (Merbs, 1983:112). The occurrence of the condition higher in the vertebral column of the Sadlermiut women is attributed to their carrying of heavy objects on the back, particularly the carrying of infants in this position while sledding.

A high frequency of vertebral compression was also observed in the skeletons of medieval Germans (Grimm, 1959), people who traveled over rough roads in springless, wooden-wheeled carts. On the other hand, the high frequency seen in the sled-riding Canadian Eskimos stands in sharp contrast to the 22.2% observed by Yesner (1981:51) in the nonsledding Aleuts of Alaska.

Stress Fractures

Unlike most fractures, which are caused by distinct episodes of acute trauma, stress fractures (also commonly known as fatigue fractures) result from sustained stress or repeated microtrauma. Stress fractures occur in individuals who have normal-appearing bone form and structure, but an apparent susceptibility to fracturing under conditions of unaccustomed stress and physical activity. Beginning as "incomplete" fractures that generally run at right angles to the long axis of the bone, stress fractures may proceed to "complete" fractures if the recurring stress is not eliminated.

Stress fractures were first described in 1855 by Breithaupt (Cohen et al., 1974), a Prussian military surgeon, who noted that army recruits frequently complained of foot pain and swelling after long marches. In 250 consecutive cases of stress fracturing observed in 219 military trainees at Fort Benning, Georgia, by far the largest number, more than 87%, involved

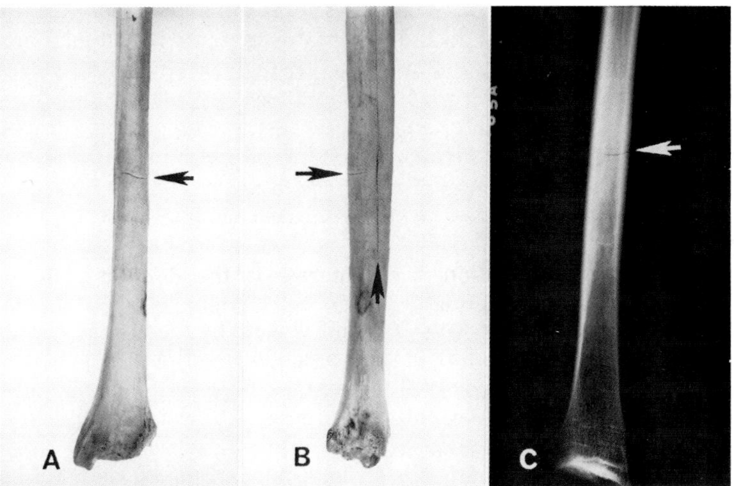

Fig. 5. Longitudinal and horizontal (arrows) postmortem breaks resembling stress fractures caused by drying and cracking. Right tibia (ASU M-165-A); Semna South, Sudan. **A:** Posterior view. **B:** Lateral view. **C:** Radiograph, anteroposterior view. (Photos courtesy of ASU.)

a metatarsal (88), calcaneus (70), or tibia (60) (Wilson and Katz, 1969:481). Also affected were ribs (14), the fibula (8), and the neck of the femur (7), with one case each involving a femoral shaft, a pubic ramus, and a third lumbar vertebra (spondylolysis). When two stress fractures occurred in the same individual, the second frequently involved the same bone on the opposite side, this being particularly true of the calcaneus.

Initially, stress fractures may be difficult to discern. In 17% (43/250) of the cases studied by Wilson and Katz (1969:482), for example, no evidence of fracture was apparent on radiographs taken soon after the onset of symptoms. In this respect, anthropologists have an advantage over radiologists because even the smallest fractures are more easily detected on bare bones than in standard radiographs. In the case of spondylolysis, for example, it may be possible to identify even the earliest stages of separation in the interarticular region. Anthropologists, on the other hand, have to be wary about postmortem changes, such as bone splitting due to weathering, that could be confused with stress fracturing (Fig. 5).

Initially referred to as a "march" fracture because of its frequent appearance in army recruits and other groups that engage in marching, stress fractures are now also associated with other activities. The carrying of a heavy knapsack or backpack over the shoulders may result in stress fracturing of the first rib, while repeated coughing from an upper respiratory infection has been implicated in stress fractures of other ribs (Wilson and Katz, 1969:484). Stress fractures tend to be more prevalent in athletes such as runners, jumpers, and ice skaters, in people who spend considerable time on their feet such as nurses and salesmen, and in people carrying extra weight such as pregnant women (Savoca, 1971). Stress fractures of the tibia (and sometimes the fibula) have also been reported in ballet dancers (primarily male) (Burrows, 1956), and those of the metatarsals in members of the Hare Krishna sect (Cohen et al., 1974).

Spondylolysis

Spondylolysis is a fracture related to erect posture and the presence of a lumbar curve, and it is thus uniquely human in distribution. Translated literally, "spondylo" refers to the vertebral column and "lysis" to dissolution or separation. The most common manifestation of the condition is complete bilateral separation between the superior and inferior articular processes (pars interarticularis) of the fifth lumbar vertebra. Other vertebrae may be affected, but occurrences outside the lumbosacral region are rare. Additional variations of the condition include 1) the part of the vertebra affected, with involvement of pedicles or laminae occasionally seen; 2) the extent of the lysis, which can range from a barely detectable cleft to complete separation; and 3) whether just one side or both sides of a vertebra are affected. Although frequently referred to as "separate neural arch," the lysis must be complete and bilateral for the arch to be actually separated from the body.

Although still occasionally referred to as a "congenital disorder" (Ubelaker, 1978:84), the fracture etiology of spondylolysis is now well established (Roberts, 1947; Wiltse et al., 1975). Its presence at birth has never been documented, and the medical literature contains only two instances of its occurrence in infants before the age of walking (Borkow and Kleiger, 1971; Wiltse et al., 1975). The condition also appears to be uniquely human, suggesting that the erect posture and bipedal locomotion of our species is a significant factor of its occurrence (Neugebauer, 1881; Thieme, 1950). Supporting this idea is the apparent absence of spondylolysis in nonambulatory individuals (Rosenberg et al., 1981).

Even before the turn of the century, Lane (1893) noted that spondylolysis occurred most frequently "in people doing heavy labor," and Friberg (1939) observed that those engaging in strenuous work showed symptoms earlier and more frequently than those in light work. Its greater frequency in males than females has also been long established. Spondylolysis was a common occurrence in the U.S. military during World War II, especially in new recruits undergoing strenuous training (Newman, 1959), and it is associated in modern orthopedic practice with stressful athletic activities, such as rowing, gymnastics, and football, and strenuous occupations, especially those involving heavy lifting (Goldberg, 1980; Semon and Spengler, 1981; Stallard, 1980; Wiltse et al., 1975). Stewart (1956) attributed the unusually high frequency of the condition in Eskimos to their habit of extending the legs (standing or sitting) while the hips and back are hyperflexed. This posture, according to Stewart, would reduce the lumbar curve, thus tending to concentrate stress in the interarticular region of the lower lumbar vertebrae.

The idea that spondylolysis is due to stress (or fatigue) fracturing rather than acute trauma was first advanced by Roberts in 1947. Some of the best support for the stress fracture hypothesis now comes from orthopedic cases involving vertebral fusion, cases such as that reported by DePalma and Marone (1959) where lysis occurred in L4 after the intentional fusion of L5 to the sacrum to correct a separation involving L5. The stress that caused the L5 problem appears simply to have been shifted one unit upward by the fusion. Examples of partial separation identified in archaeological specimens, such as a fifth lumbar vertebra from the Eskimo site of Kulaituijavik, Northwest Territories (Fig. 6), also support a stress fracture etiology for spondylolysis (Merbs, 1983:121; Stewart, 1953). Nevertheless, acute trauma must also be responsible for some share of the spondylolysis seen, particularly in cases where the pedicle is involved (Stewart, 1953).

Attempts at repair in spondylolysis are clearly frustrated by any continuation of the stresses that originally produced the separation and by difficulties in immobilizing the affected bone. As already noted in the discussion of ununited fractures, some rare cases of union have been documented, some spontaneous, but most often after immobilization of the lower back with an elaborate corset, brace, or cast (Wiltse et al., 1975). Two possible examples of union after natural immobilization, both involving the sacrum and both in 18–19-year-old males, have been reported for the Sadlermiut Eskimos (Merbs 1983:127, 175–176). In each case, lysis of the first sacral vertebra appears to have occurred while this unit was still separate from the unit below, with some movement between these two vertebrae thus being possible. With the fusion of S1 with S2, movement ceased. The incomplete separation seen in the interarticular region of S1 thus appears to represent an attempt at reunion of the lysed parts, an attempt that was terminated by death.

An additional factor making the repair of spondylolysis difficult is the forward slippage (olisthesis) that often accompanies complete bilateral separation. This slippage produces a gap ranging from several millimeters to a centimeter or more between the separated parts. A fairly rare condition known as pseudospondylolisthesis—olisthesis without lysis (Stewart,

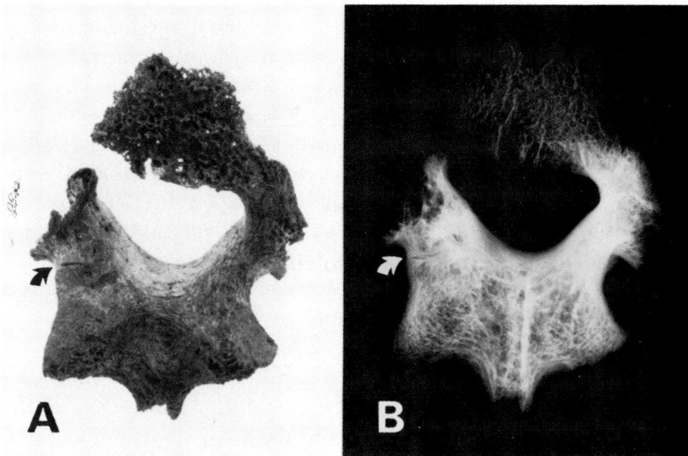

Fig. 6. Spondylolysis; partial separation (fatigue fracture) through right pars interarticularis (arrow). **A:** Anterior view. **B:** Radiograph; anteroposterior view. Third lumbar vertebra (CMC XIV-C-709); Kulaituijavik, Northwest Territories, Canada. (Photos courtesy of ASU.)

1935)—may represent spondylolytic repair subsequent to mild olisthesis.

Spondylolysis is unusual among fractures in having a distinctly familial pattern of occurrence (Wiltse, 1957), leading some researchers to even speculate on its "mode of inheritance" (Shahriaree et al., 1979; Wynne-Davies and Scott, 1979). It seems clear that what is being inherited is not spondylolysis itself, but some aspect of anatomy that predisposes an individual to the fracture. Several anatomical features have been investigated in this context, including the thickness of the interarticular region and the size of the articular processes impinging upon it from above and below (Nathan, 1959), number of presacral vertebrae, presence of transitional lumbosacral vertebrae, level of the sacral promontory, inclination of the sacrum, and extent of lumbar lordosis (Stewart, 1956). Interestingly, a bone mineral study of Koniag Eskimo and Aleut skeletons indicated that, in general, individuals with spondylolysis had significantly higher bone mineral values than individuals without the condition (Gunness-Hey, 1980). This observation, taken along with the positive correlation between vertebral compression fracturing and reduced bone mineral values in Eskimos (Thompson et al., 1985), suggests that vertical forces may produce two very different kinds of fractures in vertebrae—spondylolysis in individuals with normal bone mineral and compression of the body in individuals with deficient bone mineral.

DENTAL TRAUMA

Dental trauma can be accidental or intentional, and it can result in tooth loss, a fractured tooth, or simply an alteration in tooth shape. The trauma itself can originate from many sources, such as an accidental fall or a blow delivered in anger. It can also be intentional but nonhostile, such as the removal of teeth for curative purposes or as a social signal. The intent of the trauma may simply be to alter their shape, producing notched, grooved, or inlaid teeth for the sake of beauty or to denote status, or it may involve drilling and filling to treat caries. The identification of intentionally altered teeth is generally not difficult, but problems may arise in distinguishing between teeth missing congenitally or lost through disease and teeth lost through trauma, intentional removal, or accidental loss.

The healing of the wound created by a tooth extraction closely resembles that of a bone fracture. All extraction wounds may be considered "compound" in the sense that they communicate with the oral cavity, thus leaving the alveolar tissues open to infection. The rarity with which such infection actually occurs seems to be due to the antibacterial and cleansing action of the saliva. The healing of an extraction wound proceeds as follows: 1) a blood clot forms and fills the socket, 2) the clot becomes organized by proliferating young connective tissue, 3) the connective tissue is replaced by coarse fibrillar bone, 4) the alveolus undergoes reconstruction through resorptive activity and replacement of the immature bone by mature bone, and 5) epithelization and healing of the surrounding wound occurs simultaneously with the other reparative processes (Weinmann and Sicher 1955:332). Because the clot represents a perfect culture medium for the proliferating cells of the young connective tissue and, at the same time, serves to protect the more or less exposed surface of the bony socket, failure of formation or early removal of the blood clot, the condition known as "dry socket," leads to complications in the healing process, which include localized inflammation, extreme pain, and delayed healing.

Ritual tooth removal is well documented ethnographically in some areas such as East Africa (Singer, 1953). The African patterns appear to be entirely symmetrical and limited to one jaw, and they are tribal specific. The age of removal varies from group to group, but three "clusters" can be identified: 8 to 10 years, "puberty," and around 16 years. The usual reasons given for removal are to increase the beauty of the individual, to serve as a mark of manhood, or to be a sign of ability to withstand pain. Where the process of removal in Africa is known, it consists of loosening the tooth with a chisel and levering it out of the alveolus. No mention is made of alveolar fracturing, although it seems quite likely that this occasionally occurs. It is interesting that among one group at least, the A-Kamba, accidental loss of teeth is viewed quite differently than intentional removal, and the accidentally lost tooth is replaced by a false one (Singer, 1953:118).

One of the most convincing archaeological cases for intentional removal of anterior teeth involves skeletal material from northwest Africa dating to the Mesolithic (Briggs, 1955:82–84). The sample is small (42 intact crania) and heterogeneous, but the pattern of tooth loss is striking. All but two specimens had at least one incisor or canine missing with symmetrical loss patterns making up 86% of the affected sample. The most frequently occurring pattern, seen in 62% of the affected crania, is bilateral loss of the maxillary medial incisors. Based upon tooth wear, the removal is thought to have taken place in the 8–11-year-old age range (Briggs, 1955:83), a conclusion supported by the degree of mesial migration seen in teeth adjacent to those that were removed and the overeruption of teeth opposing those that were removed. Removal of the teeth resulted in considerable resorption (Briggs, 1955:82), but in only two cases were there signs of serious infection.

Hrdlička (1940) studied the dentitions of over 8,000 skulls and came to two important conclusions: 1) anterior tooth loss occurred with unusually high frequency in Eskimos and other Arctic Mongoloids and 2) this loss was due to intentional removal for "ritual" purposes. His first conclusion appears correct as high frequencies of anterior tooth loss have now been found in other Eskimo series (Costa, 1980; Curzon, 1978; Merbs, 1968). However, his second conclusion, that the removal was intentional, is open to serious question. Hrdlička's (1940) data fail to meet his own criteria for distinguishing between accidental loss and intentional ritual removal, criteria such as symmetry and repetition of loss patterns and mention of the practice in myths and legends (Merbs, 1983:43–45). An examination of Eskimo ethnography and folklore (Merbs, 1968), for example, produced no references to intentional tooth removal. Hrdlička's notion that the teeth were lost during youth appears to be based on the degree of alveolar remodeling he observed rather than actual observation of missing teeth in young individuals. He appears to have been operating under the premise that this remodeling takes place over a period of years, when in actuality it can occur in a matter of weeks. In his study of Sadlermiut Eskimo crania, Merbs (1983:133) found no missing teeth in subadults, while the frequency in adults increased with age. Missing anterior teeth were also found to correlate with age in Ipiutak and Tigara Eskimos (Costa, 1980).

The high frequency of anterior tooth loss in Eskimos does not appear to be due to ritual removal, but rather to tooth use and accidental trauma (Merbs, 1983:156–157). The extensive use by Eskimos of their teeth as tools is so well known that their dentition has come to be

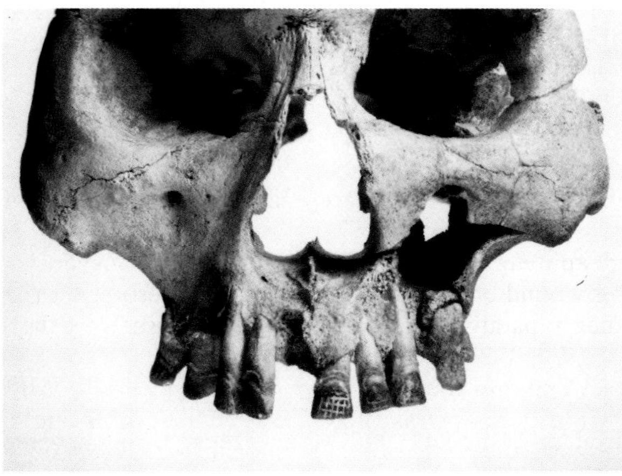

Fig. 7. Cross-hatch pattern filed into labial surfaces of incisors. Cranium; Guam. (Photo courtesy of ASU.)

called a "third hand." Employed primarily as a vise or pliers, Eskimo men use their teeth to hold a fish or line while other fish are being pursued with a leister, to tow a seal behind a kayak while the hands are engaged in propelling the boat, to hold the wooden rib of a kayak while the hands are used to bend it into shape, and to grasp the mouthpiece of a bow drill while one hand moves the bow and the other holds the object being drilled (Merbs, 1983:156). They also use their teeth to crush the heads of birds and crack seal bones and to tighten and untie lines. Eskimo women use their teeth primarily in the softening of skins for clothing and in the stretching of skin while it is being sewn (Merbs, 1983:156–157). According to Hall (1865:122), Eskimo women also strip waterfowl by "taking a duck and drawing the knife once around the outer joint of each wing and the head." They then "seized the cut part with their teeth, and stripped the fowl entire." Mayhall (1977), in his study of living Canadian Eskimos, attributes the tooth loss to these and other activities that produced low levels of trauma that loosened the teeth and led to extraction or exfoliation. The teeth could also have been lost in a single event of acute trauma (Merbs, 1983: 178), as in a wrestling match, a football game, or, presumably, a simple fall on the ice.

Cook (1981), in her examination of Koniag Eskimo children less than 10 years of age, found 12 skulls containing evidence of traumatic loss of deciduous teeth. Although favoring intentional removal, she acknowledges that traumatic loss due to childhood accidents is difficult to exclude. The tooth loss in these children may simply be analogous to that in their elders, the children perhaps mimicking the tooth-use activities of their parents. If these deciduous teeth were purposefully removed, the intent may have been therapeutic rather than ritual. The removal may have been carried out to allow for better eruption of the permanent dentition, a procedure used in modern orthodontia.

The intentional "mutilation" of teeth by notching, grooving, grinding, or drilling for inlay is well known in Mesoamerica, Africa, Southeast Asia, and Oceania. Among the prehistoric inhabitants of Guam, for example, the filing of cross-hatch patterns on the lingual surfaces of incisors was a common practice (Fig. 7). In a study carried out in 1973, Pindborg et al. (1975) found high frequencies of dental mutilation among the residents of two Indonesian villages. Limiting the sample to individuals 15 years of age and older, 99.2% of the females and 81.1% of the males of Wonosari, Central Java, and 96.6% of the females and 91.3% of the males of Kintamani, Bali, were found to have had their teeth abraded (ground or filed). Both the occlusal and buccal surfaces of maxillary incisors and canines were subjected to the abrasion, and a dark stain was then applied to the abraded teeth. Usually accomplished before 15 years of age, particularly among the females, the dental mutilation appears to serve as an initiation ritual. Another reason given for such mutilation is that the shortening and darkening of the teeth make them less doglike in appearance.

The drilling of teeth for inlays to beautify the dentition is well known, particularly in Mesoamerica (Romero, 1958), but its use as a curative technique in prehistoric times appears quite rare. A fairly convincing example of curative drilling in the tooth of an adult male from a Neolithic passage grave at Hulbjerg, Denmark, has recently been described by Bennike (1985: 175–182). A right maxillary second molar, still in position in the skull, has a conical hole drilled into its two buccal roots. A possible reason for the drilling is the presence of large caries in this tooth, as well as the adjacent first molar, which resulted in infection through the root canal with formation of an apical abscess. An experimental boring in a newly extracted tooth, carried out with a reconstructed bow drill bearing a flint tip and requiring only $5\frac{1}{2}$ minutes of labor, showed striking similarity, even under scanning electron microscopy, to the Neolithic example. Despite a thorough cleaning of the Hulbjerg tooth before scanning, a little calculus was found on the surface of the borehole, important evidence to indicate that the intervention had taken place while the individual was still alive. The presence of a partially healed trephination in another skull from this passage grave confirms a tradition of invasive medical treatment in this culture.

WEAPON WOUNDS

Certainly among the most dramatic specimens in all of human osteology is one with a weapon still firmly embedded in bone. Even without a weapon still in place, the matching of a bone lesion with the type of weapon that produced it can be a useful endeavor, allowing for significant interpretation in an archaeological context and sometimes providing key forensic evidence in a modern homicide case.

Brothwell (1965:122, 125) divided weapon injuries to the skull into four categories: 1) gross crushing, 2) less extensive fracturing, 3) piercing, and 4) cutting. Gross crushing injuries would be caused by large blunt weapons such as stones and clubs. Injuries in Brothwell's "less extensive fracturing" category would be produced by smaller clubs, maces, and sling-driven pellets. Particularly lethal in this regard was the metal-spiked mace of medieval Europe, whose mark has been identified on a skull from the Sedlec Ossuary, Czechoslovakia, which dates to the Hussite wars of the fifteenth century (Courville, 1965b), and the stone or metal star mace of Peru, which left its distinctive imprint on numerous skulls of that region (Fig. 8A). Weapons producing piercing injuries would include daggers, spears, javelins, and arrows; also included would be sling pellets if small enough and driven with enough velocity to pierce the skull and, of course, modern bullets (Fig. 8B). Brothwell's final category, cutting injuries, would be produced by weapons with sharp blades such as swords and axes. Sword wounds are generally narrower than those caused by an ax and may include sections of bone, usually circular, sliced completely away. The effect that the sword can have on human bones is clearly indicated by the numerous lesions found on skeletons of Gotland warriors who died in 1361 at the Battle of Visby (Courville, 1965a). The distribution of the lesions, primarily on the legs rather than the arms and primarily on the left side rather than the right, is indicative of face-to-face combat, the use of fairly effective upper-body armament, and perhaps a stategy of directing most of the blows to the legs.

As far as embedded weapons are concerned, one of the most impressive cases involves two bone points in the skeleton of an early Neolithic adult male found at Porsmose, Denmark (Bennike, 1985:111). One point, measuring 106 mm in length and 7 mm in diameter, entered through the nasal aperture, becoming firmly embedded in the hard palate with 45 mm of its length protruding into the back of the mouth. The second point, measuring 127 mm in length and 8 mm in diameter, penetrated the manubrium, its free end protruding 55 mm into the soft tissue behind the sternum. While the point in the face was probably not fatal, that through the sternum may well have penetrated the aorta, causing rapid death.

Several examples of a point embedded in the anterior portion of a vertebra have been reported, an example being a stone point in the

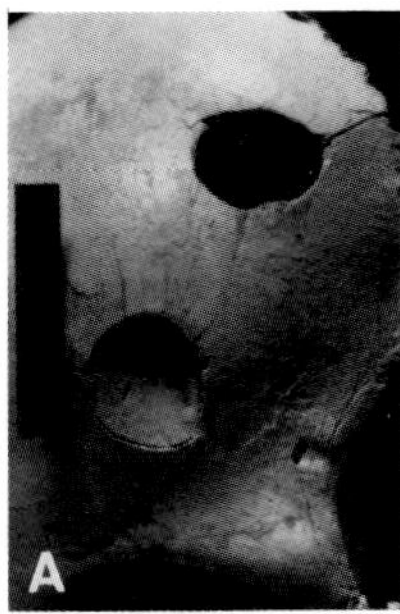
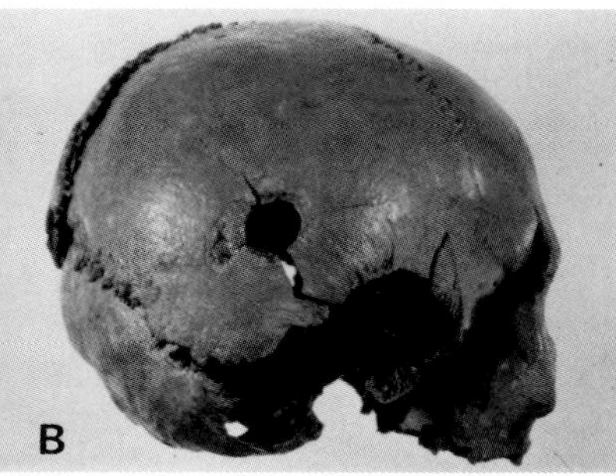

Fig. 8. **A:** Circular depression fracture and perforation, probably caused by a star mace. Cranium (SDMM 1915-2-20); Huacho, Peru. (Photo courtesy of SDMM.) **B:** Circular perforation caused by bullet (miniball). Seen here is the exit hole, the bullet having entered the skull through the left side. Cranium (UW H343/2049); Civil War soldier. (Photo courtesy of ASU.)

fifth lumbar vertebra of an Illinois Indian (Ortner and Putschar, 1981:73). This point had clearly penetrated important organs before becoming lodged in the vertebra. In a similar case from the French Neolithic site of Grotte de la Tourasse, Wells (1964:264) speculates that a flint arrowhead perforated the abdominal aorta before becoming embedded in a lumbar vertebra. The resultant hemorrhage would have led to rapid death. Murad and Mertz (1982:212) describe a skeleton recovered from the Sierra Mountains of northeastern California with three points embedded in various vertebrae. In reconstructing the trajectory and resultant damage of each point, the authors conclude that any of the three were capable of causing death.

Although not actually embedded in bone, the location of a weapon relative to skeletal parts in a grave can indicate the nature of the trauma it produced. For example, a bone arrow point was found lodged between the second and third cervical vertebrae of a male skeleton from the Mesolithic site of Bøgebakken, Denmark (Bennike, 1985:102–104). Presumably this point was buried in soft tissue at the time the individual was buried, and its passage through organs and blood vessels was the cause of death.

Weapons or parts thereof have also been found in the skeletons of individuals who obviously survived the trauma. An example is a small stone point embedded in the left third cuneiform of a Hohokam Indian from southern Arizona (Fig. 9). The point had clearly entered the foot from below, the victim either stepping on it or being shot while the bottom of his foot was exposed. Some bone resorption had taken place in the area of entry, but no indication of infection is discernible. In a modern example of this phenomenon, a 32-caliber bullet was found embedded in the rib of a 66-year-old man (Fig. 10). The bullet wound was superficial, and healed bone in the area clearly indicates that the individual survived the event.

Although the weapon itself may not be recovered, its effects on the skeleton may be ob-

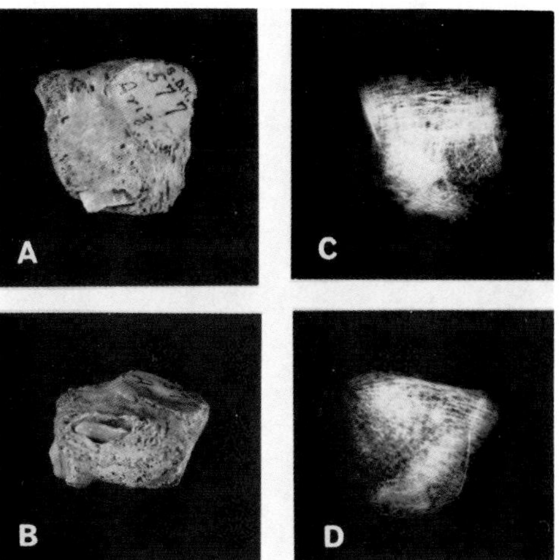

Fig. 9. Stone projectile point embedded in foot bone. **A:** Lateral view. **B:** Inferior view. (Photos courtesy of SDMM.) **C:** Radiograph; lateral view. **D:** Radiograph; medial view. (Note faint outline of point on radiographs.) (Photos courtesy of ASU.) Left third cuneiform (SDMM 1915-2-577); Hohokam, Arizona.

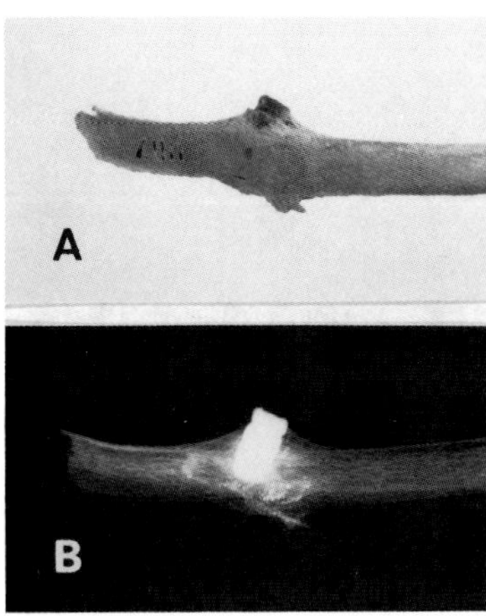

Fig. 10. **A:** Thirty-two caliber lead bullet embedded in rib. **B:** Radiograph. Right middle rib (SDMM 1981-30-50); recent Caucasian. (Photos courtesy of ASU.)

vious. An aperture into the frontal sinus of a skull from the Sundown site in Arizona has been interpreted as a partially healed wound produced by an untipped arrow (Merbs and Vestergaard, 1985). The arrow (7 mm in diameter) appears to have penetrated the outer wall (but not the inner wall) of the left sinus while on a downward trajectory with reduced velocity. Evidence of inflammation is present in the sinus on the side of the perforation, but not the opposite side. This individual clearly lived for some period of time following the injury.

Perhaps the most dramatic form of intentional life-ending trauma is decapitation. Clear-cut evidence of this act consists of cut marks on or through the cervical vertebrae and burial with the skull separated from the remainder of the skeleton. The skeletons of two Viking males excavated at Kalmergården, Denmark, are a good example. The head of one had been severed from the body by a horizontal cut through the second cervical vertebra, while the other had a cut extending from the base of the skull in the back to just below the eyes in front (Bennike, 1985:108). In both cases the heads had been placed between the legs when the bodies were buried. Another Danish Viking burial in which the skull had been separated from the rest of the skeleton, this one from Lejre, showed evidence of the hands and feet having been tied (Bennike, 1985:108). A decapitated head may also serve as a symbol to discourage certain kinds of behavior, as in the case of a Danish farmer who was convicted of attempting to murder his wife with rat poison. The man was decapitated and his head riveted to a stake as a warning to others (Bennike, 1985:118).

Remarkable soft tissue evidence of execution dating back approximately 2,000 years can be found among the so-called "bog bodies" of Europe. Examples from Denmark include women from Roum and Stidsholt who had been beheaded, men from Tollund and Borremose who had been hanged or strangled, and a man from Grauballe who had his throat cut from ear to ear (Bennike, 1985:119–121). A particularly gruesome example, found in 1984 at Lindow Moss, Cheshire, England, is described as follows:

> . . . the injuries . . . suggest that Lindow Man was killed as part of some ritual sacrifice, with a possible sequence of wounding being two blows to the head, followed by the garrotting, and then the incision in the neck—although this was possibly performed before the garrotte was tightened sufficiently to break the neck. (West, 1986:80)

DISLOCATIONS

Joint dislocation includes "subluxation," a partial loss of contact between joint components, but no distruption of the capsule, and "luxation," where the joint components are out of contact and the joint capsule is disrupted (Ortner and Putschar, 1981:85). Most joints are vulnerable, but to be detected in an archaeological specimen the dislocation must have taken place some time before death to allow recognizable bone modifications to occur.

Dislocation of the hip can be congenital rather than traumatic. Since the acetabulum is never occupied by a femoral head in a congenital dislocation, it tends to be small, shallow, and triangular in shape. In a dislocation due to trauma, on the other hand, the acetabulum will be fully developed, but usually remodeled through new bone development. A secondary acetabulum may be recognizable on the ilium posterior to the primary acetabulum (Ortner and Putschar, 1981:89), its degree of definition due in large extent to the duration of the dislocation and the extent to which biomechanical stresses in the new joint have produced degenerative changes.

Because of its anatomy and greater mobility, shoulder dislocations occur with greater frequency than those of the hip. Although the anatomy of the shoulder joint prevents spontaneous reduction of a dislocation, methods for achieving reduction are fairly simple and go back at least to the time of Hippocrates (Ortner and Putschar, 1981:87). It is perhaps for this reason that shoulder dislocations are not as common in archaeological specimens as might be expected. As with the hip, congenital shoulder dislocations, or later dislocations of this joint due to congenital abnormalities, are also a possibility (Bennike et al., 1987). In the classic case of shoulder luxation (Ortner and Putschar, 1981:88), a new articular facet (Bankhart lesion) develops on the anterior surface of the scapular blade while the glenoid fossa undergoes degenerative changes.

SCALPING

Scalping is a practice usually associated with the collecting of human trophies, and as such it can be placed in the same category as the taking of heads, including the famous "shrunken heads" of the South American Jivaro. One obvious difference is that in scalping the victim sometimes survives the event. Scalping was practiced by the Scythians in ancient times, according to Herodotus (Friederici, 1907), and by the Germans and French until at least A.D. 870 (Burton, 1864). One of the earliest accounts of scalping by Indians in the Americas is by Hernando De Soto in 1540, one of his men having been a victim near Appalachicola Bay, Florida (Friederici, 1907). Although popularly believed to have been introduced into the Americas by Europeans, the archaeological record indicates that scalping was practiced in this area long before their arrival (Allen et al., 1985; Hoyme and Bass, 1962; Neumann, 1940). That is not to say, however, that it was as common in prehistoric as in historic times, the taking of scalp bounties having been greatly encouraged by the English, French, and American governments (Mooney, 1910).

Although the size of the scalp removed and the method of removal varied, the following procedure described by Nadeau (1944) is typical. Incisions were made in the skin in a series of short parallel cuts across the forehead, over and around one ear, across the back of the head near the nuchal crest, and over and around the other ear. Ear ornaments were sometimes included by cutting the scalp below rather than above the ears. The hair was then given a sharp tug to loosen the skin from the head and the scalp was peeled off. If the individual had closely cropped hair or was bald, the edge of the scalp was raised with the fingers and pulled loose with the teeth. The cut marks seen on an Indian skull from Illinois (Steinbock, 1976:28) and ten Indian skulls from Arizona (Allen et al., 1985) correspond closely with Nadeau's description.

An interesting alternative to trophy taking as an explanation for the ten Arizona examples is presented by Allen et al. (1985). Using the Mausuwu society of the Hopi Indians for analogy, the "scalpings" may be viewed as a primitive kind of autopsy carried out to investigate causes of head ailments. Members of the Mausuwu supposedly had the power to cure "head swellings" and severe headaches, and six of the scalped skulls show clear evidence of cranial pathology that would have been capable of producing "swellings" or headaches. Three of the crania exhibit healed depression fractures of the frontal, one shows signs of severe infection involving most of the frontal, one shows signs of severe infection involving most of the frontal, and two appear to have experienced severe trauma with no evidence of healing (Fig. 4A). The "scalpings" may thus represent an attempt by members of a society like the Mausuwu to get a closer look at the skull to learn more about the effects of healed and death-causing trauma as well as other kinds of cranial pathology. It is interesting to note that in order to be initiated into the Mausuwu as a "real" warrior, and thus, presumably, as an effective healer of "head swellings" and severe headaches, one first had to take a scalp (Allen et al., 1985:31–32).

Hamperl and Laughlin (1959) report on the skull of a historic male Arikara Indian from near Mobridge, South Dakota, who apparently survived a scalping. The area of involvement, elliptical in shape and measuring 7×10 cm, is centered to the left of lambda. Its surface is smooth but very uneven, showing many flattened depressions. Whereas the normal thickness of the skull is 4 to 5 mm, in the affected area it amounts to only 2 to 3 mm. The authors conclude that in the affected area all normal bone of the outer table and most if not all of the diploe had entirely disappeared to be imperfectly replaced by new bone of different structure. A similar case exhibiting evidence of osteitis and new bone formation was reported by Morse (1973) in a Mississippian adult male from Arkansas. These two cases closely match one described by R.C. Moore (Reese, 1940:18–19) in which an employee of the Union Pacific Railroad was scalped by Cheyenne Indians near Plum Creek Station, Nebraska, in 1867. The scalp had been entirely removed, including, presumably, the periosteum of the cranial bones. In about three weeks the outer table began to exfoliate, but eventually the surface presented the appearance of a healthy wound and the patient, "being strong," survived.

SURGERY

Trephination

Among the most impressive aspects of trauma is trephination (trepanation), the process of removing a portion of the calvarium without disrupting the underlying blood vessels, meninges, and brain. Evidence of trephination goes back to the Mesolithic of Europe and North Africa, and the procedure is clearly well established in this area by Neolithic times (Bennike, 1985:93). Evidence of trephination has also been reported in other areas such as the Middle East, India, China, southern Siberia, and Melanesia (Lisowski, 1967:652). Although well-documented cases from North America are rare (Cybulski, 1980; Wilkinson, 1975), trephination achieved a particularly high level of skill and diversity of technique in the Andean region of South America before the Spanish conquest (Stewart, 1958). The procedure is also well known ethnographically in East Africa (Margetts, 1967).

Trephination begins by cutting the skin overlying the bone to be excised and reflecting it away from the area or removing it entirely. Sometimes the area from which the skin was removed can be identified by the presence of scratches from the cutting or discoloration of the denuded bone, if they have not been obliterated by healing (Stewart, 1958:483). Lisowski (1967) describes five methods by which the bone itself is cut. In the first, referred to as "scraping," the area of bone to be removed is gradually scraped or abraded away; the external table and diploe are removed, and then, with great care, the abrading is extended through the internal table to expose the dura mater (Lisowski, 1967:662). The opening produced is characterized by wide, beveled edges (Fig. 11A), and the removed part has necessarily been reduced to dust.

In the second or "grooving" method of trephination, curvilinear lines are abraded into the bone with a sharpened instrument until a circular section of bone becomes loose and can be removed (Lisowski, 1967:663). Characteristic of this method is the more circular appearance of the lesion and the lesser degree of edge beveling. A roundel of bone is produced and it has sometimes been found still in position. Lisowski's fourth method, making use of an instrument called a "trephine" (or "trepan") for removing a disk of bone, might be thought of as a more sophisticated variant of his second method. A "crown" trephine, referred to as a *prion* by the Greeks (Majno, 1975:196) and a *modiolus* by the Romans (Lisowski, 1967:664), consisted of a hollow iron cylinder with a toothed edge that could cut through bone. A center pin held the instrument in place during the surgery.

The third method described by Lisowski (1967:664), referred to as "boring-and-cutting," involves the drilling of a nearly continuous circle of small holes (Fig. 11C) that are then connected by cutting until the enclosed section of bone is released and can be levered out. Probably limited to Peru, the most obvious features of this method are the serrations produced by the drill holes on the periphery of the lesion and the roundel.

Lisowski's (1967:664–665) final method consists of cutting four straight incisions joined at right angles and levering out the rectangular fragment thus released (Fig. 11B). Lesions produced by this method sometimes contained five or more sides, and several individual lesions might be joined to produce an extremely complex final outline. Characteristic of this method are the straight edges produced and the crossing of cut marks at the corners of the lesions. Employed extensively in ancient Peru, the primary tool for this method of trephina-

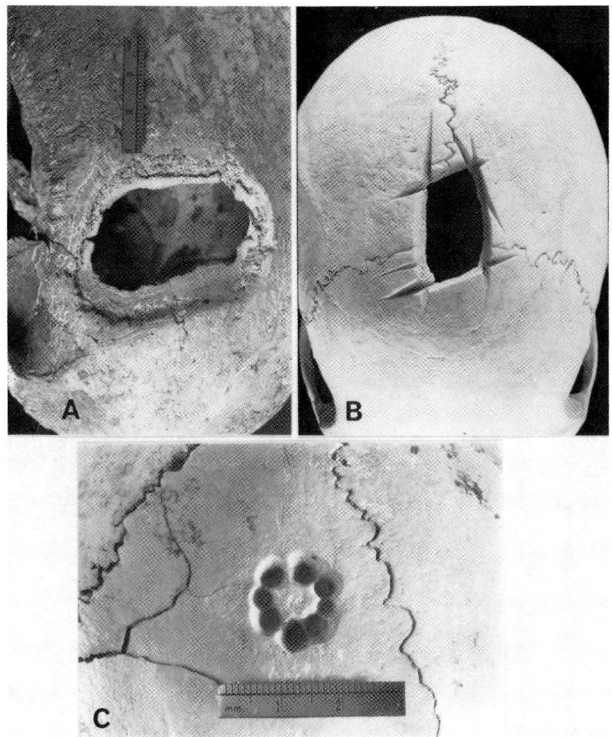

Fig. 11. **A:** Trephination with little if any healing; scraping or abrading technique. Cranium (SDMM 1915-2-479); Lovosice (Neolithic), Czechoslovakia. **B:** Complete trephination with no healing; straight cutting. Cranium (SDMM 1915-2-308); San Damian, Peru. **C:** Incomplete trephination; boring technique. Cranium (SDMM 1915-2-283); Matucana, Peru. (Photos courtesy of SDMM.)

tion was the *tumi,* a copper or bronze knife with a vertical handle and curved horizontal blade. The handles of some of these knives contain figures. One at the San Diego Museum of Man, for example, contains two figures, one presumably the patient, wearing what appears to be a bandage around its head, and the other, probably the surgeon, wearing an ornate headdress. A trephination in progress is represented on a *tumi* at the Museum für Völkerkunde, Hamburg (Thorwald, 1962:307). Three individuals are present—a surgeon (standing), an assistant, and the patient (both seated). Trephination is also the subject of a Peruvian Mochica period ceramic vessel at the National Museum in Lima (Thorwald, 1962:305). In this case the patient is in a prone position and the surgeon appears to be sitting on his back.

Both healed and unhealed trephinations may be confused with other phenomena, probably resulting in an assumed higher frequency of this surgery than is warranted. For example, a circular lesion may represent a roundel of bone sliced away by a sword, while a straight-sided lesion may be due to the removal of a fragment from a comminuted fracture. If no healing has taken place, the cutting may have occurred after death to secure a roundel of bone for a talisman, a practice still seen today in parts of Africa (Oakley et al., 1959). Holes found cut into a cranium could have served merely to hang it from something. Some of the "unhealed" trephinations may actually represent practice surgery carried out on cadavers. It takes little imagination, for example, to see the work of several would-be surgeons on a skull from Lupo, Peru (Fig. 12A).

Trephination-like lesions can also be produced through rock abrasion or the action of acid in the grave (Pales et al., 1952) or by the activities of organisms such as beetles, rodents, and porcupines (Brothwell, 1965:128). Various

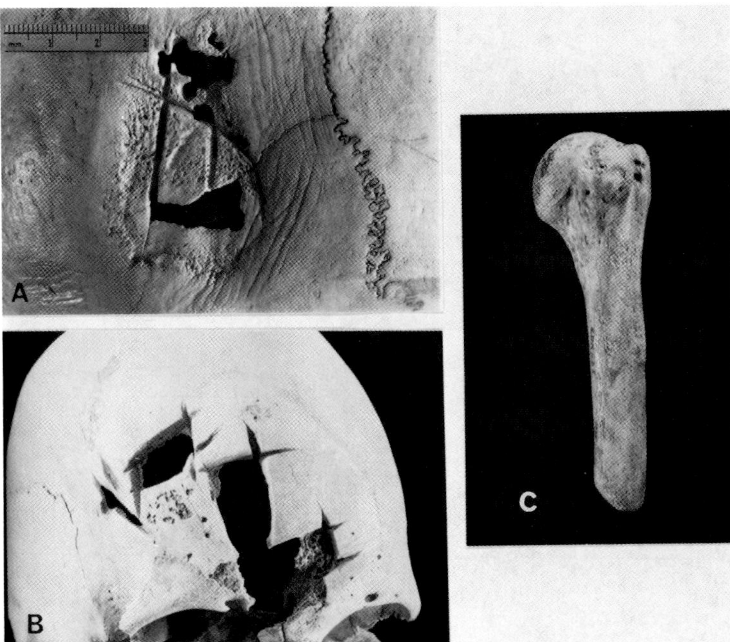

Fig. 12. **A:** Crude multiple trephination with no healing; possibly performed as practice on an individual already dead. Cranium (SDMM 1915-2-284); Lupo, Peru. **B:** Multiple trephination with evidence of bone reaction following the earliest cutting. Cranium (SDMM 1915-2-309); Cinco Cerros, Peru. **C:** Amputation. Left humerus (SDMM 1915-2-668); Lupo, Peru. (Photos courtesy of SDMM.)

congenital, neoplastic, and infectious conditions may be misinterpreted as "healed" trephinations. An example of a congenital condition with this potential is the so-called "Catlin mark," named for the family in which it was observed, a condition consisting of bilateral apertures in the parietals (Goldsmith, 1945).

The reasons for performing this difficult surgical procedure are probably quite varied. Trephining among the Kisii of South Nyanza, Kenya, is said to be done to alleviate headache resulting from injury to the head, with or without fracture of the skull (Margetts, 1967:683). Prehistoric trephined skulls from Peru frequently show evidence of injury, and in many instances the surgery has been centered directly over the site of the trauma. Trephination in this region likely originated from a practice of carefully removing bone fragments judged to be dangerous from such injuries and cutting or abrading away sharp edges. In many cases depressed fractures could have created internal cranial pressures that resulted in headache and possibly aberrant behavior, whereas other fractures, not necessarily depressed, could have had the same effect through the development of blood clots. The discovery that these conditions could sometimes be alleviated by the removal of the offending agents would certainly have given credibility to this surgical procedure.

Although he found no evidence of trephination in his study of Danish skeletons from medieval Aebelholt, Møller-Christensen (1958) did discover that cranial lesions associated with wounds occurred with a much greater frequency in males than females (32 to 2) and were mostly on the left side of the skull. This pattern, he concluded, was produced by hand-to-hand combat among men, the blows being delivered primarily by right-handed combatants standing face-to-face with their victims. This is the same pattern found by Bennike (1985:66, 94) in her study of 18 trephined skulls from Denmark dating from the Early Neolithic (4200 B.C.) through the Iron Age (500 B.C.). Only one of the affected individuals was female, and most of the lesions were located on the left side. Thus, as in Peru, trephination in Denmark appears to be associated with head wounds, particularly cranial fractures sustained in battle. Unlike in Europe, however, trephination in Peru frequently involved women and even children (Stewart, 1958:481), most of the latter showing clear evidence of fracture prior to trephination.

Trephination may also have been employed for other problems involving the cranium, such as treponemal infection (Rytel, 1962), otitis media and mastoid inflammation (Oakley et al., 1959), and possibly even metastatic carcinoma (Moodie, 1929:720). It may also have been employed for strictly magical purposes, such as to release evil spirits thought to reside in the skull (Lisowski, 1967:657–658). Head pain was presumably caused by these spirits, and its alleviation following trephination might be considered a clear indication of the operation's effectiveness. The large number of trephined skulls found in the chambered tombs in the Seine-Oise-Marne region of France, for example, are thought to have ritual significance (Oakley et al., 1959).

In most specimens where some healing has occurred before death, an area of osteitis surrounds the lesion. This inflammation has been attributed to infection caused by either the original wound or the surgical procedure itself (Ortner and Putschar, 1981:98). In some instances the inflammatory reaction had not proceeded far before a new area of bone was removed, this time leading to quick death (Fig. 12B). A successful operation with complete healing is indicated by a closed diploe and relatively smooth borders (Moodie, 1929). Since new bone formation in the trephined area is slight, the aperture remains open.

Potential complications in trephination that could cause death are a tearing of the meninges or injury to the brain and infection due to septic conditions. Nevertheless, success seems to have occurred more often than failure. Stewart (1958:486) reports that of 214 Peruvian trephinations he studied, 55.6% show complete healing, 16.4% show beginning healing, and 28% show no healing. Similarly, Rytel (1962) found evidence of healing in 62.5% of the 400 trephined Peruvian crania he studied. In some cases death was obviously due to the original trauma that prompted the surgery and not to the surgery itself. The rate of success would also be greater if some of the "unhealed" specimens actually represented practice operations on cadavers.

Amputation

Examples of amputation are known from the archaeological record, but they are not numerous. Limbs may be lost in battle, or they may be surgically removed for medical reasons, as punishment for a crime, or as a sign of grief. Identification of amputation in the osteological record is complicated by other conditions, particularly ununited fractures where the distal fragment is not recovered. In a true amputation, callus will begin to develop approximately two weeks after the event to narrow the exposed medullary cavity (Steinbock, 1976:36). After several weeks (or months), a bony cap, not always complete, forms over the cavity, and there is a rounding and smoothing of the stump. Disuse atrophy may later lead to osteoporosis.

An interesting example of apparent amputation involves the mummy of an elderly male Egyptian dating from the Ptolemaic period (330–30 B.C.). The hand of this individual had been removed several centimeters above the wrist and replaced, presumably at time of burial, by an artificial limb complete with digits (Gray, 1966). A humerus from an adult, probably male, buried at Lupo, Peru, also shows evidence of apparent amputation (Rogers, 1973). This bone terminates cleanly at the level of the deltoid tuberosity (Fig. 12C), and its light weight suggests disuse osteoporosis.

Amputation of the right foot 10 cm above the ankle joint has been reported for a skeleton dating from the late Middle Ages (ca. A.D. 1500) recovered from the churchyard in Odense, Denmark (Jakobsen, 1979). The amputation stumps are rounded and their marrow cavities are closed by a condensed cap of bone. Osteophytes surround the stump of the fibula in a cuplike manner and firmly unite the stumps along their interosseous margins, indicating that a firm amputation stump had been obtained. A roughening of shaft surfaces suggests a previous periosteal infection, and the cortices are thin and osteoporotic, changes that indicate that the person survived the amputation for at least several weeks and probably much longer.

In addition, the extended position of the leg in the grave indicates that contractures of the hip and knee had been prevented. This skeleton also includes two other examples of trauma, a badly healed comminuted fracture of the left femur and healed fractures of the left radius and ulna that had formed an arthrosis between the bones.

Amputation may also be observed in ancient art. What appear to be amputated legs and feet, complete with indications of suturing, for example, are represented on Mochica period ceramic pieces from Peru (Thorwald, 1962: 296–297).

An remarkable example of self-amputation observed in a living Canadian Eskimo is illustrated by de Poncins (1949:68–69). Having lost the soft tissue surrounding the terminal phalanx of all four fingers (not the thumb) of his left hand through freezing, this individual simply cut away most of the exposed bone. A small stump of bone was left protruding from each finger, however, carefully carved into the shape of a fingernail "with which he scratched himself with the greatest of ease." It would have been interesting to see how these phalanges would have been interpreted if found in an archaeological context.

Other Surgery

One of the most curious forms of primitive surgery is the so-called "sincipital T" scarring of the skull vault first described by Manouvrier in 1895 (see Ortner and Putschar, 1981:102–103; Steinbock, 1976:35–36). In its classic form, the condition consists of a depression in the shape of a T extending into the diploe. The vertical portion of the T usually begins near the center of the frontal squama and extends along the sagittal suture to near the oblionic foramina, and the horizontal part then passes down the sides of the skull between the parietal bosses and the lambdoidal suture. The sincipital T mutilation is seen primarily on skulls of women and children dating from the Neolithic of France, but it has also been reported in Hungary, central Asia, the Canary Islands, Peru, and Africa. Examples are scarce, however, and it is not certain that what is being reported is always the same phenomenon. The condition appears to have begun as damage to the scalp that interrupted the blood supply to the vault. This in turn produced inflammation, which, upon healing, left behind the observed scarring. The reasons for performing sincipital T mutilation remain obscure.

Evidence of ancient surgery other than trephination, amputation, or sincipital T mutilation will necessarily be scarce because of the rarity of skeletal involvement. One indication of this missing part of the picture, however, comes from a *tumi* dating to the Mochica period of Peru (Tyson and Alcauskas, 1980). Two individuals are represented at the top of the handle, one a surgeon, clearly identified by the inverted *tumi* motif worn as a headdress, and the other his patient, lying supine before him. The surgeon is gripping a *tumi* with his right hand and guiding it with his left. What is particularly interesting about this scene is that the surgery is taking place not on the cranium or a limb, but in the abdominal region, a clear indication that the skills of the prehistoric Peruvian surgeon transcended trephination and amputation.

PERIMORTEM CUTS AND BREAKS

Human bones sometimes contain cut marks or show signs of having been broken, which can be interpreted as caused violence at time of death or intentional mutilation, dismemberment, or even cannibalism following death. Interpretations such as these are fraught with problems, which in some cases have produced considerable skepticism. In the case of broken bones, for example, the first question that must be asked is whether the breakage occurred at or soon after death or much later as a result of ground pressure. The possibility of breakage occurring during excavation or while being curated in a museum must also be considered. Even when it is possible to attribute breakage to human activity, the actual intent of the act may prove elusive. Similarly, if it can be demonstrated that cut marks on bones were produced at or soon after death rather than later, through animal activity or careless excavation, the question of intent may still be difficult to answer in a convincing manner. Given that the question includes the emotion-laden subject of cannibalism, interpretation requires a particularly careful, bias-free analysis of the evidence.

Several Thule culture Eskimo skeletons recovered from stone cairn graves located north-

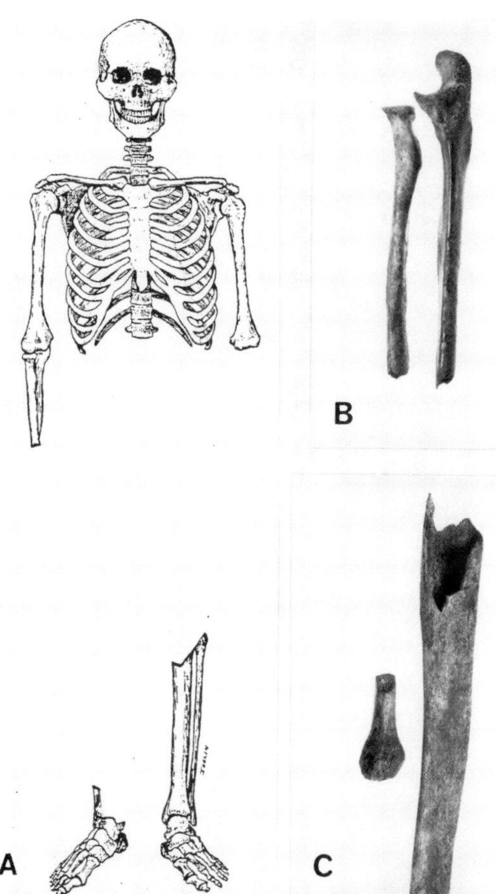

Fig. 13. Probable polar bear victim. **A:** Parts included in grave. **B:** Fractured right radius and ulna. **C:** Fractured right fibula and left tibia. Skeleton (CMC XIV-C-685); Kulaituijavik, Northwest Territories, Canada. (Drawing and photos courtesy of ASU.)

west of Hudson Bay, for example, show severe breakage with many missing parts (Fig. 13). The bone in these cases is well preserved and can, even today, be broken only with great difficulty. Also, the graves at the time of excavation showed no sign of disturbance whatsoever. These conditions, plus the occasional presence of deep indentations as from large canines, indicate that these individuals had been the victims of polar bears. It is interesting that in each case the friends and relatives of the deceased not only collected the remains, but accorded them a full-size grave, even placing the parts in the structure where they would have been had the body been intact.

In the American Southwest, a number of human bone collections showing extensive perimortem damage have been analyzed by Turner (1983). Although exhibiting some intergroup variation, these collections as a whole are characterized by the representation of multiple individuals, massive breakage (particularly of the cranium, including the face, and long bones), systematically missing parts (particularly vertebrae), and some evidence of cutting and burning. The argument that this condition was caused by humans and was quite intentional seems irrefutable, but its purpose is more difficult to discern. Given the exotic treatment some groups accord their own dead, to say nothing of the treatment (short of cannibalism) accorded the remains of enemies, particularly individuals thought to be witches, Turner's conclusion that the Southwest remains represent cannibalism is bound to be met with some skepticism.

Cut marks have also been found on ancient fossil remains. The Bodo cranium dating from the middle Pleistocene of Ethiopia, for example, contains cut marks that, according to White (1986:503), ". . . closely resemble experimental damage caused by the application of stone tools to fresh bone." White sees this as the "earliest solid evidence of intentional defleshing" in a hominid. The skull of Engis 2, a juvenile Neandertal from Belgium, has also been observed to contain "several series of incised striations" (Russell and LeMort, 1986:317). Here again an interpretation of intentional hominid activity has been suggested, this based primarily on "the number, straightness, orderliness, and length of the marks over the left orbit and those running down the center of the frontal squama" (Russell and LeMort, 1986:321).

It was both cut marks and breakage among the Neandertal remains from Krapina, Yugoslavia, that led to the interpretation that they had been victims of cannibalism (see Russell, 1987b:381). An estimated 43 individuals are represented by 650 bone specimens at Krapina, with most limb bone shafts broken cross-sectionally and larger limb bone diaphyses split longitudinally. Trinkaus (1985) noted, however, that the pattern of fractures in the Krapina material closely resembles that seen in other Neandertal skeletons that had been crushed in situ by the weight of sediment. Most likely to collapse under transverse pressure, reasoned Trinkaus, were bones with large diameters and relatively thin cortices like femora and tibiae, not bones with narrow diameters and relatively thick cortices like ulnae, radii, and fibulae, and this is the pattern generally observed. Oblique or spiral fracturing, sometimes attributed to human activity, can in fact be produced by many nonhuman taphonomic agents whenever relatively "green" bone is involved (Bonnichsen, 1979). Similarly, longitudinal splitting of the diaphysis, also sometimes attributed to human activity, has been shown to be a natural response to transverse pressures of any kind, the fractures following the orientation of haversian systems and collagen fiber bundles (Trinkaus, 1985). On the basis of microscopic inspection of all Krapina specimens, Russell (1987a) feels that all the breakage in this series was caused by sedimentary pressure and/or rock falls or occurred during the quarrying and excavation of the site.

The cut marks seen on the Krapina bones, more likely the result of human activity, were nevertheless found to differ significantly from Mousterian butchery marks on reindeer bones (Russell, 1987b). On the other hand, they closely match cut marks on 22 modern human skeletons that show convincing evidence of having been defleshed with stone tools in preparation for secondary burial. The evidence for cannibalism at Krapina thus seems quite weak.

More recently, clusters of human bone fragments found at the Neolithic cave site of Fontbregoua in southeastern France have been attributed by Villa et al. (1986) to butchery and cannibalism. Also found at the site were features containing the bones of animals, primarily domestic sheep and wild boars. Twenty-five marks on human fragments and six on animal bones from Fontbregoua were confirmed as cut marks when examined by scanning electron microscopy. The marks also show features, established through experimentation, that indicate that they had been produced shortly after death rather than a year or more later. These results, plus the "unceremonial patterns of discard in a domestic setting" seen at the site, led Villa et al. (1986:233) to reject the idea that the cuts represented preparation for secondary burial and to conclude instead that the residents of Fontbregoua had consumed "human meat." Changes in collagen chromatographs and microscopic changes in surface morphology, both indicators of cooking that might be found on bone, are lacking in the Fontbregoua remains. The absence of these indicators, plus the nature and location of the cut marks found on the bones, led Villa et al. (1986:436) to conclude that the flesh had been filleted from the bones before being roasted or otherwise prepared for consumption. This may be the most convincing osteological evidence for cannibalism reported to date.

INDIVIDUAL PROFILES

The record of trauma imprinted upon an individual skeleton may contain fascinating information, not always easily decipherable, about a lifetime of encounters with the environment and fellow humans. The partial skeleton of an adult male Neandertal, found in Shanidar Cave, Iraq, and known as Shanidar I, is a good example (Trinkaus and Zimmerman, 1982). The pattern of trauma seen in Shanidar I involves fractures of the cranium, a humerus, and a metatarsal, and degenerative changes, thought to be trauma related, in the right knee, ankle, and first metatarsal joint. All of these changes appear to have occurred at least a number of years before death. The humerus had undergone at least two fractures, a transverse fracture across the olecranon fossa and a diagonal fracture of the diaphysis approximately one-third of the way from the distal end, and the right clavicle exhibits an osteomyelitic lesion probably produced by an injury to adjacent soft tissue. The bone in the region of the diaphyseal fracture exhibits a slightly sinuous curve that was formed by the deposition of callus and extensive resorption of cortical bone around the fracture site. This fracture also produced a angular deformity that turned the distal diaphysis about 20° medially. The fracture through the trochlea shows evidence of nonunion. Because neither the distal fragment of the humerus nor anything distal to it was recovered, the possibility of amputation must also be considered. In any event, the entire bone has undergone extensive hypotrophy (during growth) or atrophy (in adulthood). The right fifth metatarsal exhibits a well-healed fracture of its diaphysis, and degenerative changes are apparent in joints of the right knee, ankle, and foot. The cranium also shows evidence of injury, the most significant being a crushing injury to the lateral side of the left orbit.

Trinkaus and Zimmerman (1982:70) consider three alternate scenarios to explain the pattern of pathology observed in Shanidar I. According to one of these, Shanidar I suffered a crushing fracture to the left orbital region that probably caused blindness in that eye. It may also have damaged the left cerebral motor cortex directly or indirectly through a localized disruption of cerebral circulation. Such an injury to the brain could cause hemiplegia to the right side of the body, affecting motor innervation to the upper limb and possibly also the lower limb. Once weakened by partial paralysis, these limbs would have been vulnerable to the trauma, infection, and degenerative pathology observed in the skeleton of Shanidar I. The very fact that he lived for many years with a severe disabling condition implies "that the Neandertals had achieved a level of societal development in which disabled individuals were well cared for by other members of the social group" (Trinkaus and Zimmerman, 1982:75).

The evidence of trauma observable on a medieval skeleton from Cox's Lane at Ipswich, England, presents a very different picture than that seen at Shanidar. Based on the appearance and location of the various lesions, Wells (1963) attempts to reconstruct the last moments of life of this individual, a well-built adult male. Assumed to have been a horseman (based on a jagged exostosis where the adductor longus inserts into the left femur and other evidence) and mounted at the time of initial contact, the first blow appears to have been delivered by sword to the pelvis (cut mark on left ilium). This was followed by a far more serious thrust to the left thigh (cut mark on left femur) delivered from below upwards as by an adversary on foot. The wound probably resulted in a severing of the main extensor muscles of the knee, rendering the leg useless and toppling the man from his horse. At this point he received a blow to the right shoulder (end of acromion sliced away) that severed his deltoid muscle so that he could no longer raise his sword arm. An attacker next cut down on his right wrist (cut and broken ends of radius and ulna), virtually amputating his hand. This was followed by a blow to the top of the head (cut mark on skull with fractures extending from each end) and what appears to have been the coup de grace, a dagger thrust deep into the chest (cut marks on adjacent borders of two ribs as the weapon passed between them). Unfortunately, there is no way to verify the accuracy of this vivid reconstruction of a medieval warrior's violent death, but it certainly is consistent with the skeletal evidence.

POPULATION STUDIES

The subject of trauma seems to lend itself better to the study of individual cases than it does to the study of populations. Sample size data is often presented in a fashion that makes it difficult to determine actual frequencies of trauma, and entire categories of trauma may be omitted or lost under inappropriate headings. Neither of these problems is easy to deal with, the first because postmortem damage and missing parts makes the determination of sample size in a skeletal series very difficult, and the second because an etiology of trauma may in some cases be difficult to establish or because of a lack of agreement on what should be included under a particular heading. Fracture is among the easier categories of trauma to deal with in a reliable and precise manner, but even here there may be difficulties in making correct identifications and establishing precise frequency rates.

An excellent attempt to deal with some of these problems is Lovejoy and Heiple's (1981) study of fractures in a Late Woodland population from the Libben site in northern Ohio. Taking great care in establishing total sample size for each of seven bones, rates of fracturing at Libben were established as follows: clavicle, 15/260 (5.8%); radius, 20/369 (5.4%); fibula, 9/257 (3.5%); ulna, 11/351 (3.1%); femur, 9/347 (2.6%); tibia, 5/349 (1.4%); and humerus, 3/450 (0.7%). Two age groups were found to be at highest risk, adolescents and young adults (15–25 years) and the elderly (45+ years). The absence of a sex factor in the younger group suggests that the fractures were more likely the result of "high activity levels (frequent and/or repetitive physical behaviors which expose the individuals to trauma, e.g., play, hunting, etc.)" rather than of warfare (Lovejoy and Heiple, 1981:539). The Libben series also lacks so-called "battered" individuals displaying multiple fractures, and only two fractures were observed in the 0–5 year age group. Almost every case of fracture had healed without marked angulation or significant reduction in length, prompting Lovejoy and Heiple (1981:540) to conclude that the people of Libben possessed "considerable knowledge and ability to care for traumatic lesions."

Fracture rates may also be studied relative to settlement patterns and means of subsistence. Making use of published data on American Indian groups, Steinbock (1976:23) observes a decreasing frequency of postcranial fractures with time, going from 9.6 to 10.7% (number of fractures/number of individuals) during the Archaic period (4000–1000 B.C.) to 5.0 to 5.4% during the Woodland period (1000 B.C.–A.D. 1000) to 1.2 to 3.9% during the Mississippian period (A.D. 1000–1600). This sequence parallels a change from a more migratory hunting-gathering way of life to a more sedentary agricultural existence. Another temporal/cultural approach to trauma, a comparison of Colonial and post-Colonial skeletons with those of modern middle-class Americans, found that "bone breaking violence has increased in America, that females are less involved, and that head and face injuries have increased" (Angel, 1976).

Evidence of trauma may also be used to reconstruct behavior at the population level, as illustrated by a study of the Sadlermiut (Merbs, 1983). This study does not limit its interest to simple counting of bone fractures, but looks at a variety of trauma-produced conditions and tries to relate them to specific activities, known or reconstructed, and environmental hazards that could have produced them. A total of 91 adults, 50 females and 41 males, were found to exhibit just ten "typical" fractures, the bones involved being the clavicle (three examples), a manual phalanx, spinous processes of two vertebrae (C7–T1), an ossified first costal cartilage, the femur, the fibula, and a metatarsal (two examples). All but two of these fractures, both involving the clavicle, occurred in males, and the only localized example of severe osteoarthritis, affecting the navicular-cuneiform articulation, was also in a male. The fractured costal cartilage, vertebral spinous processes, and clavicle in the males most likely occurred during the violent wrestling matches engaged in by the Sadlermiut, whereas the fractured clavicles in the females were more likely due to falls. The finger fracture may also have occurred during a wrestling match or on a hunting trip, the finger possibly becoming entangled in a harpoon line during retrival of a large seal or walrus. The metatarsal fractures and navicular-cuneiform osteoarthritis are seen in individuals who subject their feet to great stress. Here they may relate to some particularly hazardous terrain in the area occupied by the Sadlermiut, old beach ridges composed of sharp limestone plates. The femoral fracture, an incomplete longitudinal separation of the shaft that appears to have occurred in childhood, resulted in a distinct broadening of the shaft. It may represent a chronic stress fracture that later healed, or a "green-stick" separation resulting from pronounced torsion, but in either case it is difficult to pinpoint a specific Sadlermiut activity as the cause. The individual experiencing the fracture of the distal fibula may have been hit by the platform of his sled, an accident occasionally seen among Eskimos today. The height of the fracture corresponds exactly with the height of the sled platform. Other aspects of the total picture of trauma seen among the Sadlermiut involve tooth use, posture, riding on sleds, and a variety of other activities.

CONCLUSIONS

Trauma has clearly played a significant role in the epic of humanity, a role that can frequently be deciphered through a careful analysis of the skeleton. The evidence may be dramatic as in the case of a compound, comminuted fracture that resulted in gross bone deformity, or it may be subtle as in the case of a stress fracture just beginning to develop. It may represent nothing more than a passing annoyance as in a well-healed long bone fracture, or it can indicate the termination of life as in minute cut marks on a cervical vertebrae produced during decapitation. The most commonly noted category of skeletal trauma is fracturing of the bone with such fracturing taking a wide variety of forms. Dealing with fractures in skeletal remains must begin with a clear description of the location and nature of the fracture. The effects of fracturing must also be considered. To what extent, for example, might a fracture have disabled the person affected making it difficult or impossible to engage in normal activities? If those activities involved hunting as the sole means of providing food for a family, the effects of a disabling fracture could be catastrophic for others as well as the person actually affected. Fractures can also produce skeletal changes such as degenerative joint pathology or disuse atrophy that must be considered as part of the total picture of trauma.

The medical aspects of trauma such as "bonesetting" must also be considered. Although generally viewed as a negative phenomenon, trauma itself has also been employed as a curative technique. The most dramatic example of this is surgery, often quite skillful, performed on the skull. The techniques are now well understood, but important questions remain regarding the intent of this surgery. Trauma certainly affects the living, and it may cause death, but even the dead may be subjected to trauma. This could involve the disarticulation of the skeleton to meet the needs of particular burial practices, the smashing of bones as a form of insult or to deprive them of magical powers, or the cutting or smashing of bones to accommodate the consumption of human flesh. Serious problems may arise in distinguishing between intentional and accidental bone damage, and even when the damage is convincingly intentional, the actual intent may not be obvious. This is particularly true with respect to cannibalism, a subject in which emotionalism sometimes appears to take precedence over rational science.

Traumatic effects on the skeleton go back to the origin of the skeleton itself, and they have been a significant part of the total picture of human pathology ever since our hominid ancestors evolved from their anthropoid and prosimian forebears. Trauma due to hostile encounters with the environment and other humans, and as increasingly significant medical procedures, will also be with us as far into the future as can be foreseen.

REFERENCES

Allen WH, Merbs CF, and Birkby WH (1985) Evidence for prehistoric scalping at Nuvakwewtaqa (Chavez Pass) and Grasshopper Ruin, Arizona. In CF Merbs and RJ Miller (eds): Health and Disease in the Prehistoric Southwest. Arizona State University Anthropological Research Papers No. 34, pp 23–42.

Angel JL (1976) Colonial to modern skeletal change in the U.S.A. Am J Phys Anthropol 45:723–736.

Bennike P (1985) Palaeopathology of Danish Skeletons. Copenhagen: Akademisk Forlag.

Bennike P, Bro-Rasmussen F, and Bro-Rasmussen P (1987) Dislocation and/or congenital malformation of the shoulder joint. Observations on a mediaeval skeleton from Denmark. Anthropol Anz 45:117–129.

Bonnichsen R (1979) Pleistocene bone technology in the Beringian Refugium. National Museum of Man Mercury Series, Archaeological Survey of Canada Paper No. 89.

Borkow SE, and Kleiger B (1971) Spondylolisthesis in the newborn: A case report. Clin Ortho 81:73–76.

Briggs LC (1955) The Stone Age races of northwest Africa. American School of Prehistoric Research, Peabody Museum, Harvard University, Bulletin No. 18.

Brothwell DR (1965) Digging up Bones. London: British Museum (Natural History).

Burrows HJ (1956) Fatigue infraction of the middle of the tibia in ballet dancers. J Bone Joint Surg [Br] 38:83–94.

Burton R (1864) Notes on scalping. Anthropol Rev 2:49–52.

Cohen HR, Becker MH, and Genieser NB (1974) Fatigue fracture in Hare Krishna converts. NY State J Med 74: 1998–1999.

Cook DC (1981) Koniag Eskimo tooth ablation: Was Hrdlička right after all? Curr Anthropol 22:159–163.

Costa RL Jr (1980) Age, sex, and antemortem loss of teeth in prehistoric Eskimo samples from Point Hope and Kodiak Island, Alaska. Am J Phys Anthropol 53:579–587.

Courville CB (1965a) War wounds of the cranium in the Middle Ages. 1. As disclosed in the skeletal material from the Battle of Visby (1361). Bull Los Angeles Neurol Soc 30:27–33.

Courville CB (1965b) War wounds of the cranium in the Middle Ages. 2. As noted in the skulls of the Sedlec Ossuary near Kuttenberg, Czechoslovakia. Bull Los Angeles Neurol Soc 30:34–44.

Curzon MEJ (1978) Dental disease in Eskimo skulls in British museums. Ossa 1976–77 3/4:83–95.

Cybulski JS (1980) Skeletal remains from Lillooet, British Columbia, with observations for a possible diagnosis of skull trephination. Syesis 13:53–59.

Dart RA (1949) The predatory implemental technique of *Australopithecus*. Am J Phys Anthropol 7:1–38.

DePalma AF, and Marone PJ (1959) Spondylolysis following joint fusion. Clin Ortho 15:208–211.

Friberg S (1939) Studies on spondylolisthesis. Acta Chirop Scand 82 (Suppl 55):1–140.

Friederici G (1907) Scalping in America. Washington, DC: Annual Report of the Smithsonian Institution, 1906, pp 423–438.

Goldberg MJ (1980) Gymnastic injuries. Orthop Clin North Am 11:717–726.

Goldsmith WM (1945) Trepanation and the "Catlin Mark." Am J Antiq 10:348–352.

Gray PHK (1966) A radiographic skeletal survey of ancient Egyptian mummies. Excerpta Med Int Cong Ser 120:35–38.

Grimm H (1959) Vorgeschichtliches, fruhgeschichtliches und mittelalterliches fundmaterial zur Pathologie der Wirbesäule. Nova Acta Leopold, Band 21, Nummer 142.

Gunness-Hey M (1980) Bone mineral and histological variation with age and vertebral pathology in two human skeletal populations. Ph.D. thesis, University of Connecticut, Storrs.

Hall CF (1865) Arctic Researches and Life Among the Esquimaux. New York: Harper.

Hamperl H, and Laughlin WS (1959) Osteological consequences of scalping. Hum Biol 31:80–89.

Hilt NE, and Cogburn SB (1980) Manual of Orthopedics. St. Louis: C.V. Mosby.

Hoyme LE, and Bass WM (1962) Human skeletal remains from the Tollifero (Ha 6) and Clarksville (Mc 14) sites, John H. Kerr Reservoir Basin, Virginia. Bureau Am Ethnol Bull 182:329–400.

Hrdlička A (1940) Ritual ablation of front teeth in Siberia and America. Washington, DC: Smithsonian Miscellaneous Collections, Vol. 99, No. 3.

Jakobsen AL (1979) A cripple from the late Middle Ages. Ossa 1978 5:17–24.

Knowles AK (1983) Acute traumatic lesions. In GD Hart (ed): Disease in Ancient Man. Toronto: Clarke Irwin, pp 61–83.

Lane A (1893) Case of spondylolisthesis associated with progressive paraplegia: Laminectomy. Lancet 1:991–992.

Lisowski FP (1967) Prehistoric and early historic trepanation. In D Brothwell and AT Sandison (eds): Diseases in Antiquity. Springfield, IL: Charles C. Thomas, pp 651–672.

Lovejoy CO, and Heiple KG (1981) The analysis of fractures in skeletal populations with an example from the Libben site, Ottawa County, Ohio. Am J Phys Anthropol 55:529–541.

Majno G (1975) The Healing Hand. Cambridge, MA: Harvard University Press.

Margetts EL (1967) Trepanation of the skull by the medicine-men of primitive cultures, with particular reference to present-day native East African practice. In D Brothwell and AT Sandison (eds): Diseases in Antiquity. Springfield, IL: Charles C Thomas, pp 673–701.

Mayhall JT (1977) Cultural and environmental influences on the Eskimo dentition. In AA Dahlberg and TM Graber (eds): Orofacial Growth and Development. The Hague: Mouton, pp 215–227.

Merbs CF (1968) Anterior tooth loss in Arctic populations. Southwest J Anthropol 24:20–32.

Merbs CF (1983) Patterns of activity-induced pathology in a Canadian Inuit population. National Museum of Man Mercury Series, Archaeological Survey of Canada Paper No. 119.

Merbs CF (1985) Atlanto-occipital fusion and spondylolisthesis in an Anasazi skeleton from Bright Angel Ruin, Grand Canyon National Park, Arizona. Am J Phys Anthropol 67:381–391.

Merbs CF, and Vestergaard EM (1985) The paleopathology of Sundown, a prehistoric site near Prescott, Arizona. In CF Merbs and RJ Miller (eds): Health and Disease in the Prehistoric Southwest. Arizona State University Anthropological Research Papers No. 34, pp 85–102.

Møller-Christensen V (1958) Bogen am Aebelholt Kloster. Copenhagen: Dansk Videnskabs Forlag.

Moodie RL (1929) Surgery in pre-Columbian Peru. Studies in Paleopathology XXI. Ann Med Hist N.S. 1:698–728.

Mooney J (1910) Scalping. Bureau Am Ethnol Bull 30(2): 482–483.

Morse DF (1973) Pathology and abnormalities of the Hampson skeletal collection. In DF Morse (ed): Nodena. Arkansas Archeological Survey Public Research Series No. 4, pp 41–60.

Murad TA, and Mertz D (1982) A forensic analysis of a prehistoric vertebral column from northeastern California. Am J Phys Anthropol 57:212.

Nadeau G (1944) Indian scalping techniques in different tribes. Ciba Symp 5:1677–1681.

Nathan H (1959) Spondylolysis. J Bone Joint Surg [Am] 41: 303–320.

Neugebauer F (1881) Die Entstehung der Spondylolisthesis. Zentralbl Gynakol 5:260–261.

Neumann GK (1940) Evidence for the antiquity of scalping from central Illinois. Am Antiq 5:287–289.

Newman PH (1959) Low back pain. In R Nassim and HJ Burrows (eds): Modern Trends in Diseases of the Vertebral Column. New York: Paul E. Hoeber, pp 263–280.

Oakley KP, Brooke WMA, Akester AR, and Brothwell DR (1959) Contributions on trepanning or trephination in ancient and modern times. Man 59:93–96.

Ortner DJ, and Putschar WGJ (1981) Identification of pathological conditions in human skeletal remains. Smithsonian Contrib Anthropol 28.

Pales L, Falck E, and Lutrot J (1952) Les perforations posthumes naturelles des crânes Eskimo du Groenland. Bull Mem Soc Anthropol Paris, Serie 10 3:229–237.

Pindborg JJ, Moller IJ, and Effendi I (1975) Dental mutilations among villagers in Central Java and Bali. Community Dent Oral Epidemiol 3:190–193.

Poncins G de (1949) Eskimos. New York: Hastings House.

Reese HH (1940) The history of scalping and its clinical aspects. Yrbk Neurol Psychiatr Endocrinol, 8:3–19.

Roberts RA (1947) Chronic Structural Low Backache Due to Low-Back Structural Derangements. London: H.K. Lewis.

Roberts VL, Noyes FR, Hubbard RP, and McCabe J (1971) Biomechanics of snowmobile injuries. J Biomech 4:569–577.

Rogers SL (1973) A case of surgical amputation from aboriginal Peru. San Diego Museum of Man Ethnic Technology Notes No. 11.

Romero J (1958) Mutilaciones Dentarias, Prehispánicas de México y América en General. Mexico: Instituto Nacional de Antropologia e Historia.

Rosenberg NJ, Bargar WL, and Friedman B (1981) The incidence of spondylolysis and spondylolisthesis in nonambulatory patients. Spine 6:35–37.

Russell MD (1987a) Bone breakage in the Krapina hominid collection. Am J Phys Anthropol 72:373–379.

Russell MD (1987b) Mortuary practices at the Krapina Neandertal site. Am J Phys Anthropol 72:381–397.

Russell MD, and LeMort F (1986) Cutmarks on the Engis 2 calvaria? Am J Phys Anthropol 69:317–323.

Rytel MM (1962) Trephinations in ancient Peru. Pol Med Sci Hist Bull 5:42–45.

Savoca CJ (1971) Stress fractures: A classification of the earliest radiographic signs. Radiology 100:519–524.

Schaefer U (1957) Homo neanderthalensis (King). I. Das Skelett aus dem Neandertal. Z Morphol Anthropol 48: 268–297.

Schultz AH (1939) Notes on diseases and healed fractures of wild apes. Bull Hist Med 7:571–582.

Semon RL, and Spengler D (1981) Significance of lumbar spondylolysis in college football players. Spine 6:172–174.

Shahriaree H, Sajadi K, and Roololamini SA (1979) A family with spondylolisthesis. J Bone Joint Surg [Am] 61: 1256–1258.

Singer R (1953) Artificial deformation of teeth: A preliminary report. S Afr J Sci 50:116–122.

Stallard MC (1980) Backache in oarsmen. Br J Sports Med 14:105–108.

Steinbock RT (1976) Paleopathological Diagnosis and Interpretation. Springfield, IL: Charles C. Thomas.

Stewart TD (1935) Spondylolisthesis without separate neural arch (pseudospondylolisthesis of Junghanns). J Bone Joint Surg 17:640–648.

Stewart TD (1953) The age incidence of neural-arch defects in Alaskan natives, considered from the standpoint of etiology. J Bone Joint Surg [Am] 35:937–950.

Stewart TD (1956) Examination of the possibility that certain skeletal characters predispose to defects in the lumbar neural arches. Clin Orthop 8:44–60.

Stewart TD (1958) Stone Age skull surgery: A general review, with emphasis on the New World. Washington, DC: Annual Report of the Smithsonian Institution, 1957, pp 469–491.

Thieme FP (1950) Lumbar breakdown caused by erect posture in man. Anthropological Papers of the Museum of Anthropology, University of Michigan No. 4.

Thompson DD, Laughlin SB, Laughlin WS, and Merbs CF (1985) Bone core analysis and vertebral pathologies in Sadlermiut Eskimo skeletons. Ossa 1982–84 9/11:189–197.

Thorwald J (1962) Science and Secrets of Early Medicine. New York: Harcourt, Brace and World.

Trinkaus E (1985) Cannibalism and burial at Krapina. J Hum Evol 14:203–216.

Trinkaus E, and Zimmerman MR (1982) Trauma among the Shanidar Neandertals. Am J Phys Anthropol 57:61–76.

Turner CG II (1983) Taphonomic reconstructions of human violence and cannibalism based on mass burials in the American Southwest. In GM LeMoine and AS MacEachern (eds): A Question of Bone Technology. Proceedings of the 15th Annual Conference, Archaeological Association, University of Calgary, pp 219–240.

Tyson RA, and Alcauskas ESD (1980) Representations of surgery in ancient Peruvian art. Paper presented at the Annual Meeting of the Southwestern Anthropological Association, April 10–12, San Diego.

Ubelaker D (1978) Human Skeletal Remains. Chicago: Aldine.

Villa P, Bouville C, Courtin J, Helmer D, Mahieu E, Shipman P, Belluomini G, and Branca M (1986) Cannibalism in the Neolithic. Science 233:431–437.

Walker PL (1981) Cranial injuries as evidence for the evolution of prehistoric warfare in southern California. Am J Phys Anthropol 54:287.

Weidenreich F (1943) The Skull of *Sinanthropus Pekinensis*. Palaeontologica Sinica, New Series D. No. 10. Pehpei, Chungking: Geological Survey of China.

Weinmann JP, and Sicher H (1955) Bone and Bones: Fundamentals of Bone Biology. St. Louis: C.V. Mosby.

Wells C (1963) The human skeleton from Cox Lane, Ipswich. Proc Suffolk Inst Archaeol 29:329–333.

Wells C (1964) Bones, Bodies and Disease. London: Thames and Hudson.

West IE (1986) Forensic aspects of Lindow Man. In IM Stead, JB Bourke, and D Brothwell (eds): Lindow Man: The Body in the Bog. Ithaca: Cornell University Press, pp 77–80.

White TD (1986) Cut marks on the Bodo cranium: A case of prehistoric defleshing. Am J Phys Anthropol 69:503–509.

Wilkinson RG (1975) Techniques of ancient skull surgery. Nat Hist 84:94–101.

Wilson ES, and Katz FN (1969) Stress fracture: An analysis of 250 consecutive cases. Radiology 92:481–486.

Wiltse LL (1957) Etiology of spondylolisthesis. Clin Orthop 10:48–58.

Wiltse LL, Widell EH Jr, and Jackson DW (1975) Fatigue fracture: The basic lesion in isthmic spondylolisthesis. J Bone Joint Surg [Am] 57:17–22.

Wynne-Davies R, and Scott JHS (1979) Inheritance and spondylolisthesis. A radiographic family survey. J Bone Joint Surg [Br] 61:301–305.

Yesner DR (1981) Degenerative and traumatic pathologies of the Aleut vertebral column. Arch Calif Chirop Assoc 5:45–57.

Reconstruction of Life From the Skeleton

Chapter 10

Infectious Disease

Marc A. Kelley
Department of Sociology and Anthropology, University of Rhode Island, Kingston, Rhode Island 02881

INTRODUCTION

Perhaps more than any other category of disease, infectious disease offers the skeletal biologist insight into the interplay of disease, diet (including weaning practices), ecology, social structure, settlement pattern, plant and animal domestication, warfare, sanitation level, immunological resistance, and psychological stress. Anthropological studies of infections have tended to adopt one or more of the following complementary perspectives: 1) differential diagnosis of lesions detected in the skeletal remains of modern and ancient human beings; 2) the origin, evolution, and spread of infectious diseases, specific and general; 3) synergistic interactions between infectious disease and nutrition, medical technologies, and various other cultural practices; and 4) ecological studies of the relation of infectious diseases to the physical environment.

OSTEOPATHOLOGICAL DIAGNOSIS

The first perspective is represented by a large body of medical studies by modern clinicians outlining the key characteristics of infectious lesions in bone (e.g., Jaffe, 1972; Aegerter and Kirkpatrick, 1975; Greenfield, 1975). Paleopathologists have contributed to osteopathological diagnosis by studies of dry bone remains from modern and ancient skeletal collections (e.g., Cassidy, 1972; Buikstra, 1976, 1977; Steinbock, 1976; Buikstra and Cook, 1978; Morse, 1978; Kelley, 1979; Perzigian and Widmer, 1979; Kelley and El-Najjar, 1980; Ortner and Putschar, 1981; Jackes, 1983; Elting and Starna, 1984; Pfeiffer, 1984; Eisenberg, 1986). Studies based on dry bone remains have both advantages and disadvantages in comparison with modern clinical studies including autopsies. Many subtle bone lesions (e.g., the subtle periostitis of internal rib surfaces associated with pulmonary tuberculosis; Kelley and Micozzi, 1984) are radiographically invisible to clinicians treating living patients and are likely to be overlooked during routine autopsies. Consequently, published clinical findings on the frequency and percentage of bone involvement for a given infectious disease may not agree with frequencies detected in archaeologically derived skeletal samples. On the other hand, modern clinicians are assisted in arriving at correct diagnoses by a vast array of laboratory tests, whereas paleopathologists' diagnoses are often tentative at best (Wells, 1964). In addition, it is always possible that a pattern of inflammatory lesions encountered in an ancient sample represents an extinct clinical entity. Finally, even though bone is a very dynamic and sensitive tissue, relatively few infectious diseases produce recognizable lesions. Table 1 lists most of the infectious diseases that affect bone. Useful clinical descriptions and photographic illustrations of the bony lesions produced by these infections are avail-

TABLE 1. Major Infectious Diseases Producing Potentially Identifiable Bone Lesions

Actinomycosis	Osteomyelitis, suppurative
Blastomycosis	Periostitis, nonspecific
Brucellosis	Poliomyelitis
Coccidioidomycosis	Smallpox
Cryptococcosis	Sporotrichosis
Echinococcosis	Treponemal infection (yaws, venereal and nonvenereal syphilis)
Histoplasmosis	Tuberculosis
Leprosy	Typhoid spine
Osteomyelitis, nonsuppurative	

Selected sources: Murphy (1916), Parker (1923), Eikenbary and LeCocq (1931), Tabb and Tucker (1933), Carter (1934), Colonna and Gucker (1944), Bradlaw (1953), Hallock and Jones (1954), Meltzer et al. (1956), Cockshott and MacGregor (1958), LaFond (1958), Møller-Christensen (1961), Ganguli (1963), Huntley et al. (1963), Furcolow et al. (1966), Anderson (1969), Waldvogel et al. (1971), Jaffe (1972), Hackett (1975), Steinbock (1976), Brothwell (1981).

able in Brothwell and Sandison (1967), Steinbock (1976), Brothwell (1981), Ortner and Putschar (1981), and Zimmerman and Kelley (1982). Some of the inflammatory processes that occur in documented skeletal remains are illustrated in Figures 1–5.

EVOLUTION OF INFECTIOUS DISEASES

Infectious diseases have certainly contributed to the shaping of the hominid line over the last several million years, but, as we have seen, relatively few of them leave detectable or distinctive lesions in hard tissue. Our earliest ancestors are presumed to have been nomadic foragers living in small groups. Parasitic infestations such as body and head lice, trypanosomes, and intestinal protozoa were probably present (Polgar, 1964; Armelagos and Dewey, 1970; Cockburn, 1971; Metress, 1983). Occasional problems may have been created by diseases transmitted from wild animals to man (zoonoses) such as sleeping sickness, scrub typhus, tetanus, tularemia, and schistosomiasis (Polgar, 1964). Early foragers would have also suffered from nonspecific infections (typically those resulting from staphylococcus and streptococcus) producing identifiable periostitic and osteomyelitic lesions.

It would not have been until several million years later that the contagious diseases associated with sedentary life and large population aggregates would have posed any significant threat to our species. The first sedentary peoples, even in relatively small village settings, were exposed to human waste accumulations, and thus hepatitis and dysentery must have flourished among them. The domestication of animals would have brought exposure to anthrax, Q fever, brucellosis, psittacosis, bovine tuberculosis (Polgar, 1964; Kunitz and Euler, 1972), and perhaps echinococcosis. Agriculture would have encouraged a rise in malaria rates (Livingstone, 1958) in certain areas of the world. As population density increased, crowd-dependent pathogens such as smallpox, measles, plague, typhoid fever, influenza, diphtheria, mumps, chickenpox, and cholera emerged, often in epidemic fashion. Some of these diseases appear to require population reservoirs of 350,000 to 1,000,000 individuals (Black, 1966; Cockburn, 1967).

The placement of tuberculosis (*Mycobacterium tuberculosis*) in this evolutionary model has been controversial. Cockburn (1963:89, 1971:48) classified it as a crowd-type infection initially arising from zoonotic infection. Black (1975), however, provides evidence that tuberculosis is capable of persisting in small Amazon tribes, and McGrath's (1986) recent computer simulations support this view. Hare (1967) suggests that the tubercle bacillus *M. tuberculosis* may be a mutant of the agent of bovine tuberculosis, *M. bovis*, but the situation may be more complicated than this. Clark and associates (1987) address some of the problems concerning the evolution of mycobacteria in the New World. They stress the need for interdisciplinary collaboration among anthropologists, epidemiologists, immunologists, and microbiologists. There are at least 41 species of mycobacteria, most of which occupy watery environments. Many of the latter, known as environmental mycobacteria, may be introduced into the human body through flesh wounds, inhalation, or the drinking of infected water (host-to-host transmission is rare). The environmental mycobacteria are capable, albeit infrequently, of producing overt disease in humans. Moreover, the host may develop partial immunity or, alternatively, be rendered even more susceptible to infection by one or more of the pathogenic mycobacteria (see Clark et al., 1987, for a detailed discussion). Tuberculosis presents further complexities to medical

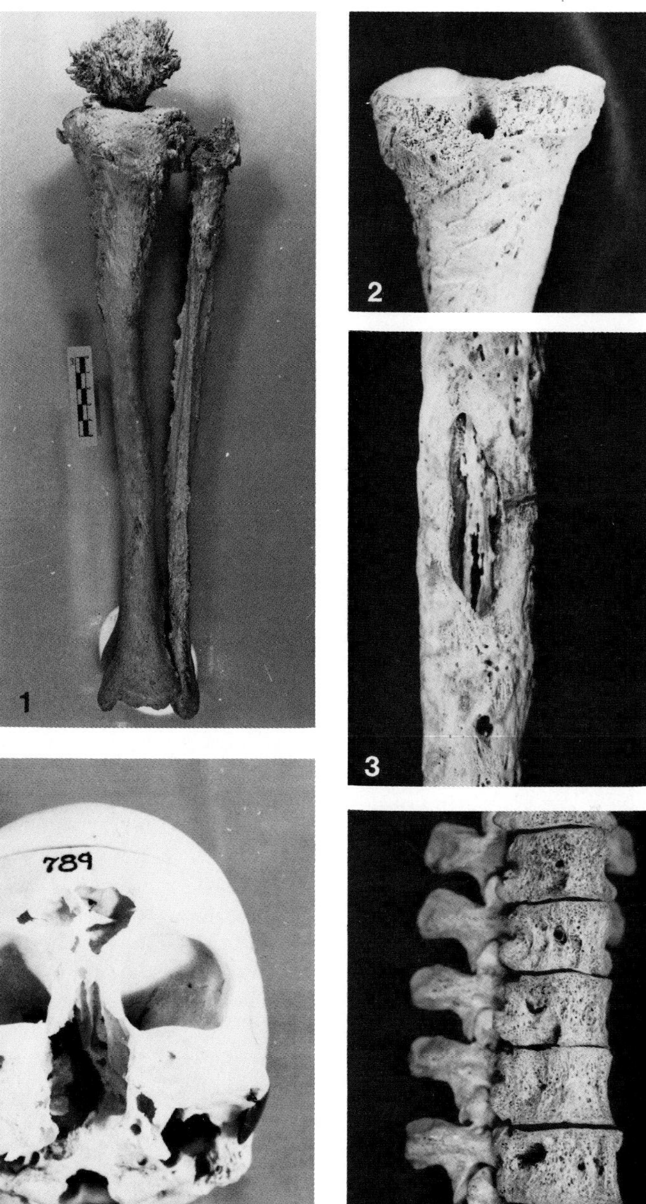

Fig. 1. Extensive nonspecific spicular periostitis of the tibia and fibula (Cleveland Museum of Natural History; Case 0.342).

Fig. 2. Chronic nonspecific suppurative osteomyelitis with large draining sinus in proximal posterior tibia (Cleveland Museum of Natural History; Case 1069).

Fig. 3. Long-standing suppurative osteomyelitis of fibular shaft. Necrotic bone fragment (sequestrum) surrounded by exuberant new bone shell (involucrum) (Cleveland Museum of Natural History; Case A1040, white male).

Fig. 4. Advanced destruction of nasal-palatal and frontal bone areas from venereal syphilis (Cleveland Museum of Natural History; white male, 54 years old).

Fig. 5. Active tuberculous involvement of multiple thoracic vertebral bodies. Smooth bone resorption and small sinuses prevail; neural arch segments are uninvolved (Cleveland Museum of Natural History; Case 1116; black male, 31 years old).

historians and paleopathologists because social disruption, alcoholism, and other variables exacerbate its incidence.

Treponemal infection has also been the subject of evolutionary study. Hudson (1963, 1965) has proposed that four syndromes—pinta, yaws, nonvenereal syphilis, and venereal syphilis—are all produced by *Treponema pallidum.* According to one scenario, yaws accompanied early foraging humans through their migrations from tropical to arid to cooler temperate environments, and the treponemes adapted by migrating to moist parts of the body. As permanent settlements appeared, endemic treponematosis in the form of nonvenereal syphilis, yaws, and pinta flourished. These infections are typically transmitted among children in a nonsexual fashion. Venereal syphilis, Hudson proposes, arose after the emergence of urban centers, when changing social patterns (including prostitution), sanitation levels, clothing, and crowding in effect altered the mode of transmission. Thus Hudson is advocating a change not in the causative treponemal microorganism (a spirochete) but in the sociocultural setting. By this logic, venereal syphilis would have emerged in various urban centers in both the Old and New Worlds. Critics of this theory ask why the treponemal syndromes produce differing degrees and patterns of skin, bone, joint, dental, vascular, and neurologic involvement.

These evolutionary models have been presented with virtually no hard data from skeletal or mummified remains to back them up; however, they probably contain a good deal of truth. By integrating findings from epidemiology, immunology, evolutionary theory, and sociocultural studies, they make an important contribution to our understanding of infectious disease.

SYNERGISTIC INTERACTIONS BETWEEN INFECTIOUS DISEASE AND CULTURAL PRACTICES

Scrimshaw (1964) suggested that episodes of acute or chronic nutritional inadequacy render the individual more susceptible to infectious disease. Conversely, infectious disease reduces the availability of nutrients, thus creating a vicious circle (Scrimshaw and Young, 1976). Detecting synergistic relationships in ancient samples is a challenging task. Mensforth et al. (1978), investigating these relationships at a prehistoric midwestern American Indian site, note a high frequency and partial overlap of periosteal reactions and porotic hyperostosis in the subadult segment of the sample. Porotic hyperostosis has been widely regarded as a bony response to iron-deficiency anemia in precontact American Indians, a conclusion with which these researchers concur. They suggest, however, that the coexistence of periosteal reactions indicates a relationship with childhood infections such as pneumonia, septicemia, otitis media, staphylococcus infection, and gastroenteritis. Thus synergism between age, diet, and infectious disease is proposed. Mensforth and associates also reach two conclusions concerning methodology: 1) age and sex assignments must be as detailed as possible and 2) skeletal lesions must be described precisely as "active" or "healed," "remodeled" or "unremodeled." Nutrition-infection synergisms may be found for adult segments of a population as well. For example, Walker (1986) suggests that pregnant and lactating females may become deficient in dietary iron or other nutrients and thus more susceptible to infection.

The interaction between infectious disease and medical care delivery systems can produce pronounced differences in disease frequency from one culture to another. Newman (1976) stresses this point in his comparison of native and introduced diseases in the New World. The pharmacopoeia of sixteenth- and seventeenth-century native Americans was probably as sophisticated as its European counterpart, but "crowd-type" introduced diseases took a staggering toll throughout the Western Hemisphere. Smallpox, measles, plague, chickenpox, and many other diseases decimated countless tribes. Newman (1976), citing Centerwall (1968), asserts that the assumed genetic susceptibility of American Indians to introduced diseases is unsubstantiated. Rather, the simultaneous affliction of young, middle-aged, and old persons in a tribe often leads to social chaos, depression, and flight of the unaffected. In this social and psychological setting, and given a medical technology ill-suited to the treatment of unfamiliar viruses and bacteria, mortality rates are often excessive.

After examining remains from a seventeenth-century Narragansett burial ground in North Kingstown, Rhode Island, in conjunction with ethnohistorical documents, I have reached similar conclusions (Kelley, 1986). New England natives suffered several devastating blows from introduced disease during the first half of the seventeenth century. William Bradford, governor of the Massachusetts Colony, described the 1633–64 smallpox epidemic that killed a large portion of the remaining Massachusett and Wampanoag Indians as follows (1970:271, emphasis mine):

> And then being very sore, *what with cold and other distempers,* they die like rotten sheep. The condition of this people was so lamentable and they fell down so generally of this disease *as they were in the end not able to help one another,* no not to make a fire nor to fetch a little water to drink, nor any to bury the dead. But would strive as long as they could, and when they could procure no other means to make fire, they would burn the wooden trays and dishes they ate their meat in, and their very bows and arrows. And some would crawl out on all fours to get a little water, and *sometimes die by the way and not be able to get in again.*

It is clear from this description that a synergism existed between smallpox and living conditions, that most tribal members fell ill simultaneously, and that they received little medical attention. Seventeenth-century European medical technology was not significantly superior to that of the native Americans, but Europeans were more knowledgeable about basic health care delivery in the case of Old World pathogens. Adequate bed rest, warmth, fluids, and emotional comfort often meant the difference between life and death; effective chemotherapy for viral infections is still wanting even today. The English eventually took pity on the ailing Indians, but it was too late.

By the mid-seventeenth century, when the North Kingstown burial ground was in use, the sweeping epidemics seem to have subsided. Instead, the Narragansetts were suffering heavily from chronic tuberculosis, pneumonia, and dysentery. Thirty percent of the individuals exhibited lesions characteristic of tuberculosis of the spine, hip, and ribs. Members of all age groups exhibited lesions, but children and adolescents appear to have been the most severely afflicted. The ethnohistorical accounts refer to pneumonia, syphilis, and dysentery (Williams, 1866). Evidence of changing diet, tobacco smoking, alcoholism, exposure to cattle, warfare with its attendant social disruption, and close contact with the colonists can also be gleaned from these documents. For example, Daniel Gookin, writing in the 1670s, remarked (1792:173, emphasis mine):

> . . . sundry of those Indian youths died, that were bred up to school among the English. The truth is, this disease is frequent among the Indians; and sundry die of it, that live not with the English. A hectick fever, issuing in a consumption, is a common and mortal disease among them. *I know some . . . have attributed it unto the great change upon their bodies, in respect of their diet, lodging, apparel, studies; so much different from what they were inured to among their own countrymen.*

It is well established that tuberculosis rates are intimately related to social and nutritional factors (Burnet and White, 1975). Thus, tuberculosis serves as a sensitive indicator of the synergism.

ECOLOGICAL STUDIES

While it must be acknowledged that culture often alters the physical environment to some degree, a focus on the role of the environment in the expression of disease is extremely important. Kunitz and Euler (1972) apply an ecological model to the pre-Columbian southwestern United States that simultaneously acknowledges the synergism between malnutrition and infectious disease. They assert that ecologic changes occurring during the twelfth and thirteenth centuries A.D. had an adverse effect on the agricultural yield of crucial proteins (beans) with eventual increases in morbidity and mortality.

Livingstone (1958) and Wiesenfeld (1967), among others, have examined the geographic distribution of the hemolytic anemias in relation to malaria and agriculture. A mutant gene producing sickled blood cells confers higher resistance to malaria for individuals with the heterozygous genotype. In West Africa, the mosquito *Anopheles gambiae* is attracted to human habitations so long as the local water supplies are not brackish, very shaded, swiftly moving, polluted, and/or alkaline (Livingstone, 1958). The clearing of forests and the introduction of agriculture provide ideal breeding grounds for these mosquitoes.

Bone changes resulting from sickle-cell anemia are generally more severe than those observed in iron-deficiency anemia. Both the cranial and postcranial bones are subject to marrow hyperplasia. The skull may exhibit the "hair-on-end" pattern, while the vertebrae often display compression of the central portions of the vertebral bodies (Steinbock, 1976). The long bones display cortical thickening and the joints, especially the hip, are vulnerable to aseptic necrosis of the femoral head.

In a similar vein, the ecological studies of May (1960) in North Vietnam illustrate the differential risk of malarial infection in the delta and in the hills. The malarial vector *Anopheles minimus* is found in the hills but poses little problem to the inhabitants, who construct their houses on stilts. The delta has no malarial vectors, and its inhabitants live in houses low to the ground. When delta people migrate to the hills and build their low-lying houses there, malaria rates increase sharply.

CASE STUDY

Ideally, anthropological research on infectious disease should incorporate elements from each of these four perspectives. Kelley and Eisenberg (1987) take such an approach to two large North American skeletal series that display similar patterns of inflammatory lesions. The series come from Mobridge, South Dakota (protohistoric Arikara, seventeenth century just prior to contact), and Averbuch, Tennessee (thirteenth and fourteenth centuries A.D.). Subsistence economies were similar at the two sites, involving horticulture, hunting, gathering, and fishing. The physical and cultural variables reconstructed for each site included mineral deficiencies, floral and faunal remains, domesticated animals, climate, shelter types, population density, occupancy patterns, and trade channels. Age and sex were ascertained for 494 individuals from Mobridge and 766 from Averbuch. All age categories from fetal remains through senescence were well represented in each series. Except for a significantly higher number of infants (neonate to 1 year) at Mobridge, the mortality profiles were quite similar.

Pathological analysis was performed for 1,260 individuals. The lesions were described with objective terminology such as "resorptive," "lytic," "proliferative," "periostitic," "fusion," "healed," and "unhealed." Fifty-nine (4.7%) individuals exhibited a pattern of inflammatory lesions. Using diagrams of the human skeleton, lesions were colored in (a different color representing resorptive, proliferative, etc.) as they occurred throughout the skeleton. The spine, ribs, tibiae, pelvis, femora, and radii were most often affected, in descending order. However, virtually any other part of the skeleton was susceptible as well. Analysis of this pathological pattern by age and sex indicates that nearly all cases occur in adults, with a peak during the third to fifth decades. Lesions predominate in males by a ratio of nearly two to one. On the basis of lesion appearance and location, differential diagnosis narrows the possible causative agents down to two: tuberculosis and blastomycosis. Figure 6 depicts the most frequent sites of skeletal inflammation for tuberculosis and blastomycosis (based on published clinical and skeletal studies) and compares these with the pattern observed at Mobridge and Averbuch. The overall pattern favors a diagnosis of blastomycosis, but a few individuals display lesions that fit the classic tuberculosis picture. It therefore seems reasonable to examine more closely the physical and cultural environmental settings at Mobridge and Averbuch.

Factors favoring tuberculosis include high population density and sedentism at Averbuch and physical crowding in Mobridge's Arikara earth lodges, which also tended to be dark, damp, and unsanitary. Other factors to be considered at Mobridge (for which there are more detailed accounts than for prehistoric Averbuch) are seasonal periods of malnutrition and close association with bison and horses, which have been known to transmit *M. bovis* to humans (Hull, 1963). Environmental factors that would have favored exposure to *Blastomyces,* a soil-borne fungus, at Averbuch and Mobridge are the location of the sites in the geographic zone for blastomycosis, the horticultural practices of these people (which would increase risk of exposure through close contact with the soil

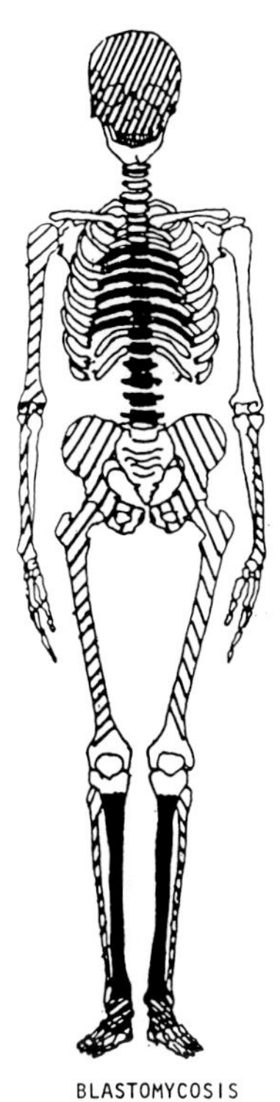

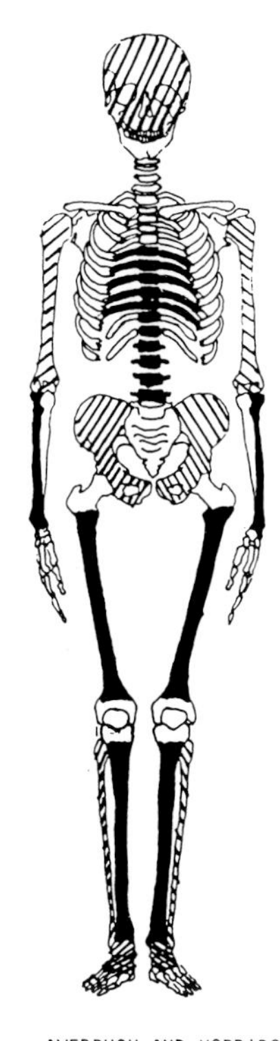

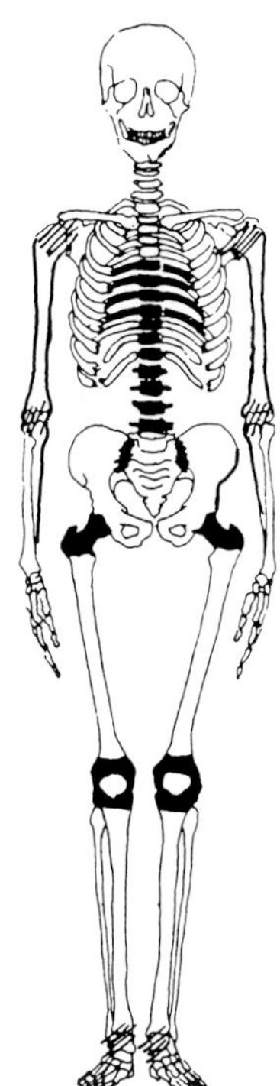

Fig. 6. Distribution of skeletal lesions. Darker shades indicate more common involvement.

and/or decaying wood), seasonal movements over extensive terrain, and, for the Arikara, the possibility of transmission from horse to man. Unlike tuberculosis, which often favors subadults, blastomycosis is age progressive, with individuals between 20 and 50 years old most often being affected. In modern clinical studies, males are affected six to ten times more often than females.

Thus environmental data offer support for the possible existence of both diseases. The skeletal remains favor blastomycosis, but it is certainly possible that some cases of tuberculosis are "hidden" in the sample. Placing all 59 individuals under one etiological heading, therefore, may be too parsimonious; both blastomycosis and tuberculosis were probably contributing to morbidity and mortality at these sites.

CONCLUSIONS

In summary, the anthropological study of infectious disease, both in modern times and, especially, in antiquity, is complex and challenging. The interplay of many variables—host resistance, pathogen virulence, cultural practices, ecological settings, malnutrition, crowding—needs to be considered. Accurate interpretation is dependent on proper methodology: adequate sample size, accurate age and sex determination, use of objective terminology for lesions, careful recording of lesion location and distribution, and reconstruction of the physical and cultural environments as completely as is possible.

REFERENCES

Aegerter E, and Kirkpatrick JA Jr (1975) Orthopedic Diseases. Philadelphia: W.B. Saunders.

Anderson JG (1969) Studies in the mediaeval diagnosis of leprosy in Denmark. Dan Med Bull 16(Suppl):1–142.

Armelagos GJ, and Dewey JR (1970) Evolutionary response to human infectious diseases. Bioscience 157: 638–644.

Black FL (1966) Measles endemicity in insular populations: Critical community size and its evolutionary implication. J Theor Biol 11:202–211.

Black FL (1975) Infectious diseases in primitive societies. Science 187:515–518.

Bradford W (1970) Of Plymouth Plantation 1620–1647. New York: Alfred A. Knopf.

Bradlaw RV (1953) The dental stigmata of prenatal syphilis. Oral Surg 6:147–158.

Brothwell DR (1981) Digging Up Bones, 3rd Ed. Ithaca: Cornell University Press.

Brothwell DR, and Sandison AT (eds) (1967) Diseases in Antiquity. Springfield, IL: Charles C Thomas.

Buikstra JE (1976) The Caribou Eskimo: General and specific disease. Am J Phys Anthropol 45:351–367.

Buikstra JE (1977) Differential diagnosis: An epidemiological model. Yrbk Phys Anthropol 20:316–328.

Buikstra J, and Cook DC (1978) Pre-Columbian tuberculosis: An epidemiological model. MCV Quarterly 14(1):32–44.

Burnet M, and White DO (1975) Natural History of Infectious Disease, 4th Ed. New York: Cambridge University Press.

Carter RA (1934) Infectious granulomas of bones and joints, with special reference to occidioidal granulomas. Radiology 23(1):1–16.

Cassidy CM (1972) A comparison of nutrition and health in pre-agricultural and agricultural Amerindian skeletal populations. Ph.D. dissertation, University of Wisconsin.

Centerwall WR (1968) A recent experience with measles in a "virgin-soil" population. PAHO Science Publication No. 165.

Clark GA, Kelley MA, Grange J, and Hill MC (1987) The evolution of mycobacterial disease in human populations. Curr Anthropol 28(1):45–62.

Cockburn TA (1963) The Evolution and Eradication of Infectious Diseases. Baltimore: Johns Hopkins University Press.

Cockburn TA (ed) (1967) Infectious Diseases: Their Evolution and Eradication. Springfield, IL: Charles C Thomas.

Cockburn TA (1971) Infectious diseases in ancient populations. Curr Anthropol 12:45–62.

Cockshott P, and MacGregor M (1958) Osteomyelitis variolosa. Q J Med 27:369–387.

Colonna PC, and Gucker T (1944) Blastomycosis of the skeletal system. J Bone Joint Surg [Am] 26:322–328.

Eikenbary CF, and LeCocq JF (1931) Osteomyelitis variolosa. JAMA 96:584–587.

Eisenberg LE (1986) Adaptation in a "marginal" Mississippian population from middle Tennessee: Biocultural insights from paleopathology. Ph.D. dissertation, New York University.

Elting JJ, and Starna WA (1984) A possible case of pre-Columbian treponematosis from New York State. Am J Phys Anthropol 65:267–273.

Furcolow ML, Balows A, Menges RW, Pickar D, McClellan JT, and Saliba A (1966) Blastomycosis. JAMA 198:529–532.

Ganguli PK (1963) Radiology of Bone and Joint Tuberculosis. New York: Asia Publishing House.

Gookin D (1792) Historical collection of Indians of New England. Mass Hist Soc Coll Series 1:141–226.

Greenfield GB (1975) Radiology of Bone Diseases, 2nd Ed. Philadelphia: J.B. Lippincott.

Hackett CJ (1975) An introduction to diagnostic criteria of syphilis, treponarid and yaws (treponematoses) in dry bones, and some implications. Virchows Arch [Pathol Anat] 368:229–241.

Hallock H, and Jones JB (1954) Tuberculosis of the spine. J Bone Joint Surg [Am] 36:219–240.

Hare R (1967) The antiquity of diseases caused by bacteria and viruses, a review of the problem from a bacteriologist's point of view. In DR Brothwell and AT Sandison (eds): Diseases in Antiquity. Springfield, IL: Charles C Thomas, pp 115–131.

Hudson EH (1963) Treponematosis and anthropology. Ann Intern Med 58:1037–1048.

Hudson EH (1965) Treponematosis and man's social evolution. Am Anthropol 67:885–901.

Hull TG (1963) Diseases Transmitted from Animals to Man, 5th Ed. Springfield, IL: Charles C Thomas.

Huntley BE, Phillip RN, and Maynard JE (1963) Survey of brucellosis in Alaska. J Infect Dis 112:100–106.

Jackes MK (1983) Osteological evidence for smallpox: A possible case from seventeenth century Ontario. Am J Phys Anthropol 60:75–81.

Jaffe HL (1972) Metabolic, Degenerative, and Inflammatory Diseases of Bones and Joints. Philadelphia: Lea and Febiger.

Kelley MA (1979) Skeletal changes produced by aortic aneurysms. Am J Phys Anthropol 51:35–38.

Kelley MA (1986) Disease, warfare and population decline among seventeenth century New England Indians. Paper presented at Peoples in Contact: Indians and Europeans in the Seventeenth Century, Haffenraffer Museum of Anthropology, Bristol, RI, September 27.

Kelley MA, and Eisenberg LE (1987) Blastomycosis and tuberculosis in early American Indians: A biocultural view. Midcont J Archaeol 12:89–116.

Kelley MA, and El-Najjar MY (1980) Natural variation and differential diagnosis of skeletal changes in tuberculosis. Am J Phys Anthropol 52:153–167.

Kelley MA, and Micozzi MS (1984) Rib lesions in chronic pulmonary tuberculosis. Am J Phys Anthropol 65:381–386.

Kunitz SJ, and Euler RC (1972) Aspects of southwestern paleoepidemiology. Tucson, AZ: Prescott College Anthropology Reports No. 2.

LaFond EM (1958) An analysis of adult skeletal tuberculosis. J Bone Joint Surg [Am] 40:346–364.

Livingstone FB (1958) Anthropological implications of sickle cell gene distribution in West Africa. Am Anthropol 60:533–562.

May J (1960) The ecology of human disease. Ann NY Acad Sci 84:789–794.

McGrath JW (1986) A computer simulation of the occurrence of tuberculosis in prehistoric North America. Am J Phys Anthropol 69:238 (abstract).

Meltzer HL, Kovacs L, Oxford T, and Matas M (1956) Echinococcus in North American Indians and Eskimos. Can Med Assoc J 75:121–128.

Mensforth RP, Lovejoy CP, Lallo JW, and Armelagos GJ (1978) The role of constitutional factors, diet, and infectious disease in the etiology of porotic hyperostosis and periosteal reactions in prehistoric infants and children. Med Anthropol 2(1):1–59.

Metress SP (1983) The changing patterns of human disease. Collegium Anthropol 7:189–194.

Møller-Christensen V (1961) Bone Changes in Leprosy. Copenhagen: Munksgaard.

Morse D (1978) Ancient Disease in the Midwest, 2nd Ed. Springfield, IL: Charles C Thomas.

Murphy JB (1916) Bone and joint disease in relation to typhoid fever. Surg Gynecol Obstet 23:119–125.

Newman MT (1976) Aboriginal New World epidemiology and medical care and the impact of Old World disease imports. Am J Phys Anthropol 45:672–677.

Ortner DJ, and Putschar WGJ (1981) Identification of pathological conditions in human skeletal remains. Smithsonian Contrib Anthropol 28.

Parker CA (1923) Actinomycosis and blastomycosis of the spine. J Bone Joint Surg 5:759–777.

Perzigian AJ, and Widmer L (1979) Evidence for tuberculosis in a prehistoric population. JAMA 241:2643–2646.

Pfeiffer S (1984) Paleopathology in an Iroquoian ossuary, with special reference to tuberculosis. Am J Phys Anthropol 65:181–189.

Polgar S (1964) Evolution and the ills of mankind. In S Tax (ed): Horizons of Anthropology. Chicago: Aldine, pp 200–211.

Scrimshaw NS (1964) Ecological factors in nutritional disease. Am J Clin Nutr 14:112–122.

Scrimshaw NS, and Young VR (1976) The requirements of human nutrition. Sci Am 235 (September):51–64.

Steinbock RT (1976) Paleopathological Diagnosis and Interpretation. Springfield. IL: Charles C Thomas.

Tabb JL, and Tucker JT (1933) Actinomycosis of the spine. Am J Roentgenol Radium Ther 29:628–634.

Waldvogel FA, Medoff G, and Schwartz MN (1971) Osteomyelitis. Springfield. IL: Charles C Thomas.

Walker PL (1986) Porotic hyperostosis in a marine-dependent California Indian population. Am J Phys Anthropol 69:345–354.

Wells C (1964) Bones, Bodies, and Disease: Evidence of Disease and Abnormality in Early Man. London: Thames and Hudson.

Wiesenfeld SL (1967) Sickle-cell trait in human biological and cultural evolution. Science 157:1134–1140.

Williams R (1866) A key into the language of America. In JH Trumbull (ed): Publications of the Narragansett Club, 1st series, 1. Providence. (First published in London, 1643.)

Zimmerman MR, and Kelley MA (1982): Atlas of Human Paleopathology. New York: Praeger.

Reconstruction of Life From the Skeleton

Chapter 11

Nutritional Deficiency Diseases: A Survey of Scurvy, Rickets, and Iron-Deficiency Anemia

P. L. Stuart-Macadam
Department of Anthropology, University of Toronto, Toronto, Ontario M5S 1A1, Canada

INTRODUCTION

Nutrition is a critical factor in the dynamic interrelationship between a population and its environment. However, assessing the nutritional status of archaeological populations can be particularly difficult. The comprehensive data required by modern clinicians are simply not available, and the nature of bone means that its response to stress can be quite limited. Despite this challenge, anthropological research over the past few years has increasingly focused on methods and techniques for determining the nutrition of past human populations (Hush-Ashmore et al., 1982; Martin et al., 1985). Researchers have utilized a number of skeletal indicators of dietary stress to assess nutritional status. While this is an important approach, much can also be gained by comprehensive analyses of specific nutritional deficiencies, which would include consideration of the physiology and metabolism of the relevant nutrient as well as examination of historical, clinical, radiographic, and archaeological data. This approach can stimulate new ideas and insights into the interaction between a population and its environment. To illustrate this approach, a comprehensive survey of three deficiency diseases—scurvy, rickets, and iron-deficiency anemia—is presented in this chapter.

Scurvy, rickets, and iron-deficiency anemia are often thought of as simple dietary deficiency diseases. The true story, however, is much more complex and intriguing and illustrates how diseases are woven into the fabric of a sociocultural context. These three diseases owe more to ideas, customs, or circumstance than they do to undernutrition. Certainly nutrition is involved, but the end product of the disease is the result of a complex interaction of cultural, physiological, and dietary factors. All three diseases can leave their mark on bone, making it possible for the physical anthropologist to assess how past populations were affected. All three diseases also have a fascinating history, which can be traced from the time of the first written documents. This chapter presents the story of scurvy, rickets, and iron-deficiency anemia, using historical, medical, and anthropological information to create a picture of each disease and its effect on people in the past.

SCURVY

Scurvy is produced by a deficiency of ascorbic acid (vitamin C). Vitamin C is necessary for a number of metabolic processes, but it is particularly important in the formation of collagen, the major structural protein of the body. Scurvy is a condition that can affect all age groups, but throughout history, as a direct result of social and cultural factors, those most commonly affected have been infants and men. It is unusual for scurvy to develop under "normal" living conditions; usually it is associated with natural or social disasters or specific culturally derived behaviors. Because the body is able to store the vitamin, it can take an adult several months on a vitamin C-deficient diet to develop the symptoms of scurvy. In children, however, because of the demands of growth, symptoms develop much more rapidly.

Vitamin C is the only vitamin required in the diet of humans that is not required by most other animal species. Only humans and other primates, guinea pigs, a fruit-eating bat from India, the red-vented bulbul of Turkey, and several species of trout and salmon do not have the enzyme necessary to synthesize vitamin C (Hodges, 1980). Vitamin C protects, regulates, and facilitates the catalytic and biologic processes of other enzyme systems (Hodges, 1980). Its most important function is its role in collagen formation: vitamin C is necessary for the hydroxylation of proline to hydroxyproline, one of the important amino acids in collagen. Collagen is the main protein component of connective tissue, including skin, cartilage, and bone. A deficiency of vitamin C leads to a reduction in the formation of osteoid, the organic matrix of bone, a general weakness of connective tissues, and a hemorrhagic diathesis. This weakness of the connective tissues is vividly described in a 1748 account of a circumnavigation by the ship's chaplain, Richard Walter (Bourne, 1971):

> At other times the whole body, but more especially the legs, were subject to ulcers of the worst kind, attended with rotten bones, and such a luxuriance of fungous flesh, as yielded no remedy. But a most extraordinary circumstance, and what would be scarcely credible upon any single evidence, is that the scars of wounds which had for many years healed, were found open again by this violent distemper: of this, there was a remarkable instance in one of the invalids upon the Centurian who had been wounded about fifty years earlier in the Battle of Boyne (1690); for although he was cured soon after, and had continued well for a great number of years past, yet on his being attacked by the scurvy, his wounds, in the progress of his disease, broke out afresh, and appeared as if they had never been healed. Nay, what is still more astonishing, the callous of the broken bone, which had been completely formed for a long time, was found to be hereby dissolved, and the fracture seemed as if it had been consolidated.

Clinical and Radiographic Picture

Scurvy in infants commonly occurs when they are between 5 and 24 months of age, with a peak between 8 and 11 months (Goodhart and Shils, 1980). Predisposing factors are prematurity or twin birth, infections, and, above all, feeding with prepared infant foods and condensed milk. The signs of infantile scurvy are pain and tenderness of the extremities, immobility, crying when touched or even approached, and the drawing up of the legs in a froglike position (Park et al., 1935). The lower limbs, especially the thighs, are particularly affected (Fig. 1). There is also pallor, wasting, edema of limbs, fretfulness, irritability, and disruption of the dentition. Other signs are bruising, prominence of the ribs at the costochondral junction (beading), enlargement of the joints, especially the wrists and ankles, and swelling of the gums if the teeth have erupted (Holmes et al., 1973). In advanced cases there can be infraction (incomplete fractures) and fractures at the metaphyses of the long bones. Hemorrhage can occur in the subcutaneous tissues, intestinal tract, gums (if the teeth have erupted), and particularly over the bones. The subperiosteal hemorrhages tend to occur more at the rapidly growing ends of the long bones of the lower limbs, the ribs, and occasionally the skull vault and orbit (Harris, 1933). Enlargement of cartilage at shaft junctions, especially at wrists and ankles, can also occur. The hemorrhages and bone changes that occur are usually symmetrical in distribution. Children with vitamin C deficiency are especially susceptible to infections, resulting in otitis media, pneumonia, diphtheria, and other problems such as digestive disturbances and general debility (Jaffe, 1972).

The earliest sign in adult scurvy is a change in the complexion, which becomes sallow or

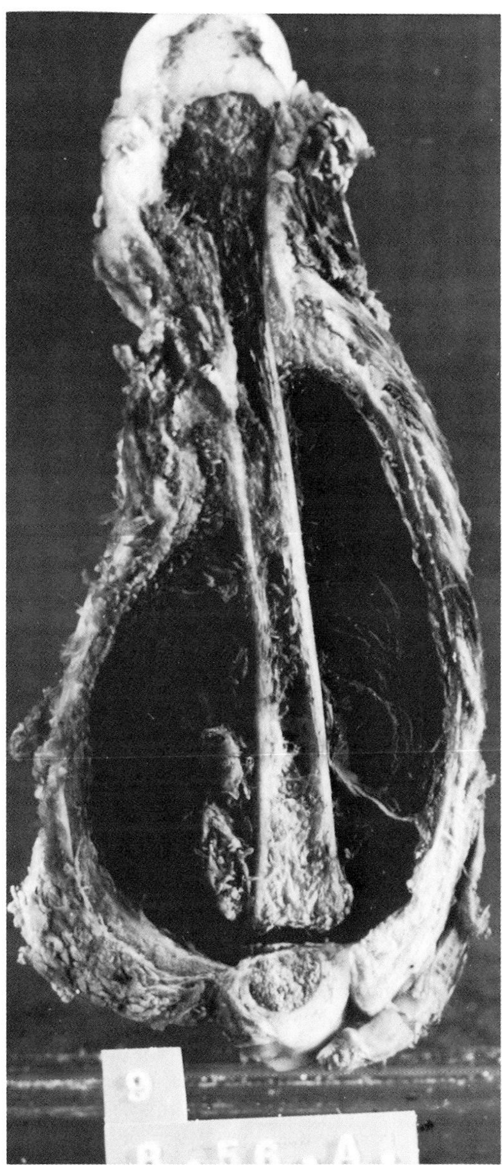

Fig. 1. Infant scurvy, right femur. (Photo courtesy of Dr. Don Ortner, Smithsonian Institution.)

muddy. There is general malaise and fleeting pains in the joints and limbs, especially the legs (Hess, 1920). A few minute hemorrhagic spots appear on the skin (petechiae), followed by swanlike deformities of hairs (follicular hyperkeratosis), mainly on the buttocks, thighs, and calves (Goodhart and Shils, 1980). The gums become sore, spongy, and bleed easily, and the teeth may loosen and fall out. Hemorrhages may occur anywhere on the body, but are most common in the gums (if the teeth are present), on the skin, and beneath the periosteum of bones and synovia of joints (Holmes et al., 1973). The sites of minor trauma are more vulnerable, so subperiosteal hemorrhages are more commonly found on the tibia, femur, and ramus of the lower jaw (Hess, 1920). Subperiosteal hemorrhages are less common in adults than they are in children; in one study they were found in only 10% of cases of adult scurvy (Harris, 1933).

A description by Father Antonia de la Ascension in 1602 gives a graphic account of adult scurvy (Carpenter, 1986):

> The first symptom they notice is a pain in the whole body which makes it so sensitive to touch . . . After this, all the body, especially from the waist down, becomes covered with purple spots larger than great mustard seeds . . . The sensitiveness of the bodies of these sick people is so great that . . . the best aid which can be rendered them is not even to touch the bed clothes . . . the upper and lower gums of the mouth in the inside of the mouth and outside the teeth, become swollen to such a size that neither the teeth nor the molars can be brought together. The teeth become so loose and without support that they move while moving the head . . . they come to be so weakened in this condition that their natural vigor fails them, and they die all of a sudden, while talking.

Radiographic changes in both infantile and adult scurvy reflect a pattern of reduced formation, but continued resorption of bone matrix, as well as hemorrhage. Bone undergoing active growth is much more vulnerable, so the child experiences more severe bone change than the adult.

In infantile scurvy the bones most affected are those involved in rapid growth; these are the sternal ends of the ribs, distal ends of the femur, proximal end of the humerus, both ends of the tibia and fibula, and distal ends of the radius and ulna (Caffey, 1978). Changes include generalized bone atrophy and a thickening and increased density of the provisional zone of mineralization of the metaphyses, which may appear as bone spurs. Caffey (1978) considers these bone changes to be pathognomonic of juvenile scurvy. The increased brittleness of the metaphyseal zone may result in infraction, giving an appearance of metaphyseal cupping (Greenfield, 1975). The primary spongiosa of the metaphyses become sparse and appear as a zone of radiolucence known as the Trummerfeld zone or scurvy line. The trabeculae of the shaft and the cortex atrophy, sometimes resulting in a cortex one-quarter or one-fifth of its original thickness (Caffey, 1985). The ossification centers of the epiphyses and small bones show a dense, sharply demarcated ring of mineralization called the Wimberger's sign. Enlargement of the costochondral junction also occurs and is most marked in the fifth, sixth, and seventh ribs (Park et al., 1935).

With healing of the disease, there is increased thickening of the cortex as well as increased definition of the trabeculae. The thickened provisional zone of mineralization becomes progressively buried within the shaft as growth proceeds; it appears as a transverse line of density. The epiphyseal ossification center may exhibit a central area of osteopenia (lack of density) that persists for years after the onset of healing (Caffey, 1985). New periosteal bone, which has been stimulated by the presence of the hematomas, settles onto the shaft and thickens the cortex. This thickening may remain for many years, particularly on the concavities of the posterior aspects of the femur (Caffey, 1985).

In adults, radiographic findings of scurvy include osteoporosis and periosteal bone formation as the result of hemorrhage (Jaffe, 1972). The osteoporosis is most prominent in the axial skeleton, and in the long bones of the lower limbs. The changes in the vertebral column simulate clinical osteoporosis, and compressional collapse of one or more vertebrae is common (Jaffe, 1972). In the long bones there may be cortical thinning associated with slight periosteal new bone growth.

History

The word "scurvy" first appeared in English publications in the 1580s, where it was referred to as "scarby" or "skurvie." In 1582 the secretary of an expedition to the West Indies wrote in his diary that "the more exercise within reason the better, for if you once fall to laziness and sloth, then the scarby is ready to catch you by the bones and will shake out every tooth in your head" (Carpenter, 1986). The word can be traced back further to *scorbutus,* a Latinized version of the Danish word *scorbuck,* to even earlier Scandinavian forms of *skjoerbug* and *skörbjugg,* and finally to the Old Icelandic *skyrbûgr,* which is believed to mean "cut (or ulcerated) swellings" (Carpenter, 1986).

Scurvy, as a clinical entity, was not known to Greek, Roman, or Arab physicians, although in retrospect it is possible to recognize some early descriptions of the disease. One of the earliest recorded episodes of scurvy is thought to have affected French soldiers who spent the winter of 1249–1250 in Egypt fighting the Saracens. By the end of the Middle Ages, sailors began to make long voyages of discovery from western Europe to unknown lands, and it was at this time that definite references to scurvy began to appear. In 1497 Vasco da Gama led an expedition to the West Indies. After about six months at sea, many of the men fell ill, "their hands and feet swelling, and their gums growing over their teeth so they could not eat" (Carpenter, 1986). By the sixteenth century, scurvy began to be mentioned more frequently, mainly in connection with wars, sea voyages, or institutions such as orphanages and prisons. Between 1560 and 1600 a number of Dutch and German physicians wrote about scurvy. It seemed to be a common disease at that time in the damper parts of Holland, especially during the rainy season. At sea it became a problem of immense proportions. In 1590 an English sea captain, Sir Richard Hawkins, said that in his 20 years at sea he could give account of 10,000 men consumed with scurvy (Carpenter, 1986). It was not uncommon for as many as one-half to four-fifths of a crew to die of scurvy during a single long voyage (Henschen, 1966).

James Lind was a Scot who served as surgeon's mate in the Royal Navy and who for nine years observed the horrors of scurvy firsthand (Evans, 1982). He tested six different treatments on a group of 12 sailors with scurvy, concluding that oranges and lemons were the most effective remedy. This fact seems to have been known, but repeatedly forgotton or ignored, since the earliest recorded cases of scurvy. Lind became famous for his treatise on scurvy, which was published in 1753. He discussed some of the many suspected causes of scurvy, which included heredity, an infected nurse, tobacco smoking, salted foods, cold wet climates, or the immoderate use of sugar.

Thousands of cases of scurvy occurred in Britain during the great potato famine of 1845 to 1848, and it was prevalent among miners in the California gold rush of 1848 to 1850. One of the cures favored by the miners was burial up to the neck in the earth; it was believed that because sailors were miraculously cured when they reached land there must be some curative property inherent in the earth itself. Scurvy was also common during the Crimean War and the American Civil War.

Scurvy in children did not receive much attention in the early medical literature. It could have been that there were problems in recognizing the condition as a distinct clinical entity, or perhaps it was simply not common. Between 1590 and 1640 scurvy was reported in children in French charitable institutions, and in 1596, in children in a London hospital (Carpenter, 1986). The first clear description of infantile scurvy was given by Francis Glisson in 1650. He was also the first to differentiate between scurvy and rickets, a disease that was often associated with scurvy. Over the next 200 years there were only a few references to infantile scurvy. In 1883 Barlow wrote a classic paper that differentiated scurvy from rickets and gave a good description of the clinical symptoms of scurvy. At about this time, infantile scurvy became an increasing problem in Europe and North America (Follis, 1958); this was directly related to the introduction of milk pasteurization and proprietary baby foods. Babies who were not breast-fed, but were instead given condensed or pasteurized milk and other processed baby foods, were very susceptible to scurvy. These infants were mainly the offspring of well-off parents who could afford such products. Infantile scurvy again became a health problem between 1945 and 1965, particularly in Canada. At that time it affected infants of lower-income, poorly educated parents, who were feeding their infants evaporated milk. Scurvy is now seen mainly in old men with monotonous diets that do not include fresh fruits and vegetables; in individuals with general undernutrition, perversions of appetite, or who are following dietary fads; or in association with some other disease such as chronic diarrhea.

Archaeological Evidence

Evidence for scurvy in the paleopathological literature is rare. Møller-Christensen (1958) diagnosed the condition in 28 of 800 skeletons from the Aebelholt monastery in Denmark on the basis of bone and tooth lesions. He found scurvy to be present in men three times as often as in women (cf. Wells, 1975). Wells (1975) found some evidence for scurvy in seven of 350 (2.0%) of individuals from an Anglo-Saxon site in East Anglia, England. He felt that there were many examples of scurvy in medieval cemeteries in Britain, based on the presence of edentulous jaws and alveolar osteitis (Wells, 1964). Saul (1972) diagnosed scurvy in a number of individuals from the pre-Columbian Mayan site of Altar de Sacrificios in Guatemala. His criterion was the combination of premortem tooth loss and periostitis of long bone diaphyses. Ortner (1984) described a probable case of scurvy in a child of about 8 years of age from Metlatavik, on the Seward Peninsula of Alaska (Fig. 2). The site was dated to somewhere between the late nineteenth and the early twentieth centuries. Ortner suggested that the late date of this specimen would have meant that contact with whites had occurred. The changing of food patterns that resulted would have upset the normal balance between vitamin C requirements and the evolved diet of the Eskimos. Roberts (1987) describes a possible case of scurvy in a young child from a late Iron Age/early Roman site in Worcestershire, England.

A study by Maat (1982) provides a unique opportunity to understand skeletal changes in scurvy. He was able to examine the skeletal remains of 50 Dutch whalers who had been excavated from a cemetery on the Arctic island of Zeeusche Uytkyck. This cemetery had been in use from 1642 until the end of the eighteenth century, and because of the polar conditions bone preservation was excellent and the effects of scurvy could still be observed even after a

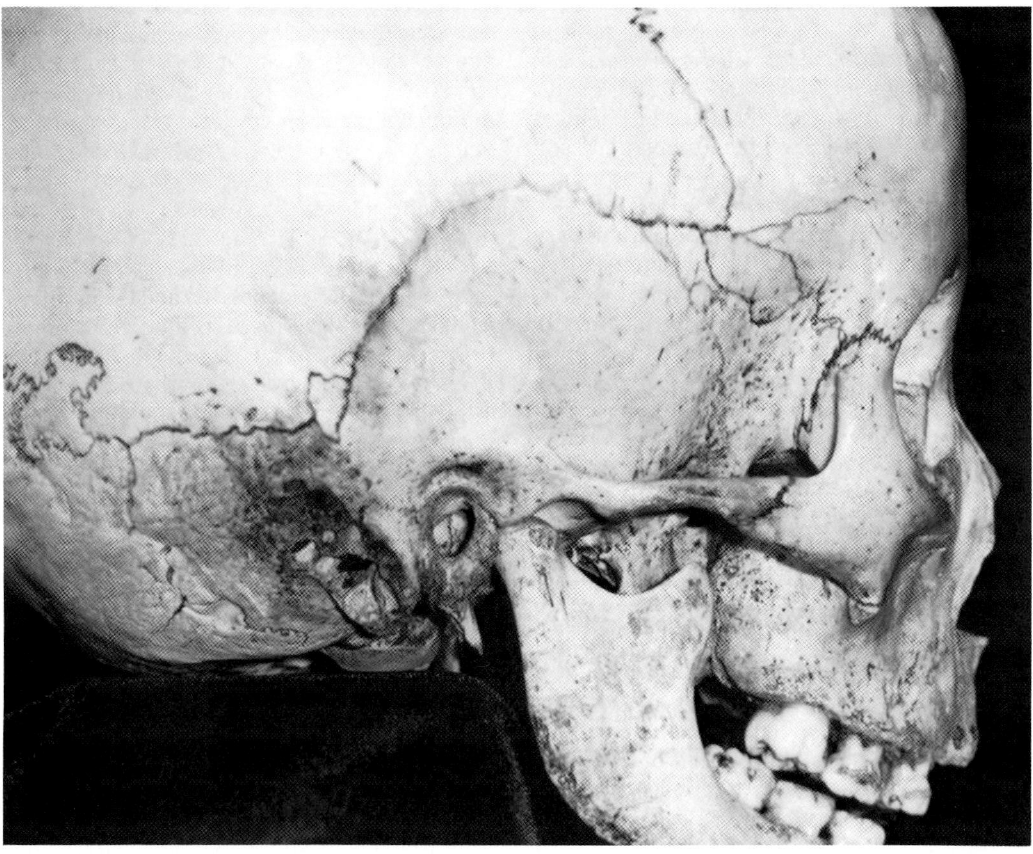

Fig. 2. Possible scurvy in 8-year-old child, Metlatavik, Alaska. (Photo courtesy of Dr. Don Ortner, Smithsonian Institution.)

time lapse of 200 to 350 years (Maat, 1982). Historical records indicate that scurvy had been a major problem for the men on these whaling expeditions; scurvy would begin to appear seven to eight months after leaving Holland. Maat was able to observe hemarthroses (bleeding into a joint), infractions with subperiosteal hematomas, periodontal bleeding, and resorption of alveolar bone. Thirty-nine of the 50 whalers showed features of scurvy; of these, all 39 showed hemarthroses of the lower ex tremities, particularly the ankles and knees. The tibia and fibula were the most common bones to exhibit infractions with subperiosteal hematoma. Usually these features were bilateral in distribution.

Only one individual showed obvious signs of healed scurvy; there were many bilateral depositions of periosteal bone. Because Maat found that alveolar resorption was present in some individuals without obvious scurvy, he did not consider that this feature could be accepted as a reliable diagnostic feature. Infractions with subperiosteal hematoma were most often found at areas that were subject to physical stress, such as the insertions of muscles and fascias.

RICKETS

Rickets is a disease of infancy and childhood that is characterized by mineralization failure in growing cartilage and bone. It is caused mainly by insufficient vitamin D, either because of a dietary inadequacy or because of a lack of exposure to short ultraviolet rays of sunlight. Studies have shown that the most important source of vitamin D is exposure to sunlight (Poskitt et al., 1979), not dietary intake. It is thought that as much as 90% of the vitamin in our bodies is produced by photosynthesis in the skin (Passmore and Eastwood, 1986). There are few sources of vitamin D in foods, especially in the winter, with the exception of some dairy products and fish. The best dietary source is fish oil. Fish, unlike mammals, birds, reptiles, and amphibians, can synthesize vitamin D without ultraviolet light (Loomis, 1970). There are many factors involved in any one individual's susceptibility to rickets, including growth velocity, ray-filtering power of the atmosphere (latitude, pollution levels), customs (type of clothing, time spent outdoors), quantities and ratios of calcium and phosphorous in the diet, and unknown constitutional factors (Caffey, 1978).

There are two principal types of vitamin D—calciferol (D2) and cholecalciferol (D3)—as well as a number of metabolites. D2 is produced by ultraviolet irradiation of ergosterol and is of plant origin, whereas D3 is produced by the action of ultraviolet light on 7-dehydrocholesterol and is of animal origin (Mankin, 1974). 7-Dehydrocholesterol is synthesized in the human body and deposited in the skin, where it can then undergo photosynthesis to produce vitamin D3. However, it is the metabolites of vitamin D2 and D3, produced by conversion of D2 and D3 in the liver and kidneys, that are biologically active and critical in bone metabolism. One of these metabolites, 1,25-dihydroxycholecalciferol, has been identified as the principal hormone acting in the intestine and possibly in bone cells. It is of crucial importance in calcium and phosphate transport in the body and their absorption by the intestine (Mankin, 1974). Parathormone and calcitonin are two other hormones responsible for maintenance of normal calcium and phosphorous levels in the body.

The sequence of events that occurs in the absence of sufficient vitamin D, for whatever reason, proceeds as follows. Without the precursors of the biologically active metabolites of vitamin D, insufficient 1,25-dihydroxycholecalciferol is produced. This results in a diminished absorption and transport of calcium and phosphates, eventually triggering a negative feedback that results in an increased production of parathormone (Mankin, 1974). Parathormone increases serum levels of calcium and phosphorous by activating bone cells (osteoclasts) to destroy bone, thus liberating the bone mineral. Bone formation is also increased in a futile attempt to substitute quantity for quality. However, with insufficient vitamin D, the osteoid (organic matrix of bone) produced by the bone cells (osteoblasts) and the cartilage produced by the cartilage-forming cells (chondroblasts) are not properly mineralized. This results in an excess of unmineralized cartilage at the growing ends of bones as well as bones that are smaller, lighter, and susceptible to deformation under pressure.

Clinical and Radiographic Picture

Clinically, rickets is most commonly seen during periods of rapid growth; that is, between the ages of 6 months and 3 years and during puberty (Passmore and Eastwood, 1986). It also occurs frequently and at an early age in premature infants, again as a result of rapid growth and other factors (Caffey, 1978; Park, 1923). Babies that are breast-fed are less likely to develop rickets (Park, 1923). Normally, only a small percentage of cases of rickets are found at puberty, and it is under exceptional circumstances that it occurs. For example, there were hundreds of cases in young boys in central Europe after World War I, when there was undernutrition and heavy physical strains. Rickets also occurs in girls of high caste in India, who marry young and go into purdah.

The clinical signs of rickets include restlessness, irritability or apathy, and flabby, toneless muscles (Mankin, 1974). The skin may be pallid and pasty, and excessive sweating on the head may occur. Gastrointestinal upsets and diarrhea are common, and the child is prone to respiratory infections. General development is delayed, and the child is often shorter than normal for its age. At times the disease can be so severe that a young child is unable to walk, stand, or sit without support (Mankin, 1974).

There are two types of rickets, depending on the nutritional status of the child (Jaffe, 1972). If there is general undernourishment (atrophic or porotic form), then the bones have thin and porous cortices with wide marrow spaces and relatively few and thin spongy trabeculae. The bones are very fragile and susceptible to fractures. More well-nourished children develop the "hypertrophic" or "hyperplastic" form. Here the bone cortices are porous but are thick because of excessive deposition of osteoid, and the marrow spaces become narrowed because of abundant spongy osteoid trabeculae (Jaffe, 1972). In this form fractures are less common, but the bones can become very distorted in shape. Rickets is very much a disease of growth, and if growth is severely retarded, then bone changes will not be so evident. This explains the "paradox of rickets": as the disease becomes more severe and the child more ill, changes in the epiphyseal plate become milder and may even disappear (Mankin, 1974). It has been observed in the past that children with rickets who became infested with body parasites, which interfered with growth, frequently exhibited a dramatic regression of the bone lesions (Harris, 1933). In experimental studies, florid or severe rickets developed more frequently in well-fed animals. In children also, the most severe deformities are found in those who are relatively well nourished.

The earliest bone change is often seen in the skull and involves widening of the sutures and persistence of the anterior and posterior fontanelles. Craniotabes, or areas of softened and poorly mineralized bone, also develop (Jaffe, 1972). Often there is marked flattening and thinning due to pressure on the side of the head on which the infant normally lies (Jaffe, 1972). The vault is abnormally thickened in other areas, leading to asymmetric contours. The thickening is not always evenly distributed and is particularly common on the frontal bone (frontal bossing), although the parietals can also be affected. This thickening is due to bone deposition on the external table of bone rather than a thickening of the diploë. Dental development is often affected, with delay in eruption of deciduous teeth, eruption of teeth out of sequence and poor mineralization. Hypoplastic defects and caries can be frequent and severe.

On either side of the sternum, rounded nodular prominences can develop between the junction of the costal cartilage and the rib; this is referred to as the rachitic rosary. Harrison's groove (a groove along the lower border of the thorax) can also develop because of ribs giving way to the muscle pull exerted by the diaphragm (Engfeldt and Njertquist, 1961). A thoracic kyphosis (increased convexity in curvature) or, more rarely, scoliosis (lateral curvature) of the spine can also occur. If the child is able to walk, a waddling gait and marked accentuation of the lumbar lordosis (forward curvature) may also be present. Enlargement of the joints of the wrist and ankle, and less commonly the elbow and knee, can also been seen and palpated. Deformities of the pelvis can sometimes occur and may include a retardation of growth, disproportionate growth of parts leading to a decrease in the anteroposterior diameter of the pelvic cavity, or deformation (Hess, 1929). Bowing deformities can occur as the result of weight on the softened bone or by epiphyseal displacement and fracturing (Fig. 3). These deformities often take the form of exaggerations of the normal bone curvatures. Before the child can walk, these deformities are usually limited to the upper limbs, such as humeri, clavicles, radii, and ulnae. After the child is able to walk, bowing deformities of the lower limbs, including the tibiae, fibulae, and femora, can occur. The most common forms of lower-limb deformity are knock knee, bowleg, and saber shin (Caffey, 1978). These occur mainly in the first two years of life, but a small percentage occurs at puberty. It is important to be aware that these deformities occur only in infants who have good muscle tone and are ambulant (Swischuk and Hayden, 1979). An infant who has good muscle tone but is not ambulant will show mild or no deformity, whereas an infant who has poor muscle tone and is not ambulant will not show bowing deformities.

The earliest radiographic changes usually occur at the distal ends of the radius and ulna, particularly the ulna. These changes consist of a loss of bone density and the development of an irregular, frayed appearance of the metaphyses. The metaphyses may also develop a concave central depression (cupping) and become slightly widened or flared (Caffey, 1978). Changes usually do not occur at the proximal ends of the bones, where bone growth is slower. Cupping is common at both ends of the fibula and in the distal ends of the ulna and

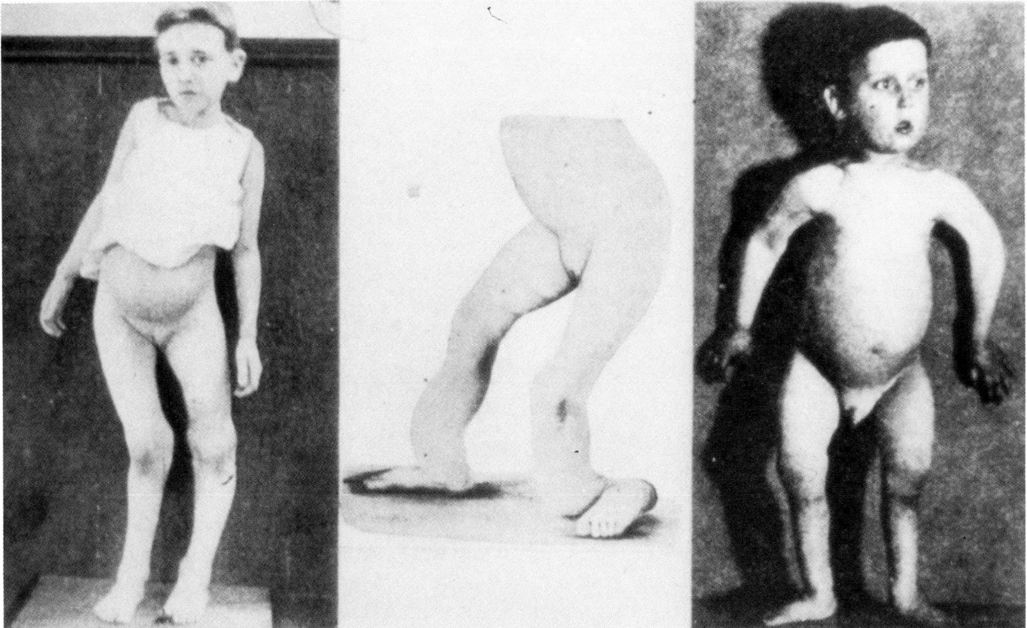

Fig. 3. Limb deformities in rickets. (Photos courtesy of Dr. Keith Manchester, Calvin Wells Laboratory, University of Bradford.)

tibia; it is rarely found in the bones of the elbows or knees. These cupping and spreading deformities of the metaphyses do not occur in cases of rickets that are so severe that growth is retarded. It is in well-nourished infants with relatively good muscle tone and mobility that metaphyseal cupping and flaring are commonly seen. In rickets occurring in older children, the medial segments of the femoral and tibial metaphyses at the knees are often affected, even when there is no change in other parts of the skeleton (Caffey, 1978).

Changes in the shafts of the bone develop slightly later than changes at the ends. There is loss of density accompanied by thinning of the cortex, whose outline becomes fuzzy and indistinct, as well as a coarsening of the overall texture of bone (Caffey, 1978; Mankin, 1974). Green-stick fractures can occur, as can milkman's pseudofractures (*umbauzonen* or Looser's lines), which are symmetrical, transverse, ribbonlike zones of decreased density (Mankin, 1974). Milkman's pseudofractures are seen more commonly in older children with active rickets, particularly in the forearms. These zones of decreased density disappear as healing progresses.

With the onset of healing, the cupping and flaring deformities can become much more severe and obvious radiographically. With complete healing, the gross bone structure can usually be restored. However, distortion and sclerosis of spongiosa in areas affected during the active phase are common and usually remain visible in the shaft for years (Caffey, 1985). Caffey (1978) states that cortical thickening of the bone affected during the active stage of rickets may persist for years after healing, especially on the concave surfaces of curvature deformities. Mineralization of the thick osteoid layers can result in a diffuse cortical envelope that may be of uniform density or lamellated, similar to changes occurring in syphilis. Caffey (1978) also noted that skull thickening on the frontal and parietal bones can remain throughout childhood, and in some cases into adulthood. Beading of ribs may also persist throughout childhood and, in extreme cases, even into adulthood (Hess, 1929). In a longitudinal study it was shown that bowing of long bones usually disappeared by 6 years of age, but in 10% of cases it persisted throughout childhood (Hess, 1929).

History

The word "rickets" is believed to be derived from either *wrick* (Old English for twist), *wiggates* (crooked gait), *rucket* (Dorset dialect meaning to breathe with difficulty), *riquets* (Norman for hunchback), or *rachitis* (derived from the Greek word for spine) (Hess, 1929; Engfeldt and Njertquist, 1961; Findlay, 1919; Mankin, 1974). The first adequate description of rickets is attributed to Soranus Ephesus, who lived between A.D. 98 and 138 and practiced as a physician in Rome and Alexandria (Findlay, 1919). He wrote that "the legs become twisted at the thighs when the child wishes to walk about," and that the disease was "observed more in the neighborhood of Rome than in other places." Soranus did not mention seeing rickets in Egypt, and he specifically stated that it did not affect Greek children. Several centuries passed before the disease again came into prominence in medical writings, and it was European physicians who began writing about the disease, notably Whistler in 1645, Bootius in 1649, and Glisson in 1650 (cited in Hess, 1929). Glisson was the first to give a detailed description of rickets and is credited with writing a classic account of the disease (Engfeldt and Njertquist, 1961).

In the seventeenth century, rickets was known as "the English disease," either because it had been extensively described in England or because of its high incidence there. However, its prevalence during medieval and postmedieval times is difficult to assess, because the disease was often not differentiated from others affecting the skeleton of the child. Nevertheless, it has been suggested that a number of paintings from the fifteenth and sixteenth centuries depict children who show signs of clinical rickets (Foote, 1927). A textbook written in 1764 emphasized the bad influence of damp and dark living quarters in the development of the disease (Vahlquist, 1975), but it was not until the nineteenth century that there was much information on demographic factors relating to rickets. Early in the nineteenth century, Wendelstadt wrote *Endemic Diseases of Wezlar,* which described a German town of 8,000 that was infamous for rickets (Hess, 1929). This town had exceptionally narrow streets and dark alleys and there were entire streets of houses with people crippled from the disease.

> The children must sit indoors . . . which ends in death, or if they continue to live, they develop thick joints, cease to be able to walk or have deformed legs. The head becomes large and even the vertebral column bends. It comes to pass that such children sit often for many years without being able to move; at times they cease to grow and are merely a burden to those about them. If they recover they often develop into monstrosities, or if things go well they become deformed individuals.

A study in 1889 illustrated the relationship between rickets and cities when the British Medical Association surveyed the prevalence of the disease in the British Isles (Owen, 1889). The differences in prevalence between the country and city were striking, with rickets being common in large towns and thickly populated districts, especially where there was industrialization, and rare in rural districts. In England and Wales there were five main areas of rickets clustered around the heavy industrial and coal-mining cities (Owen, 1889). In London, rickets was rare in the wealthier residential districts like Mayfair and Belgravia, but common everywhere else. The farther away from the center of London, the less prevalent the disease. The prevalence of rickets appeared to be directly related to the density of the population. Almost all large towns had a high incidence of rickets; the incidence was slightly lower in towns of moderate size and much lower in small market towns of 4,000–5,000 people. Rickets was virtually absent in villages and village towns.

In 1890 Theobald Palm, a medical missionary to Japan, reported on the incidence of rickets in different parts of the world. He found that it was present in Europe and North America, especially in the middle latitudes. It was rare in the United States except for large cities such as Philadelphia, where it was as common as in the large cities of Europe. In the rest of the world, the disease was seldom seen, except in unique cases such as the upper classes in Egypt or shawl weavers in towns in Kashmir. Reports that Palm received from doctors all over India, China, and North Africa, and his own observations in Japan, indicated that rickets was almost unknown in those countries, even though hygiene was poor and diet was minimal in many areas (Palm, 1890); however, clear skies and abundant sunshine were common factors in these countries. Of England, Palm states:

> The fact that poorer classes suffer more than the rich, the townborn and bred children more than those in the country, and those in manufacturing towns more than in small towns, point to those climatic conditions which are intensified by poverty and residence in large manufacturing cities . . . It is in the narrow alleys, the haunts and play-grounds of the children of the poor, that this exclusion of sunlight is at its worst, and it is there that the victims of rickets are to be found in abundance.

Hess (1929) also found that urbanization and lack of sunlight were the main factors in the etiology of rickets. He compared the incidence of rickets with the average hours of sunlight per year in cities around the world. The two cities that had the highest incidence and severity of rickets, London and Glasgow, also had the least number of hours of sunshine per year. He concluded that "in general, a map of incidence of rickets is the practical equivalent of a map of deficiency of sunlight."

Hutchinson and Shah (1921) found no rickets among poor Hindus who had inadequate diets but who worked outdoors all day with their babies and children nearby. However, it was quite common among the well-fed Moslems and upper-caste Hindus who practiced purdah. Girls often married at age 12 and went into seclusion, while infants usually remained with their mothers for the first six months of life in a room in the interior of a house. Wilson (1931) noticed a tendency for rickets to occur more frequently in overcrowded cities in India, among women and girls observing purdah, and among the lower social classes. Fifty-four percent of the girls from a city school had clinical evidence of rickets as opposed to 18% from a suburban school (Wilson, 1931).

The severity of rickets gradually began to decline after 1900 with the advent of pollution controls and the use of cod liver oil and vitamin-enriched food products. By 1935, about 20% of all children under 2 years of age who were admitted to a pediatric clinic in Uppsala, Sweden, showed clinical signs of rickets; at the present time it is rarely found (Vahlquist, 1975). What was once a disease of the temperate regions is now found more commonly in the tropics and the subtropics of Third World countries (Vahlquist, 1975). Salimpour (1975) reported on 200 cases of rickets in Iran, a country with plenty of sunshine throughout the year. However, these children were from lower socioeconomic groups who lived in high-walled, sunless houses, and the children were kept indoors for most of their first year of life. In North America and England, rickets is now found primarily in certain ethnic groups, mainly those from Asia. The primary factors are not known, but it is thought that an interaction of climate, diet, type of clothing, seclusion indoors, and genetic constitution is responsible (Holmes et al., 1973).

Archaeological Evidence

It is rare to find archaeological evidence for rickets. As Wells (1964) says, "the disease was a rarity everywhere and at all times in the prehistoric and early historic periods." A few cases do start to appear from the Neolithic period, particularly in northern Europe. Nielsen (cited in Wells, 1975) diagnosed six cases in Danish Neolithic material and three from the Danish Iron Age. Gejvall (1960) stated that rickets was rare in Swedish material from the Neolithic period to the late Middle Ages. He found only one unequivocal case among 364 individuals from Västerhus, a chapel dating from A.D. 1100 to 1300. Møller-Christensen (1958) found nine cases among 800 skeletons from Aebelholt, a Danish monastery that was occupied from A.D. 1250 to 1550. In Hungary, two cases from the Roman period and two from medieval times have been recorded (Regöly-Mérei, cited in Wells, 1975). Nemeskéri and Harsányi (cited in Wells, 1975) found a gradual increase in frequency from 0.7% to 2.5% from the tenth to thirteenth centuries in Hungarian material. However, Wells (1975) feels that these frequencies should be even lower, as some of the diagnoses were based on features such as plagiocrany (asymmetry of the skull) or tooth irregularities that are nonspecific.

Rickets appears to have been even more uncommon in other parts of the world. Hrdlička (1907) stated that rickets did not occur in the prehistoric peoples of North America. Snow (1948) described a possible case in an infant from Indian Knoll, Kentucky, but Ortner and Putschar (1981) did not think that the evidence was conclusive. Elliot-Smith and Dawson (1924) and Wood-Jones (1910) did not consider that there were any definite cases in ancient Egyptian skeletal material.

There does appear to have been a very gradual increase in the occurrence of rickets during the European Middle Ages, at least in the cities. Ortner and Putschar (1981) describe a case of healed rickets in a child from the Winchester Saxon collection in the British Museum (Natural History) that showed anterior bowing of the femur and tibia. They also describe another case from the medieval period in Switzerland, a male with deformities of the tibiae. Manchester (1983) describes a classic example of rickets in a child from the medieval cemetery of St. Helen-on-the-Walls, York, with typical bowing of the leg bones. An infant from a medieval site in Chapstow, England, shows the widening of epiphyses and bowing of long bones typical of rickets (Manchester, personal communication). However, it was only with increasing urbanization and the rise of the industrial era in Europe and North America that rickets became common. Distortion of the lower extremities is seen in an adult from Ludgate Hill, London, a postmedieval site (Manchester, 1983). A 7-year-old child from the nineteenth-century First African Baptist Church site in Philadelphia (Angel et al., 1985) shows typical bowing of all long bones of the lower extremities (Fig. 4). Wells (1967) found that 25% of an eighteenth- to nineteenth-century Norwich population had evidence of rickets. Many of these individuals showed the classic changes, including severe bowing of femora and tibiae and widened epiphyses.

IRON-DEFICIENCY ANEMIA

Anemia can be broadly defined as a reduction below normal in concentration of hemoglobin or red blood cells (Wintrobe, 1974). Iron-deficiency anemia is one of many types of anemia; it develops when there is insufficient iron for the hemoglobin in the newly forming red blood cells of the bone marrow. As a result, the cells become pale in color (hypochromic) and small in size (microcytic). Iron-deficiency anemia is the most widespread type of anemia; it is said to be the most common organic malady of humankind (Fairbanks and Beutler, 1972).

Iron was named *sideros* (star) by the Greeks, who believed that it was a special gift sent to earth by one of the gods (Liebel et al., 1979). It is one of the essential body minerals and is involved in processes that regulate the transfer of oxygen to body cells, immunocompetence, and possibly neurotransmission and collagen synthesis (Liebel et al., 1979). Although iron is found in a number of foods, there are particularly rich sources in organ meats, egg yolk, legumes, shellfish, and parsley (Prasad, 1978). It is absorbed from food by the mucosa of the small intestine, from which it is either moved immediately into the blood or stored in the mucosal cell as ferritin. The exact mechanism by which the intestinal mucosa regulates the amount of iron absorbed is still not known (Hoffbrand and Lewis, 1981). What is known, however, is that it is a complex and highly adaptable system. For example, iron of animal origin is more easily absorbed by the intestine than iron of plant origin. Some substances, such as the phytates found in grains, can actually inhibit absorption, whereas others, such as vitamin C, can facilitate absorption. In any one individual, depending on the circumstances, more or less iron can be absorbed from exactly the same diet. Iron absorption is decreased if the body becomes overloaded with iron or is suffering from acute or chronic infections. Absorption is increased during infancy and childhood, in women in general, particularly during the later stages of pregnancy, and if body reserves of iron become depleted. The more iron there is in the diet of a normal person, the less of the total amount the body absorbs; the body actually seems to be more concerned with preventing excess iron absorption.

The causes of iron-deficiency anemia are many and varied, including blood loss (hemor-

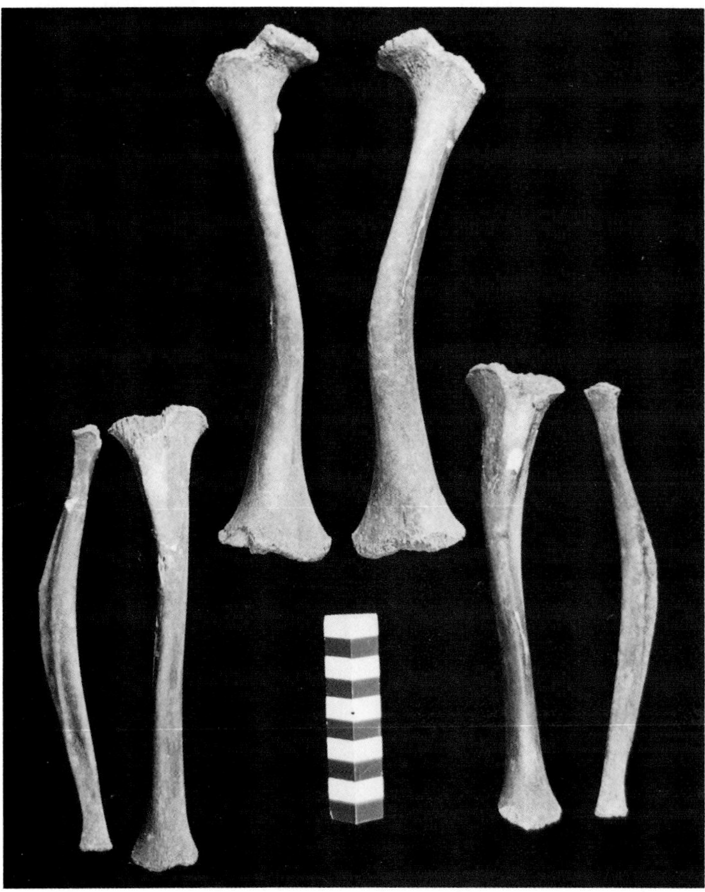

Fig. 4. Lower limb bones of ca. 7-year-old child from the First African Baptist Church Cemetery site, Philadelphia. (Photo courtesy of Dr. Don Ortner, Smithsonian Institution.)

rhage, parasite infestation), deficiency in the diet during periods of accelerated demand, inadequate absorption of iron (diarrhea), or nutritional deficiencies (Robinson, 1972). It appears that iron deficiency caused only by an inadequate diet is not very common; according to Passmore and Eastwood (1986), "it is unusual for anemia to arise in an otherwise healthy person solely as a direct result of poor diet." A study by Davidson et al. (1933) showed that those people who developed iron-deficiency anemia had exactly the same diet as others who did not develop anemia. Generally, the body can adjust its absorption of iron to compensate for decreased amounts in the diet, and other factors are more important in precipitating the state of iron-deficiency anemia. For example, in tropical countries, malaria and hookworm infestation contribute very significantly to its development. In infants and children there are a number of predisposing factors, including premature clamping of the umbilical cord, low birth weight, and sex (Liebel et al., 1979; Woodruff, 1958).

Clinical and Radiographic Picture

A clear clinical picture is obscured by conflicting evidence on the specificity of signs and symptoms as well as differences of opinion concerning the definition of iron-deficiency anemia. The signs and symptoms can be varied and contradictory. For example, it is not unusual to find a patient who is completely asymptomatic, even in severe cases of iron-deficiency anemia. This is particularly true if the anemia has developed gradually (Fairbanks et al., 1971). The symptoms also show a poor correlation with the severity of the anemia, at least above hemoglobin levels of 6 to 7 g/100 ml of blood. This seems to be the critical level, below which pathological changes occur (Wadsworth, 1975). There are no proven significant organic disturbances in otherwise healthy individuals with moderate reductions in hemoglobin (Liebel et al., 1979).

Some of the more frequently reported symptoms of iron-deficiency anemia are fatigue, weakness, light-headedness, headaches, dyspnea, palpitations, and paresthesias (abnormal spontaneous sensations). Gastrointestinal disturbances such as loss of appetite, flatulence, diarrhea, constipation, nausea, and vomiting are not uncommon (Fairbanks and Beutler, 1972). When the iron-deficiency anemia is severe and chronic, other changes such as koilonychia (spoon-shaped nails), angular stomatitis (cracks at the corner of the mouth), glossitis (sore tongue), flattening of the lingual papillae, atrophic gastritis (stomach inflammation with atrophy of the mucous membranes), and bone changes in children may occur (Hoffbrand and Lewis, 1981). The bone changes are thought to be related to a hyperactive bone marrow that creates pressure on surrounding bone, thus increasing the width of the marrow space and decreasing the outer table of bone.

In the past, some of the severe signs were often seen, perhaps because cases were more advanced or were associated with other deficiencies or diseases. Today, however, often there are no abnormal physical findings that may be attributed to iron deficiency (Fairbanks et al., 1971). This apparent difference in the clinical picture could also be explained by a different understanding of the definition of iron-deficiency anemia. In 1967 the World Health Organization set up criteria for adequate levels of hemoglobin. They concluded that in a healthy population 95% of individuals should *exceed* the following hemoglobin levels: 1) 6 months–6 years, 11 g/100 ml; 2) 6 years–14 years, 12 g/100 ml; 3) adult males, 13 g/100 ml; 4) adult females, 12 g/100 ml; 5) pregnant women, 11 g/100 ml. The diagnosis of iron-deficiency anemia is made on the basis of these figures. However, it has been argued that these figures may result in a great overrepresentation of iron-deficiency anemia and that in fact there has been little study of hemoglobin levels and normal variability in healthy populations (Wadsworth, 1975). It is certainly true that hemoglobin levels are variable and adaptable, depending on age, season of the year, and other factors. If the WHO's standards are used, then it would appear that many millions of the world's population are suffering from the effects of iron-deficiency anemia. It seems more likely, however, that in some cases the true lower limits of normality are lower than the standards that are now in use (Wadsworth, 1975). In any population, the groups most susceptible to iron-deficiency anemia will be those involved in faster rates of growth and development, resulting in higher nutritional requirements per unit of body weight. Those groups whose nutrient needs are relatively greatest are infants, children at puberty, and women during pregnancy and lactation, and it is just these groups whose normal lower limits of hemoglobin concentration seem to be lower than those that are generally accepted. Surveys have shown that the probable lower limit of normality in hemoglobin concentration is about 9 g/100 ml in infants and young children, 11 g/100 ml in normal women of childbearing age, 10 g/100 ml in pregnant women in temperate climates, and 8 g/100 in pregnant women in tropical climates (Wadsworth, 1975).

Women, infants, and children are more susceptible to developing iron-deficiency anemia, but the picture is a complex one, especially with regard to infants and children. In infants, an apparent or "physiological" iron deficiency is present between the ages of about 6 and 18 months of age. As it occurs in all infants, regardless of conditions, and also in animals in comparable periods of their life, this deficiency is considered to be normal. It may be associated with the development of the body's defense mechanism (Stuart-Macadam, 1987a). In chronic infections and inflammatory states, the body's natural response is to decrease intestinal absorption of iron, prevent the release of iron into the blood from the reticuloendothelial system, and increase the amount of iron stored in the liver. Apparently the assimilation of iron is a requirement for microbial growth; in fact, microbes synthesize substances that bind iron. Studies have shown that if iron is depleted, the host defense is strengthened, and if iron is added, the microbial growth is enhanced (Weinberg, 1974). It is definitely to the advantage of the host to be transiently hypoferremic in the situation of microbial invasion. It follows that in the period of immunological vulnerability for the infant, when it has lost the immunity conferred by the mother and is exposed to a number of pathogens, that it is advantageous to be iron deficient. There is a large body of data that lends further support to the concept that iron deficiency may not always be detrimental, but may increase the body's defense against infections (Liebel et al., 1979; Lukens, 1975; Strauss, 1978). It is only when additional factors are present that iron deficiency may pass over the critical threshold into an iron-deficiency anemia that could interfere with the health of the child.

It is only in the last 30 years that researchers have recognized that iron-deficiency anemia can produce changes in bone. In 1936 Sheldon described a case of iron deficiency with skull alterations, but this was largely ignored. It was not until the 1950s that attention was again drawn to bone change as the result of iron-deficiency anemia (Eng, 1958; Girdany and Gaffney, 1952). In a case of iron-deficiency anemia associated with parasitic infestation, Eng (1958) demonstrated skull changes that included widening of the diploic space, thinning of the outer table, and a "hair-on-end" type of trabeculation. This pattern closely resembled that seen in the genetic anemias, particularly thalassemia.

There are few radiographic studies of large numbers of patients with iron-deficiency anemia. However, two studies that include over 100 and 90 patients respectively (Agarwal et al., 1970; Reimann et al., 1976) indicate that it is not uncommon to find bone change associated with iron-deficiency anemia. Most of the cases described in the clinical literature are of infants and young children, with the earliest documented bone changes occurring in a child 10 months old (Burko et al., 1961).

In the skull (Fig. 5), bony alterations range from outer table thinning or a widening of the diploic space to severe granular osteoporosis and the presence of "hair-on-end" trabeculation (Aksoy et al., 1966; Britton et al., 1960; Burko et al., 1961; Lanzkowsky, 1968; Moseley, 1961; Ryan, 1962; Sax, 1963; Shahidi and Diamond, 1960). The frontal and parietal bones are most frequently affected; the occipital bone rarely so. The radiographic pictures can vary greatly among patients of the same age and with the same severity of anemia. A reliable estimate of incidence of bone change is not available, because so few large samples of patients have been studied. In a study of 12 patients, Aksoy et al. (1966) found that five showed bony alterations. Agarwal et al. (1970) found outer table atrophy in 95% of 100 cases, diploic widening in 2%, and "hair-on-end" trabeculation in 4%. Reimann and Kuran (1973) found that 5% of a sample of 80 patients exhibited "hair-on-end" trabeculation.

Moseley reported that up until 1971 no studies of iron-deficiency anemia reported interference of paranasal sinus development similar to that seen in thalassemia. However, a more recent study by Reimann et al. (1975) indicated that the paranasal sinuses can be affected. In their study of 88 patients, 38% showed deficiencies in form, size, or aeration of the frontal sinus, and 50% showed abnormalities of the maxillary sinuses.

Less information is available on postcranial changes related to iron-deficiency anemia. Initially it was suggested that a lack of postcranial alterations was an important diagnostic factor in differentiating between iron-deficiency anemia and the genetic anemias (Moseley, 1963). This statement was challenged (Agarwal et al., 1970; Aksoy et al., 1966; Lanzkowsky, 1968) as increasing numbers of cases were studied radiographically. It now appears that postcranial changes do occur, but with less severity and lower frequency than those seen in the genetic anemias.

Only one study describes changes in the axial skeleton. Aksoy et al. (1966) found that three of 11 patients had mild to severe osteoporosis of the pelvic bones and three of ten patients had changes in the lumbar vertebral bodies. These investigators also found osteoporosis

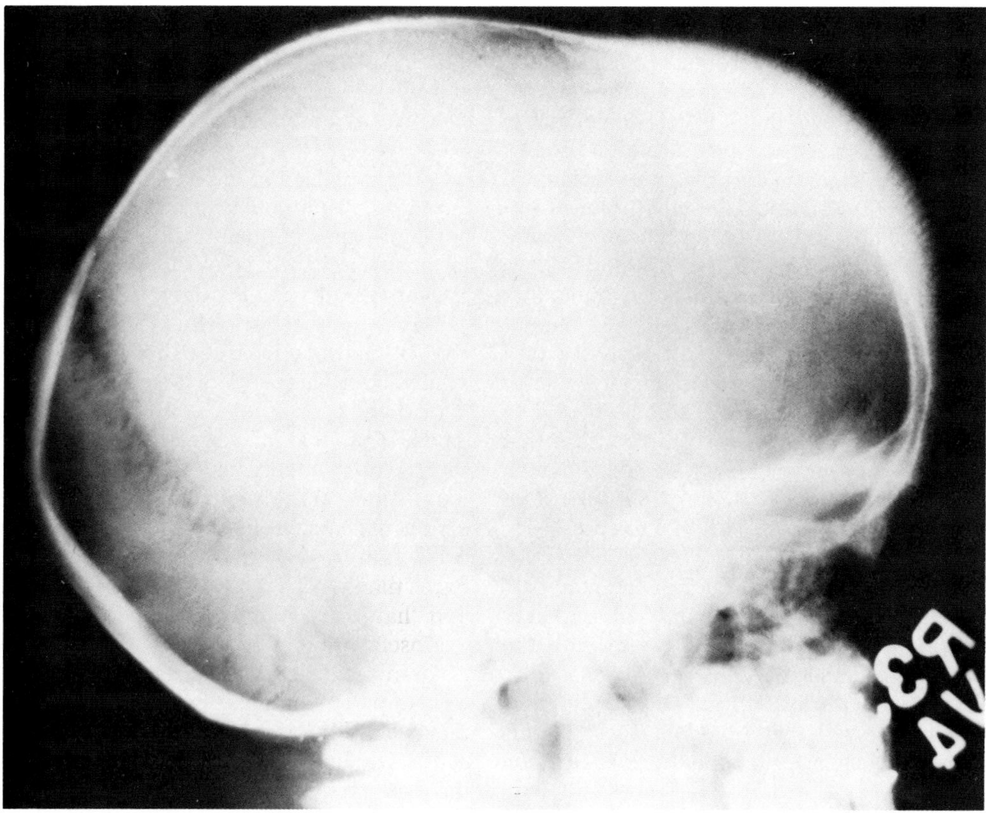

Fig. 5. Radiograph of child with iron-deficiency anemia. (Photo courtesy of Dr. S. Bhargava, India.)

and coarse trabecular striation in 11 of 12 patients with chronic iron-deficiency anemia. They noted that this was the most frequently encountered radiographic finding in their patients. Nine of 12 patients showed alterations in the hand bones: coarsened trabeculae were observed in both metacarpals and phalanges. Lanzkowsky (1968) found that seven of 15 children exhibited widening of hand bones due to an expansion of the medullary space, as well as a thinning of the cortices.

History

The history of iron-deficiency anemia remains obscure. Fairbanks et al. (1971) stated that "for centuries the etiology, pathogenesis, and clinical expressions of this disorder were poorly delineated." Apparently, iron-deficiency anemia or a similar condition was known as early as 1500 B.C. An Egyptian manual of therapeutics from that time, the *Papyrus Ebers,* describes a disease that is characterized by pallor, dyspnea, and edema (Fairbanks and Beutler, 1972). In subsequent medical literature prior to the nineteenth century, articles and monographs dealing with iron-deficiency anemia and other blood disorders are found only infrequently. One of the reasons may be that the symptoms are very nonspecific in nature (Vahlquist, 1975). In addition, clinical syndromes of what is now recognized as a single entity, iron-deficiency anemia, were often considered to be separate diseases. This led to a profusion of terms, including "chlorosis," "mild anemia," "essential hypochromic anemia," and "anemia of chronic blood loss."

"Chlorosis" or "green sickness" was first described in 1554 and was well known to European physicians after the middle of the sixteenth century (Fairbanks and Beutler, 1972). By 1640 Lazarus Riberus had recommended the use of iron as a remedy for chlorosis. His description of the symptoms included pallor, edema, dyspnea (breathlessness), palpitation, headache, and cessation of menses (Prasad, 1978). By the beginning of the twentieth century, it was realized that chlorosis was associated with a decrease in the iron content of blood. It was recognized to be a disease that was more common in women, particularly those living in cities, the poor, and those people with deprived diets.

The true picture of iron-deficiency anemia in the past may never be known. Only with the advent of modern laboratory methods has it become possible to learn about the prevalence and severity of the condition. Reliable methods for hemoglobin determination were not introduced until the 1870s and were not widely used until even later (Vahlquist, 1975). With the use of these methods a demographic pattern has emerged, showing higher frequencies in infants, children, and women of childbearing age, in individuals from lower socioeconomic groups, and in both urban and rural areas of the tropics. However, it is very likely that iron-deficiency anemia is a condition that has existed throughout human history, simply varying in incidence and severity depending upon the circumstances.

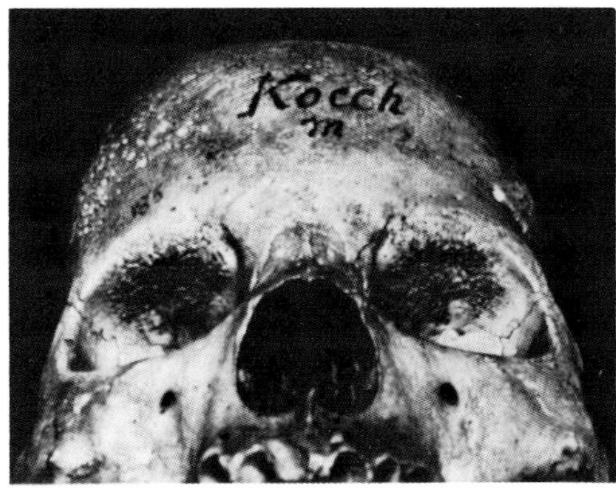

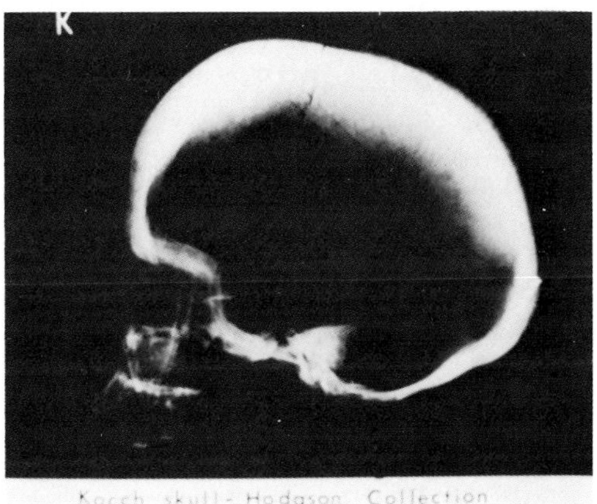

Fig. 6. Macroscopic and radiographic appearance of porotic hyperostosis. (Photos courtesy of British Museum [Natural History].)

Archaeological Evidence

The archaeological evidence for iron-deficiency anemia is ambiguous for a number of reasons. First, there are still questions remaining as to exactly what the archaeological evidence for anemia, and in particular iron-deficiency anemia, actually is. It is extremely difficult to differentiate the type of anemia on the basis of skeletal remains alone. Because of the nature of bone and bone marrow physiology, it appears probable that iron-deficiency anemia may produce bone change only in young children (Stuart-Macadam, 1985). This means that it may never be possible to determine the effect of anemia on adults of past populations. Furthermore, over the years, researchers have applied different methodologies and descriptive techniques to their investigations, leading to problems in data comparison. However, the following review may clarify the situation.

Porotic bone lesions of the skull have been recognized and commented on by researchers since the mid-nineteenth century. These lesions are characterized by pitting of the compact bone, usually associated with an increase in the thickness of the adjacent diploic bone (Fig. 6). The lesions can vary in size from less than 1 mm in diameter to large, coalescing apertures, and are found on the orbital roof and skull vault, particularly the frontal, parietal, and occipital bones. Although a number of descriptive terms have been applied, the most commonly used at present are cribra orbitalia (after Welcker, 1888) for lesions of the orbit and porotic hyperostosis (after Angel, 1966) for lesions of the vault and/or orbit.

A number of etiologies have been suggested over the years, but in 1929 two researchers, Moore and Williams, independently suggested that anemia was responsible for the development of lesions. Recent work supports this hypothesis and verifies the relationship between orbital and vault lesions (Stuart-Macadam, 1982, 1986, 1987b). At first it was thought that the anemia was genetic in origin (Angel, 1964, 1966, 1967; Zaino, 1964, 1967), but later researchers implicated an acquired iron-deficiency anemia (Hengen, 1971; Moseley, 1961). More recent studies indicate that the iron-deficiency anemia hypothesis has gained wide recognition (Carlson et al., 1974; El-Najjar et al., 1976; Lallo et al., 1977; Mensforth et al., 1978). It is possible that genetic anemias such as sickle-cell anemia and thalassemia could have been a factor in groups from areas of the world where these anemias are now common. However, if calculations are made based on the very highest gene frequencies seen today, it is evident that the probability of finding individuals in archaeological collections with skeletal alterations due to genetic anemia is quite low (Stuart-Macadam, 1982). It would not explain the high levels of porotic hyperostosis seen worldwide or in groups from northern Europe and North America where genetic anemias did not exist in the past. On the basis of this, and the lack of the more severe bone changes associated with genetic anemias, it is likely that the porotic hyperostosis occurring in most skeletal collections is the result of an iron-deficiency anemia.

Porotic hyperostosis has been observed in skeletal collections around the world and throughout the past. It appears to have been rare in Paleolithic and Mesolithic times, but to have increased in frequency from the Neolithic period, suggesting that the appearance of iron-deficiency anemia is associated with agriculture and/or settlement and increasing population densities (Angel, 1984; Lallo et al., 1977; Rathbun, 1984; Smith et al., 1984). However, the fact that Ubelaker (1984) found no porotic hyperostosis in a Ecuador highland site where there was intensive agriculture suggests that other factors were operative. The frequency of porotic hyperostosis varies considerably depending on the geographic area, but it does seem to have decreased in the recent past, at least in Europe. Hengen (1971) found that there was a statistically significant decrease in incidence of porotic hyperostosis in Germany from the twelfth century (38.5%) to the late nineteenth and early twentieth centuries (15.5%). In a study of Swedish skulls, Henschen (1961) found cribra orbitalia to be present in the mid-nineteenth century, but absent in 2,000 skulls collected since 1930. However, Hengen found that in tropical and subtropical areas porotic hyperostosis still occurred in the nineteenth and twentieth centuries. He observed that it is more common the nearer the country of origin is to the equator.

Porotic hyperostosis has been found to occur in skeletal collections from every continent. However, its incidence can vary from site to site in the same general area and time period, depending on ecological and environmental conditions. Hrdlička (1914) found that porotic hyperostosis was much more common in individuals from coastal areas in Peru than in those from highland areas. Møller-Christensen (1953) observed that individuals from a medieval leper hospital at Naesteved had twice as much cribra orbitalia as those from a monastery located on the same island during the same time period. In the Southwest American sites of the Anasazi Indians, El-Najjar et al. (1975, 1976) found that cribra orbitalia was more common in crania from canyon bottom sites than sage plain sites.

Speculation on the factors that might have contributed to the development of the anemia represented by porotic hyperostosis has led to several lines of thought. As early as 1929, Williams suggested that nutritional deficiencies might be responsible for the porotic hyperostosis. In 1961 Henschen stressed this possibility, as did Nathan and Haas in 1966. Hengen (1971) was the first to suggest that parasitic infestation was an important factor:

> Changes of the hygienic conditions and of the incidence of iron deficiency anemias in former times

depended without doubt largely on deviations of the climate, differences in the habits of daily life, procuring and preparation of food, types of housing, keeping of domestic animals, disposal of excrements and so on.

Carlson et al. (1974) speculated that poor diet, parasitic infection, and weanling diarrhea contributed to the development of iron-deficiency anemia in Nubian populations. El-Najjar et al. (1975, 1976) considered that nutritional deficiencies as the result of a maize-dependent diet explained the higher incidence of porotic hyperostosis in individuals from canyon bottom sites compared with those from sage plain sites in the American Southwest. Lallo et al. (1977), however, suggested that diet was not the major factor in the etiology of porotic hyperostosis at Libben, a prehistoric site in Ohio; it seems that available protein was adequate. Instead they considered that there was a synergistic relationship between microbial infection, reduced iron absorption due to weanling diarrhea, and nutrient depletion that occurs with rapid growth. Walker (1986) found a high incidence of porotic hyperostosis in a group from the Santa Barbara Channel Islands in spite of the fact that they subsisted on iron-rich, high-protein marine resources. He felt that diarrheal infections were the main contributing factor and suggested that this might be a more accurate explanation for the higher incidence of porotic hyperostosis seen in southwestern American sites than nutritional inadequacies as the result of a maize-based diet.

CONCLUSIONS

A synthesis of medical knowledge, history, and archaeology of scurvy, rickets, and iron-deficiency anemia provides several insights. It emerges that these three diseases are not primarily diseases of undernutrition. Environmental or cultural factors have had a much greater impact on their occurrence throughout the past. It is faulty nutrition as the result of ideas or circumstances rather than undernutrition that has been responsible for much of the past suffering from these three diseases. All three conditions became common only with "civilization" and the associated changes in customs, diet, and settlement patterns. Scurvy appeared when long sea voyages began, and was later associated with wars, famine, institutionalization and increasing urbanization, and the introduction of processed foods and pasteurization of milk. Rickets occurred increasingly with industrialization and increasing urbanization and the adoption of certain customs of dress and living. Iron-deficiency anemia began appearing in the Neolithic period, with increasing settlement of people and a correspondingly greater exposure to pathogens.

Scurvy, rickets, and iron-deficiency anemia all have their greatest effect, especially in terms of bone change, on children. This is due to the fact that the young child, particularly in the first two to three years of life, is going through a period of greatly accelerated growth and increased demands for nutrients. It is at this time that all the body systems, including the skeletal system, are most vulnerable to environmental stress. This explains why all three conditions have their greatest effect on young children between the ages of 6 months and 2 years. It also explains why premature or multiple-birth infants, with their even greater growth demands, are particularly susceptible to all three conditions and accounts for the fact that in scurvy and rickets it is the most rapidly growing parts of the skeleton that are affected most. There is an interrelationship between the three conditions, in the sense that if one is present, one or both of the others can also be present. Scurvy is often associated with anemia, scurvy and rickets often occur simultaneously, and rickets and iron-deficiency anemia also occur together. This can complicate the interpretation of bone changes seen in archaeological collections. However, in terms of frequency, it appears that iron-deficiency anemia was much more common in the past than scurvy or rickets. Scurvy did not appear with any frequency until medieval times, and rickets not until the Industrial Revolution.

The human body has developed a flexible, efficient system of nutrient acquisition and use that is the result of millions of years of evolution. Safeguards have been developed that maximize the availability of nutrients. For example, vitamin C can be obtained from both plants and animals and stored in the body for a number of months; it takes four to five months on a completely vitamin C-deficient diet for an adult to develop scurvy. There is some indication that the human body can even manufacture its own supply of vitamin C in times of need. Babies born of mothers in starvation situations are rarely scorbutic, and the breast milk contains many times the amount of vitamin C that the mother has access to in the diet. Vitamin D can be obtained from two sources, the diet and the sun. The diet is only a secondary source since 90% of the active vitamin D comes from photosynthesis induced by the sun. It is thought that vitamin D can also be stored in the body for a number of months. Iron can be obtained from both plant and animal sources. Iron metabolism is a very efficient system, as most of the iron needed by the body is obtained by the recycling of iron from senescent red blood cells.

It is true that nutrition is an important aspect of the relationship between a population and its environment. However, a comprehensive survey of scurvy, rickets, and iron-deficiency anemia illustrates the importance of other culturally and environmentally determined factors involved in this relationship. There are complex adaptations between the human body, its nutrient requirements, and its environment. It is vital to have an appreciation of these complexities in any consideration of a "nutritional deficiency" disease.

REFERENCES

Agarwal KN, Dhar M, Shah M, and Bhardwaj OP (1970) Roentgenologic changes in iron deficiency anemia. Am J Roentgenol Radium Ther 110:635–637.

Aksoy M, Camlı NM, and Erdem S (1966) Roentgenographic bone changes in chronic iron deficiency anaemia. Blood 27(5):677–686.

Angel JL (1964) Osteoporosis: Thalassemia? Am J Phys Anthropol 22:369–374.

Angel JL (1966) Porotic hyperostosis, anemias, malarias and the marshes in prehistoric eastern Mediterranean. Science 153:760–762.

Angel JL (1967) Porotic hyperostosis or osteoporosis symmetrica. In D Brothwell and AT Sandison (eds): Diseases in Antiquity. Springfield, IL: Charles C Thomas, pp 378–389.

Angel JL (1984) Health as a crucial factor in the changes from hunting to developed farming in the eastern Mediterranean. In MN Cohen and GJ Armelagos (eds): Paleopathology at the Origins of Agriculture. New York: Academic Press, pp 51–73.

Angel JL, Kelley JO, Farrington M, and Pinter S (1985) Stresses of first freedom: 19th century Philadelphia. Am J Phys Anthropol 66(2):140 (abstract).

Barlow T (1883) On cases described as 'acute rickets' which are possibly a combination of rickets and scurvy, the scurvy being essential and the rickets variable. Med Chir Trans 66:159–220. (Reprinted in Arch Dis Child 1935, 10:223–252.)

Bourne G (1971) Vitamin C and bone. In G Bourne (ed): The Biochemistry and Physiology of Bone, Vol. 1. New York: Academic Press, pp 231–279.

Britton HA, Canby JP, and Kohler CM (1960) Iron deficiency anaemia produces evidence of marrow hyperplasia in the cranium. Pediatrics 25:621–628.

Burko H, Mellins H, and Watson J (1961) Skull changes in iron deficiency anemia simulating congenital hemolytic anemia. Am J Roentgenol Radium Ther 86(3):447–452.

Caffey J (1978) Pediatric X-ray Diagnosis, 7th Ed. Chicago: Year Book Medical Publishers.

Caffey J (1985) Pediatric X-ray Diagnosis, 8th Ed. Chicago: Year Book Medical Publishers.

Carlson D, Armelagos G, and van Gerven D (1974) Factors influencing the etiology of cribra orbitalia in prehistoric Nubia. J Hum Evol 3:405–410.

Carpenter K (1986) The History of Scurvy and Vitamin C. Cambridge: Cambridge University Press.

Davidson LSP, Fullerton HW, Howie JW, Croll JM, Orr JB, and Godden W (1933) Observations on nutrition in relation to anaemia. Br Med J 1:685–690.

Elliot-Smith G, and Dawson WR (1924) Egyptian Mummies. London: Allen and Unwin.

El-Najjar MY, Lozoff B, and Ryan DJ (1975) The paleoepidemiology of porotic hyperostosis in the American Southwest: Radiological and ecological considerations. Am J Roentgenol Radium Ther 25:918–924.

El-Najjar MY, Ryan DJ, Turner CG II, and Lozoff B (1976) The etiology of porotic hyperostosis among the prehistoric and historic Anasazi Indians of the southwestern U.S. Am J Phys Anthropol 44:477–488.

Eng L (1958) Chronic iron deficiency anaemia with bone changes resembling Cooley's anaemia. Acta Haematol 19:263–268.

Engfeldt B, and Njertquist S-O (1961) Vitamin-D deficiency and bone and tooth structure. World Rev Nut Diet 2:189–208.

Evans P (1982) Infantile scurvy: The centenary of Barlow's disease. Br Med J 287:1862–1863.

Fairbanks VF, and Beutler E (1972) Erythrocyte disorders. In W Williams (ed): Haematology. New York: McGraw-Hill, pp 305–317.

Fairbanks VF, Fahey J, and Beutler E (1971) Clinical Disorders of Iron Metabolism. New York: Grune and Stratton.

Findlay L (1919) Rickets: An historical note. Glasgow Med J 91:147–155.

Follis R (1958) Deficiency Disease. Springfield, IL: Charles C Thomas.

Foote J (1927) Evidence of rickets prior to 1650. Am J Dis Child 34:443–452.

Gejvall N-G (1960) Westerhus. Lund: Ohlssons.

Girdany BR, and Gaffney PC (1952) Skull changes in nutritional anemia of infancy. Proc Soc Pediatr Res p 49 (abstract).

Goodhart RS, and Shils ME (1980) Modern Nutrition in Health and Disease. Philadelphia: Lea and Febiger.

Greenfield GB (1975) Radiology of Bone Diseases. Philadelphia: J. B. Lippincott.

Harris HA (1933) Bone Growth in Health and Disease. London: Oxford Medical Publications.

Hengen OP (1971) Cribra orbitalia: Pathogenesis and probable etiology. Homo 22:57–75.

Henschen P (1961) Cribra cranii—A skull condition said to be of racial or geographical nature. Pathol Microbiol 24: 724–729.

Henschen F (1966) The History of Diseases. London: Camelot Press.

Hess AF (1920) Scurvy, Past and Present. Philadelphia: J. B. Lippincott.

Hess AF (1929) Rickets Including Osteomalacia and Tetany. Philadelphia: Lea and Febiger.

Hodges RE (1980) Vitamin C. In RB Alfin-Slater and D Kritchevsky (eds): Nutrition and the Adult. New York: Plenum Press.

Hoffbrand AV, and Lewis SM (1981) Postgraduate Haematology. London: William Heinemann.

Holmes AM, Enoch BA, Taylor JL, and Jones ME (1973) Occult rickets and osteomalacia amongst the Asian immigrant population. Q J Med, New Series, XLII, 165:125–149.

Hrdlička A (1907) Handbook of American Indians. Bureau Am Ethnol Bull 30:540–541.

Hrdlička A (1914) Anthropological work in Peru in 1913, with notes on pathology of ancient Peruvians. Smithsonian Misc Coll 61:1–69.

Hush-Ashmore R, Goodman AH, and Armelagos GJ (1982) Nutritional inference from paleopathology. In MB Schiffer (ed): Advances in Archeological Method and Theory, Vol. 5. New York: Academic Press, pp 395–473.

Hutchinson HS, and Shah SJ (1921) The aetiology of rickets, early and late. Q J Med 15:167–194.

Jaffe HL (1972) Metabolic, Degenerative and Inflammatory Diseases of Bones and Joints. Philadelphia: Lea and Febiger.

Lallo J, Armelagos GJ, and Mensforth RP (1977) The role of diet, disease and physiology in the origin of porotic hyperostosis. Hum Biol 49(3):471–483.

Lanzkowsky P (1968) Radiological features of iron deficiency anemia. Am J Dis Child 116:16–29.

Liebel RL, Greenfield AB, and Pollitt E (1979) Iron deficiency: Behavior and brain biochemistry. In M Winick (ed): Nutrition, Pre- and Postnatal Development. New York: Plenum Press.

Loomis WF (1970) Rickets. Sci Am 223:77–91.

Lukens J (1975) Iron deficiency and infection. Am J Dis Child 129:160–162.

Maat GJR (1982) Scurvy in Dutch whalers buried at Spitsbergen. Proceedings of the Palaeopathology Association 4th European Meeting, Middleberg/Antwerpen, pp 82–93.

Manchester K (1983) The Archaeology of Disease. Leeds: Arthur Wigley and Sons.

Mankin H (1974) Rickets, osteomalacia, and renal osteodystrophy. J Bone Joint Surg [Am] 56:101–128.

Martin DL, Goodman AH, and Armelagos GJ (1985) Skeletal pathologies as indicators of quality and quantity of diet. In RI Gilbert and JH Mielke (eds): The Analysis of Prehistoric Diets. New York: Academic Press, pp 227–279.

Mensforth R, Lovejoy C, Lallo J, and Armelagos G (1978) The role of constitutional factors, diet, and infectious disease in the etiology of porotic hyperostosis and periosteal reactions in prehistoric infants and children. Med Anthropol 2(1):1–59.

Møller-Christensen V (1953) Ten Lepers from Naestved in Denmark. Copenhagen: Danish Science Press.

Møller-Christensen V (1958) Bogen om Aebelholt Kloster. Copenhagen: Dansk Videnskabs Forlag.

Moore S (1929) Bone changes in sickle cell anemia with note on similar changes observed in skulls of ancient Mayan Indians. J Missouri State Med Assoc 26:561–564.

Moseley JE (1961) Skull changes in chronic iron deficiency anemia. Am J Roentgenol Radium Ther 85(4):649–652.

Moseley JE (1963) Bone Changes in Hematologic Disorders. New York: Grune and Stratton.

Moseley JE (1971) Hematologic disorders. In T Newton and DG Potts (eds): Radiology of the Skull and Brain. St. Louis: C.V. Mosby, pp 697–715.

Nathan H, and Haas N (1966) "Cribra orbitalia." A bone condition of the orbit of unknown nature. Isr J Med Sci 2:171–191.

Ortner DJ (1984) Bone lesions in a probable case of scurvy from Metlatavik, Alaska. MASCA J 3:79–81.

Ortner DJ, and Putschar W (1981) Identification of Pathological Conditions in Human Skeletal Remains. Washington, DC: Smithsonian Institution Press.

Owen S (1889) Geographical distribution of rickets, acute and subacute rheumatism, chorea, cancer, and urinary calculus in the British Islands. Br Med J 19:113–116.

Palm T (1890) The geographical distribution and aetiology of rickets. Practioner 4:270–342.

Park E (1923) The etiology of rickets. Physiol Rev 3:106.

Park E, Guild H, Jackson D, and Bond M (1935) The recognition of scurvy with especial reference to the early x-ray changes. Arch Dis Child 10:265–294.

Passmore R, and Eastwood MA (1986) Human Nutrition and Dietetics. London: Churchill Livingstone.

Poskitt EME, Cole TJ, and Lawson DEM (1979) Diet, sunlight, and 25-hydroxy-vitamin D in healthy children and adults. Br Med J 1:221–223.

Prasad A (1978) Trace Elements and Iron in Human Metabolism. New York: Plenum Press.

Rathbun TA (1984) Skeletal pathology from the Paleolithic through the Metal Ages in Iran and Iraq. In MN Cohen and GJ Armelagos (eds): Paleopathology at the Origins of Agriculture. New York: Academic Press, pp 137–167.

Reimann F, Kayhan V, Talasli V, and Gökman E (1975) X-ray and clinical study of the nose, sinuses and maxilla in patients with severe iron deficiency diseases. Laryngol Rhinol Otol 54(11):880–890.

Reimann F, and Kuran S (1973) The course, origin and nature of the "brush-like" symptom on the skull in severe blood disorders. Virchows Arch [Pathol Anat] 358:173–191.

Reimann F, Talasli V, and Gökman E (1976) Radiological determination of skull thickness and skull thickness increase in patients with severe blood dyscrasias and hyperplasia of the red marrow. Fortschr Rontgenstr 125(6):540–545.

Roberts C (1987) Case Report No. 9. Paleopathol Newsletter 57:14–15.

Robinson CH (1972) Normal and Therapeutic Nutrition. New York: Macmillan.

Ryan B (1962) Skull changes associated with chronic anaemias in Papuan children. Med J Aust 49:844–847.

Salimpour R (1975) Rickets in Tehran. Arch Dis Child 50:63–66.

Saul F (1972) The human skeletal remains of Altar de Sacrificios. Papers Peabody Museum Archeol Ethnol 63(2):3–75.

Sax B (1963) Roentgen manifestations of iron deficiency anemia in the skull of infants and children simulating those seen in Cooley's and sickle cell hemolytic anemia. Germantown Hosp J 4:72–75.

Shahidi N, and Diamond L (1960) Skull changes in infants with chronic iron-deficiency anaemia. N Engl J Med 262(3):137–139.

Smith P, Bar-Yosef O, and Sillen A (1984) Archaeological and skeletal evidence for dietary change during the late Pleistocene/early Holocene in the Levant. In MN Cohen and GJ Armelagos (eds): Paleopathology at the Origins of Agriculture. New York: Academic Press, pp 101–136.

Snow CE (1948) Indian Knoll skeletons. University of Kentucky Reports in Anthropology 4:371–545.

Strauss R (1978) Iron deficiency, infections, and immune function: A reassessment. Am J Clin Nutr 31:660–666.

Stuart-Macadam PL (1982) A correlative study of a palaeopathology of the skull. Ph.D. thesis, Department of Physical Anthropology, University of Cambridge.

Stuart-Macadam P (1985) Porotic hyperostosis: Representative of a childhood condition. Am J Phys Anthropol 66: 391–398.

Stuart-Macadam P (1986) Porotic hyperostosis: Relationship between orbital and vault lesions. Paper presented at the Sixth European Meeting of the European Palaeopathology Association, Madrid.

Stuart-Macadam P (1987a) Nutrition and anaemia in past human populations. Proceedings of the 19th Annual Chocmool Conference, 1986. Diet and Subsistence: Current Archaeological Perspectives. Calgary: University of Calgary.

Stuart-Macadam P (1987b) Porotic hyperostosis: New evidence to support the anemia theory. Am J Phys Anthropol 74:521–526.

Swischuk LE, and Hayden CK (1979) Rickets: A roentgenographic scheme for diagnosis. Pediatr Radiol 8:203–208.

Ubelaker D (1984) Prehistoric human biology of Ecuador: Possible temporal trends and cultural correlations. In MN Cohen and GJ Armelagos (eds): Paleopathology at the Origins of Agriculture. New York: Academic Press, pp 491–513.

Vahlquist B (1975) Two century perspective on some major nutritional deficiency diseases of childhood. Acta Paediatr Scand 64(2):161–171.

Wadsworth GR (1975) Nutritional factors in anemia. World Rev Nutr Diet 21:75–150.

Walker PL (1986) Porotic hyperostosis in a marine-dependent California Indian population. Am J Phys Anthropol 69(3):345–354.

Weinberg E (1974) Iron and susceptibility to infectious disease. Science 184:952–956.

Welcker H (1888) Cribra orbitalia, ein ethologisch-diagnostisches merkmal am schadel mehrerer menschrassen. Arch Anthropol 17:1.

Wells C (1964) Bones, Bodies and Disease. London: Thames and Hudson.

Wells C (1967) Weaver, tailor or shoemaker? An osteological detective story. Med Biol Illus 17:39–47.

Wells C (1975) Prehistoric and historical changes in nutritional diseases and associated conditions. Prog Food Nutr Sci 1(2):729–779.

Williams H (1929) Human paleopathology. Arch Pathol 7: 839.

Wilson DC (1931) Osteomalacia (late rickets) studies: Osteomalacia in Kangra district. Indian J Med Res 18:951–958.

Wintrobe M (1974) Clinical Hematology. Philadelphia: Lea and Febiger.

Wood-Jones F (1910) The pathological report. Bull Archaeol Surv Nubia 2:55–69.

Woodruff C (1958) Multiple causes of iron deficiency in infants. JAMA 167(6):715–720.

Zaino E (1964) Paleontologic thalassemia. Ann NY Acad Sci 119:402–412.

Zaino E (1967) Symmetrical osteoporosis, a sign of severe anemia in the prehistoric Pueblo Indians of the S.W. In WD Wade (ed): Miscellaneous Papers in Paleopathology 1, Technical Series No. 7:40–47. Flagstaff: Museum of Northern Arizona.

Reconstruction of Life From the Skeleton

Chapter 12

Stable Isotope Analysis of Prehistoric Diet

William F. Keegan
Department of Anthropology, Florida Museum of Natural History, University of Florida, Gainesville, Florida 32611

INTRODUCTION

Anthropologists have long recognized the prominent role of subsistence in the organization and evolution of human cultures (Harris, 1979; Malinowski, 1944; Morgan, 1879; White, 1949). In fact, with the adoption of an ecological or adaptational paradigm (Binford, 1968; Cohen, 1977; Flannery, 1972; Kirch, 1980), most archaeological studies have come to place a major emphasis on the distribution of humans in relation to food resources and on the strategies employed to capture those resources (e.g., Earle, 1980; Keene, 1982; Winterhalder and Smith, 1981).

The significance of subsistence activities is immediately apparent in the diversity of approaches that archaeologists have developed to study prehistoric diet. Empirical approaches include studies of floral (paleoethnobotany) and faunal (zooarchaeology) remains, subsistence technology, skeletal pathology (paleopathology), trace element analysis, and stable isotope analysis. In addition, formal models from economics and ecology and inferences from ethnographic analogy are frequently used to interpret the empirical categories of evidence (Ambrose, 1987; Buikstra et al., 1987; Keegan, 1987; Wing and Brown, 1979).

The incomplete nature of the archaeological record dictates the need for a rigorous, integrated research methodology for reconstructing past subsistence activities. Such a methodology must include three general lines of investigation that correspond to the three primary sources of knowledge concerning prehistoric diets. The first approach uses formal economic and/or ecological models of food choice. These models, expressed in terms of a common denominator or currency and tested with reference to extant subsistence economies, are required to identify the types of data to be collected and the techniques by which the data should be analyzed (Earle, 1980; Keegan, 1986; Smith 1983; Winterhalder, 1981). These models are also used to generate testable hypotheses concerning past subsistence activities.

The second approach utilizes the archaeological record. This record provides evidence of subsistence activities in many forms, including bones, plant remains, food production and processing equipment, skeletal remains, and skeletal pathological lesions resulting from known or suspected dietary causes. The recovery and identification of subsistence remains provides hard evidence of what was being consumed. However, the archaeological site formation processes that result in preservational biases make it difficult to transform such species lists or prehistoric menus into a reconstructed picture of prehistoric diet (Cohen and Armelagos, 1984; Hastorf and DeNiro, 1985; Wing and Brown, 1979). To overcome such biases a third line of investigation must be pursued. This third approach is the direct measurement of actual long-term consumption. It is accomplished with techniques such as trace element analysis and stable isotope analysis (Bumstead, 1984, 1985; DeNiro and Epstein, 1978, 1981; Farnsworth et al., 1985; Katzenberg, 1984; van der Merwe, 1982).

By considering what we would expect people to eat, the debris that survives from what they ate, and the hard tissue (bone) evidence of what they did eat, a more complete understanding of prehistoric subsistence practices can be developed. This chapter examines the use of stable isotope analysis as one component of an integrated research methodology designed to reconstruct past subsistence practices. Because the interpretation of isotopic compositions is based on the comparison of values measured in human bone collagen with those measured for items identified as having been consumed, and because isotopic compositions can only be used to distinguish certain food groups rather than individual food items, it is important to remember that this technique is not an independent method of diet reconstruction. Rather, it is a technique that requires inputs from other lines of investigation, and it provides one means for resolving certain deficiencies in those other approaches. In sum, stable isotope analysis provides a method for testing and refining dietary reconstructions that are generated from the interpretation of other sources of evidence.

This chapter begins with a historical overview of the development and anthropological applications of stable isotope analysis. Stable isotopes and their distributions are then discussed. Isotopic methods are reviewed, leading to the presentation of a model of dietary analysis. The chapter closes with a brief summary of conclusions.

HISTORICAL OVERVIEW

The use of stable isotope analysis and other osteochemical techniques to evaluate prehistoric food consumption are recent innovations in bioarchaeology. In the 1960s, radiocarbon workers noticed that dates obtained from samples of corn cobs and kernels were usually too young compared to companion dates from wood samples (Bender, 1968). Geochemical studies had already documented the discrimination of the heavier isotope ^{13}C by plants during photosynthesis (Craig, 1953, 1954; Wickman, 1952), and Bender (1968, 1971) demonstrated that such discrimination included the heaviest isotope of carbon, ^{14}C. The younger dates observed for corn samples were thus the result of enrichment in ^{14}C in corn relative to wood. Subsequent studies have generated calibrations that can be used to correct for the effects of isotopic discrimination of carbon in plants when these plants are used for radiocarbon dating (Creel and Long, 1986).

The research on plants identified a significant difference in the isotopic compositions of C_3 and C_4 plants. Since both animals and humans ultimately derive their carbon from plants, it was logical to expect that differences between classes of plants could be observed at higher levels of the food chain (Burleigh and Brothwell, 1978; DeNiro and Epstein, 1978). Among the earliest applications of this technique to human diet were efforts to identify the introduction of corn, a C_4 plant, into temperate regions in which C_3 plants predominate and C_4 plants are not common (Bender et al., 1981; Vogel and van der Merwe 1977; see Teeri and Stowe, 1976; Teeri et al., 1980).

The successes of these initial applications of stable isotope analysis to the study of human diet stimulated an increase in both the range of applications and efforts to refine the technique. With regard to applications, it has been observed that marine plants have isotopic compositions that are intermediate to those of C_3 and C_4 plants. The recognition of this difference between marine and terrestrial plants prompted efforts to identify the relative contributions of marine and terrestrial food sources in the diets of coastal human populations (Chisholm et al., 1982; Keegan and DeNiro, 1988; Schoeninger et al., 1983; Sealey and van der Merwe, 1985; Tauber, 1981).

Efforts to refine the technique include the general study of "nutritional ecology" (Kuhnlein, 1981). In its broadest sense, nutritional ecology refers to the biochemical reactions that convert food sources into organic tissues (Bumstead, 1985). It has been shown that the isotopic compositions of tissues vary as a result of the reactions that produced them (Schimmelmann, 1985; van der Merwe, 1982). Of immediate significance is the need to relate the isotopic composition of human bone collagen to the isotopic compositions of dietary items. In some cases it is also necessary to relate the bone collagen ratios of prehistoric fauna to the ratios of their flesh, the flesh being that which the prehistoric humans actually consumed (Keegan and DeNiro, 1988; Vogel and van der Merwe, 1977). Bone collagen is enriched in ^{13}C during the process of collagen formation (i.e., there is an isotopic fractionation), so it is necessary to estimate the fractionation factor in order to identify the isotopic composition of the food source(s).

A final area of investigation concerns the possible postmortem modification of carbon isotope ratios. DeNiro (1985) has demonstrated that bone collagen and other tissues may be subject to diagenic effects that shift their isotope ratios (DeNiro and Hastorf, 1985; DeNiro et al., 1985). Such shifts may result in isotope ratios that no longer reflect the diet of the individual, as discussed below.

Their success with carbon isotope studies led DeNiro and Epstein (1981:341) to suggest that "it might be possible to study other aspects of diet by isotopic analysis if it could be shown that the isotopic ratios of other elements that comprise animal tissue also reflect the isotopic composition of the diet." Building upon research that identified significant differences in the isotopic compositions of nitrogen-fixing and nonfixing plants (Delwiche and Steyn, 1970; Delwiche et al., 1979), DeNiro and Epstein (1981) reexamined the diet of prehistoric humans in the Tehuacan Valley of Mexico (cf. MacNeish, 1967). That study has been followed by other attempts to identify the contribution of nitrogen-fixing legumes in terrestrial-based diets (Farnsworth et al., 1985; Schwarcz et al., 1985). Unfortunately, the relatively minor contribution of nitrogen-fixing plants to prehistoric human diets and the modern use of fertilizer nitrogen, which reduces the difference between $\delta^{15}N$ values of legumes and nonlegumes, limit the potential applications of the nitrogen isotope method (DeNiro and Epstein, 1981; DeNiro and Hastorf, 1985).

In contrast to terrestrial ecosystems, aquatic ecosystems receive a much greater contribution of nitrogen from nitrogen-fixing species (Burns and Hardy, 1975; Capone and Carpenter, 1982; Carpenter and Capone, 1983). The study of nitrogen isotope distributions in marine environments has shown them to be useful for evaluating the contributions of marine and terrestrial foods to the diets of some coastal human populations (Keegan and DeNiro, 1988; Schoeninger and DeNiro, 1984; Schoeninger et al., 1983).

In sum, stable isotope analysis has developed to the point at which differences between plants in their carbon source, photosynthetic mode, and their use of fixed or nonfixed nitrogen provide significant dimensions for evaluating the diets of higher-order consumers. These differences have proved especially useful for evaluating marine vs. terrestrial contributions to human diet and for examining trophic level differences within ecosystems. Specific applications of the isotopic method of diet analysis are discussed in the sections that follow. The delta values for plants at the base of food webs and their significance for diet analysis are summarized in Table 1. The distributions of stable carbon and nitrogen isotopes in food webs are represented in Figure 1.

STABLE ISOTOPES AND THEIR DISTRIBUTIONS

An isotope is a form of an element with the same chemical properties but a different atomic mass. Atomic mass is a function of the number of neutrons in an atom, with heavier isotopes possessing a greater number of neutrons. In chemical and kinetic reactions, the isotopically heavier forms move at a slower rate, which results in mass-dependent differences in organic tissues. It is these mass-dependent differences in organic tissues that are used to distinguish feeding relationships. Since the absolute differences in isotopic abundances between sources are relatively small, these differences are expressed in parts per thousand (i.e., per mil or ‰) relative to a standard.

Isotopes occur in both stable and unstable (radioactive) forms. The breakdown of unsta-

TABLE 1. Delta Values of Plants at the Base of Food Webs and Their Significance for Diet Analysis

Plant group	δ-Value range (0/00)	Significance
C_3 plants (e.g., temperate grasses, wheat, rice, trees, nuts, fruits, root crops)	−25 to −21	Characterizes most plants
C_4 plants (e.g., tropical grasses, maize, *Setaria,* sugarcane, sorghum)	−15 to −5	Identifies introduction of tropical cultigens
Seagrasses (e.g., *Thalassia testudinum*)	−13 to −4	Gives seagrass food webs a distinct isotopic signature
Marine particulate organic carbon (e.g., phytoplankton and zooplankton)	−22 to −16	Gives pelagic fishes and marine mammals distinct values
N_2-fixing plants (e.g., blue-green algae)	+0 to +6	Gives coral reef habitats a distinct signature; should distinguish legumes
Non-N_2-fixing plants (e.g., most plants)	> +6	Characterizes most plants
Nitrogen fertilizers	+3 depletion	Lowers δ-values by about +3 0/00; can affect diet studies when modern equivalents are used to approximate values

ble isotopes at regular intervals (half-life) has facilitated their use as a dating technique, but they are unsuited for dietary analysis because the process of breakdown commences with the death of the plant or animal. In contrast, the relationship between stable isotopes in certain organic tissues remains constant (stable) even after the plant or animal dies. This stable ratio facilitates their use as a means for estimating dietary inputs.

Stable isotopes are used in a variety of scientific studies. For instance, oxygen isotopes ($^{18}O/^{16}O$) are sensitive to temperature differences and have therefore been used to study annual periodicity in mollusc growth (Wefer and Killingley, 1980); sulfur isotopes ($^{34}S/^{32}S$) have been used to study nutrient uptake by plants that grow in coastal locations (Fry et al., 1982b); carbon ($^{13}C/^{12}C$) and nitrogen ($^{15}N/^{14}N$) isotopes are commonly used to study the movement of nutrients through food chains (e.g., DeNiro and Epstein, 1978, 1981; Fry and Sherr, 1984; Schoeninger and DeNiro, 1984).

Isotopic studies of human diet have relied on differences in mass in the stable isotope ratios of carbon and nitrogen in the food sources. This emphasis on carbon and nitrogen reflects their roles as the building blocks of organic molecules. Isotopes of other elements may someday contribute to the study of human diet. However, the list of potential contributors is limited by the following requirements: 1) the element must be light enough to facilitate the mass-dependent discrimination of the isotopes in chemical and kinetic reactions in organic tissues; 2) the element must exhibit sufficiently large isotopic differences between major food classes (e.g., differences between nitrogen fixers and nonfixers for nitrogen and C_3 and C_4 photosynthetic modes for carbon); and 3) the isotopic ratios of the element must be amenable to measurement. The remainder of this chapter will focus on the current use of carbon and nitrogen isotopes to study diet.

Carbon Sources

The atmosphere provides a single, homogeneous source for almost all carbon in food chains. Carbon occurs in the atmosphere in two isotopically stable forms, ^{12}C and ^{13}C, which make up approximately 99% and 1%, respectively, of atmospheric carbon. Unstable radiocarbon, ^{14}C, makes up about 10^{-12}% of the carbon in the atmosphere (van der Merwe, 1982). The global uniformity of the carbon source for food chains greatly simplifies interpretations and interregional comparisons (Ambrose, 1987).

Atmospheric carbon enters food chains through plants, which obtain carbon in several ways. The primary distinction is between plants that employ the Calvin or C_3 photosyn-

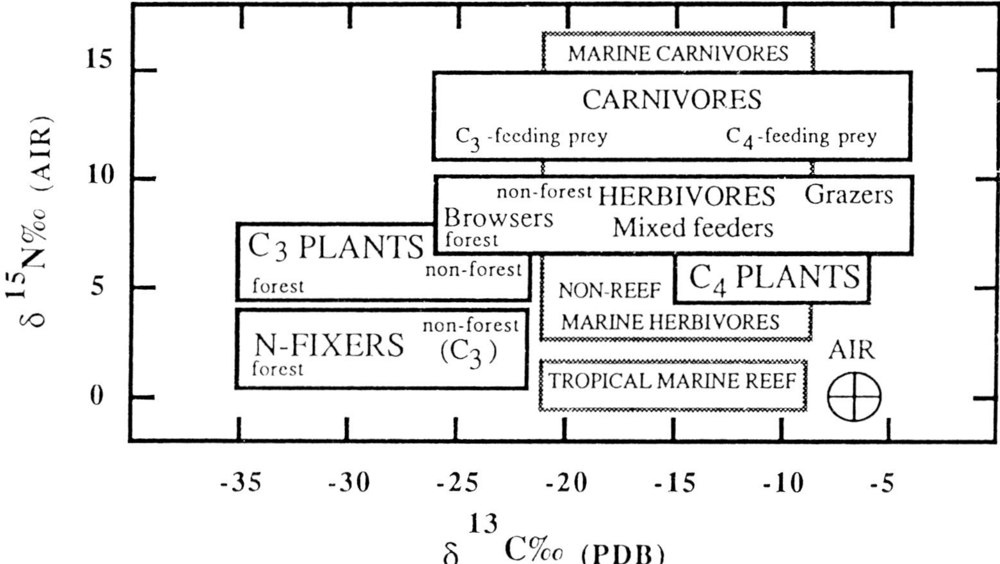

Fig. 1. An idealized representation of the distribution of stable carbon and nitrogen isotopes in terrestrial and marine ecosystems. The herbivore $\delta^{13}C$ values are shifted +5‰ from the plants they consume because of an observed isotopic enrichment between these trophic levels (Krueger and Sullivan, 1984; van der Merwe, 1982; Vogel and van der Merwe, 1977). Enrichment in $\delta^{13}C$ values between the herbivore and carnivore trophic levels has not been conclusively demonstrated, but may be only +1‰ (Ambrose and DeNiro, 1986a). Figure from Ambrose (1987). © 1987 by the Board of Trustees, Southern Illinois University. Reprinted by permission of the Center for Archaeological Investigations.

thetic pathway and those that employ the Hatch-Slack or C_4 photosynthetic pathway (van der Merwe, 1982; Vogel and van der Merwe, 1977). The labels C_3 and C_4 represent the number of carbon atoms in the molecule formed in the first step of photosynthesis. Because C_3 plants discriminate against the slower-moving ^{13}C, they have about 2% or 20‰ less ^{13}C than the atmospheric CO_2 source. In contrast, C_4 plants fix virtually all available atmospheric CO_2, which makes their isotopic values closer to that of atmospheric CO_2 (see Ambrose, 1987). Atmospheric CO_2 has a $\delta^{13}C$ value of −7‰, C_3 plants have $\delta^{13}C$ values averaging −27‰, and C_4 plants have $\delta^{13}C$ values averaging −12‰. The distribution of $\delta^{13}C$ values for C_3 and C_4 plants is bimodal with virtually no overlap between them. C_3 plants include temperate grasses, all trees and shrubs, all fruits and nuts, and cultivated roots and tubers; C_4 plants are predominately tropical grasses (e.g., corn, sugarcane, sorghum, some amaranths, and some chenopods) and other pioneering weeds (Ambrose, 1987; Teeri and Stowe, 1976; Teeri et al., 1980).

A third, less-widespread pathway has been identified for another class of terrestrial plants. Succulents and cacti adapted to xerophytic conditions use the crassulacean acid metabolism (CAM) for CO_2 fixation. This pathway produces $\delta^{13}C$ values that are similar to those for C_4 plants under certain conditions (i.e., averaging −12‰) (van der Merwe, 1982). A well-known example of a CAM plant is the pineapple.

The isotopic compositions of classes of plants are a function of both photosynthetic pathway and carbon source. In forest environments, in which only C_3 plants grow, isotopic differences between the upper and lower canopies can occur due to the addition of CO_2 from the decomposition of C_3 plant matter on the forest floor. This "canopy effect" results from the release of CO_2 with a $\delta^{13}C$ value of −26‰ to the atmosphere of the lower canopy (van der Merwe, 1982; Vogel, 1978; Wickman, 1952).

Plants in the understory thus obtain carbon from a source reduced in ^{13}C relative to plants in the upper canopy. Ambrose and DeNiro (1986b) have shown that animals feeding on forest floor plants have $\delta^{13}C$ values up to 5‰ lower than those feeding in the upper canopy.

Aquatic plants exhibit much greater variability in their isotopic compositions than their terrestrial counterparts. For instance, the reported $\delta^{13}C$ range for marine macroalgae is 30‰ (Fry and Sherr, 1984). The variability exhibited by marine plants appears to result from the isotopic composition of the dissolved inorganic carbon pool, the intracellular concentration of CO_2 or HCO_3^- that is the active species fixed by the decarboxylating enzyme, and the isotopic discrimination of the enzyme responsible for carbon fixation (Farquhar et al., 1982). Average $\delta^{13}C$ values are given below as examples of the differences between classes of marine plants. These values should not, however, be used in diet analysis without first consulting or conducting studies on local marine plants.

Most marine plants use a C_3 photosynthetic pathway. However, their seawater source of carbon is enriched in ^{13}C relative to atmospheric CO_2, and this enrichment is reflected in their $\delta^{13}C$ values. Phytoplankton, which are measured as particulate organic carbon (POC), have the most negative $\delta^{13}C$ values, averaging −21‰ for temperate marine phytoplankton (Fry and Sherr, 1984). Most marine plants occupy habitats in which the seawater carbon source is enriched in ^{13}C by about 7‰ relative to atmospheric CO_2, and their $\delta^{13}C$ values average −19‰ (Ambrose, 1987; Smith, 1972). In coral reef environments the ^{13}C enrichment is even more pronounced, with seagrasses and algae exhibiting $\delta^{13}C$ values averaging −10‰ (Bender, 1971; Benedict et al., 1980; Fry and Sherr, 1984; Fry et al., 1982a). Another source of carbon that has been identified in the study of human diet is that contributed by autotrophic sulfur bacteria through invertebrate symbionts (Berg et al., 1985; Capone and Taylor, 1980; Fry et al., 1982a; Guerinot and Patriquin, 1981; Keegan and DeNiro, 1988). Autotrophic sulfur bacteria have $\delta^{13}C$ values in the range −38 to −20‰.

To summarize, a total of seven carbon pathways and the canopy effect have been introduced as the sources of carbon for food chains. These sources are the C_3 and C_4 photosynthetic pathways, the CAM pathway, ^{13}C enrichment in aquatic and especially coral reef environments, the POC of phytoplankton, and autotrophic sulfur bacteria. This large number of carbon pathways can greatly complicate the analysis of diet for animals that feed at high-order trophic levels. Although most human diets involve inputs from a limited number of these carbon sources, Keegan and DeNiro (1988) have identified two terrestrial and three marine carbon sources in the diet of prehistoric Bahamians. Given the cultivation of pineapples, the use of aquatic species, and the tropical forest canopy in the Greater Antilles, it is possible that all of the carbon sources discussed above made some contribution to the diet of the Taino peoples who prehistorically occupied the Greater Antilles (Keegan, 1987).

Nitrogen Sources

As with carbon, the atmosphere provides the single, globally homogeneous, and ultimate source of nitrogen in most food chains. With regard to nitrogen isotope distributions, the primary distinction is between those plants and bacteria that fix nitrogen directly from air (nitrogen fixers) and those plants that rely on soil nitrogen.

Nitrogen-fixing species include bacteria and blue-green algae, and these species have $\delta^{15}N$ values that are close to that of their atmospheric source. Other plants and animals obtain fixed nitrogen through close association with bacteria and blue-green algae. For instance, legumes that form symbioses with bacteria, and certain marine invertebrates with similar symbioses, have $\delta^{15}N$ values that are also close to the atmospheric value (Capone et al., 1977; Delwiche and Steyn, 1970; Delwiche et al., 1979; Guerinot and Patriquin, 1981; Postgate, 1983; Waterbury et al., 1983). In addition to symbioses, nitrogen fixers may have a more general effect on their surrounding environment. Nitrogen fixation in the phyllosphere and rhyzosphere of marine seagrasses (e.g., *Thalassia testudinum*) may account for the less-positive $\delta^{15}N$ values of other plants and animals that inhabit seagrass and coral reef environments (Capone and Taylor, 1977, 1980; Keegan and DeNiro, 1988; Schoeninger et al., 1983).

Soil nitrogen is enriched in ^{15}N relative to air. Therefore, plants that rely on soil nitrogen also have higher levels of ^{15}N. The predominance of blue-green algae in seagrass/coral reef environments also influences the habitat as a whole. In the same way, the lower rates of nitrogen fixation in hot, open environments (Bate, 1981; Granhall, 1981), along with lower rates of ammonium volatilization (Stevenson, 1986), tend to increase $\delta^{15}N$ values in open ecosystems relative to closed ecosystems (Ambrose, 1987). In addition, the use of animal fertilizers tends to increase soil $\delta^{15}N$ values, whereas chemical fertilizers tend to decrease these values (DeNiro and Hastorf, 1985).

Finally, the environment may play a further role in the distribution of nitrogen isotopes by influencing the retention of isotopes by animals. For instance, Heaton et al. (1986) have noted a climate effect. Of greater significance is the suggested relationship between physiological mechanisms of water conservation and nitrogen isotopic mass balance (Ambrose and DeNiro, 1986b, 1987). The major form of excreted nitrogen in animals is urea in urine. Urea has lower $\delta^{15}N$ values (Steele and Daniel, 1978), which may result in interindividual differences where water balance is critical and urea recycling occurs (Ambrose and DeNiro, 1986b).

Although carbon isotope distributions have proved useful for examining the consumption of specific species (e.g., the introduction of corn), nitrogen isotope distributions seem better suited to distinguishing habitat-specific differences in diet. With the possible exception of legumes, which as yet have not been identified in isotopic analyses (but see DeNiro and Epstein, 1981; Farnsworth et al., 1985; Schwarcz et al., 1985), human populations did not rely very heavily on nitrogen-fixing plants. In contrast, important differences are apparent in the relative abundances of fixed nitrogen in marine and terrestrial environments. In this regard, nitrogen isotope analysis appears to provide an important method for distinguishing marine from terrestrial dietary inputs, as well as providing a possible method for distinguishing trophic levels within food chains (Ambrose, 1987; Keegan and DeNiro, 1988; Schoeninger and DeNiro, 1984).

Food Chains, Individual Variations, and Trophic Relations

The use of stable isotopes to analyze the diet of herbivores and higher-order consumers is based on several assumptions. First, the technique would not be applicable unless the isotopic composition of the consumer's tissues reflected the isotopic composition of the consumer's diet. Studies of the stable isotope ratios of carbon and nitrogen in bone collagen have demonstrated that these do indeed reflect the isotopic composition of the animal's diet (Bender et al., 1981; Burleigh and Brothwell, 1978; DeNiro and Epstein, 1978, 1981; Vogel and van der Merwe, 1977).

Second, in the analysis of human diet it typically is necessary to generalize about a population's diet from the analysis of a small sample of the population's members. Sampling problems in most archaeological situations influence the size and composition of the sample available for isotopic study. It is therefore necessary to establish the degree to which differences in the isotopic compositions of different bones, differences between males and females, and the relationship between individuals and the population mean affect the interpretation of isotopic measurements. In other words, the influence of diet must be distinguished from other possible variables that may have affected an individual's isotopic composition. Laboratory studies of populations that were raised on monotonous diets have demonstrated that the differences due to sex, bone sample, and small sample size are small (Bender et al., 1981; DeNiro and Epstein, 1978, 1981; DeNiro and Schoeninger, 1983). These studies make it reasonable to assume that differences in the isotopic composition of bone collagen between individuals are a reflection of differences in their diets and not the result of some other variable.

Finally, bioarchaeological studies rely on the analysis of preserved tissues. It is therefore necessary to establish the relationship between the isotopic composition of the tissue(s) and the consumer's diet. Three effects can influence the interpretation of a sample's isotopic composition: fractionation effects, trophic effects, and diagenic effects; these effects are discussed in turn.

In the course of metabolism, the isotope ratios obtained from food may be changed before they are stored in the consumer's tissues. Bumstead (1985) has suggested that differences between an individual's tissues may reflect isotopic bias, in which the carbon source for each tissue has a different isotope ratio, and isotope fractionation, in which an enzyme or other chemical process alters the ratio between source and tissue. Such separation and discrimination of isotopes during the manufacture of tissues has been shown to result in slight differences in the isotopic values of flesh, fat, bone, hair, and chitin. Previous studies have indicated a +5 ± 1‰ fractionation for $\delta^{13}C$ and about +2.5‰ fractionation for $\delta^{15}N$ for bone collagen relative to diet (Burleigh and Brothwell, 1978; DeNiro and Epstein, 1978, 1981; van der Merwe, 1982).

The isotopic composition of an animal is dependent upon its position in the food chain (Schoeninger, 1985). The distribution of stable isotopes of carbon and nitrogen in natural ecosystems has been reported in previous studies (Ambrose, 1987; Fry and Sherr, 1984; Schoeninger and DeNiro, 1984; Smith, 1972; van der Merwe, 1982).

As isotopes progress through a food chain along the continuum from plants to herbivores to primary carnivores and finally to secondary carnivores, $\delta^{13}C$ and $\delta^{15}N$ values become more positive (McConnaughy and McRoy, 1979; Minagawa and Wada, 1984; Miyake and Wada, 1967; Pang and Nriagu, 1977; Wada and Hattori, 1976). Laboratory experiments indicate an average +1‰ $\delta^{13}C$ and +3‰ $\delta^{15}N$ values of animal tissues relative to those of the animal's diet (Bender et al., 1981; DeNiro and Epstein, 1978, 1981; Macko et al., 1982). Despite difficulties in documenting trophic effects in natural ecosystems, recent field studies support the more positive trends identified in laboratory studies (Ambrose and DeNiro, 1986a; Fry and Sherr, 1984; Keegan and DeNiro, 1988; Schoeninger and DeNiro, 1984).

Trophic effects have an important influence over the distribution of $\delta^{15}N$ values (Schoeninger and DeNiro, 1984). For instance, Keegan and DeNiro (1988) found a high degree of overlap among coral reef food chains that began from different nitrogen sources. Trophic effects make it necessary to consider the isotopic compositions of all food sources that contributed to a human diet.

Finally, the postmortem processes that may have altered bone chemistry must be considered (Ambrose, 1987; Bumstead, 1985; DeNiro, 1985; DeNiro and Hastorf, 1985). Fresh bone contains two phases, a collagen or bone protein phase and an apatite or bone mineral phase. Because the carbonate in the apatite phase is reactive with the carbonate in the burial environment, apatite cannot be used for dietary analysis (Schoeninger and DeNiro, 1982, 1983; contra Sullivan and Krueger, 1981, 1983). In theory, the protein (collagen) phase of bone should not be reactive with the burial environment. Therefore, the most important diagenic effect would seem to be the loss of bone collagen such that sufficient quantities do not remain for isotopic analysis. Although the loss of collagen prevents the isotopic analysis of interesting populations, it is not as severe as problems that can arise when the isotope ratios that are obtained do not reflect in vivo dietary values.

To obtain accurate values it is first necessary to obtain a purified collagen sample (Bumstead, 1984, 1985). To determine whether or not the collagen sample is sufficiently pure to permit its use in dietary analysis, DeNiro (1985) has suggested that the atomic carbon-to-nitrogen (C/N) ratio of the sample be measured. C/N ratios in the range of 2.9 to 3.6, values that characterize collagen from fresh bone, retain their in vivo $\delta^{13}C$ and $\delta^{15}N$ values. Samples whose C/N ratios fall outside that range may not reflect the composition of the individual's diet. DeNiro et al. (1985) have shown that heating bone, as in cooking or cremation, is one process that can result in C/N ratios outside the acceptable range. However, heating does not appear to be the only possible diagenic process, because it could not be demonstrated that all of DeNiro's aberrant samples were heated. Since collagen samples with C/N ratios that fell outside the range of fresh bone had $\delta^{13}C$ and $\delta^{15}N$ values that were shifted by as much as 5‰, dietary inferences for which C/N ratios or other measures of sample purity are not reported must be evaluated with due caution.

In summary, as with all scientific techniques, stable isotope analysis is based on a variety of observations and assumptions. It is possible to analyze the diet of herbivores and higher-order consumers because the consumers' tissues reflect the isotopic composition of their diet. The isotopic composition of a subset of the population, without regard to bone or sex, can be generalized to characterize the diet of the population as a whole because the diet is the predominant variable being measured. The diet of deceased individuals can be estimated because fossil remains preserve a record of the individual's diet. This logic of isotopic analysis is not, however, without constraints. The bone collagen sample must be purified, and some measure of that purity must be reported; possible postmortem diagenic processes must be considered; and the isotopic composition of food sources must be measured to account for possible trophic effects.

ISOTOPIC METHOD OF DIET ANALYSIS

The isotopic method of diet analysis can be divided into two stages: the first stage involves the preparation of samples and the measurement of their isotopic compositions; the second stage is the interpretation of diet.

Sample Preparation

The isotopic composition of any organic tissue can be measured. In studies of human diet the samples tend to be of two types. One type of sample is examples of the food items that were consumed prehistorically. These samples tend to be modern examples of the edible portions of the food items (e.g., flesh, tubers, leaves, seeds). However, it is sometimes necessary to include hard tissue samples (e.g., bone collagen, chitin) when the food items are extinct or when samples of their flesh are unavailable. The second type of sample is typically bone collagen extracted from the skeletons of the prehistoric population. These samples are selected to reflect dietary items on the one hand and the consumers of those items on the other.

Samples of the edible portions of plants and animals are prepared by freeze-drying and grinding to a fine powder prior to combustion. An alternative procedure for terrestrial plants is to carbonize the plant to ensure the preservation of its isotope ratios. DeNiro and Hastorf (1985) have shown that carbonization does not change the carbon and nitrogen isotope ratios of plants by substantial amounts. With marine plants and invertebrates it may be necessary to wash them in dilute HCl to remove associated inorganic carbon-containing phases (Fry et al., 1982a). In all cases, the prepared sample is a freeze-dried or carbonized fine powder.

In their study of prehistoric Bahamian diets, Keegan and DeNiro (1988) found it necessary to measure the isotopic compositions of chitin from crab exoskeletons and bone collagen from extinct or endangered animals for which flesh samples were not available. Chitin preparation and analysis has been described by Schimmelmann (1985), and bone collagen preparation is described below.

"Bone collagen" is the term used by stable isotope and radiocarbon workers for the proteinaceous fraction extracted from bone by treatment with dilute acid at elevated temperatures. The material extracted has the same chemical and amino acid composition as collagen as it exists in bone. Thus, the use of "bone collagen" to describe it is justified. Although the process used in the extraction is the same as that used in the production of gelatin from bone, most workers refer to it as bone collagen.

Bumstead (1985) has suggested that existing preparation procedures are not sufficient to completely separate soil organic material from the bone organic material.

> The problem is one of separating a large, water-soluble molecule (humic-fulvic acid) from a large, water-soluble molecule (bone gelatin); both behave in chemically similar ways. Fortunately, complete separation of soil and bone protein is not required in any case where the contributing soil isotopic ratio does not differ from that of the bone samples or where purification has proceeded to the extent that contamination cannot be detected. (Bumstead 1985:546)

Bumstead (1984) has suggested specific purification techniques to eliminate possible soil contamination and has cautioned investigators against assuming that their sample is bone protein (i.e., collagen) without first checking the sample for possible contamination.

Another source of sample contamination results from the production of organic material during postmortem heating and/or diagenesis (DeNiro, 1985). To account for all possible sources of sample contamination, DeNiro (1985) has suggested that the C/N ratios of every sample be measured. Samples whose C/N ratio exceeds the range for fresh bone, 2.9–3.6, exhibit evidence of contamination, whereas those within the range are probably sufficiently pure samples of bone collagen.

The author has adopted DeNiro's (1985: 808) operational definition of bone collagen as "that fraction solubilized by treatment with 0.001 M HCl at 90° C for 10 h after bone powder is treated with 1.0 M HCl at room temperature for 20 min, washed to constant *p*H, treated with 0.125 M NaOH at room temperature for 20 h, and again washed to constant *p*H" (see DeNiro and Epstein, 1981; Schoeninger and DeNiro, 1984). The bone powder referred to in this preparation is produced by grinding the bone to less than 0.71 mm following ultrasonic cleaning. Other investigators may prefer to consult Bumstead's (1984) procedures, although both produce comparable samples.

Following sample preparation, all of the samples are combusted (Northfelt et al., 1981; Stump and Frazer, 1973). The volumes and isotopic ratios of the resulting CO_2 and N_2 are then determined by manometry and mass spectrometry, respectively. The volumes of CO_2 and N_2 are used to calculate C/N ratios (DeNiro, 1985). The isotope ratios measured by mass spectrometry relate the sample to a standard and are expressed in the δ notation

$$\delta^{13}\text{C} = \left[\frac{(^{13}\text{C}/^{12}\text{C})_{\text{SAMPLE}}}{(^{13}\text{C}/^{12}\text{C})_{\text{STANDARD}}} - 1\right] \times 1{,}000‰$$

$$\delta^{15}\text{N} = \left[\frac{(^{15}\text{N}/^{14}\text{N})_{\text{SAMPLE}}}{(^{15}\text{N}/^{14}\text{N})_{\text{STANDARD}}} - 1\right] \times 1{,}000‰$$

with Peedee belemnite (PDB) carbonate from South Carolina used as the δ^{13}C standard and atmospheric nitrogen (AIR) as the δ^{15}N standard.

The precision of the measurements is evaluated through the replicate analysis of a single sample performed intermittently throughout the study. The gas collection and measurement techniques developed by DeNiro have a precision of measurement of +0.2‰ for δ^{13}C and +0.4‰ for δ^{15}N values (DeNiro and Epstein, 1981; Schoeninger and DeNiro, 1984).

Interpretation of Diet

Most investigators who have used stable isotope analysis to analyze prehistoric diets have called this procedure "diet reconstruction." In many respects the use of such terminology is unfortunate, because it carries with it the unwarranted expectation that isotopic techniques can be employed without corroborating evidence and that the results are sufficient to provide a reconstruction of the relative percentages of each food item that was consumed. As discussed previously, isotopic methods require contributions from a variety of sources before the methods can be applied to diet analysis. Furthermore, since isotopic methods are not able to distinguish between every individual food type in the diet, interpretations must be limited to distinctions between food groups. In this regard, osteochemical techniques do not provide a direct reconstruction of diet in the sense that a diet is the sum of contributions from individual food types. Rather, these techniques identify consumption profiles, which reflect the relative contributions of different food groups.

"Food groups" are here defined as food items whose isotopic signatures are sufficiently similar to permit their clustering as a discrete group and whose group-isotopic signature is sufficiently different from other food groups to distinguish between these groups. For instance, plant food groups have been identified on the basis of whether they employ a C_3 or C_4 photosynthetic mode. "Consumption profiles" are defined as the isotopic signatures of the consumer, which reflect the contributions to diet from different food groups.

The first step in diet analysis involves the identification of the stable isotope ratios of carbon and nitrogen in a consumer's diet. The stable isotope ratios of dietary items are obtained through the direct measurement of the consumed tissues (e.g., flesh, tubers, leaves, seeds) or by estimating the isotope ratios of consumed tissues from measurements made on other tissues. For instance, it is necessary to measure the isotopic composition of bone collagen for extinct vertebrates. Because bone collagen values are enriched in ^{13}C relative to flesh, it is necessary to convert bone collagen values to the values of the consumed tissue with the appropriate fractionation factor (DeNiro and Epstein, 1978, 1981; van der Merwe, 1982). Finally, the isotopic compositions of dietary items can be estimated with reference to values published in previous studies. It is important to remember that the purpose of this step is to characterize the isotopic compositions of the food items and food groups that were consumed.

The second step involves the measurement of the isotopic compositions of bone collagen for the human consumers. To determine the isotopic composition of their diet it is necessary to convert bone collagen isotope values to diet isotope values. This conversion is accomplished by subtracting the fractionation factors for $\delta^{13}C$ and $\delta^{15}N$ from the bone collagen values. Fractionation factors between human bone collagen and diet have not been measured directly, but indirect estimates in previous studies suggest a $+5 \pm 1‰$ increase in $\delta^{13}C$ and about a $+2.5‰$ increase in $\delta^{15}N$ values for bone collagen relative to diet (Burleigh and Brothwell, 1978; DeNiro and Epstein, 1978, 1981; van der Merwe, 1982).

The final step involves interpreting what the human isotope ratios mean by comparing them to the values of food groups. Such interpretations are based on significant differences in the isotopic compositions of food groups. At the simplest level of analysis, the investigator may seek only to determine whether a particular food group made a contribution to human diet; for example, whether or not C_4 plants had been consumed in an area dominated by C_3 food groups (Bender et al., 1981; Lynott et al., 1986; van der Merwe et al., 1981; Vogel and van der Merwe, 1977). More complicated analysis can be accomplished by predicting the relative contributions of different food items with economic models and then determining the degree to which the human consumption profile conforms to the predicted diet. This final step is the most difficult. It is based upon the question being asked by the investigator, and it is limited by the ability of stable isotope analysis to distinguish between food items and food groups.

CONCLUSIONS

It has only been a decade since stable isotope analysis was first applied in the study of prehistoric human subsistence (Vogel and van der Merwe, 1977). Yet despite its recent introduction, there has been a dramatic expansion of its applications, and the method is assuming a major role in the study of prehistoric diet. Contributing to its utility are its relatively straightforward procedures, a relatively low cost, and the absence of significant conflating variables. It is therefore likely that the technique will come to assume an ever-increasing role in archaeological and bioarchaeological studies.

Starting from a globally homogeneous atmospheric source, stable isotope ratios of carbon and nitrogen provide effective tracers for the movement of these elements through food chains. This technique is limited by the similarity of isotopic signatures within classes of plants at the base of food chains, but it affords sufficient distinctions to permit the identification of the contributions to human diets from certain food groups and environments. When used in conjunction with other ethnobiological techniques, stable isotope analysis provides a valuable tool for testing and refining reconstructions of past human diets (Keegan, 1987). In this regard, it is invaluable as a independent means of hypothesis testing.

ACKNOWLEDGMENTS

It is impossible to adequately express my debt to Michael DeNiro for introducing me to the isotopic method and for supporting my research. Whether they realize it or not, Henry Aje, Stanley Ambrose, Bruno Marino, Arndt Schimmelmann, Margaret Schoeninger, and Leo Sternberg have also provided valuable assistance. Stanley Ambrose and Yaşar İşcan commented on an earlier draft; their comments were used to improve the organization and the content of this chapter. Finally, I am especially grateful to M. Yaşar İşcan and Patricia Miller-Shaivitz for inviting me to participate in their 1986 American Anthropological Association symposium, where a version of this paper was originally presented.

REFERENCES

Ambrose SH (1987) Chemical and isotopic techniques of diet reconstruction in eastern North America. In WF Keegan (ed): Emergent Horticultural Economies of the Eastern Woodlands. Carbondale: Southern Illinois University, Center for Archaeological Investigations, Occasional Paper No. 7, pp 87–107.

Ambrose SH, and DeNiro MJ (1986a) Reconstruction of African human diet using bone collagen carbon and nitrogen isotope ratios. Nature 319:321–324.

Ambrose SH, and DeNiro MJ (1986b) The isotopic ecology of East African mammals. Oecologia 69:395–406.

Ambrose SH, and DeNiro MJ (1987) Bone nitrogen isotope composition and climate. Nature 325:201.

Bate GC (1981) Nitrogen cycling in savanna ecosystems. In FE Clark and T Rosswall (eds): Terrestrial Nitrogen Cycles. Stockh Ecol Bull 33:463–475.

Bender MM (1968) Mass spectrometric studies of carbon-13 variations in corn and other grasses. Radiocarbon 10: 468–472.

Bender MM (1971) Variations in $^{13}C/^{12}C$ ratios of plants in relation to the pathway of photosynthetic carbon dioxide fixation. Phytochemistry 19:1239–1244.

Bender MM, Baerris DA, and Steventon RL (1981) Further light on carbon isotopes and Hopewell agriculture. Am Antiq 46:346–353.

Benedict CR, Wong WWL, and Wong JHH (1980) Fractionation of the stable isotopes of inorganic carbon by seagrasses. Plant Physiol 65:512–517.

Berg CJ Jr, Krzynowek J, Alatalo P, and Wiggin K (1985) Sterol and fatty acid composition of the clam, *Codakia orbicularis,* with chemoautotrophic symbionts. Lipids 20: 116–120.

Binford LR (1968) Some comments on historical versus processual archaeology. Southwest J Anthropol 24:267–275.

Buikstra JE, Bullington J, Charles DK, Cook DC, Frankenberg SR, Konigsbert L, Lambert JB, and Xue L (1987) Diet, demography, and the development of horticulture. In WF Keegan (ed): Emergent Horticultural Economies of the Eastern Woodlands. Carbondale: Southern Illinois University, Center for Archaeological Investigations, Occasional Paper No. 7, pp 67–85.

Bumstead MP (1984) Human variation: $\delta^{13}C$ in adult bone collagen and the relation to diet in an isochronous C_4 (maize) archaeological population. Los Alamos, NM: Los Alamos National Laboratory Report LA-10259-T.

Bumstead MP (1985) Past human behavior from bone chemical analysis—Respects and prospects. J Hum Evol 14:539–551.

Burleigh R, and Brothwell D (1978) Studies on Amerindian dogs, 1: Carbon isotopes in relation to maize in the diet of domestic dogs from Peru and Ecuador. J Archaeol Sci 5:535–538.

Burns RC, and Hardy RWF (1975) Nitrogen Fixation in Bacteria and Higher Plants. New York: Springer.

Capone DG, and Carpenter EJ (1982) Nitrogen fixation in the marine environment. Science 217:1140–1142.

Capone DG, and Taylor BF (1977) Nitrogen fixation (acetylene reduction) in the phyllosphere of *Thalassia testudinum.* Mar Biol 40:19–26.

Capone DG, and Taylor BF (1980) N_2 fixation in the rhyzosphere of *Thalassia testudinum.* Can J Microbiol 26: 998–1005.

Capone DG, Taylor DL, and Taylor BF (1977) Nitrogen fixation (acetylene reduction) associated with macroalgae in a coral-reef community in the Bahamas. Mar Biol 40: 29–32.

Carpenter EJ, and Capone DG (eds) (1983) Nitrogen in the Marine Environment. New York: Academic Press.

Chisholm BS, Nelson DE, and Schwartz HP (1982) Stable-carbon isotope ratios as a measure of marine versus terrestrial protein in ancient diets. Science 216:1131–1132.

Cohen MN (1977) The Food Crisis in Prehistory. New Haven: Yale University Press.

Cohen MN, and Armelagos G (eds) (1984) Paleopathology at the Origins of Agriculture. New York: Academic Press.

Craig H (1953) The geochemistry of the stable carbon isotopes. Geochim Cosmochim Acta 3:53–92.

Craig H (1954) Carbon 13 in plants and the relationships between carbon 13 and carbon 14 variations in nature. J Geol 62:115–149.

Creel D, and Long A (1986) Radiocarbon dating of corn. Am Antiq 51:826–837.

Delwiche CC, and Steyn PL (1970) Nitrogen isotope fractionation in soils and microbial reactions. Environ Sci Technol 4:929–935.

Delwiche CC, Zinke PJ, Johnson CM, and Virginia RA (1979) Nitrogen isotope distribution as a presumptive indicator of nitrogen fixation. Bot Gaz 140(Suppl):565–569.

DeNiro MJ (1985) Postmortem preservation and alteration of in vivo bone collagen isotope ratios in relation to palaeodietary reconstruction. Nature 317:806–809.

DeNiro MJ, and Epstein S (1978) Influence of diet on the distribution of carbon isotopes in animals. Geochim Cosmochim Acta 42:495–506.

DeNiro MJ, and Epstein S (1981) Influence of diet on the distribution of nitrogen isotopes in animals. Geochim Cosmochim Acta 45:341–351.

DeNiro MJ, and Hastorf CA (1985) Alteration of $^{15}N/^{14}N$ and $^{13}C/^{12}C$ ratios of plant matter during the initial stages of diagenesis: Studies utilizing archaeological specimens from Peru. Geochim Cosmochim Acta 49:97–115.

DeNiro MJ, and Schoeninger MJ (1983) Stable carbon and nitrogen isotope ratios of bone collagen: Variations within individuals, between sexes, and within populations raised on monotonous diets. J Archaeol Sci 10:199–203.

DeNiro MJ, Schoeninger MJ, and Hastorf CA (1985) Effects of heating in the stable carbon and nitrogen isotope ratios of bone collagen. J Archaeol Sci 12:1–7.

Earle TK (1980) A model of subsistence change. In TK Earle and AL Christenson (eds): Modeling Change in Prehistoric Subsistence Economies. New York: Academic Press, pp 1–29.

Farnsworth P, Brady JE, DeNiro MJ, and MacNeish RS (1985) A re-evaluation of the isotopic and archaeological reconstructions of diet in the Tehuacan Valley. Am Antiq 50:102–116.

Farquhar GD, Ball MC, Von Caemmerer S, and Roksandic Z (1982) Effect of salinity and humidity on $\delta^{13}C$ value of halophytes—Evidence for diffusional isotope fractionation determined by the ratio of intercellular atmospheric partial pressure of CO_2 under different environmental conditions. Oecologia 52:121–124.

Flannery KV (1972) The cultural evolution of civilization. Annu Rev Ecol Syst 3:399–426.

Fry B, Lutes R, Northam M, Parker PL, and Ogden F (1982a) A $^{13}C/^{12}C$ comparison of food webs in Caribbean seagrass meadows and coral reefs. Aquatic Bot 14:389–398.

Fry B, Scanlon RS, Winters K, and Parker PL (1982b) Sulphur uptake by salt grasses, mangroves, and seagrasses in anaerobic sediments. Geochim Cosmochim Acta 46: 1121–1124.

Fry B, and Sherr EB (1984) $\delta^{13}C$ measurements as indicators of carbon flow in marine and freshwater ecosystems. Contrib Mar Sci 27:13–47.

Granhall U (1981) Biological nitrogen fixation in relation to environmental factors and functioning of natural ecosystems. In FE Clark and T Rosswall (eds): Terrestrial Nitrogen Cycles. Stockh Ecol Bull 33:131–144.

Guerinot ML, and Patriquin DG (1981) N_2-fixing vibrios isolated from the gastrointestinal tract of sea urchins. Can J Microbiol 27:311–317.

Harris M (1979) Cultural Materialism. New York: Holt, Rinehart and Winston.

Hastorf CA, and DeNiro MJ (1985) Reconstruction of prehistoric plant production and cooking practices by a new isotopic method. Nature 315:489–491.

Heaton THE, Vogel JC, von la Chevallerie F, and Collett G (1986) Climatic influence on the isotopic composition of bone nitrogen. Nature 322:822–823.

Katzenberg MA (1984) Chemical analysis of prehistoric bone from five temporally distinct populations in southern Ontario. National Museum of Man Mercury Series, Archaeological Survey of Canada Paper No. 129.

Keegan WF (1986) The optimal foraging analysis of horticultural production. Am Anthropol 88:92–107.

Keegan WF (1987) Evolutionary ethnobiology: Behavioral models of foraging efficiency and their prehistoric Caribbean correlates. Paper presented at the 10th Annual Ethnobiology Conference, Gainesville, FL, March 5–8, 1987.

Keegan WF, and DeNiro MJ (1988) Stable carbon and nitrogen isotope ratios of bone collagen used to study coral reef and terrestrial components of prehistoric Bahamian diet. Am Antiq 53:320–336.

Keene AS (1982) Prehistoric Foraging in a Temperate Forest: A Linear Programming Model. New York: Academic Press.

Kirch PV (1980) The archaeological study of adaptation: Theoretical and methodological issues. In MB Schiffer (ed): Advances in Archaeological Method and Theory, Vol. 3. New York: Academic Press, pp 101–156.

Krueger HW, and Sullivan C (1984) Models for carbon isotope fractionation between diet and bone. In JE Turnlund and PE Johnson (eds): Stable Isotopes and Nutrition. ACS Symposium Series 258. Washington, DC: American Chemical Society, pp 205–220.

Kuhnlein HV (1981) Dietary mineral ecology of the Hopi. J Ethnobiol 1:84–94.

Lynott MJ, Boutton TW, Price JE, and Nelson DE (1986) Stable carbon isotopic evidence for maize agriculture in southeast Missouri and northeast Arkansas. Am Antiq 51: 51–65.

Macko SA, Lee WY, and Parker PL (1982) Nitrogen and carbon isotope fractionation by two species of marine amphipods: Laboratory and field studies. J Exp Mar Biol Ecol 63:145–149.

MacNeish RS (1967) A summary of subsistence. In DS Byers (ed): The Prehistory of the Tehuacan Valley, Vol. I: Environment and Subsistence. Austin: University of Texas Press, pp 290–309.

Malinowski B (1944) A Scientific Theory of Culture and Other Essays. Chapel Hill: University of North Carolina Press.

McConnaughy T, and McRoy CP (1979) Food-web structure and the fractionation of carbon isotopes in the Bering Sea. Mar Biol 53:257–262.

Minagawa M, and Wada E (1984) Stepwise enrichment of ^{15}N along food chains: Further evidence and the relation between $\delta^{15}N$ and animal age. Geochim Cosmochim Acta 48:1135–1140.

Miyake Y, and Wada E (1967) The abundance ration of $^{15}N/^{14}N$ in marine environments. Recent Oceanogr Works Jpn 9:32–53.

Morgan LH (1879) Ancient Society. Chicago: Charles H. Kerr.

Northfelt DW, DeNiro MJ, and Epstein S (1981) Hydrogen and carbon isotopic ratios of cellulose nitrate and saponifiable lipid fractions prepared from annual growth rings of a California redwood. Geochim Cosmochim Acta 45: 1895–1898.

Pang PC, and Nriagu JO (1977) Isotopic variations of the nitrogen isotopes in Lake Superior. Geochim Cosmochim Acta 41:811–814.

Postgate J (1983) A zoocoenotic symbiosis? Nature 306: 19–20.

Schimmelmann A (1985) Stable isotopic studies on chitin. Doctoral dissertation, Department of Earth and Space Sciences, University of California, Los Angeles. Ann Arbor, MI: University Microfilms.

Schoeninger MJ (1985) Trophic level effects of $^{15}N/^{14}N$ and $^{13}C/^{12}C$ ratios in bone collagen and strontium levels in bone mineral. J Hum Evol 14:515–525.

Schoeninger MJ, and DeNiro MJ (1982) Carbon isotope ratios of apatite from fossil bone cannot be used to reconstruct diets of animals. Nature 297:577–578.

Schoeninger MJ, and DeNiro MJ (1983) Reply to Sullivan and Krueger (letter). Nature 301:177–178.

Schoeninger MJ, and DeNiro MJ (1984) Nitrogen and carbon isotopic composition of bone collagen from marine and terrestrial animals. Geochim Cosmochim Acta 48: 625–639.

Schoeninger MJ, DeNiro MJ, and Tauber H (1983) Stable nitrogen isotope ratios of bone collagen reflect marine and terrestrial components of prehistoric human diet. Science 220:1381–1383.

Schwarcz HP, Melbye PJ, Katzenberg MA, and Knyf M (1985) Stable isotopes in human skeletons of southern Ontario: Reconstructing paleodiet. J Archaeol Sci 12: 187–206.

Sealey JC, and van der Merwe NJ (1985) Isotope assessment of Holocene human diets in Southwestern Cape, South Africa. Nature 315:138–140.

Smith BN (1972) Natural abundance of stable isotopes of carbon in biological systems. Bioscience 22:226–231.

Smith EA (1983) Anthropological applications of optimal foraging theory: A critical evaluation. Curr Anthropol 24: 625–651.

Steele KW, and Daniel RMJ (1978) Fractionation of nitrogen isotopes by animals: A further complication to the use of variations in the natural abundance of ^{15}N for tracer studies. J Agric Sci 90:7–9.

Stevenson F (1986) Cycles of Soil: Carbon, Nitrogen, Phosphorus, Sulfur, Micronutrients. New York: John Wiley.

Stump RK, and Frazer JW (1973) Simultaneous determination of carbon, hydrogen and nitrogen in organic compounds. Nucl Sci Abstr 28:746.

Sullivan CH, and Krueger HW (1981) Carbon isotope analysis of separate phases in modern and fossil bone. Nature 292:333–335.

Sullivan CH, and Krueger HW (1983) Carbon isotope ratios of bone apatite and animal diet reconstruction. Nature 301:177.

Tauber H (1981) ^{13}C evidence for dietary habits of prehistoric man in Denmark. Nature 292:332–333.

Teeri JA, and Stowe LG (1976) Climatic patterns and the distribution of C_4 grasses in North America. Oecologia 23:1–12.

Teeri JA, Stowe LG, and Livingstone DA (1980) The distribution of C_4 species of Cyperaceae in North America in relation to climate. Oecologia 47:307–310.

van der Merwe NJ (1982) Carbon isotopes, photosynthesis and archaeology. Am Sci 70:596–606.

van der Merwe NJ, Roosevelt AC, and Vogel JC (1981) Isotopic evidence for prehistoric subsistence change at Parmana, Venezuela. Nature 292:536–538.

Vogel JC (1978) Recycling of carbon in a forest environment. Oecologia Plantarium 13:89–94.

Vogel JC, and van der Merwe NJ (1977) Isotopic evidence for early maize cultivation in New York State. Am Antiq 42:238–242.

Wada E, and Hattori A (1976) Natural abundance of ^{15}N in particulate organic matter in the North Pacific Ocean. Geochim Cosmochim Acta 40:249–251.

Waterbury JB, Calloway CB, and Turner RD (1983) A cellulolytic nitrogen-fixing bacterium cultured from the gland of Deshayes in shipworms (Bivalvia: Teredinidae). Science 221:1401–1402.

Wefer G, and Killingley JS (1980) Growth histories of strombid snails from Bermuda recorded in their O-18 and C-13 profiles. Mar Biol 60:129–135.

White LA (1949) The Science of Culture. New York: Farrar, Straus.

Wickman FE (1952) Variations in the relative abundance of the carbon isotopes in plants. Geochim Cosmochim Acta 2:243–254.

Wing ES, and Brown AB (1979) Paleonutrition. New York: Academic Press.

Winterhalder B (1981) Optimal foraging strategies and hunter-gatherer research in anthropology: Theory and models. In B Winterhalder and EA Smith (eds): Hunter-Gatherer Foraging Strategies. Chicago: University of Chicago Press, pp 13–35.

Winterhalder B, and Smith EA (eds) (1981) Hunter-Gatherer Foraging Strategies. Chicago: University of Chicago Press.

Reconstruction of Life From the Skeleton

Chapter 13

Chemical Analysis of Skeletal Remains

Arthur C. Aufderheide
Department of Pathology, University of Minnesota–Duluth, Duluth, Minnesota 55812

INTRODUCTION

Although occasional investigators used "wet" laboratory methods on ancient materials as early as the 1920s, the development of the radiocarbon dating technique is often viewed as an event that ushered in the era of chemical archaeometry. Initially, the laboratory approach was directed at traditional archaeological questions, for example, analysis of artifacts to trace the source of the ore, stone, or clay from which the artifact had been fashioned. The proliferation of laboratory instrumentation following World War II, however, resulted in a progressively greater efficiency in detection and quantitation of elements and compounds in a variety of matrices. Application of some of these methods to skeletal remains has generated information that is supplemental to traditional archaeological evidence.

This chapter presents an overview of such applications, with emphasis on those that have accumulated a usable data base. The discussion begins with the application of trace element analysis. This has been employed principally in an effort to reconstruct the diet of ancient populations, but more recently has also been used to attempt demonstration of status in a population with social stratification and to identify residence site and other more "peripheral" applications. Because accumulation of lead in bone is primarily the result of anthropogenic manipulations of that metal, the utility of bone lead content to identify an increasingly wide range of social or occupational behavioral variables is becoming evident. Immunochemical methods, limited for many years to identification of the A and B antigens of the red blood cell, are finding a wider array of applications. Dating methods that are based on certain cumulative protein or mineral alterations have now evolved. The increasing utility of isotopes other than those of strontium are not included in this review because they are the focus of a separate chapter in this book. In the discussions that follow, an effort has been made to concentrate on the types of information of anthropological interest that can be generated by the utilization of the various available methods and the degree of certainty of each method. Typical examples of archaeological applications are demonstrated. Particular emphasis is placed on those metabolic aspects of the measured chemical that influence its accumulation in bone as well as the special circumstances that limit interpretative reliability of the analytical values.

USE OF TRACE ELEMENT ANALYSIS IN ANTHROPOLOGY

General Principles

Elements composing the bulk of human tissue (nitrogen, carbon, hydrogen, and oxygen) were easily measured by the relatively simple laboratory instrumentation available a generation ago, but those present in milligrams per kilogram quantities were not, causing food chemists to refer to them as "trace elements." The ease of their precise quantitation with modern measurement methods has lead current workers to prefer the term "micronutrients." These elements have little in common other than their low concentration in body tissues. The simplicity and accuracy of their laboratory quantitation has resulted in substantial medical interest during the past two decades, but the effects of both deficiencies and excesses of some of these elements have left a legacy reaching back into antiquity: the smelting of galena ore by ancient Greeks in pursuit of its silver content caused industrial poisoning from exposure to its lead by-product, and the ancient symbol for copper—ankh—was used by Egyptian priests as the symbol of life (Bhandari, 1983).

More than a dozen trace elements (Table 1) are clearly necessary for maintenance of health. A deficiency of these elements, which are known as "essential trace elements," is accompanied by negative health effects (growth retardation, specific organ dysfunctions, etc.) that are correctable by administration of the deficient element (Sandstead and Prasad, 1982). Thyroid enlargement and hypofunction secondary to iodine deficiency constitute one such well-known example. Another element may have minimal or no known useful function, but may exert a toxic effect if present in sufficient quantities. Lewis Carroll's Mad Hatter reflects the neurotoxic effect of absorbed mercury used for its depilatory effect on fur in felt production for hat manufacture. Although it is conceivable that almost any element, if absorbed in sufficiently large quantities, could produce toxic effects, those that do so in amounts small enough to be encountered in "ordinary" human experiences are sometimes grouped under the term "toxic trace elements." Lead, mercury, arsenic, and sometimes copper are included in this category. Little is known about the nutritional role of many of the other elements, which contributes to the limitations of their value to the anthropologist.

Archaeological or anthropological interest in trace elements centers principally on the prediction of 1) health effects secondary to either deficient or surplus amounts of specific trace elements in human or animal tissues and 2) social correlates of varying quantities of trace elements in body tissues.

Appropriate interpretation of measured values can only be carried out if various metabolic features often unique to each element are appreciated. Among these features, the following are often of importance to anthropologists employing trace element studies.

Exposure. The strontium content of marine shellfish is many times greater than that of the meat of a terrestrial carnivore. An unglazed, lead-free ceramic receptacle obviously will impart no lead to its contained liquid, but a pewter ewer may poison its contents. Zinc is present in high concentrations in certain meats highly prized by populations suffering protein energy malnutrition, and those food items may be more accessible to the elite of these populations. Such differences can be exploited by the investigating anthropologist.

Absorption. Dietary ingestion is not necessarily equivalent to exposure of the body tissues to the ingested element. Absorption may be profoundly influenced by competing or enhancing substances in the diet, by physiological regulation of absorption, or by the chemical state of the element. The phytate content of some cereals, for example, may bind zinc, rendering it unabsorbable; oxalates in some plants, such as rhubarb and spinach, may precipitate calcium, thus preventing its absorption; lead absorption, however, is enhanced in a low-calcium diet, while the mammalian intestine actively (but not absolutely) discriminates against strontium absorption in favor of calcium. These and other similar factors should be of major concern to those interpreting trace element concentrations in tissues.

Distribution. Trace elements are not present in equal amounts in every body organ; furthermore, various trace elements are partitioned differently. Iodine is particularly concentrated in the thyroid, which uses it as an essential element in the manufacture of thyroid hormone; its virtual absence in bone renders it valueless to the skeletal paleopathologist. Lead and strontium, however, share sufficient physicochemical properties with calcium so that the body deposits most of these elements in the same storage site as calcium, bone, a fact that is of prime importance in their employment as anthropological indicators.

Metabolism. Detoxification mechanisms may reduce the noxious effects of some elements: cadmium is bound by the metallothio-

TABLE 1. Representative Examples of Trace Elements

Element	Symbol	Function	Recommended daily allowance (mg)	Normal bone content (ppm, ash)	Dietary deficiency symptoms/signs
Essential trace elements					
Iron	Fe	Principally oxygen transport	10–20	?	Anemia; infection
Zinc	Zn	Metalloenzymes; energy and RNA metabolism	15	200	Growth retardation; infections; sexual immaturity
Copper	Cu	Metalloenzymes; hemoglobin synthesis	2–3	25	Anemia, hypoproteinemia in infants; not seen in adults
Iodine	I	Thyroid hormone synthesis	0.15	0	Hypothyroidism; goiter

Element	Symbol	Usual bone content without symptoms (ppm, ash)	Toxic symptoms
Toxic trace elements			
Lead	Pb	0–50	Abdominal colic; neuropathy; convulsions
Mercury	Hg	0.7–0.9	Brain, kidney, and liver symptoms
Arsenic	As	0.006	Liver, heart, nerve, and skin symptoms

Element	Symbol	Function	Usual bone content (ppm, ash)	Toxic symptoms
Nonessential, nontoxic trace elements				
Strontium	Sr	Unknown	100–200	None
Barium	Ba	Unknown	2	None

nein protein whose production it induces; the placenta readily permits the passage of lead, exposing the fetus to its potentially teratogenic effect, but it is quite effective in blocking the transmission of cadmium. The attraction of some tissues for certain elements (iron in muscle, zinc in bone and muscle) can be so high that the elements cannot be mobilized, even in states of deficiency, without catabolism (metabolic destruction) of the tissue.

Retention. Current interpretation of the meaning of a tissue's trace element content is possible only if the period of time during which that element was accumulated is known. This is a direct product of its tissue turnover rate, usually expressed as "half-life" ($T\frac{1}{2}$, the period required for 50% of a given amount of element to disappear from a tissue site). Such rates are quite variable among the different elements and even for the same element in different organs. The $T\frac{1}{2}$ of lead in adult brain is only a few weeks, whereas that of lead in bone is decades.

Excretion. Principal excretory routes are the urine and feces; the lungs and skin play a role in only exceptional circumstances. However, excretory efficiency varies enormously among the trace elements. Iron is so important to the body that most of it is recycled, with only a small fraction of the total being excreted in the feces. Similarly, the body's ability to excrete lead is so low that modern urban exposure inevitably results in cumulative retention. On the other hand, the potential osteopenic (reduced amount of bone per unit volume) effect of aluminum deposited in bone is normally prevented by its prompt urinary excretion following absorption. To be useful to the anthropologist, the dynamics of each trace element measured must be known.

Symptoms. The complexity of the above-listed mechanisms could be expected to produce a pathological effect unique to each element, and this is generally true. The effects of lead poisoning (colic, nerve paralysis, and convulsions), zinc deficiency (infections), or strontium accumulation (none) differ dramatically. Unfortunately, prediction of such effects based on bone content of a trace element is complicated by a dearth of reported correlations between symptoms and element concentrations in bone, by biological variation in individual susceptibility, and by the fact that human circumstances leading to trace element deficiency (such as seasonal malnutrition) rarely produce an isolated deficiency limited to only one trace element. Most of our knowledge of trace element deficiency effects is derived from laboratory animal studies rather than human experience. Indeed, for most of the trace element deficiency states identified in animals, we have little or no information regarding the fluctuations of the respective element's bone concentrations in the equivalent human state. Not surprisingly, then, the prediction of specific deficiency states based on trace element analysis of archaeological bones, logical as it might otherwise seem, is the least-attempted anthropological application of trace element studies.

From the above discussion it should be clear that all of the specifications desired by the investigating anthropologist will not be available for any of the trace elements. Furthermore, measuring additional trace elements in an attempt to overcome the uncertainties of interpretation presented by one trace element usually compounds rather than resolves the uncertainties. Nevertheless, cautious application of trace element studies in appropriately selected situations has generated information not otherwise available.

Anthropological applications. General archaeological uses made of trace element studies include the following:

1. Diet reconstruction. Archaeological evidence can frequently identify which foods were available ("menu"), but only rarely the actual selections of food consumed ("diet"), the amounts of each item selected, and its health value ("nutrition"). In appropriate circumstances trace element studies can help make such estimates, which, in turn, are useful in the prediction of time of introduction of agricultural practices in a culture, seasonal population movements, or food trading practices.

2. Health effect predictions. Elevated bone lead content has been useful in the prediction of lead poisoning in some circumstances (Handler et al., 1986), but few have attempted prediction of specific element deficiency syndromes based on archaeological trace element levels.

3. Behavioral correlations. The prediction of status (based on the presence of certain trace elements in foods considered more desirable and more available to the elite in a stratified society), subsistence pursuits (based on dietary reconstruction), and catchment delineation (based on

a *pattern* of multiple trace elements that reflects a similar pattern of the catchment area soil) are only some of the social correlates predicted by trace element study of archaeological skeletal tissue.

To be useful for archaeological purposes, therefore, a trace element 1) must accumulate in bone, 2) its amount in bone must correlate with at least one variable of anthropological interest in a known and predictable manner, and 3) its amount in archaeological bone must reflect its antemortem concentration. This last criterion is one of the most limiting of such studies. For example, iron deficiency is one of the most common and serious afflictions in the world today. Yet the assessment of iron deficiency in past populations has been frustrated by the nearly ubiquitous presence of iron in soil and its free movement from the soil into interred bone ("diagenesis"), which prevents prediction of the antemortem bone iron content. Diagenetic action is unique to each element and is poorly understood for most of them.

Specific archaeological applications of several of the more commonly measured trace elements follow; the diagenetic characteristics of each is individually discussed.

Methods of Measurement

Older, purely chemical methods did not permit precise measurements of trace element amounts, but instrumental introductions and advances during the past several decades now offer the analyst multiple options with acceptable sensitivity. A brief survey of their operational principles and varying characteristics are presented here to assist the investigator in making appropriate selections.

Electroanalysis. Movement of an ion in a liquid environment charged with an electrical field is dependent on certain physical characteristics of the ion, principally its mass and electrical charge. Anodic stripping voltammetry is a method employing ion characteristics for trace element measurement. Quantitation is achieved by first collecting the dissolved sample's ions on a cathodic electrode, then "stripping" them from it by a rapid voltage decrease. Integration of the resulting anodic current curve permits quantitation (Skoog, 1985c). Samples such as bone, with a complex matrix (elements other than the one of interest, present in the sample), can reduce the sensitivity significantly below that achievable in pure solutions of the ion. The method can be adapted for multiple element measurements. One useful application is the measurement in a large number of samples of a single element demonstrated to lend itself to sensitive detection in the sampled matrix; population screening for blood lead levels is such an application. Not all trace metals possess electrochemical characteristics appropriate to this method. Its most common application is to the "toxic metal" group.

Light (optical) spectrometry. Atoms of the solution to be tested are rendered unstable ("excited") by supplying them with energy sufficient to move an inner shell electron to an outer shell. The energy source is heat (flame or electrothermal), and the height of the temperature elevation is a significant factor in the method's sensitivity. In the absorption form of the method, a beam of light of a wavelength unique to the element to be measured is passed through a cloud of excited atoms in the test solution (Van Loon, 1980); the degree of absorption of this beam is proportional to the number of excited ions, permitting their quantitation. In the emission form, the displaced electron in the excited ion returns to its original orbit, releasing an amount of energy (in the form of emitted light radiation) unique to the atom and the electron's shell; measurement of the intensity of this emitted radiation permits quantitation (Evenson, 1984). These two methods are simple, relatively inexpensive, and require only readily taught technical skills. They do require individual element measurements. The electrothermal ("graphite furnace") form of the absorption method is considerably more sensitive than the flame emission form and, because of its sensitivity, economy, and availability, is probably the most commonly used method for trace element measurements in biological tissues today. If, however, it is necessary to measure more than one element, a modification of such instrumentation, termed "inductively coupled plasma" (ICP), is becoming increasingly popular. This method injects the atoms of the test solution into a chamber of argon gas at an extremely high temperature, and multiple detectors (one for each element) monitor the light emitted from the excited atoms of the various elements. Recent modifications provide a monochromator that scans a spectral continuum and whose detector output is stored in a computer for individual element recall. ICP sensitivity is about equal to or better than that of single element flame emission methods (Skoog, 1985a).

X-ray. Atoms to be tested are excited by supplying the energy in the form of x-rays, electrons, or protons. These methods lend themselves particularly to measurements of trace elements in solid samples. Atoms above the atomic number 10 are measurable, but sensitivity is significantly reduced with the lighter elements. When coupled with scanning electron microscopy, the distribution of the element of interest can be demonstrated (Goldstein et al., 1981). Lambert et al. (1983) have used this technique to demonstrate the location of trace elements in a femur cross section, seeking distribution patterns expected in antemortem (diffuse) or postinterment (concentrated at the periphery) accumulations.

Radioactive isotope (neutron activation analysis—NAA). When isotopically stable atoms of a trace element are bombarded by a flow of neutrons in a nuclear reactor, some of them will absorb one or more neutrons. The surplus absorbed neutrons render the isotope atom unstable, resulting eventually in a spontaneous rearrangement of the atom to a stable state, achieved and accompanied by an expulsion of the surplus energy in the form of photons (gamma rays), electrons, alpha particles, etc. The nature and energy level of these expelled energy forms are unique to each atom, and their detection and measurement result in identification and quantitation of the trace element (Skoog, 1985b). The sensitivity varies enormously, depending upon the element of interest, the competing radiation induced in other matrix elements, and the discriminating power of the detector. Simultaneous measurement of multiple elements is easily carried out with this method. Minimal or absent sample preparation is an especially attractive feature of this technique, depending upon the matrix effect (not a major problem with many elements in a bone matrix). Its limiting factor is availability of access to a nuclear reactor or other neutron source.

Mass spectrometry. Mass spectrometry is capable of identifying ionized particles of varying mass, such as the difference in atomic weight between various atoms differing in their neutron content ("isotopes"). Separation and quantitation are achieved by first permitting an energy source to react with the vaporized or gaseous form of the sample. The resulting ions are accelerated by an electrical field and then led into an analyzing chamber where a magnet's influence causes them to deviate from their original flight path, the degree of which is a function of individual ions' differences in their ratio of mass to charge. These in turn are secondary to the weight differences of the two isotopes composing those ions. Such magnet-induced flight path differences are great enough to cause the ion stream of one isotopic mass to impact the far wall of the analyzing chamber at a location different from that of the other isotope. Two different, appropriately placed detectors identify and quantitate the arriving ions of each isotope (Rose and Johnstone, 1982). Although initial instrumental purchase costs can be enormous (limiting their availability), subsequent individual measurement costs are modest, and the method is capable of an enviably high sensitivity. The method is frequently employed when it is desirable to know which of several possible different sources served as the origin of a certain trace element in situations where the ratio of that element's stable isotopes varies among the possible sources. A common example in archaeology is the estimation of the fractions of a bone sample's strontium content that originated from marine animal and terrestrial food sources, because the ratios of the strontium isotopes are frequently, though not invariably, different in those two locations.

From the above it will be apparent that the investigator's needs and resources will determine the method used. Occasional need for quantitation of a single element with considerable sensitivity and precision on a limited budget can often be met by atomic absorption spectrometry using the graphite furnace form. If the element is quite abundant (strontium in human bone, for example) the simpler flame emission form would be acceptable. Where multiple elements need to be measured in each sample, inductively coupled plasma methods may satisfy the need (although variation of the different elements' detection sensitivity may be limiting with this method), unless ready access to a nuclear reactor is available, in which case the minimal sample preparation may attract the investigator to neutron activation methodology. Where geographical distribution within the specimen is of interest, x-ray fluorescence technique with a microprobe coupled to a scanning electron microscope can provide the desired information. Characteristics of interest for these methods are summarized in Table 2.

Strontium

Strontium is one of the trace elements first used for dietary reconstruction by chemical analysis of archaeological bones. Its use is based on the principle that mammalian intestine preferentially absorbs more calcium than strontium from ingested food.

Metabolism. Strontium has no known function in the human body and little toxicity (Sillen and Kavanagh, 1982). Once absorbed, however, it may compete with calcium's often vital physiological functions; hence it is not surprising that the mammalian intestine is so constructed as to absorb more calcium than strontium, a process referred to as "calcium biopurification" or "strontium discrimination."

The food chain involved may be viewed as soil–soil water–plants–herbivore–carnivore–human. The different steps in this chain are termed "trophic levels," and, with the exception of the soil water–plants stage, each step reduces the amount of strontium (relative to calcium) that is passed on (Price et al., 1985). The first reduction (soil–soil water) occurs because of the generally greater solubility of calcium than strontium salts of rocks, and the strontium reduction at this step ranges up to twofold (Elias et al., 1982). Plants absorb calcium and strontium from soil water equally (Comar et al., 1957), but subsequent step reductions may be as much as fivefold (Price et al., 1986); at the final trophic level (human), the total reduction in Sr/Ca ratio from that of rocks may be as much as 60-fold (Elias et al., 1982). Clearly a human diet consisting primarily of plants will contain more strontium than one composed mostly of carnivore meat. Various factors affect the degree of intestinal discrimination, the principal one of interest to anthropologists being the observation that low-calcium diets enhance strontium absorption. Marine strontium concentrations are uniform throughout the world (and have been since at least the Paleozoic), but rock and soil strontium content vary widely with geography (Odum, 1951; Sillen and Kavanagh, 1982), imposing some constraints on intersite comparisons. Dietary interpretations based on this scheme must incorporate possible modifications produced by ingestion of shellfish (which may concentrate strontium up to 750-fold; Ophel, 1963; Schoeninger and Peebles, 1981) and dairy products (low in strontium; Sillen and Kavanagh, 1982).

Nearly 100% of body strontium is stored in bone, where it is associated entirely with the mineral phase (Klepinger, 1984; Schroeder et al., 1972; Tanaka et al., 1981). There is an early age effect, the bone strontium content rising until subadult or young adult stage but with little change thereafter, arguing for the limitation of comparison studies to adults (Tanaka et al., 1981). Common adult skeletal strontium concentrations are in the range of 150 to 250 ppm (ash) (Hamilton et al., 1972/1973; Hodges et al., 1950; Nusbaum et al., 1965; Spadaro and Becker, 1970). During pregnancy and lactation states, more strontium accumulates in bone because of increased intestinal absorption but continued placental discrimination against strontium transfer to the fetus (Sillen and Kavanagh, 1982). The very low levels of strontium in human milk are responsible for low infant bone strontium content, the latter rising with the addition of solid food—a phenomenon exploited to estimate weaning age (Sillen and Smith, 1984) in archaeological populations. Skeletal bone differences have been found to be absent in some studies (Sowden and Stitch, 1957) and usually do not exceed 50% in most. Within-bone differences are not great (diaphyseal concentrations exceed those of the ends of bones) (Tanaka et al., 1981), but are enough to encourage standardizing the sample site (long bone mid-diaphysis) when possible and avoiding microsamples. Because tooth enamel does not remodel, its strontium content reflects strontium levels at the time it was formed. For this reason, and because eruption times vary, use of teeth for skeletal strontium evaluation in adults should be avoided if possible or used only with elaborate controls (Sillen and Kavanagh, 1982).

Measurement methods. Atomic absorption spectrometry (AAS) in the flame mode has the

TABLE 2. Characteristics of Measurement Methods for Trace Elements

Method	Acronym or symbol	No. of measurable elements[a]	Variables relative to AAS			
			Complexity of sample preparation	Sensitivity[b]	Initial instrumental cost	Subsequent cost—individual measurement
Electrochemical						
Anodic stripping voltammetry	ASV	M	Same	Higher	Same	Same
Optical spectrometry						
Emission	AES	M	Same	Less	Less	Same
Absorption	AAS	S	—	—	—	—
Inductively coupled plasma	ICP	M	Same	Same	Higher	Less
X-ray spectrometry						
X-ray fluorescence	XF	M	Less	Less	Higher	Less
Electron microprobe	EMP	M	Less	Less	Higher	Less
Proton-induced x-ray emission	PIXE	M	Less	Less	Higher	Less
Radioisotope						
Neutron-activated analysis	NAA	M	Less	Varies with element; many higher	Higher	Less
Mass spectrometry	MS	M	More	Higher	Higher	Same

Table data is derived partly from information supplied in narrative form by Plantin (1984).
[a] S, single; M, multiple.
[b] Consult element of interest; individual variation is often substantial.

virtue of simplicity, economy, and availability as well as sensitivity, but it can only measure elements individually. Neutron activation analysis (NAA) has about equal sensitivity and is free from matrix interference, although access to instrumentation is usually limited. Inductively coupled plasma spectrometry (ICPS) requires a relatively expensive initial instrument purchase, but once acquired it possesses the desirable quality of measuring many trace elements simultaneously. Selection of method is individualized, based on the above factors.

Diagenetic considerations. Initial studies suggested that little exchange occurs between the strontium in soil and that in interred bone. Parker and Toots (1970, 1979, 1980) found equal concentrations of strontium in bone, dentine, and enamel, concluding that no diagenesis had occurred; Sillen and Kavanagh (1982) suggested that this conclusion was incorrect because enamel in vivo has lower concentrations than bone. Lambert et al. (1979) demonstrated that strontium content in excavated and modern bones were equal, and in 1982 they found no differences in strontium concentrations in ribs and femurs. Since rib contains more cancellous bone (porous, with a high surface area) than the compact femur diaphysis, the rib could be expected to yield more readily to exchange with metals in soil water. Equal concentrations found in both bones were considered supportive of a conclusion of no diagenetic effect. In 1983 Lambert and coworkers used x-ray fluorescence electron microprobe study to demonstrate diffuse distribution of strontium throughout the cross-sectional surfaces of femurs. In a field sampling study, Lambert et al. (1984) were also unable to show strontium migration from skeletal tissue into soil. All of these findings were interpreted as being consistent with no evidence of strontium diagenesis.

However, Boaz and Hampel (1978) found fossil bone strontium to correlate better with soil strontium levels than with known fossil diets, and Wessen et al. (1978) demonstrated more strontium in terrestrial herbivores than in normally high-strontium marine animals. Sillen and Kavanagh (1982) also noted that skeletal strontium concentrations in Aurignacian herbivores were equal to those of carnivores at an Israel cave site and felt the anticipated difference between the two had been obliterated by diagenesis.

After burial, the small, relatively soluble apatite crystals may dissolve, releasing their biogenic strontium content, which then mixes with the diagenetic strontium in ground water. Subsequent precipitation of ground water ions as apatite crystals can incorporate strontium of both biogenic and diagenetic origin. Diagenesis resulting in bone apatite crystal dissolution with subsequent recrystallization may be detected by scanning electron microscopy because of the larger size of the recrystallized apatite (Baud et al., 1985). Sillen argued that if some of the in vivo apatite crystals survive in an archaeologically recovered bone, then their biogenic strontium signature may be recoverable by exploiting the solubility differences between the in vivo apatite crystals and those of diagenetic origin. Using an acetate buffer at pH 4.5, he demonstrated a biogenic Sr/Ca ratio in East African animal fossils whose biogenic mineral patterns had been obliterated by diagenesis (Sillen, 1986). Application of this somewhat cumbersome method to South African fossils was partially successful, suggesting constraining variables that require further elaboration (Sillen, 1988).

Strontium's two stable isotopes—^{87}Sr and ^{86}Sr—have proved to be useful for detecting the presence and degree of diagenesis. Their ratio in sea water is 0.7091 and is constant in all oceans. This ratio, however, is altered in many terrestrial rocks and soils, especially in young volcanic rocks. The amounts of each isotope are measured by mass spectrometry, and values are very reproducible ($\pm$0.02% at the 95% confidence level). Nelson et al. (1983) successfully exploited the differences in the ^{87}Sr/^{86}Sr ratio of sea water and that of many soils. In the skeleton of a soil-interred marine mammal (seal), they demonstrated that diagenesis had increased that ratio (to 0.7460) substantially above its anticipated antemortem value, which was near that of sea water (0.7091). The difference between two such values conceivably could be used to estimate quantitatively the fraction of total strontium present in human bone from the same site that is of diagenetic origin.

From these studies it is evident that at least some circumstances can result in strontium diagenesis, requiring controls for its detection (and "correction"?). Sillen and Kavanagh (1982) urge the use of both herbivores and carnivores (preferably more than one species) from the same site and period as controls, while Elias et al. (1982) suggest comparing the Sr/Ca ratio of both modern and ancient herbivores at a particular site. The hazard of diagenetic effect currently is the major constraint on the use of strontium content for dietary reconstruction.

Anthropological applications. *Change in diet with time.* Gilbert (1975, 1977) studied strontium (and other elements) in Late Woodland Mississippian populations and found an increasing strontium concentration consistent with a dietary shift from a meat-predominant, hunter-gatherer diet to maize cultivation. A similar pattern was identified by Price and Kavanagh (1982) in Late Archaic, Middle Woodland, and Mississippian cultures. Connor and Slaughter (1984) studied northern Alaskan sites (A.D. 100 to the late nineteenth century) and discovered a progressive decrease in strontium concentrations, suggesting a shift from a marine diet (high in strontium) to one incorporating more terrestrial meat (caribou, lower in strontium), using the largely seal-eating polar bear and the grazing caribou as controls.

Detection of status differences. Studies of status differences are based on the assumptions that meat is a preferred food choice over plants and that access to meat in a society with social stratification will be greater for the elite group. Such studies are vulnerable to the validity of the assumption in the particular population of interest, and even if valid, variations in consumption of meat by different status subgroups can be expected only if meat abundance in the population is marginal. Brown (1973) suggested that higher strontium levels in females from several North American Indian sites were the result of status differences, but Sillen and Kavanagh (1982) pointed out that an equally valid interpretation could view those differences as the result of pregnancy and lactation effects. Using multiple trace elements, including strontium, Geidel (1982) compared bone levels of a group of mound burials (whose archaeological characteristics suggested they were elite) with those of nearby villagers and felt that the results suggested subadults and males had greater status than females. A similar arrangement at an A.D. 1000 Mississippian site in Georgia was studied by Blakely and Beck (1981); they found no strontium concentration differences (or those of zinc, copper, or magnesium) between the mound and the village burials. Since there appeared to be definite archaeological evidence of status for the mound burials, they concluded that such status was "earned," not ascribed (inherited), because the latter situation would have resulted in preferential access to meat since childhood, which would have decreased bone strontium content.

Delineation of catchment basin or premarital residence site. Total strontium, and especially strontium isotope ratios, may vary in different geographical settings. Measurement of numerous other trace elements may further characterize the individuality of a particular site. Such an elemental pattern may be reflected in the skeletal tissue of such a site's residents. Collective immigrant populations at a new site, or specific individuals such as might occur with individual translocation secondary to marriage, could then be identified in a burial site where such persons are commingled with natives. Decker (1986) demonstrated that such patterns (involving beryllium, vanadium, scandium, and nickel as well as strontium) at a fourteenth-century A.D. Grasshopper Pueblo site in Arizona suggested sufficient differences among burials in different areas within and extramural to the pueblo so as to imply origin from different catchment sites, a finding consistent with the archaeological evidence.

Zinc

A vast amount of medical information is available regarding zinc deficiency, but data relating to archaeological interests are sparse. The anthropologist's special interest in this metal lies in the known clinical relationship of infection to zinc deficiency states and its abundance in several food items believed to have been considered especially desirable by members of ancient populations exhibiting social stratification.

Metabolism. Although zinc is present to some extent in most food items, high levels found in meats, seafoods, and certain crustaceans (Sandstead, 1984) attracts anthropological interest because of its potential as a dietary marker. While readily absorbed by the mammalian intestine, its absorption is antagonized by calcium, and it can be bound firmly into an unabsorbable state by phytate (inositol hexophosphate), a substance commonly present in certain cereal proteins and legumes. Much of the body's zinc is found in skeletal muscle and also in bone, where it is incorporated into the apatite crystal. The zinc content of different bones in the skeleton can vary up to twofold: vertebra highest, long bone diaphysis lowest (Strehlow and Kneip, 1969). The mean of normal bone zinc content values in several different studies was about 200 ppm (ash) (Hamilton et al., 1972/1973; Nusbaum et al., 1965). It is important to recognize that the bulk of bone and muscle zinc is so tightly bound that it can be mobilized in deficiency states only by catabolism of the tissue in which it is deposited (Calhoun et al., 1974). It is equally important to understand that, while decrease in bone zinc has been demonstrated repeatedly in rats and pigs fed zinc-deficient diets under special laboratory conditions (Prasad et al., 1967, 1969; Swenerton and Hurley, 1968; Williams and Mills, 1970), we have minimal to no data regarding *human* bone zinc levels in zinc deficiency states (Calhoun et al., 1974; McBean et al., 1972). Zinc is a vital element in a host of physiological reactions; more than 200 metalloenzymes involving zinc have been described. Of these, those dealing with RNA and nuclear synthesis are of greatest interest (Oberleas and Prasad, 1970; Prasad et al., 1971). Zinc also appears to participate at the earliest stage of osteogenesis.

Measurement methods. Atomic absorption spectrometry and neutron activation analysis are sufficiently sensitive for the measurement of zinc levels, but matrix interference may prevent the application of inductively coupled plasma spectrometry (Klepinger et al., 1986).

Clinical deficiency states. Most of our knowledge about zinc deficiency in humans is derived from a genetic disease. Acrodermatitis enteropathica is a rare congenital condition characterized by zinc malabsorption. Shortly after birth, infants become ill with gastrointestinal symptoms, skin rashes, alopecia, growth retardation, emotional lability, and eye inflammation. Affected children with severe forms of this condition develop malnutrition and fatal infections. Plasma and urine zinc levels are low and laboratory findings reflecting defective cellular immunity are common, but there is no information on skeletal zinc content in these patients (Walravens, 1982). Acquired forms of zinc deficiency include protein energy malnutrition, which may be accompanied by decreased stature (Hambridge et al., 1979; Van den Hamer and Cornelisse, 1985). Growth retardation also occurs in a syndrome involving Iranian and Egyptian children described by Sandstead and Prasad (1982), believed to be the result of a high phytate diet with resulting failure to absorb ingested zinc. Alcoholics may have a negative zinc balance (Spencer et al., 1984). Data on skeletal zinc levels are minimal to absent for these conditions.

Diagenetic considerations. Although, like every other tested metal, zinc was able to penetrate a bone sample that had been immersed in an acid solution of metal ions during an in vitro simulation of possible soil conditions (Lambert et al., 1985a), most other observations testify to the relatively inert behavior of soil zinc. Nelson and Sauer (1984) measured the levels of zinc and magnesium of bones and the soil in which they were buried at an Archaic (Black Earth, Illinois) site and found the concentrations in the two locations (bone and soil) to vary independently. Jaworowski et al. (1984) demonstrated no change in bone zinc content in a series of skeletal samples over the past 5,000 years. Zinc was also demonstrated by x-ray fluorescence electron microprobe study to be diffusely distributed throughout the cross-sectional surface of excavated femurs without excessive accumulation at the cortical or endosteal surfaces, suggesting no diagenetic effect (Lambert et al. 1983). While a total absence of zinc diagenesis may be too much to hope for, to date there has been little demonstration of such a process.

Anthropological applications. Although zinc is often included in archaeological bone trace element studies when instrumention is used that is capable of generating simultaneous analyses of multiple elements, conclusions that are based on zinc levels alone are uncommon. Thus, in the status studies by Blakely and Beck (1981) and Geidel (1982) described above, zinc levels alone would probably have been considered insufficient support for the conclusions offered. In another study (Beck, 1985), the high values of zinc and strontium found in the bones of a preagricultural population were attributed to nuts. In a transitional, Late Woodland group of primarily hunter-gatherers with limited cultigens, zinc and strontium values were reversed, as would be expected in a population consuming a diet high in meat (Beck, 1985). Fornaciari et al. (1984) compared the zinc levels of skeletons found in a family mausoleum in Rome (whose associated archaeological findings suggested high social status) with those of a nearby skeletal population in a paleo-Christian basilica (whose archaeological features implied a low status); they found higher bone zinc levels of 221 ppm (ash) in the mausoleum population compared with 160 ppm (ash) for those in the basilica, confirming status differences. Simultaneous skeletal lead measurements paralleled the zinc concentrations, also confirming the suggested status differences.

Lead

In industrialized nations, lead is ubiquitous. Residents of such countries become exposed to lead in amounts exceeding their very limited ability to excrete it. The consequent accumulation of lead in human tissues, principally skeletal, is related to the degree of such exposure. This accumulation provides a unique research opportunity to predict human behavior, related to lead exposure, from the lead content of archaeological bones. Maximization of such predictions requires a working knowledge of the more common methods of human exposure to lead and its metabolism, toxicity, and diagenetic vulnerability.

Metabolism. *Exposure.* Prehistoric man probably enjoyed the low-lead air still found in some remote areas (0.004 $\mu g/m^3$ in Nepal; Piomelli et al., 1980), but with world production now exceeding a million tons annually (Settle and Patterson, 1980), the modern inner-city dweller is exposed to lead concentrations a hundredfold greater (Rabinowitz et al., 1975). From this high-lead air as much as 15 μgPb/day may be absorbed, contributing half of the lead found in the blood (Bogen et al., 1976), to which an additional 7 μgPb/day from 20–30 cigarettes may be added.

Away from ore outcroppings, most soils reveal an average lead content of only about 16 ppm (De Treville, 1964). Depending upon soil pH, only a part of this is dissolved by the soil water bathing the plant roots. Plant discrimination against lead absorption by their root systems can vary by as much as 18-fold (Elfving et al., 1978). Except for the circumstance of the use of lead arsenate as an insecticide for certain crops (e.g., potatoes) in the past, food contamination results not so much from soil uptake by plants but rather from food processing after harvest (Settle and Patterson, 1980). Ingestion of lead-contaminated soil (pica) constitutes a hazard for modern inner-city children.

Unless a local source of lead contaminates them, fresh-water streams contain relatively small quantities of lead. Patterson (1965) found an average of only 8 μgPb/liter when the federal legislation definition of potability was 50 μgPb/liter, and much less in sea water: 0.005 μgPb/liter. Common modern sources of contamination include lead solder in water distribution pipes and food cans (Settle and Patterson, 1980) and filters in beer manufacture (producing product concentrations of 10 to 290 μgPb/liter) and wine manufacture (50–510 μgPb/liter).

Lead exposure of archaeological populations varied enormously depending on time and place. Pre-Columbian North American populations rarely had exposure to natural high lead sources, nor did most of them have significant lead technology, though later groups utilized lead-glazed ceramics. The Greeks, even before the classical period, operated lead-silver mines at Lavrion near Athens, harvesting the smelted lead for water distribution pipes and other industrial applications. The Romans greatly broadened the use of this utilitarian metal, not only for pipes but also as aqueduct liners, weights, rain gutters on houses, and food containers. Especially dangerous were those containers used in wine production (McCord, 1954). Gilfillan (1965) even suggested that lead may have contributed in a major way to the rapid decline of the Roman aristocracy apparent in the first and second centuries A.D. by its gonadal toxicity and the resulting decreased fertility of affected individuals. The popularity of expensive pewter tableware and storage containers during the American colonial period so heavily exposed the wealthy class of that era that their resulting bone lead content has been utilized as a status marker (Aufderheide et al., 1981, 1985).

Absorption. Up to 40% of inhaled lead is absorbed (Bogen et al., 1976), and in urban areas this can be the origin of half the entire body lead burden. Chronic skin contact such as lead dust-contaminated clothing or lead-containing cosmetics can result in absorption, but this is only occasionally a source of substantial quantities. Intestinal absorption is a factor of age, with adults absorbing about 10% of ingested lead (Rabinowitz et al., 1975; Smith and Hursh, 1977), whereas children commonly absorb as much as 50% (Fielding and Russo, 1977). Other factors operating to increase lead absorption include alcohol, a diet low in calcium or iron, a high-fat diet, and small particle size (Angle and Stelmark, 1975; Barltrop and Khoo, 1975; Barltrop and Meek, 1979; Pfeiffer, 1977). The total daily lead retention from air, intestine, and skin in the average North American adult is 25 to 50 μg.

Transport, storage, and excretion. Once absorbed, the blood rapidly distributes lead throughout the body. Because the body deals with the lead ion much as it does with calcium, storage sites are quite predictable. Only about 5 to 10% is stored in the soft tissues, whereas the skeleton may store 95% or more (Barry, 1975; Schroeder and Tipton, 1968). Total excretion is only about 25 μgPb/day, of which 90% is via the urine and the remainder through the feces.

Kinetics. Within bone the lead ion enters the hydroxyapatite crystal (Neuman and Neuman, 1953), from which it is dislodged in vivo only with considerable difficulty. The utility of skeletal lead content in archaeological bone as a predictor of human behavior is dependent on the fact that, while the half-life ($T\frac{1}{2}$) of lead in blood and soft tissue is measurable in weeks, the $T\frac{1}{2}$ of lead in bone is estimated at three to 30 years (Batschelet et al., 1979; Rabinowitz, 1976; Rabinowitz et al., 1975). Continuing lead absorption can thus be expected to result in continuing accumulation in bone. While assumptions inherent in kinetic models will affect the precision of such estimates, the order of magnitude of bone lead residence time in adults is so long that it justifies attempts to use adult bone lead content as a reasonable reflection of lifetime lead exposure.

Quantitation. Compulsive attention to detail is necessary to avoid contamination by lead from air, sample handling, glassware, reagents, and other sources during analysis (Patterson, 1965). Instrumental methods have included colorimetry, neutron activation analysis, x-ray fluorescence, and, more recently, inductively coupled plasma, all with some degree of success (usually least with the latter). Atomic absorption spectrometry, however, remains the most commonly used method primarily because of its sensitivity and availability. In the graphite furnace mode it contributes substantially increased sensitivity over that of flame emission. Interference from bone matrix is a limiting factor and previously led to sample preparation involving extraction of lead from the powdered bone, but recent use of lanthanum ion addition to dissolved bone ash results in sufficient matrix suppression to permit direct measurement of milligram sample quantities (Wittmers et al., 1981).

Values are usually reported as micrograms of lead per gram of bone (μgPb/g) or parts per million (ppm), but it is essential to note whether the gram of bone is expressed as wet bone, dry bone, or bone ash. Wet bone is equivalent to a sample from a living individual, dry bone is a wet bone sample from which the water has been removed, while bone ash represents the mineral that has been separated from the organic bone components by heat or acids. The same sample may have a numerical value expressed as bone ash, which is more than twice that expressed as wet bone. The past tendency to express archaeological bone lead content as dry bone is gradually yielding to the popularity of bone ash expression.

Expected bone lead content will obviously be dependent upon the lead exposure of the studied individual or population. When lead is found to be present unexpectedly in skeletal tissues of prehistoric populations who resided in areas of average soil and water lead content and with no evidence of lead technology, it is usually most probably explainable as a methodological artifact. Mean skeletal lead values found by many different investigators (Barry, 1975; Hamilton et al., 1972/1973; Nusbaum et al., 1965; Spadaro and Becker, 1970; Wittmers et al., 1981) studying members of industrialized nations averaged about 40 ppm (ash). Distinct age progression from near zero at birth is evident with the curve's apogee at about the sixth or seventh decade. In other studies, however, quantities continued to increase even into later decades (Barry, 1965; Schroeder and Tipton, 1968; Strehlow and Kneip, 1969). Modern male values generally exceed those of females by about 25%.

Differences between bones of the same skeleton may be substantial and need to be addressed. Physiologically, "lead follows calcium," and the lead distribution during the growing years can be expected to be very different from that of the homeostatic, middle-aged adult. In children, significantly more lead is deposited in the actively growing long bone ends than in the diaphyses. Because the magnitude of the water and organic components are different for cancellous and trabecular bone, lead content expressed as wet bone values (and even to a lesser extent as dry bone values) will vary as the cancellous/compact bone ratios of the studied bones differ. In one such study (Gross et al., 1975), lead values expressed as wet bone varied more than threefold, with cancellous vertebral bone revealing a mean of 4.4 and compact tibial diaphysis bone 14.1 ppm wet bone. Expressing skeletal lead in terms of bone ash tends to mask this variation, generally reducing the differences to less than 25%. Variations within the same bone are substantially smaller. If only a single bone is to be sampled, the mid-diaphyseal portion of a long bone, preferably tibia, will minimize the variable factors, while the larger content of cancellous bone in the vertebra or rib will maximize them (Wittmers et al., 1987).

Teeth can be used as a sample site, but only if great care in sample collection is used. Enamel cannot be trusted to represent only absorbed lead because lead in oral cavity liquids can penetrate directly into the enamel. Secondary (peripulpal) dentine does reflect absorbed lead, and its turnover rate seems to be minimal, resulting in values substantially greater than bone (Shapiro et al., 1972).

Diagenetic considerations. Previously, considerable reassurance was generated by the observation that the mobility of soil lead was pH dependent, lead being tightly bound to alkaline soils, which also tended to best preserve skeletal tissue (Bolter et al., 1975). Initially it appeared this was supported by widely disparate values for lead content between a bone and the soil adherent to it (Waldron et al., 1979), suggesting no exchange between the two had occurred. Grandjean and Holma (1973), however, found a general correlation between such samples, though the relationship of bone lead to that in its adherent soil was "far from simple." Later it became clear that, at least under certain circumstances, there were limitations to lack of soil mobility when Waldron et al. (1979) reported unphysiologically high amounts of lead in Romano-British bones—up to 2,219 ppm (dry bone); two years later, Waldron (1981) identified lead levels up to 10,000 ppm (dry) in skeletons buried in lead coffins. Furthermore, by examining a femur cross section using a microprobe with an x-ray fluorescence technique, Waldron (1981, 1983) also demonstrated much of the lead was present on the cortical surface of the compact bone, precisely where it could be expected to be deposited if it were of soil origin. A similar amount and distribution were present in two skeletons found buried in the high-lead (16,000 ppm ash) tailings of the lead-silver mine at Lavrion, Greece (Aufderheide, unpublished data). However, when Sieber (1936) fed lead carbonate to guinea pigs and stained their bones, he detected a similar distribution of subperiosteal and subendosteal lead concentration. Studying bones of a cleric from the eleventh century A.D., stored indoors in a sarcophagus that had never been buried, Specht and Fischer (1959) also found a similar surface concentration of lead, suggesting that such distribution may at times be physiological (although the above-quoted quantities certainly are not). Other efforts at detection of diagenesis include a microprobe study of pre-Columbian North American bones (Lambert et al., 1983) showing a homogeneous distribution of lead, implying no diagenetic effect. However, in an in vitro study (Lambert et al., 1985b) carried out by immersing excavated bone tissue in an acid solution of various metals, Lambert and associates demonstrated that all studied metals under such circumstances were capable of entering bone tissue, the degree depending on the pH of the immersing solution.

Appropriate interpretation of analyzed values obviously requires detection of such diagenetic effects. Grandjean et al. (1979) proposed the detection of lead diagenesis by measuring the lead content ratio of bone/tooth on the assumption that the more porous bone would absorb soil lead more readily, altering the expected ratio. Waldron (1981) speculated on the possible value of measuring various lead isotope ratios in bone and soil, whereas Ericson et al. (1979) used barium/calcium ratios of Peruvian bones to detect diagenesis, assuming that demonstrated barium contamination of bone would imply probable lead contamination as well. Preliminary work by Patterson et al.

(1987) suggests that diagenetic barium and lead covary with a consistency sufficient to permit not only detection of diagenesis but its quantitative estimation, allowing prediction of the biogenic lead content in lead-contaminated archaeological bone. If subsequent confirmation and refinement of these results can demonstrate that this method is predictably applicable to a wide variety of geographic areas with appropriate consistency and sensitivity, many current diagenetic problems with this element may be resolved.

It is clear that under certain conditions significant lead diagenesis may occur, but the conditions themselves and the quality of the various suggested methods for its detection and assessment have not been established. Because bacterial degeneration of bone collagen can induce a local acidity within bone, even an alkaline pH of soil in which such bone is buried cannot guarantee an absence of metal exchange between soil and bone. Fortunately, however, when soil pH is not below 6, bone lead content usually correlates with known behavioral patterns (Aufderheide et al., 1981, 1985), though it remains vital to be alert for exceptional circumstances. Whenever possible, at least soil lead content and pH should be measured, and dense cortical bone should be selected as a sample site.

Toxicity. Although some recent laboratory animal studies have generated findings suggesting some possible, undefined physiological role of lead (Kirchgessner and Reichlmayr-Lais, 1981), there is no convincing evidence that lead serves any known useful purpose in the human body. In sufficient amounts, however, it can be toxic to almost any human organ. Of great public concern presently (and of interest to the anthropologist) is whether small quantities can interfere with intellectual development in children. The clinical studies of Needleman et al. (1979) demonstrate such a relationship. Although their findings have been challenged, these findings have served as a catalyst to federal regulation of air pollution. Hemoglobin synthesis is especially sensitive to lead, resulting in anemia with all of its effects, including weakness and growth retardation. Somewhat larger accumulations cause painful intestinal spasm ("colic"). Later, weakness or paralysis of nerves can lead to wrist drop or foot drop (Hernberg, 1980). Gradual leaching of stored lead from bone into the blood over a period of many years and subsequent excretion in the urine can damage the kidney (Wedeen et al., 1975). In animals (but not conclusively in humans) suppression of gonadal function with decreased fertility has been demonstrated. Cerebral symptoms can vary from mood changes to convulsions, coma, and death (Haley, 1971). Unfortunately, the medical literature generally relates symptoms to the amount of lead in blood or urine, but recently noninvasive (x-ray fluorescence) methods of bone lead measurement in living humans have been developed. These have provided a limited body of data, making it possible to estimate blood lead (and, hence, probability of symptoms) from the measured skeletal lead content of archaeological bones (Christoffersson et al., 1984; Scott et al., personal communication).

Anthropological applications. The prolonged residence time of lead in bone (measurable in decades) permits the pragmatic assumption that adult skeletal lead content reflects an individual's lifetime exposure to lead. Continual remodeling of adult bone results in liberation and loss of some stored lead, but in a population living under conditions of continuous lead exposure the rate of such loss is frequently so low that it does not obviate this assumption. Since accumulated lead exposure is only rarely from natural lead sources, exposure to anthropogenic sources will be related to certain specific activities of the examined individual, such as lead-related occupational activity or consumption of lead-contaminated foodstuffs. Knowledge of some basic characteristics of the studied culture may then assist the investigator in using the bone lead content to reconstruct aspects of the individual's activities that resulted in the lead exposure (Aufderheide et al., 1981, 1985).

Assessment of the extent of a population's lead technology. When an excavation reveals only a limited number of lead items, the question arises whether these reflect an endogenous industry or whether they were trade items. If endogenous, at least some of the population's members can be expected to have suffered a degree of lead exposure sufficient to result in bone lead accumulation. A study of over 100 burials of an Archaic North American Indian population and of a South American pre-Columbian mummy group (Chile) failed to demonstrate any detectable lead in the skeletal tissues, nor is there any archaeological evidence of lead production or use in these cultures (Aufderheide et al., 1988). In contrast, modern North Americans are so extensively exposed to lead that adult bone lead values average over 40 ppm (ash) (Hamilton et al., 1972/1973; Nusbaum et al., 1965).

Identification of status differences. During the North American colonial period of the seventeenth and eighteenth centuries, pewter and other lead products were so expensive that their use on plantations was largely restricted to the wealthy owners and managers. Their slaves' household goods, however, were of vegetable or unglazed earthenware construction and their water was drawn from wells as needed; these afforded little opportunity for lead exposure. Mean skeletal lead content of the wealthy owner's family members on an A.D. 1700 plantation was found to be 185 ppm (ash), whereas that of their largely black slave labor group interred in a segregated cemetery was only 35 ppm (ash) (Aufderheide et al., 1981). Historical records for this plantation confirm the prediction of status in this group suggested by the bone lead content differences.

Identification of specific individuals' unique social or occupational activity. One of the skeletons buried with those of the labor force in the above-described plantation was that of a young white male. His bone lead content was precisely that of the otherwise black labor force, whose mean value was 35 ppm (ash). Historical records of this plantation indicate the employment of white indentured servants until about A.D. 1700; this seems to be the most plausible explanation for this individual. Note that, had the labor force cemetery not been segregated, this individual's place in the plantation society would have been predicted more precisely by his bone lead content than by his race. In addition, an 18-year-old black female in the labor force skeletal group revealed a high bone lead concentration of 98 ppm (ash), suggesting she may have been functioning as a cook or servant in the plantation owner's home.

Change in lead exposure over time. Grandjean and Holma (1973) determined lead content of skeletal tissues in 111 Danish individuals between 4000 B.C. and A.D. 1972. They found only trace levels of lead until A.D. 1350; levels then rose to 6.8 ppm (ash) in the eighteenth century, rising to 19.0 in the 1940s and subsiding again to 1.4 in 1972. Jaworowski et al. (1984) found a similar pattern in Poland, though there the peak level was reached during the Middle Ages. The chronologic levels of drill cores in the Greenland ice cap can be dated, and determinations of lead content in these as far back as 800 B.C. also reveal a pattern of only trace levels until the industrial revolution (Murozumi et al., 1969).

Assessment of Roman lead exposure. Historical records indicate that the Romans were exposed to lead sources to an extent suspected of reaching levels of serious lead toxicity (Gilfillan 1965; Nriagu, 1983). In a series of skeletal lead measurements of excavated Romano-British bones, Waldron et al. (1979) confirmed elevated bone lead content; typical of their findings were values of 74 to 385 ppm (dry) in ribs from a Poundbury, England site. Confirmation from sites within Italy has been hindered by the popularity of cremation among Romans. In the relatively small number of available skeletal populations, there is also difficulty in securing provenience data sufficient to establish socioeconomic status of the studied groups. Recent discoveries of numerous skeletons at Herculaneum have provided a rare opportunity in this area, and the publication of their measured lead content after analyses have been completed is expected to make a useful contribution to this field of study.

Prediction of health effects. The black slave population of a colonial Barbados sugar plantation was found to harbor very high skeletal lead concentrations, ranging up to 424 ppm (ash) with a mean of about 120. The source was apparently lead contamination of the plantation's sugar product during its processing and its final distillation into rum using lead stills, accompanied by extensive consumption of the rum by the slaves. Confirmation of the presence of the expected symptoms was found in reports by contemporary physicians, even though they did not recognize them as those of a lead poisoning epidemic (Handler et al., 1986).

Miscellaneous applications. Skeletal lead content studies have been useful in helping separate individual bones accidentally commingled during excavation and on several occasions contributed to forensic identification of recovered skeletal tissues by revealing the presence of significant amounts of bone lead, proving their modern (post-Columbian) origin (Aufderheide et al., 1988).

PALEOSEROLOGY

The most common application of serological techniques to archaeological skeletal tissue has been in identification of blood cell antigens. Blood groups consist of genetically controlled polymorphic antigen systems, lending themselves to population genetics studies capable of demonstrating relationships between populations or, sometimes, even individuals (Race and Sanger, 1975). The ABO and, to a lesser extent, the MN systems are the best studied. The HLA system antigens are present on most blood and tissue cells other than the red blood cells. These studies are more technically difficult (Rodey, 1976) and have not been carried out on skeletal tissue, although a few reports of their demonstration in mummy soft tissues are in the literature (Allison and Gerszten, 1982; Hansen and Gurtler, 1983; Stastny, 1974). The problems with these techniques include reactions with extraneous substances capable of producing false-positive results, such as reaction of the test antibody with plant material containing substances similar to red blood cell antigens (Micle et al., 1982; Thieme and Otten, 1957). False-negative results can be the result of antigen destruction by contaminating bacterial enzymes.

Methods

Agglutination—inhibition (AI). The principle upon which the AI method is dependent is reduction in the amount of a test serum's antibody concentration brought about by action of the appropriate antigen in the test sample. This is the most commonly used technique, but it is especially vulnerable to false-positive results (Allison and Gerszten, 1982; Allison et al., 1976, 1978).

Serological micromethod (SM). The suspected antigen is extracted from the test material and adsorbed to the surface of group O red blood cells, which can then be tested by the usual anti-A or anti-B test sera (Connolly and Harrison, 1969). Addition of the antiglobulin technique can increase sensitivity (Hart et al., 1978).

Microelution (ME). A known test antibody is permitted to be exposed to a suspected antigen-containing sample; the antibody that becomes fixed to the sample's antigen is subsequently eluted and identified. The method is believed to be more consistent in its results than AI, but its performance requires fastidious laboratory manipulation (Hart et al., 1980).

Immunodiffusion (ID). Known antibody sera and sample extract are permitted to diffuse through an agar medium toward each other, and the resulting precipitation patterns in the agar where they meet and react are compared with those of known antigens. This is a very sensitive technique, but is most effective if quite concentrated solutions are available (Kellermann, 1971).

Immunoelectrophoresis (IE). Known antigen and sample extracts are first subjected to electrophoretic separation, after which the presence and location of the antigen is demonstrated by immunodiffusion. This is a very sensitive technique (Kellermann 1971, 1972).

Antibody induction (AInd). An extract of the sample is injected (usually with an immunizing-enhancing substance) into an appropriate animal in an effort to induce an antibody response; the latter is usually identified by conventional agglutination methods. The method is slow, cumbersome, and expensive, but may produce results when other methods fail (Allison and Gerszten, 1982; Allison et al., 1976).

Anthropological Applications

Katsunama and Katsunama (1929) first identified AB antigens in human remains, and Matson (1934) later identified these in skeletal tissue of mummies. Subsequent work by Boyd and Boyd (1937) and Candela (1936) expanded these applications.

Population genetics. Allison et al. (1978) examined 111 South American mummies. They found all groups present, but of interest was the fact that B and AB antigens were present in early pre-Columbian mummies, decreasing in frequency until they were almost absent during colonial times. Boyd (1959) suggested American Indians had brought blood group B with them when they crossed the Bering Strait but then gradually lost it; the work by Allison and colleagues seems to support this concept.

Hart et al. (1980) suggest that because individuals with blood group AB contain no anti-A or anti-B antibodies in their serum, they may be more vulnerable to infections by certain bacteria (*Salmonella, Pneumococcus*) that also display AB antigens. Subsequent selection against this combination of antigens may be responsible for the low frequency of the AB antigen combination today.

Paternity genetics. Employing the principles of paternity genetics, Harrison et al. (1969) and Connolly et al. (1980) used the ABO and MN blood group systems to help establish the kingship and paternity of the Egyptian pharaoh Tutankhamen.

The lack of consistently reliable methods to control against false-positive and false-negative results continues to hamper the field of paleoserology. In addition, it must be acknowledged that the ABO and MN systems are not sufficiently polymorphic to demonstrate very close relationships between populations.

The HLA antigen system is extremely polymorphic (more than 100 alleles at four loci) and capable of demonstrating very close relationships within families, but to date these antigens have not been demonstrated in material extracted from skeletal tissue.

Evolutionary genetics. Even fossilized tissues frequently contain antigenic proteinaceous material. DeJong et al. (1974) demineralized fossil shells, and by utilizing antibody induction with subsequent immunodiffusion methods they revealed positive reactions of the induced antibodies with three modern cephalopod species antigens, demonstrating remarkable preservation of a protein's antigenicity over 70 million years. They also speculated on possible evolutionary lineage implications of minor differences in reactions.

MISCELLANEOUS APPLICATIONS

Amino Acid Analysis

Analysis of amino acid content of bone collagen may reflect metabolic abnormalities. Porotic hyperostosis is a pathological change in the cranium characterized by patchy absence of the calvarium's outer table, exposing the porous cancellous bone of the underlying diploe, which are greatly thickened secondary to bone marrow hyperplasia. This enlargement of the bone marrow space is believed to have been responsive to a persistent anemia. The Mediterranean distribution of the condition parallels that of the congenital anemia "thalassemia," while in the American Southwest the anemia is thought to have been caused by a deficiency of iron in the maize-dependent diet common to that area. Efforts to predict antemortem iron levels from chemical measurements in archaeological bone have, however, been frustrated by iron diagenesis. von Endt and Ortner (1982) have provided indirect evidence that iron *may* be involved. Stability of the collagen molecule is dependent upon cross linkage of its molecular fibers; such cross linkage is stabilized in part by the amino acids proline and lysine in their hydroxylated forms. Iron and vitamin C (ascorbic acid) are cofactors in such enzymatic hydroxylation. Amino acid analysis of skeletal collagen from a southwestern American Indian child with porotic hyperostosis demonstrated up to a 25% reduction in such amino acids and their hydroxylation below the level in control samples. This result is consistent with a deficiency of iron, although a similar result would be expected with a vitamin C (and possibly other) deficiency.

Even calcified fossils as ancient as the Devonian period have demonstrated the presence of amino acids (Abelson, 1957; Miller and Wyckoff, 1968), although control of diagenetic effects in such specimens can be a problem. Ho (1966, 1967) analyzed demineralized Pleistocene fossils revealing a pattern of amino acids expected from animal collagen, truly a testimony to the durability of the collagen molecule, although less hydroxyproline than would be predicted did suggest some molecular deterioration. Even the electron microscopic structure of collagen was recognizable in some studied samples (Little et al., 1962; Shackleford and Wyckoff, 1964; Wyckoff et al., 1963). The substantial information potential implied by the presence of intact collagen in such ancient fossils has not been fully exploited, although Ho (1967) suggested that the known relationship between collagen molecular structure and body temperature could be employed to predict body temperatures of extinct animals.

Dating Methods Based on Chemical Analysis of Bone

Radiocarbon. The tissues of living humans and animals reflect the ratio of radioactive carbon isotope atoms to those of stable carbon isotopes in the carbon dioxide of the air they breathe. After death, this ratio is decreased by radioactive decay of ^{14}C at a predictable rate ($T\frac{1}{2}$ or half-life of ^{14}C is about 5,730 years). Determination of this ratio using radioactive energy detection methods permits calculation of the postmortem interval up to about 45,000 years. Recent application of the accelerator mass spectrometry method has reduced greatly the required sample size (Hedges and Gowlett, 1986).

Amino acid racemization (AAR). Amino acids composing body proteins are asymmetric molecules, capable of rotating a beam of plane-polarized light to the right or left. Living humans have proteins composed almost exclusively of *l* forms of asymmetric molecular structure. After death, a slow process of spontaneous conversion (called racemization) to its optically inactive *d* form occurs at a temperature-dependent rate. Determination of the *d* form/*l* form ratio of amino acids in bone collagen permits estimation of the postmortem interval. The practical range for such estimation is 1,000 to 150,000 years. Two bone samples from a California site were dated by this method at up to 48,000 years B.P. (Bada, 1975; Bada and Protsch, 1973; Bada et al., 1974), implying much earlier human occupation of the New World than traditional archaeological evidence would suggest (see Uranium Series below). Because a small amount of racemization occurs in certain tissues during life, the method has been used to estimate the age at death of an ancient Alaskan Eskimo whose body had been frozen for 1,600 years, the low temperature having so profoundly retarded the rate of racemization after death that it was justifiable to assume that the racemization observed in the body had all occurred during life (Masters and Zimmerman, 1978).

Uncertainty relating to the temperature experienced during the entire postmortem interval continues to limit the accuracy of this method, as does the intrusion into the bone of amino acids of diagenetic origin. Suggested methods to control these variables include "calibrating" the method for each site by independent radiocarbon measurements of alternative samples from the same site but of younger age within the range measurable by the ^{14}C technique, but unidentifiable variables operating at periods exceeding 50,000 years can remain undetected. These potential variables continue to introduce an undesirable degree of uncertainty into the interpretative validity of this otherwise conceptually attractive dating method.

Uranium series. Under certain specific circumstances, uranium-containing soil may enter bone defects created by degenerating collagen. If the uranium becomes "trapped" (often chemically), prompt and further entry is prevented; the enclosed uranium compounds continue their radioactive decay: $^{236}U \rightarrow {}^{230}Th$ and $^{235}U \rightarrow {}^{231}Pa$. Later quantitation of the ratio of uranium compounds to their decay products can estimate the interment interval over a range of 5,000 to 350,000 years. "Contamination" resulting from field conditions permitting later diagenesis, which render application of this method inappropriate, is a common problem limiting its usefulness. This technique was used to assess the age of the California bones previously measured by amino acid racemization. The uranium method dated them at only 8,000 to 11,000 years (Bischoff and Rosenbauer, 1981), well within the period beginning about 12,000 to 14,000 years B.P. for early New World immigration predicted by conventional archaeological theory. Currently, lack of control over diagenetic effects has discouraged most workers from applying this method to bone samples (Schwarcz, 1978).

Electron spin resonance (ESR). Irradiation of the hydroxyapatite crystal in bone creates paramagnetic foci whose ESR signals can be detected and quantitated. Natural radiation from the soil in which bones are interred can produce such an effect, the degree of which is a function of the burial interval. The ages of bones from several sites evaluated by this method have been estimated from 2,000 to 19,000 B.P., but the technique is believed capable of a useful range up to several million years (Gogte and Murty, 1986; Mascarenhas et al., 1982).

Bone fluorine content. Soil fluorine ions will exchange with the hydroxyl ions in the hydroxyapatite crystal of bone mineral after interment. The chemical determination of bone fluorine content for prediction of burial interval became well known with its employment to help expose the Piltdown Man hoax. It soon became apparent that the rate of hydroxyl ion replacement by fluorine was the result of a host of unpredictable soil variables unique to the burial site. Since, therefore, the results provide information only on the relative burial intervals whose validity is restricted to a single studied site, the method today is primarily of archaeometric historical interest.

THE FUTURE

The pace of expansion of chemical methods applied to bone tissue these past two decades has increased logarithmically. Even without introduction of totally new methods, one can anticipate development in certain areas. The remarkable durability of collagen in interred bone will surely encourage application of further studies based on protein preservation. These can be expected to include stable isotope ratios of elements other than nitrogen and oxygen. Effects of specific dietary deficiencies on the amino acid content of collagen analogous to that of ascorbic acid will certainly be investigated. An expansion of the search for temperature-dependent reactions similar to that of amino acid racemization will most likely be pursued because of the potential application to climate prediction. Irreversibly altered protein products that are cumulative will be sought to be employed as chemical measures of age at death. If methods can be found that will both identify the presence and quantitate the degree of diagenesis, permitting trace metal bone content values to be "corrected" to antemortem values, the applications of these elements will be expanded much more extensively. The potential information stored in bone fat tissue is almost unexplored and would seem to hold some promise for identification of animal species in the diet. Even though DNA has not been extracted from archaeological bones to date, the recent demonstration of intact human DNA fragments in soft tissues of desiccated Egyptian mummies (Paabo, 1985) and 8,000-year-old brain tissue of Amerindians recovered from a peat bog (Doran et al., 1986) suggests the exciting possibilities that could result from the ability to study molecular changes in this protein that is central to the course of life and evolution. Surely the acquisition and application of investigative chemical probes observed these past several decades, together with the promise of new ones, provide a bright and exciting future for bioanthropology.

SUMMARY

Except for stable isotope analysis (see Keegan, Chapter 12, this volume), the most common chemical substances quantitated today in archaeological bone are certainly trace elements. The theoretical basis supporting such analyses begins with the observation that humans enjoy a variety of options in selection of food items, occupations, social activities, and habitat. Trace metals of anthropologic interest are those of varying content in the environmental components relating to the listed options. Following modification by metabolic factors, bone mineral concentrations of such elements may reflect these variations, and their archaeological skeletal concentrations can then be useful in prediction of the specific choices exercised by the studied individual. Anthropological applications of these principles has involved chemical dietary reconstruction with quantitation of the individual dietary components, identification of native catchment basins, health effects, socioeconomic status, occupation, and other characteristics. Diagenetic movement of certain elements (e.g., iron and aluminum) completely frustrates their antemortem behavior predictive value, but may be inconstant or minimal in others (zinc, lead). Our greatest experience is with strontium. Used under appropriate conditions, it clearly can be predictive, but in other circumstances diagenesis just as clearly may invalidate its application. Similar conditions may affect bone lead concentration, but appear to do so much less frequently; the susceptibility of zinc and other elements largely remains to be defined. Efforts to combat diagenetic effects through the use of more sophisticated chemical methods, such as trace element isotope ratios or differential solubility (Sillen, 1986) may, if successful, greatly expand potential anthropological applications of trace element studies.

Paleoimmunological methods may be underused in anthropology. Repeated demonstration of antigen (but only rarely antibody) preservation in human remains is encouraging. Postmortem protease breakdown of intact proteins into polypeptides and peptides (not normally encountered in fresh human tissues) with consequent falsely reactive or nonreactive results challenges the laboratory skills of the investigator. These conditions require a much more elaborate system of controls and greater experience to produce consistently reliable results, but the information potentially available may justify the necessary effort. The ability to use such methods for identification of special infectious agents would be especially attractive. Recent demonstration of the persistence of intact DNA fragments in human remains promise the achievement of such goals through the application of DNA molecular biology methodology, especially the creation of specific DNA probes.

Methods applicable to dating a bone specimen older than 45,000 years are controversial, contain serious limitations, and do not generate an accuracy level approaching that of radiocarbon.

Widening availability of current instrumentation, expanding applications of new technology, and increasing acceptance by funding agencies of chemistry's potential anthropological contributions all promise a near-explosive future for this field of research.

REFERENCES

Abelson PH (1957) Some aspects of paleobiochemistry. Ann NY Acad Sci 69:276–285.

Allison MJ, and Gerszten E (1982) Paleopathology in South American Mummies, 3rd Ed. Richmond: Medical College of Virginia, pp 54–71.

Allison MJ, Hossaini AA, Castro N, Munizaga J, and Pezzia A (1976) ABO blood groups in Peruvian mummies. Am J Phys Anthropol 44:55–62.

Allison MJ, Hossaini AA, Munizaga J, and Fung R (1978) ABO blood groups in Chilean and Peruvian mummies. Am J Phys Anthropol 49:139–142.

Angle CR, and Stelmark KL (1975) Lead and iron deficiency. In DD Hemphill (ed): Trace Substances in Environmental Health, Vol. XI. Columbia: University of Missouri, pp 377–386.

Aufderheide AC, Angel JL, Kelley JO, Outlaw AC, Outlaw MA, Rapp G, and Wittmers LE (1985) Lead in bone III. Prediction of social correlates from skeletal lead content in four colonial American populations (Catoctin Furnace, College Landing, Governor's Land and Irene Mound). Am J Phys Anthropol 66:353–361.

Aufderheide AC, Neiman FD, Wittmers LE, and Rapp G (1981) Skeletal lead content as an indicator of lifetime lead ingestion and the social correlates in an archaeological population. Am J Phys Anthropol 55:285–291.

Aufderheide AC, Wittmers LE, Rapp G, and Wallgren J (1988) Anthropological applications of skeletal lead analysis. Am Anthropol 90:932–936.

Bada JL (1975) Amino acid racemization reactions and their geochemical implications. Naturwissenschaften 62: 71–79.

Bada JL, and Protsch R (1973) Racemization reaction of aspartic acid and its use in dating fossil bones. Proc Natl Acad Sci USA 70(5):1331–1334.

Bada JL, Schroeder RA, and Carter GF (1974) New evidence for the antiquity of man in North America deduced from aspartic acid racemization. Science 184:791–793.

Barltrop D, and Khoo HE (1975) Nutritional determinants of lead absorption. In DD Hemphill (ed): Trace Substances in Environmental Health, Vol. IX. Columbia: University of Missouri, pp 369–376.

Barltrop D, and Meek F (1979) Effect of particle size on lead absorption from the gut. Arch Environ Health 34(4): 280–285.

Barry PSI (1975) A comparison of concentrations of lead in human tissues. Br J Ind Med 32:119–139.

Batschelet E, Brand L, and Steiner A (1979) On the kinetics of lead in the human body. J Math Biol 8:15–23.

Baud CA, Bang S, Kramar C, Lacotte D, Tochon-Danguy HJ, and Very JM (1985) Some aspects of lead uptake by the bones. In ND Priest (ed): Metals in Bone. Lancaster: MTP Press Ltd.

Beck LA (1985) Bivariate analysis of trace elements in bone. J Hum Evol 14(5):493–503.

Bhandari B (1983) Trace elements in human health and disease. Q Med Rev 34:1–33.

Bischoff JL, and Rosenbauer RJ (1981) Uranium series dating of human skeletal remains from the Del Mar and Sunnyvale sites, California. Science 213:1003–1005.

Blakely RL, and Beck LA (1981) Trace elements, nutritional status, and social stratification at Etowah, Georgia. Ann NY Acad Sci 376:417–431.

Boaz NT, and Hampel J (1978) Strontium content of fossil tooth enamel and diet of early hominids. J Paleontol 52(4):928–933.

Bogen DC, Welford GA, and Morse RS (1976) General population exposure to stable lead and 210Pb to residents of New York City. Health Phys 30(4):359–362.

Bolter E, Butz T, and Arseneau JF (1975) Mobilization of heavy metals by organic acids in the soils of a lead mining and smelting district. In DD Hemphill (ed): Trace Substances in Environmental Health, Vol. IX. Columbia: University of Missouri, pp 107–112.

Boyd WC (1959) A possible example of the action of selection in human blood groups? J Med Educ 34:398–399.

Boyd WC, and Boyd LG (1937) Blood grouping tests on 300 mummies. J Immunol 32:307–319.

Brown A (1973) Bone strontium content as a dietary indicator in human skeletal populations. Ph.D. dissertation, University of Michigan. Ann Arbor, MI: University Microfilms, Publication No. 74-15,677.

Calhoun NR, Smith JC, and Becker KL (1974) The role of zinc in bone metabolism. Clin Orthop 103:212–233.

Candela PB (1936) Blood-group reactions in ancient human skeletons. Am J Phys Anthropol 21:429–432.

Christoffersson JO, Schutz A, Ahlgren L, Haeger-Aronsen B, Mattsson S, and Skerfving S (1984) Lead in finger-bone analyzed *in vivo* in active and retired lead workers. Am J Ind Med 36:473–489.

Comar CL, Russell RS, and Wasserman RH (1957) Strontium-calcium movement from soil to man. Science 126(3272):485–492.

Connolly RC, and Harrison RG (1969) Kingship of Smenkhare and Tutankhamen affirmed by serological micromethod. Nature 224:325.

Connolly RC, Harrison RG, Abdalla AB, and Ahmed S (1980) An analysis of the interrelationships between pharaohs of the 18th dynasty. Masca J 1(6):178–181 (Mummification Supplement).

Connor M, and Slaughter D (1984) Diachronic study of Inuit diets utilizing trace element analysis. Arctic Anthropol 21:123–134.

Decker KW (1986) Isotopic and chemical reconstruction of diet and its biological and social dimensions at Grasshopper Pueblo, Arizona. Paper presented at the 51st Meeting of the Society for American Archaeology, New Orleans, Louisiana.

DeJong EW, Westbroek P, Westbroek JF, and Bruning JW (1974) Preservation of antigenic properties of macromolecules over 70 Myr. Nature 252:63–64.

De Treville F 91964) Natural occurrence of lead. Arch Environ Health 8:212–221.

Doran GH, Dickel DN, Ballinger WE, Agee OF, Laipis PJ, and Hauswirth WW (1986) Anatomical, cellular and molecular analysis of 8000 year old human brain tissue from the Windover archaeological site. Nature 323:803–806.

Elfving DC, Hascheck WM, Stehn RA, Bache CA, and Lisk DJ (1978) Heavy metal residues in plants cultivated on and in small mammals indigenous to old orchard soils. Arch Environ Health 33:95–99.

Elias RW, Hirao Y, and Patterson CC (1982) The circumvention of the natural biopurification of calcium along nutrient pathways to atmospheric inputs of industrial lead. Geochim Cosmochim Acta 46:2561–2580.

Ericson J, Shirahata H, and Patterson CC (1979) Skeletal concentrations of lead in ancient Peruvians. N Engl J Med 300:946–951.

Evenson MA (1984) Principles of instrumentation. In JB Henry (ed): Clinical Diagnosis and Management by Laboratory Methods. Philadelphia: W.B. Saunders, pp 24–42.

Fielding JE, and Russo PK (1977) Exposure to lead: Sources and effects. N Engl J Med 297:943–945.

Fornaciari G, Trevisani E, and Ceccanti B (1984) Indagini paleonutrizionali e determinazione del piombo osseo mediante spettroscopia ad assorbimento atomico sui resti schelectrici di e poca Tardo-Romana (IV secolo d.C.) Della "Villa dei Goriani" (Roma). Arch Antropol Etnol 114: 149–175.

Geidel RA (1982) Trace element studies for Mississippian skeletal remains: Findings from neutron activation analysis. Masca J 2(1):13–16.

Gilbert RI (1975) Trace element analyses of three skeletal Amerindian populations at Dickson Mounds. Ph.D. dissertation, University of Massachusetts. Ann Arbor, MI: University Microfilms, Publication No. 76-5854.

Gilbert RI (1977) Applications of trace element research to problems in archeology. In RL Blakely (ed): Biocultural Adaptation in Prehistoric America. Athens: University of Georgia Press, pp 85–100.

Gilfillan SC (1965) Lead poisoning and the fall of Rome. J Occup Med 7:53–60.

Gogte VD, and Murty MLK (1986) ESR dating of Kurnool Caves, South India. Man Environ X:135–140.

Goldstein JI, Newbury DE, Echlin P, Joy DC, Fiori C, and Lifshin E (1981) Scanning Electron Microscopy and X-ray Microanalysis. New York: Plenum Press.

Grandjean P, and Holma B (1973) A history of lead retention in the Danish population. Environ Physiol Biochem 3:268–273.

Grandjean P, Nielson V, and Shapiro IM (1979) Lead retention in ancient Nubian and contemporary populations. J Environ Pathol Toxicol 2:781–787.

Gross SB, Pfitzer EA, Yeager DW, and Kehoe RA (1975) Lead in human tissues. Toxicol Appl Pharmacol 32:638–651.

Haley T (1971) Saturnism, pediatric and adult lead poisoning. Clin Toxicol 4:11–29.

Hambridge KM, Chavez MN, Brown RM, and Walravens PA (1979) Zinc nutritional status of young, middle-income children and effects of consuming zinc-fortified breakfast cereals. Am J Clin Nutr 32:2532.

Hamilton EI, Minski MJ, and Cleary JJ (1972/1973) The concentration and distribution of some stable elements in healthy human tissues from the United Kingdom. Sci Total Environ 1:341–374.

Handler JS, Aufderheide AC, and Corruccini RS (1986) Lead content and poisoning in Barbados slaves. Soc Sci Hist 10(4):399–425.

Hansen HE, and Gurtler H (1983) HLA types of mummified Eskimo bodies from the 15th century. Am J Phys Anthropol 61:447–452.

Harrison RG, Connolly RC, and Abdalla A (1969) Kingship of Smenkhkare and Tutankhamen affirmed by serological micromethod. Nature 224:325–326.

Hart GD, Kvas I, and Soots M (1978) Blood group testing of ancient material with particular reference to mummy Nakht. Transfusion 18(4):474–478.

Hart GD, Kvas I, Soots M, and Badaway G (1980) Blood group testing of ancient material. Masca J 1(5):141–145.

Hedges RE, and Gowlett JA (1986) Radiocarbon dating by accelerator mass spectrometry. Sci Am 254:100–107.

Hernberg S (1980) Biochemical and clinical effects and responses as indicated by blood contamination. In RL Singhal and JA Thomas (eds): Lead Toxicity. Baltimore: Urban & Schwarzenberg, pp 367–399.

Ho TY (1966) The isolation and amino acid composition of the bone collagen in Pleistocene mammals. Comp Biochem Physiol 18:353–358.

Ho TY (1967) The amino acids of bone and dentine collagens in Pleistocene mammals. Biochim Biophys Acta 133:568–573.

Hodges RM, MacDonald NS, Nusbaum R, Stearns R, Ezmirlian F, Spain P, and McArthur C (1950) The strontium content of human bones. J Biol Chem 185:519–524.

Jaworowski Z, Barbalat F, Blain C, and Peyre E (1984) Chronological course of the content of lead, cadmium and zinc in human bones in France. C R Acad Sci Paris 299(10):409–412.

Katsunama S, and Katsunama R (1929) On the bone marrow cells of man and animal in the Stone Age of Japan. Proc Im Acad Japan 5:388.

Kellermann G (1971) Methodological investigations on the ABO-typing of ancient bones. Humangenetik 14:50–55.

Kellermann G (1972) Further studies on the ABO-typing of ancient bones. Humangenetik 14:232–236.

Kirchgessner M, and Reichlmayr-Lais AM (1981) Lead deficiency and its effects on growth and metabolism. In JM Gawthorne, J Howell, and CL White (eds): Trace Element Metabolism in Man and Animals, Vol. 4. Canberra: Australian Academy of Science, pp 390–393.

Klepinger LL (1984) Nutritional assessment from bone. Annu Rev Anthropol 13:75–96.

Klepinger LL, Kuhn JK, and Williams WS (1986) An elemental analysis of archaeological bone from Sicily as a test of predictability of diagenetic change. Am J Phys Anthropol 70:325–331.

Lambert JB, Simpson SV, Buikstra JE, and Charles DK (1984) Analysis of soil associated with Woodland burials. In JB Lambert (ed): Archaeological Chemistry III. Washington, DC: American Chemical Society, pp 97–113.

Lambert JB, Simpson SV, Buikstra JE, and Hanson D (1983) Electron microprobe analysis of elemental distribution in excavated human femurs. Am J Phys Anthropol 62:409–423.

Lambert JB, Simpson SV, Szpunar CB, and Buikstra JE (1985a) Bone diagenesis and dietary analysis. J Hum Evol 14(5):477–482.

Lambert JB, Simpson SV, Weiner SG, and Buikstra JE (1985b) Induced metal-ion exchange in excavated human bone. J Archaeol Sci 12:85–92.

Lambert JB, Szpunar CB, and Buikstra JE (1979) Chemical analysis of excavated human bone from Middle and Late Woodland sites. Archaeometry 21:115–119.

Lambert JB, Vlasak SM, Thometz AC, and Buikstra JE (1982) A comparative study of the chemical analysis of ribs and femurs in Woodland populations. Am J Phys Anthropol 59:289–294.

Little K, Kelly M, and Courts A (1962) Studies on bone matrix in normal and osteoporotic bone. J Bone Joint Surg [Br] 44(3):503–519.

Mascarenhas S, Baffa Filho O, and Ikeya M (1982) Electron spin resonance dating of human bones from Brazilian shell-mounds (Sambaquis). Am J Phys Anthropol 59: 413–417.

Masters PM, and Zimmerman MR (1978): Age determination of an Alaskan mummy: Morphological and biochemical correlation. Science 201:811.

Matson GA (1934) A procedure for determining the distribution of the blood groups in mummies. Proc Soc Exp Biol Med 31:964–968.

McBean LD, Dove JT, Halstead JA, and Smith JC (1972) Zinc concentration in human tissues. Am J Clin Nutr 25: 672–676.

McCord CP (1954) Lead poisoning in the ancient world. Med Hist 17:391–399.

Micle S, Kobilyansky E, Nathan M, Arensburg B, and Nathan H (1982) ABO-typing of ancient skeletons from Israel. Am J Phys Anthropol 47:89–92.

Miller MF, and Wyckoff RWG (1968) Proteins in dinosaur bones. Proc Natl Acad Sci USA 60:176–178.

Murozumi M, Chow TJ, and Patterson C (1969) Chemical concentrations of pollutant lead aerosols, terrestrial ducts and sea salts in Greenland and Antarctic snow strata. Geochim Cosmochim Acta 33:1247–1294.

Needleman HL, Gunnoe C, Leviton A, Reed R, Peresie H, Maher C, and Barrett P (1979) Deficits in psychologic and classroom performance of children with elevated dentine lead levels. N Engl J Med 300:689–695.

Nelson B, DeNiro NJ, Schoeninger MJ, and DePaolo DJ (1983) Strontium isotope evidence for diagenetic alteration of bone: Consequences for diet reconstruction. Geol Soc Am Bull 15:562.

Nelson DA, and Sauer NJ (1984) An evaluation of postdepositional changes in the trace element content of human bone. Am Antiq 49(1):141–147.

Neuman WF, and Neuman MW (1953) The nature of the mineral phase of bone. Chem Rev 53:1–45.

Nriagu JO (1983) Saturnine gout among Roman aristocrats: Did lead poisoning contribute to the fall of the empire? N Engl J Med 308:660–663.

Nusbaum RE, Butt EM, Gilmour TC, and DiDio SL (1965) Relation of air pollutants to trace metals in bone. Arch Environ Health 10:227–232.

Oberleas D, and Prasad AS (1970) Metabolic aspects of zinc dependent enzymes. Conference on Trace Elements in Environmental Health. Substances in Environmental Health Proceedings, Vol. 4, pp 247–254.

Odum HT (1951) The stability of the world strontium cycle. Science 114:407–411.

Ophel IL (1963) The fate of radiostrontium in a freshwater community. In A Schultz and AW Klement (eds): Radioecology. London: Chapman and Hall, pp 213–216.

Paabo S (1985) Molecular cloning of ancient Egyptian mummy DNA. Nature 314:644–645.

Parker RB, and Toots H (1970) Minor elements in fossil bone. Geol Soc Am Bull 81:925–932.

Parker RB, and Toots H (1979) Strontium in vertebrate fossils: A cautionary tale. Am J Phys Anthropol 50(3):469–470.

Parker RB, and Toots H (1980) Trace elements in bones as paleobiological indicators. In AK Behrensmeyer and AP Hill (eds): Fossils in the Making. Chicago: University Chicago Press, pp 197–207.

Patterson CC (1965) Contaminated and natural lead environments of man. Arch Environ Health 11:344–360.

Patterson CC, Shirahata H, and Ericson JE (1987) Lead in ancient human bones and its relevance to historical developments of social problems with lead. Sci Total Environ 61:167–200.

Pfeiffer CJ (1977) Gastroenterologic response to environmental agents—Absorption and interactions. In SR Geiger (ed): Handbook of Physiology, Reactions to Environmental Agents. Baltimore: Williams and Wilkins, pp 349–374.

Piomelli S, Corash L, Corash MB, Seaman C, Mushak P, Glover B, and Padgett R (1980) Blood lead concentrations in a remote Himalayan population. Science 210: 1135–1136.

Plantin LO (1984) Analytical methods for trace elements in biological material. Acta Neurol Scand [Suppl] 100:95–99.

Prasad AS, Oberleas D, Miller ER, and Luecke RW (1971) Biochemical effects of zinc deficiency: Changes in activities of zinc-dependent enzymes and ribonucleic acid and deoxyribonucleic acid content of tissues. J Lab Clin Med 77:144–152.

Prasad AS, Oberleas D, Wolf P, and Horwitz JP (1967) Studies on zinc deficiency: Changes in trace elements and enzyme activities in tissues of zinc-deficient rats. J Clin Invest 46(4):549–557.

Prasad AS, Oberleas D, Wolf P, Horwitz JP, Miller ER, and Luecke RW (1969) Changes in trace elements and enzyme activities in tissues of zinc-deficient pigs. Am J Clin Nutr 22(5):628–637.

Price TD, and Kavanagh M (1982) Bone composition and the reconstruction of diet: Examples from the midwestern United States. Midcont J Archaeol 7(1):61–79.

Price TD, Schoeninger MJ, and Armelagos GJ (1985) Bone chemistry and past behavior: An overview. J Hum Evol 14:419–447.

Price TD, Swick RW, and Chase EP (1986) Bone chemistry and prehistoric diet: Strontium studies of laboratory rats. Am J Phys Anthropol 70:365–375.

Rabinowitz M (1976) Kinetic analysis of lead metabolism in healthy humans. J Clin Invest 58:60–70.

Rabinowitz M, Wetherill G, and Kopple J (1975) Absorption, storage and excretion of lead by normal humans. In DD Hemphill (ed): Trace Substances in Environmental Health, Vol. IX. Columbia: University of Missouri, pp 361–368.

Race RR, and Sanger R (1975) Blood Groups in Man. Oxford: Blackwell Scientific Publications, pp 8–63.

Rodey GE (1976) History and nomenclature of the HLA system. In RB Dawson (ed): HLA Typing. Washington DC: American Association of Blood Banks.

Rose ME, and Johnstone RA (1982) Mass Spectrometry for Chemists and Biochemists. Cambridge: Cambridge University Press.

Sandstead HH (1984) Trace metals in human nutrition. Curr Concepts Nutr 13:37–46.

Sandstead HH, and Prasad AS (1982) Clinical, Biochemical and Nutritional Aspects of Trace Elements. New York: Alan R. Liss, pp 83–101.

Schoeninger MJ, and Peebles CS (1981) Effect of mollusc eating on human bone strontium levels. Ann Archaeol Sci 8:391–397.

Schroeder HA, and Tipton IH (1968) The human body burden of lead. Arch Environ Health 17:965–978.

Schroeder HA, Tipton IH, and Nason AP (1972) Trace metals in man: Strontium and barium. J Chronic Dis 25:491–517.

Schwarcz HP (1978) Uranium series disequilibrium dating. Geosci Can 5:184–188.

Settle DM, and Patterson CC (1980) Lead in albacore: Guide to lead pollution in Americans. Science 207:1167–1176.

Shackleford JM, and Wyckoff RWG (1964) Collagen in fossil teeth and bones. J Ultrastruct Res 11:173–180.

Shapiro IM, Needleman HL, and Tuncay OC (1972) The lead content of human deciduous and permanent teeth. Environ Res 5:467–470.

Sieber E (1936) Histochemisch er Bleinachweiss im Knochen. Z Exp Med 181:273–280.

Sillen A (1986) Biogenic and diagenetic Sr/Ca in Plio-Pleistocene fossils of the Omo Shungura formation. Paleobiology 12:311–323.

Sillen A (1988) Solubility profiles of synthetic apatites and Swartkranz fossil fauna. Paper read at Advanced Seminar in Bone Chemistry, University of Capetown, South Africa, June 16–18.

Sillen A, and Kavanagh M (1982) Strontium and paleodietary research: A review. Yrbk Phys Anthropol 25:67–90.

Sillen A, and Smith P (1984) Weaning patterns are reflected in strontium-calcium ratios of juvenile skeletons. J Archaeol Sci 11:237–245.

Skoog DA (1985a) Emission spectroscopy based upon plasma, arc and spark atomization. In Principles of Instrumental Analysis, 3rd Ed. Philadelphia: Saunders College Publishing, pp 294–306.

Skoog DA (1985b) X-ray spectroscopy. In Principles of Instrumental Analysis, 3rd Ed. Philadelphia: Saunders College Publishing, pp 456–486.

Skoog DA (1985c) Voltammetry and polarography. In Principles of Instrumental Analysis, 3rd Ed. Philadelphia: Saunders College Publishing, pp 664–703.

Smith FA, and Hursh JB (1977) Bone storage and release. In SR Geiger (ed): Handbook of Physiology, Reactions to Environmental Agents. Baltimore: Williams and Wilkins, pp 469–482.

Sowden EM, and Stitch SR (1957) Trace elements in human tissue. Biochem J 67:104–109.

Spadaro JA, and Becker RO (1970) The distribution of trace metal ions in bone and tendon. Calcif Tissue Res 6:49–54.

Specht W, and Fischer K (1959) Toxicological study of the remains of a 900-year-old body. Arch Kriminol 124:61–84.

Spencer H, Kramer L, Osis D, and Norris C (1984) Studies of zinc metabolism during nutritional repletion following excess alcohol intake. In DD Hemphill (ed): Trace Substances in Environmental Health, Vol. XVIII. Columbia: University of Missouri, p 24.

Stastny P (1974) HL-A antigens in mummified pre-Columbian tissues. Science 183:864–866.

Strehlow CD, and Kneip TJ (1969) The distribution of lead and zinc in the human skeleton. Am Ind Hyg Assoc J 30: 372–378.

Swenerton H, and Hurley LS (1968) Severe zinc deficiency in male and female rats. J Nutr 95:8–18.

Tanaka G, Kawamura H, and Nomura E (1981) Reference Japanese man-II. Distribution of strontium in the skeleton and in the mass of mineralized bone. Health Phys 40: 601–614.

Thieme FP, and Otten CM (1957) The unreliability of blood typing aged bone. Am J Phys Anthropol 15:387–398.

Van den Hamer CJA, and Cornelisse C (1985) On zinc deficiency. Sci Total Environ 42:83–89.

Van Loon JC (1980) Analytical Atomic Absorption Spectroscopy. New York: Academic Press.

von Endt DW, and Ortner DJ (1982) Amino acid analysis of bone from a possible case of prehistoric iron deficiency anemia from the American Southwest. Am J Phys Anthropol 59:377–385.

Waldron HA (1981) Postmortem absorption of lead by the skeleton. Am J Phys Anthropol 55:395–398.

Waldron HA (1983) On the post-mortem accumulation of lead by skeletal tissues. J Arch Sci 10:35–40.

Waldron HA, Khera A, Walker G, Wibberley G, and Green CJS (1979) Lead concentrations in bones and soil. J Arch Sci 6:295–298.

Waldron T (1982) Human bone lead concentrations. In A McWhirr, L Viner, and C Wells (eds): Romano-British Cemeteries at Cirencester. Gloucester: Alan Sutton Publishing Limited, pp 203–207.

Walravens PA (1982) Zinc deficiency in infants and children. In AS Prasad (ed): Clinical, Biochemical, and Nutritional Aspects of Trace Elements. New York: Alan R. Liss, pp 129–144.

Wedeen R, Maesaka JK, Weiner B, Lipat GA, Lyons MM, Vitale LF, and Joselow MM (1975) Occupational lead nephropathy. Am J Med 59:630–641.

Wessen G, Ruddy FH, Gustafson CE, and Irwin H (1978) Trace element analysis in the characterization of archaeological bone. In GF Carter (ed): Archaeological Chemistry. Pullman, WA: American Chemical Society, pp 99–108.

Williams RB, and Mills CF (1970) The experimental production of zinc deficiency in the rat. Br J Nutr 24:989–1003.

Wittmers LE, Alich A, and Aufderheide AC (1981) Lead in bone I. Direct analysis for lead in milligram quantities of bone ash by graphite furnace atomic absorption spectroscopy. Am J Clin Pathol 75:80–85.

Wittmers LE, Aufderheide AC, Wallgren J, Rapp G, and Alich A (1988) Lead in bone IV. Distribution of lead in the human skeleton. Arch Environmental Health 43(6): 381–391.

Wyckoff RWG, Wagner E, Matter P, and Doberenz AR (1963) Collagen in fossil bone. Proc Natl Acad Sci USA 50:215–221.

Reconstruction of Life From the Skeleton
© 1989 Alan R. Liss, Inc., pages 261–286

Chapter 14

Dental Paleopathology: Methods for Reconstructing Dietary Patterns

John R. Lukacs
Department of Anthropology, University of Oregon, Eugene, Oregon 97403

INTRODUCTION

The oral cavity functions first and foremost as a food processor. The composition and consistency of foods consumed determine the kinds of microorganisms that flourish in the oral cavity and the nature of biomechanical forces affecting the teeth and jaws. Anatomical and pathological studies of the oral cavity thus provide direct evidence of type of diet.

Diagnosis and interpretation of dental diseases and their analysis in a paleodemographic framework are an indispensable part of any attempt to reconstruct past lifeways from human skeletal remains. The prevalence and distribution of dental diseases in a skeletal series, when analyzed by age, sex, and social group, may yield valuable clues regarding diet (what is eaten), nutrition (physiological adequacy of the diet), and subsistence (method of procuring the diet).

Prehistoric diets are assessed with an ever-increasing array of analytic methods, which include microscopic (stable isotopes: DeNiro, 1987; trace elements: Schoeninger, 1979; Sillen and Kavanagh, 1982; dental microwear: Grine, 1981) and macroscopic (attrition angles: Smith, 1984; skeletal pathology: Ortner and Putschar, 1981; stature: Haviland, 1967) techniques; direct evidence of dental paleopathology is especially paramount (Gilbert and Mielke, 1985; Hillson, 1979).

This chapter has three prime objectives: 1) to critically survey the literature of dental pathology and identify problem areas, 2) to suggest a standardized research methodology, which includes the Dental Pathology Profile, and 3) to illustrate results that are derived from this approach to dental pathology.

DEFINING THE FIELD OF STUDY: WHAT IS DENTAL PATHOLOGY?

A succinct response to the above question would be that dental pathology is the scientific study of the origin, nature, and course of dental diseases. The definition is adequate providing disease is recognized as an improper or abnormal function of an organ, structure, or system of the body resulting from the effect of heredity, infection, diet, or environment. Technically, then, dental pathology refers to the study of diseases of the teeth, but in practice many discussions of the subject are more inclusive and subsume diseases of the jaws as well. In order to define the field of inquiry and identify current problems in research, a survey of sourcebooks in human osteology and paleopathology was undertaken. The results of the survey are briefly summarized below; a critical evaluation of the results aided in the formulation of both a more precise definition of the discipline of dental pathology and suggestions for future research.

Systematic discussion of dental diseases is often omitted from standard texts in human osteology (Bass, 1971; Krogman and İşcan, 1986; Shipman et al., 1985; Ubelaker, 1978). These sources may provide details of dental anatomy sufficient to permit the identification of teeth to side and tooth class (Anderson, 1969; Bass, 1971; Shipman et al., 1985); some include descriptive and comparative data for particular polymorphic dental traits such as shovel-shaped incisors and Carabelli's trait (Bass, 1971). Casual reference to the value of dental diseases as part of anthropological research is made by Ubelaker (1978:86), but no guidelines are provided for acquiring these important data. Anderson (1969:91–99) provides brief statements and illustrations for the identification and recording of dental diseases as part of a general description of the skeleton. Bass (1971) and Shipman et al. (1985) do not discuss dental pathology systematically or in any detail, though the latter source mentions gross enamel hypoplasia as an example of the effect of nutritional deficiency on the teeth. The role of dental paleopathology in determining paleonutrition is briefly outlined by Wing and Brown (1979) in their discussion of human skeletal evidence.

Quoting from Walker (1981:58), Shipman et al. (1985) enumerate eight principal modes of deducing diet from fossil or skeletal remains: 1) interspecific tooth morphology, 2) biomechanical reconstruction, 3) inspection of tooth microwear, 4) isotope analysis, 5) trace element analysis, 6) application of "ecological rules," 7) analysis of "food refuse" from archaeological sites, and 8) diagnosis of metabolic diseases caused by diet. Dental pathology is conspicuous by its absence from this list, which reflects the microscopic and chemical techniques championed by Walker, Shipman, and their associates. Differential expression of dental diseases in human populations may yield valuable clues to dietary preferences and food preparation methods and is an important tool in paleoanthropological research. The superficial treatment of dental pathology in human osteology manuals could reflect either the author's prioritization of subject matter, bias in the author's training, or the topical and space constraints imposed by the publisher.

The only human osteology text that provides a basic discussion of dental diseases, including standardized scales for categorizing the expression of specific lesions, is by Brothwell (1981). Previous editions of this sourcebook in human osteology also included valuable sections on the recognition and diagnosis of dental diseases (Brothwell, 1965, 1972). Diseases of the teeth and jaws discussed by Brothwell (1981:151–160) include 1) dental caries and premortem tooth loss, 2) periodontal disease, 3) chronic dental abscess, 4) dental hypoplasia, 5) dental calculus (tartar), 6) cysts, and 7) odontomes. Notable by its absence from this discussion is severe dental attrition and pulp chamber exposure, features often included by others as dental pathology.

A survey of anthologies and textbooks on paleopathology revealed widely varying perspectives regarding dental pathology. Some texts omit the subject of dental pathology as a major topic in paleopathology, but include dental symptoms of complex diseases (Steinbock, 1976) or refer to the value of dental pathology in skeletal research (Zimmerman and Kelley, 1982). For example, Steinbock (1976:106–108) describes classic Hutchinson's incisors and mulberry molars as dental anomalies associated with, but not pathognomonic of, late congenital syphilis. Dental disease as a source of systemic infection and the dental manifestation of fluorosis are discussed by Zimmerman and Kelley (1982). The absence of a systematic discussion of dental pathology in these volumes limits their value to students of dental pathology.

Paleopathology texts by Hart (1983), Janssens (1970), Wells (1964), and Zivanovic (1982) each include a chapter or major section on dental diseases. The primary focus in each of these volumes is an analysis of dental caries, but abscesses, antemortem tooth loss, attrition, congenital genetic anomalies, crowding, enamel hypoplasia, hypercementosis, malocclusion, and periodontal disease are also discussed. A prime concern of these authors is understanding the correlation of dental diseases with dietary changes accompanying the development of civilization (Molnar and Molnar, 1985; Moore and Corbett, 1983). Topics ancillary to this central issue appear to be less focused and are not problem oriented.

"Lesions of the Teeth and Jaws" is the title of the final chapter of Ortner and Putschar's (1981) *Identification of Pathological Conditions in Human Skeletal Remains.* It provides well-illustrated documentation of paleopathologic expressions of dental caries, periodontal disease, disturbances of dental development (including hypoplasias, hyper- and hypodontia, fused teeth, enamel pearls, crowding), dental trauma, dental attrition, and dental discoloration. The primary concern of this chapter is identification and diagnosis of pathological lesions of the teeth and jaws; no discussion of trends or results of earlier studies is presented. This review is similar in its organization and content to Brabant's (1967) survey of dental disease entitled "Palaeostomatology."

Three key articles in dental paleopathology that for many years set the stage for this discipline are by Alexandersen (1967), Brothwell (1963), and Leigh (1925). All three articles focus exclusively on macroscopic dental pathology of prehistoric populations, but while Alexandersen and Brothwell provide overviews, Leigh surveys patterns of dental pathology among native American skeletal series from varied environments and food conditions.

Perhaps the most exhaustive and valuable reviews of dental pathology for the anthropologist are Pindborg's (1970) *Pathology of the Dental Hard Tissues* and Hillson's (1986) *Teeth.* Hillson's authoritative volume includes a well-balanced chapter on dental diseases that places pathological lesions of the oral cavity in a dynamic biological context. Detailed treatment of macroscopic lesions is presented in one chapter and includes sections devoted to dental plaque, dental caries, dental calculus, immunity and inflammation, periodontal disease, infections, trauma, anomalies, and odontomes. Microstructural defects of the dental tissues, including fluorosis and developmental lesions such as hypoplasia, are treated separately in another chapter.

Recent directions in dental pathology research parallel current developments in skeletal biology and include 1) refinement in the methods of data collection and analysis for macroscopic dental diseases, 2) increased attention to details of microstructural defects (histopathology), and 3) quantification of the trace element content of dental tissues. It is increasingly common that the description and analysis of dental diseases in a skeletal series will utilize all three approaches in a highly integrated manner.

More precise methods of data collection permit statistical analysis of the size, tooth surface, and location of dental caries lesions (Metress and Conway, 1975) or the number, severity, and age at onset of growth disruptions, as indicated by gross enamel hypoplasia (Goodman et al., 1980, 1984). The complex interactions between multiple factors such as dental wear and caries need to be deciphered before dietary reconstruction is feasible (Powell, 1985). Research on microstructural defects of dental tissues was begun by Clement (1963) and Sognnaes (1956) and was brought to the attention of physical anthropologists by Molnar and Ward (1975). Rose (1977) recently applied this method to prehistoric native American skeletal series from Illinois and differentiated between histologically defective and normal enamel. The use of developmental defects, hypoplasias, and Wilson's band in paleonutrition research is further discussed by Rose et al. (1985).

The trace element content of dental tissues is an important factor regulating their susceptibility to disease. The elemental content of teeth is the result of differential abundance of naturally occurring elements in the environment during the growth and formation of the teeth and to culturally and physiologically determined utilization of resources (St. Hoyme and Koritzer, 1976). The relationship between specific elements, such as fluorine and selenium, and dental caries is well documented (Hadjimarkos and Bornhorst, 1962; Leverett, 1982; National Research Council, 1983). The trace element content of prehistoric native American teeth as reported by Steadman et al. (1959), and the fluoride content of enamel of teeth from Neolithic Baluchistan was reported by Lukacs et al. (1985).

Finally, over 600 multisystem genetic syndromes have a major orofacial component. Numeric anomalies of the teeth (hypodontia, hyperdontia), delayed or accelerated eruption and exfoliation of teeth, and structural defects of dental tissues often occur as part of a multisystem genetic syndrome. Although dental agenesis (hypodontia) is generally viewed by anthropologists as either an isolated trait worthy of note or as part of the overall process of dental reduction, it may also be part of a multisystem syndrome that is either autosomal (dominant or recessive), X-linked, or of uncertain inheritance (Shapiro and Farrington, 1983).

This introductory survey and an independent review of current research in dental pathology suggests that major problems confronting the discipline can be grouped into two categories: 1) varying perceptions of what conditions constitute "dental pathology" combined with an overemphatic research focus on caries, and 2) methodological imprecision in both the descriptive and comparative phases of research. These problems are interrelated and have synergistic consequences that preclude precise comparative study of dental pathology between populations and thereby prevent further advancement in the field.

DENTAL PALEOPATHOLOGY: METHODOLOGY STANDARDIZED

Limits to progress in dental paleopathology, as discussed above, can be effectively countered by improving the precision with which pathological dental lesions are defined, described, and comparatively analyzed. Results that are not reproducible and high levels of interobserver error cannot be tolerated if comparative studies of dental pathology are to yield significant conclusions.

Three suggestions for the improvement of methods in dental paleopathology are presented: 1) a classification of dental diseases, 2) guidelines for the descriptive recording of pathological dental lesions, and 3) a method for enhancing interobserver comparability, the Dental Pathology Profile.

Classification of Dental Diseases

The first proposal is a tentative classification of dental diseases by primary etiology. The assignment of a given dental disease to one of four categories in Table 1 is based on the initial or primary causal agent. Infectious dental diseases are those that arise because of the action of a pathogenic microorganism; for example, acidogenic bacteria are involved in creating dental caries. Secondary consequences of infectious dental diseases are also listed in this category if the primary factor can be assessed as infectious.

TABLE 1. Classification of Dental Diseases

Category	Dental disease
Infectious	Antemortem tooth loss (abscess or caries induced)
	Dental abscess
	Dental caries
	Periodontal disease
	Pulp chamber exposure (caries induced)
Degenerative	Antemortem tooth loss (attrition induced)
	Periodontal disease
	Pulp chamber exposure (attrition induced)
	Calculus accumulation (tartar)
Developmental	Gross enamel hypoplasia
	Fluorosis
	Microstructural defects
	Dental crowding
	Malocclusion
	Secondary dentine deposition
	Hypercementosis
Genetic	Dental agenesis (hypodontia)
	Cleft palate
	Supernumerary teeth (hyperodontia)
	Malocclusion

Degenerative dental diseases are those that display loss of a conspicuous amount of tooth or bone surface or substance. Attrition itself is a normal process and is regarded as pathological only if it is a primary cause of pulp chamber exposure or antemortem tooth loss. Severe attrition results in improper function since the tooth is unable to biologically respond to attritional stress by disposition of secondary dentine. Abscess and caries also show loss of tooth or bone material and could be regarded as degenerative, but the unique feature shared by these conditions is their infectious causation.

Developmental diseases are those whose effect or influence occurs during the formation of dental tissues or during the developing interrelationship between teeth and their supporting structures, the jaws. Developmental dental diseases often include a prominent environmental component, but genetic influences cannot be completely excluded in their etiology (especially for malocclusion).

Genetic dental diseases are those for which a large genetic component is involved. Though

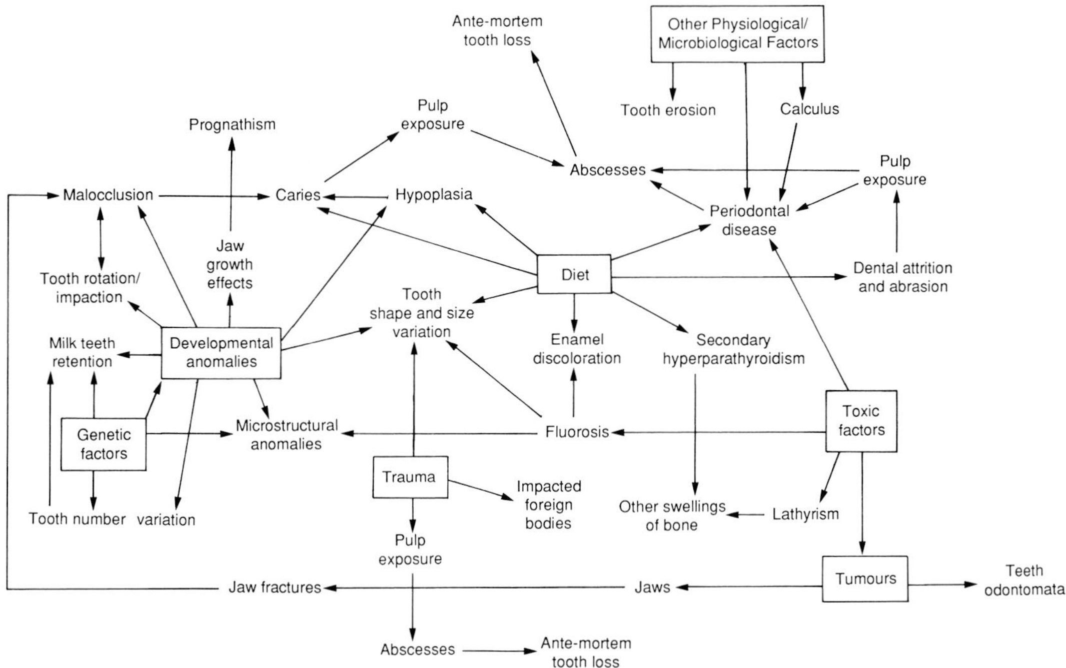

Fig. 1. Complex interactions between oral diseases and their causes. (Modified from Baker and Brothwell, 1980.)

included here for completeness, "diseases" of genetic origin shed no light on dietary or food preparation methods in prehistory. Data on numeric anomalies of the teeth are more appropriately discussed in the context of dental morphology and studies of population affinity. The complex interactions between oral diseases and their causes and consequences is depicted in Figure 1.

It may be useful to think of dental diseases or conditions as primary or secondary. For example, antemortem tooth loss (AMTL) may be caused by several different etiological pathways: 1) caries–pulp exposure-abscess–resorption–tooth loss; 2) calculus accumulation–periodontal disease–resorption–tooth loss; or 3) attrition–pulp exposure-abscess–resorption–tooth loss. In each pathway, the initial causal factor—caries, calculus, or attrition—would be the primary pathology; the other conditions along the pathway leading to tooth loss are secondary. Though the ultimate result of all three pathways is the same, being able to ascertain the etiological pathway leading to a given dental disease is especially useful in dietary reconstruction.

Diagnosis of Pathological Lesions

The second suggestion is uniform adoption of standard techniques for recognition and classification of pathological lesions of the teeth and jaws. Since guidelines are absent from many widely distributed manuals of human osteology, the following sections provide a brief definition of each pathological condition and the methods used to recognize and classify them.

Dental caries. Caries is a progressive demineralization of the tooth caused by localized fermentation of food sugars by dental plaque (Mandel, 1979). Caries is considered an infectious disease because bacterial organisms become concentrated on specific tooth sites in the form of an adherent gelatinous mat known as bacterial plaque. The presence of sucrose in association with acidogenic bacteria produces demineralization of enamel and dentine resulting in cavitation (Fig. 2). The examiner of dental

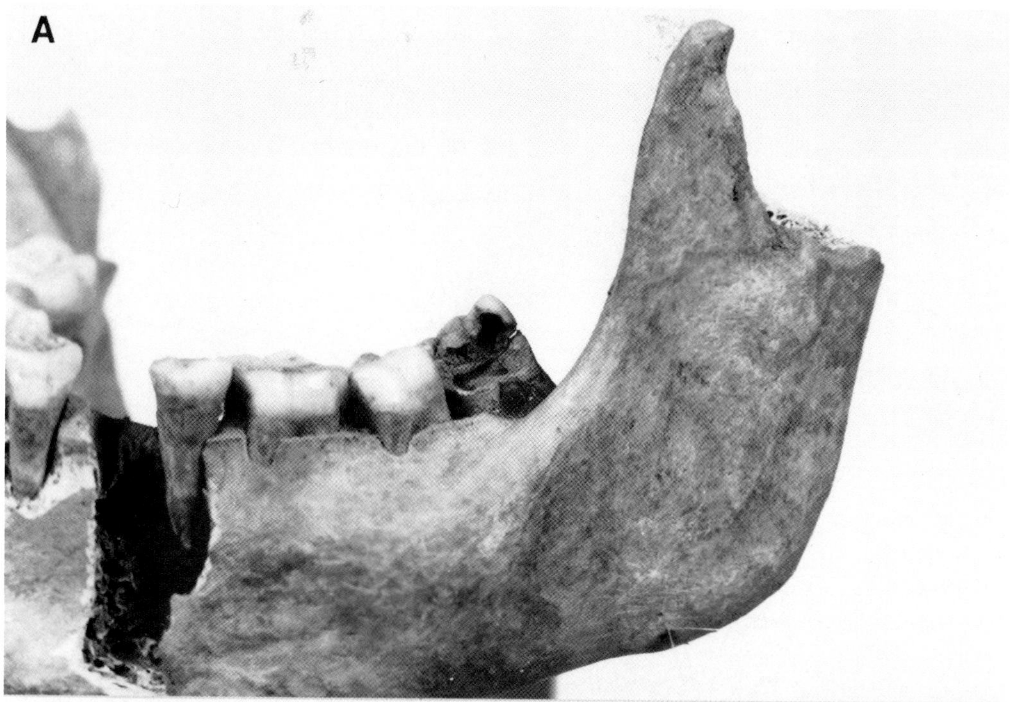

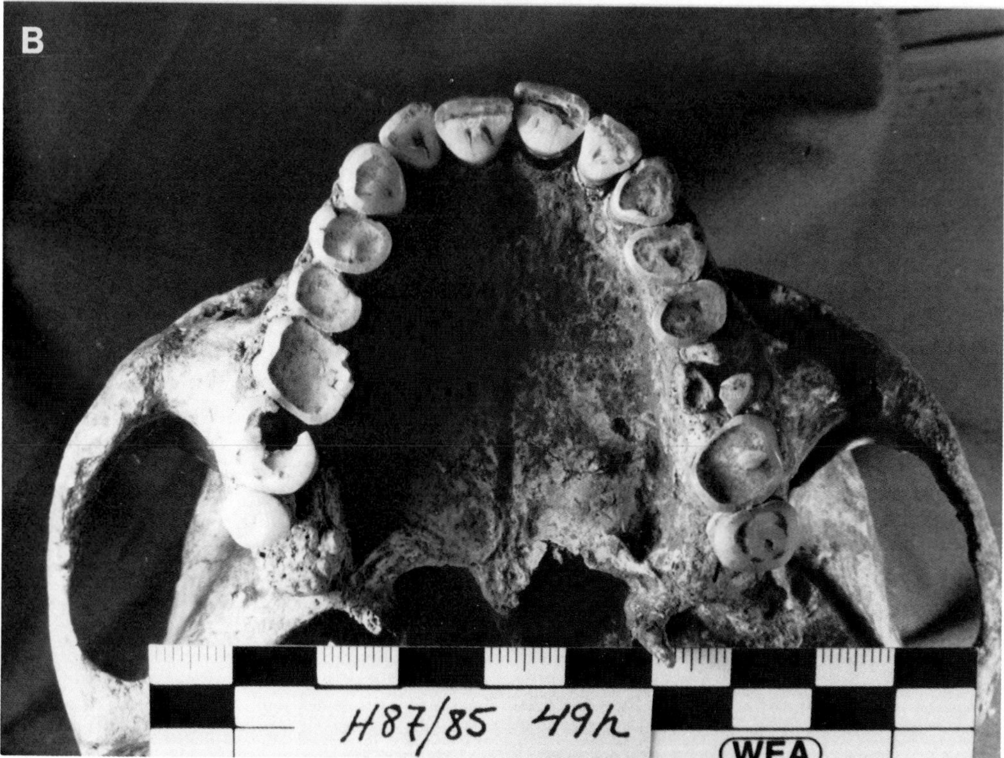

Fig. 2. Dental caries. **a:** Cervical caries exposing the pulp chamber of LM_3. **b:** Occlusal caries (RM^2) and complete carious destruction of RM^1 crown, roots remain visible.

caries in skeletal remains must carefully distinguish "true" from "false" caries (Brabant, 1967); the latter result from postmortem damage to the tooth and are a form of pseudopathology (Wells, 1967). A clear association exists between agricultural subsistence systems, soft, sticky, and sweet foods and high caries rates (Hillson, 1986; Larsen, 1983; Turner, 1978).

Each carious lesion is classified by its size and location on the tooth (Metress and Conway, 1975). Four caries size gradations are recognized: 1) pit or small fissure caries; 2) medium to large—but with less than one-half of the tooth crown destroyed; 3) large—more than one-half of the tooth crown destroyed; and 4) complete destruction of the tooth crown, with only the roots remaining. For grade 1 caries, a probe should be used to determine the presence of demineralization of the enamel surface; care must be taken *not* to count the morphological trait "buccal pit" or "foramen caecum hypoplasia" as dental caries (Pedersen, 1949).

The location of each carious lesion is noted according to which surface of the crown (or root) is primarily affected. However, in large caries (grades 3 and 4), the initial location of the carious lesion cannot always be determined. Special note of cervical caries, root caries, and buccal pit caries must be recorded.

Gross enamel hypoplasia. Gross enamel hypoplasia is "a deficiency in enamel thickness due to a disruption of ameloblast (enamel forming) activity" and is an easily identified marker of stress or growth disruption (Goodman et al., 1980). Enamel hypoplasia appears as irregular horizontal linear grooves or pits in the enamel surface, best viewed on the labial (buccal) aspect of the crown (Fig. 3).

Macroscopic hypoplastic defects provide an indelible and retrospective record of growth-disruptive stresses occurring during the period of childhood (birth to about 13 years) when tooth enamel was being formed. Multiple causal factors can produce enamel hypoplasia, including nutritional stress (Huss-Ashmore et al., 1982), vitamin D deficiency, hypoparathyroidism, and exantematous fevers (Scott and Symons, 1982). While the specific cause of a particular hypoplastic defect cannot be determined, the mere existence of a defect indicates a stress of sufficient magnitude to disrupt the normal growth process (Goodman and Armelagos, 1985).

Because the chronology of tooth formation is known, the developmental age at which a growth disruption occurred in a child can be precisely determined. Multiple hypoplasias in a single individual yield clues as to the timing or periodicity of repetitive stresses, such as recurring seasonal scarcity of nutrients. Differences in the frequency of enamel hypoplasias between sexes, social status groups, and groups with different subsistence bases can provide valuable data on the pattern of stress in a prehistoric population (Huss-Ashmore et al., 1982).

Analysis of macroscopic enamel hypoplasia is best conducted with a ×10 hand lens and dental probe. All teeth should be examined for hypoplasia and the position of the defect on the tooth crown, type of hypoplasia (linear, pitted, or both), and the surface of the crown affected should be recorded. When hypoplastic defects are linear, the height of the defect above the cement–enamel junction is measured with a needlepoint Helios dial caliper and rounded to the nearest tenth of a millimeter.

Dental calculus. Dental calculus is the mineralization of bacterial plaque. This hard inorganic mass adheres to the crown or root surface and is frequently found in archaeological skeletal remains (Fig. 4) (Ortner and Putschar, 1981). In life, calculus may irritate the gingival tissues, resulting in inflammation and periodontal disease.

In many prehistoric skeletal remains calculus is found in most or all the teeth of an individual, usually on the buccal and/or lingual aspect of the crown. The energetics of mastication generally preclude calculus deposits from accumulating on the occlusal surface of teeth (Turner, 1979), but when found, occlusal calculus suggests some form of masticatory dysfunction (Alexandersen, 1967). Three discrete grades of calculus formation are used to categorize this trait: slight, medium, and considerable, following the standard established by Brothwell (1981).

Dental crowding. The etiology of dental crowding is complex and includes both genetic and environmental factors (King, 1983). The displacement of teeth from their "normal" ana-

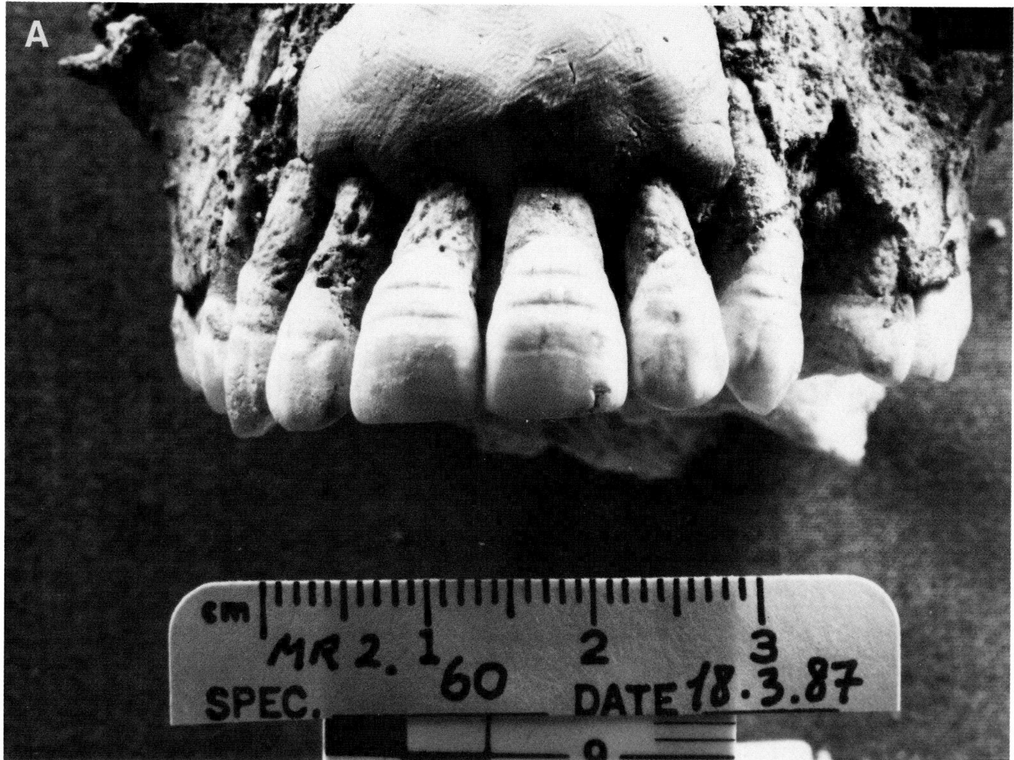

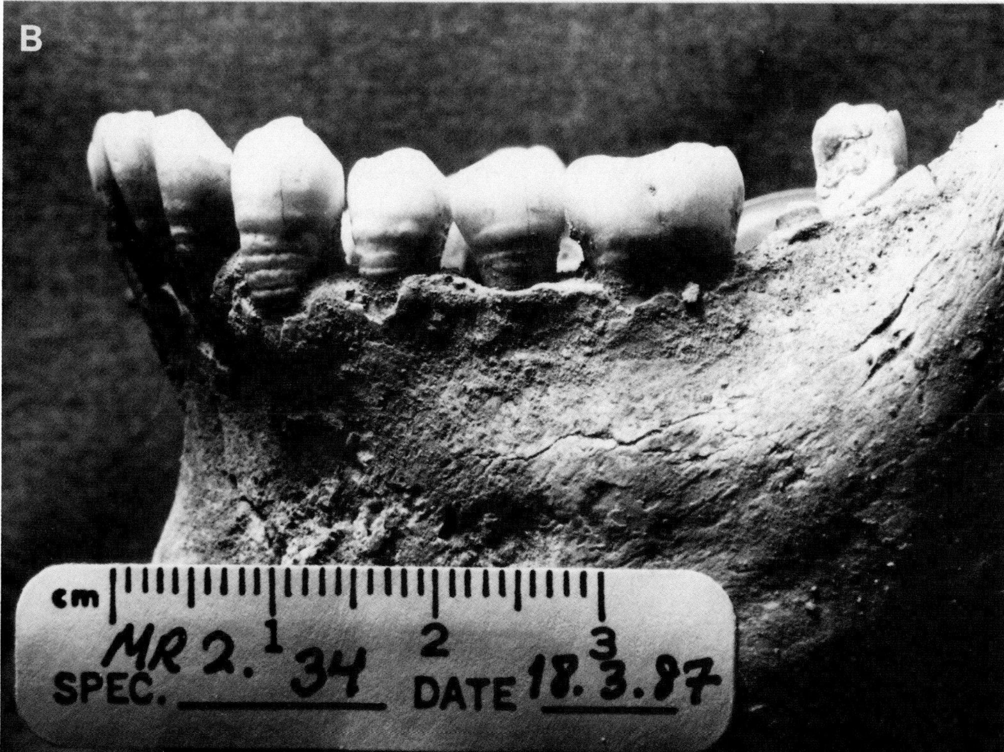

Fig. 3. Enamel hypoplasia. **a, b:** Linear enamel hypoplastic maxillary and mandibular anterior teeth. **c:** Foramen caecum hypoplasia (arrows) encircling the buccal pit of RM_2. **d:** Photomicrograph of circular hypoplastic pits on facial surface of Ldc.

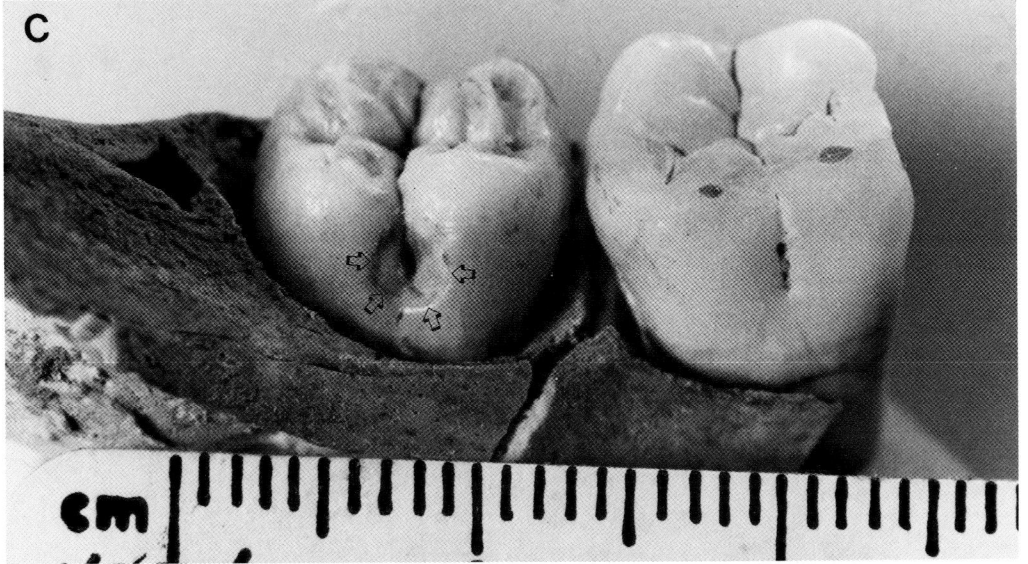
C
cm

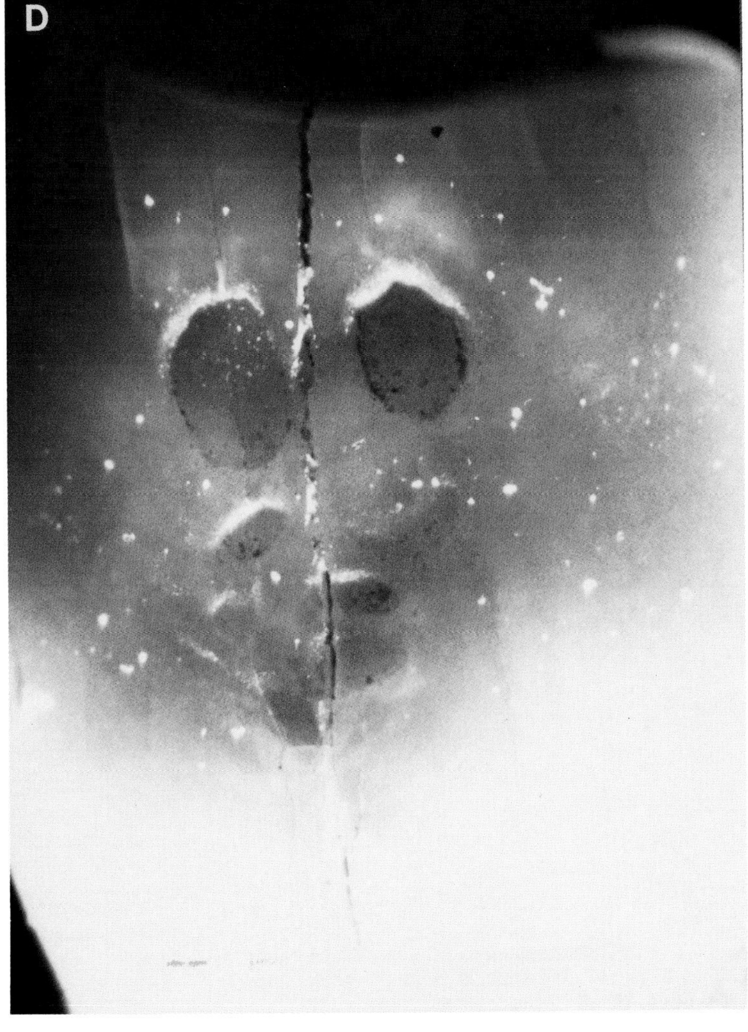
D

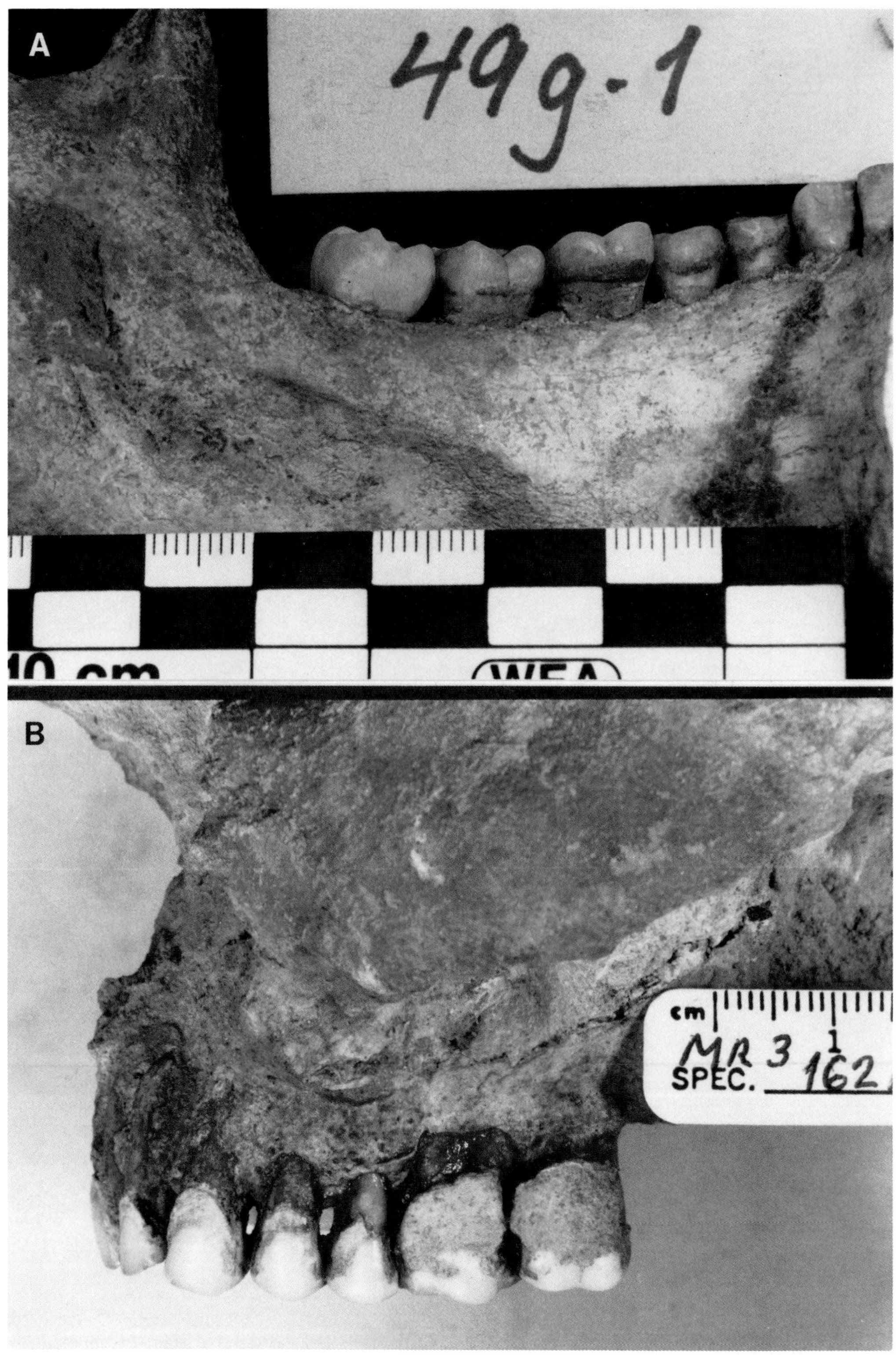

Fig. 4. Dental calculus. **a:** Small calculus deposits on the lingual aspect of the left lower molar row. **b:** Large calculus deposits covering the cement–enamel junction of LM^1 and LM^2; note associated moderate degree of alveolar resorption.

tomical relationship because of lack of adequate developmental jaw space is called dental crowding. If adequate jaw space *is* available, but the tooth is rotated from proper alignment, this is not considered as crowding.

Crowding tends to occur in certain areas of the dental arcade more than others. In modern populations third molar teeth and lower incisor teeth are especially prone to crowding. Crowding of teeth is considered to be either an indicator of nutritional stress, since dental development is less affected by stress than the growth of the jaws (Huss-Ashmore et al., 1982; Kaul and Corruccini, 1984), or suggestive of relaxed masticatory stress (Corruccini and Whitely, 1981; Oppenheimer, 1964).

The degree of crowding is qualitatively assessed by the number of malpositioned teeth and the severity of their displacement. Three grades of crowding are recognized: slight, moderate, and severe. Care must be taken *not* to include the genetic trait "maxillary incisor rotation" as evidence of dental crowding (Enoki and Dahlberg, 1958).

Antemortem tooth loss (AMTL). The loss of teeth prior to an individual's death is referred to as AMTL; it is recognizable by progressive resorptive destruction of the alveolus (Fig. 5). Teeth lost immediately before death will be confused with postmortem tooth loss. Identification of specific teeth lost antemortem is often difficult in specimens with advanced attrition and multiple instances of AMTL.

Pulp exposure and necrosis followed by periapical osteitis and alveolar resorption are commonly successive prerequisites to AMTL. Alternatively, calculus deposits of moderate to large size may cause gingival irritation, periodontal disease, and alveolar resorption that ultimately lead to AMTL. Establishing the primary causal agents that produce AMTL yields valuable information about the nature of masticatory stress in a skeletal population.

Alveolar resorption. Alveolar resorption is caused by inflammation of the gingival tissue, or periodontal disease, which produces macroscopic porosity, periostitis, and resorption of bone along the alveolar margins. Determining pathological degenerative changes in alveolar bone, as opposed to normal atrophic change associated with the aging process, is difficult (Alexandersen, 1967). Direct comparison of the degree of alveolar bone resorption is complicated by the varying standards used by dental investigators.

The grading of alveolar resorption follows a fivefold classification: 0) absent—no resorption; 1) slight—less than one-half of the root exposed; 2) moderate—more than one-half the root exposed; 3) severe—evulsion of the tooth, remnants of the alveolus discernible; and 4) complete—tooth evulsed, alveoli completely obliterated.

Periapical abscess. Exposure of the pulp chamber through severe attrition or extensive carious decay produces an inflamed or necrotic pulp. This causes infection of the periapical tissues and osteitis, but is only recognizable in skeletal remains if the spreading pathological process has destroyed the external bony surfaces of the jaw (Fig. 6) (Alexandersen 1967).

Only visually diagnosed periapical osteitic foci are generally reported in skeletal analyses, since x-ray diagnosis is not routinely used in paleodontological research. Consequently, the true frequency of periapical abscesses is unknown for most of the prehistoric populations, and figures based on macroscopic diagnosis are underestimated.

Periapical abscesses may be differentiated from postmortem damage to the jaws by their location at the apex of the dental root and by the smooth and rounded margin of the orifice of the abscess cavity, which exposes the tooth root. Pseudopathological cases of periapical abscesses may develop from postmortem erosion of the thin bony covering of the maxillary incisor roots in the subnasal region (Brothwell, 1981). All evidence of postmortem destructive activity must be carefully excluded from the count of periapical osteitis.

Periapical abscesses are arbitrarily classified on the basis of the measured diameter of the externally visible orifice—small (less than 3.0 mm), medium (greater than 3.0 mm, less than 7.0 mm), and large (equal to or greater than 7.0 mm)—and on the basis of the location of the orifice.

Data Reduction and Presentation

The results of dental pathology studies are variously presented by different investigators, and often the method of data presentation is not explicitly stated. The prime technique used

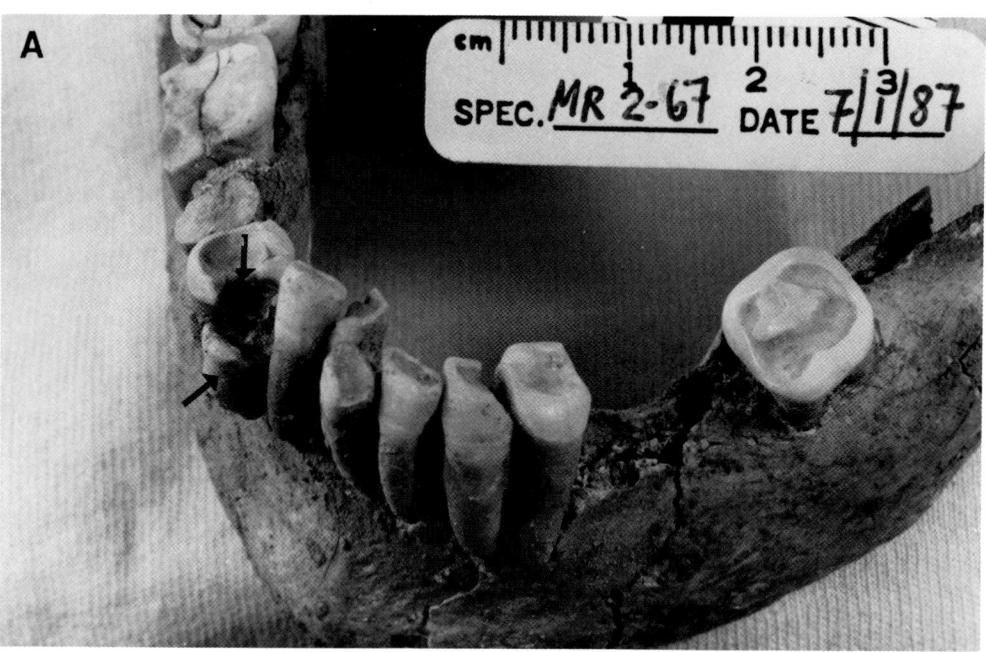

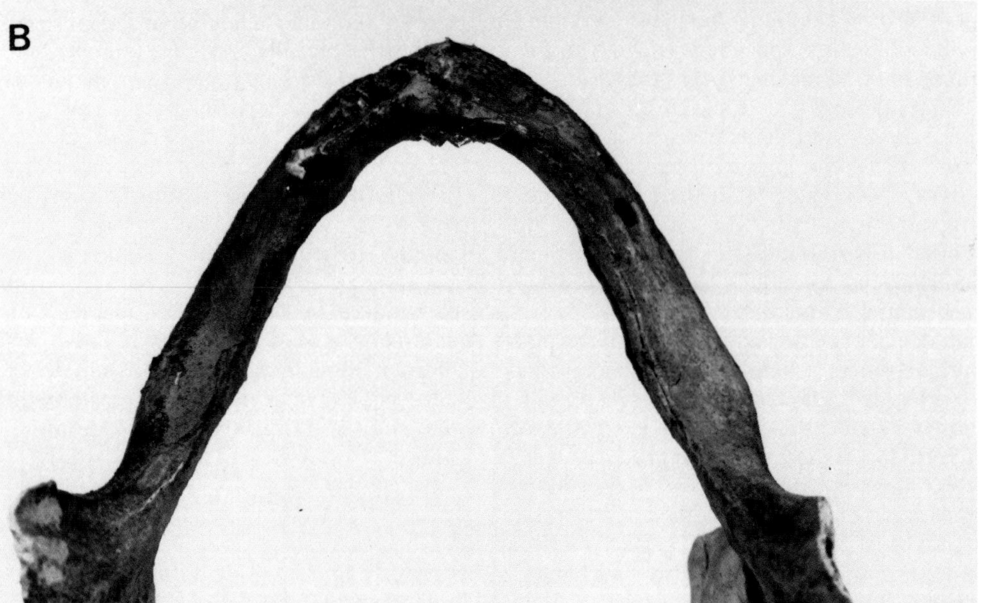

Fig. 5. Antemortem tooth loss. **a:** Antemortem loss of LP_4 and LM_1 is associated with mesial drift of LM_2; also note interproximal caries in RP_3 (arrows) and carious destruction of RC crown. **b:** Advanced antemortem tooth loss in edentulous mandible from Sarai Khola.

in this analysis is the frequency, or percentage, of individuals exhibiting a particular dental lesion or abnormality. This frequency is obtained by dividing the number of specimens with a certain disease by the number of specimens that *could* have yielded evidence of the disease (i.e., those that have the relevant parts preserved). Percentages should be reported for each sex and each subset (stratum, region, etc.) of a skeletal sample, as well as for the total skeletal series. This technique is known as the individual count method. Tables and figures based on this method must be appropriately labeled.

Since completeness of preservation differs from specimen to specimen and not all individuals can potentially yield evidence of every disease, the sample size used in computing the percentage occurrence of dental lesions normally differs from disease to disease. For certain diseases, an individual count is less useful than a record of the percentage of teeth in the total dental sample that are affected. This method of presentation, often used for reporting the prevalence of caries, is called the tooth count method. Another method of presentation, often used for dental caries only, is recording the mean number of carious lesions per specimen. Expressing caries prevalence in this way permits a broader comparative survey of this condition among living and prehistoric study samples.

Adoption of the standards outlined above for the descriptive recording of dental pathology should ensure a greater degree of comparability among the results of different investigators. However, there are several additional guidelines, the use of which should contribute to still greater comparability of dental pathology data sets. These include 1) placing the dental pathology data in demographic perspective, 2) clearly specifying the method of reporting disease prevalence, and 3) reporting on as many pathological conditions as possible using the Dental Pathology Profile.

The age and sex composition of the skeletal series must be known for dental pathology prevalence statistics to have any anthropological or comparative value. An observation of low antemortem tooth loss would be quite normal in a sample whose age structure is predominately adolescent or young adult, but would be unusual and require explanation in a sample comprising individuals 50 years old and older. Unless dental pathology data sets are normalized for variations in age and sex composition, comparisons should only be made between skeletal series with comparable age and sex structures.

Individual count, tooth count, and per specimen count methods are the primary alternatives for reporting prevalence of dental lesions. The tendency to report results without clearly and explicitly stating the procedure employed in calculating prevalence rates is unfortunately common. The imprecision that arises from comparing prevalence rates based on different reporting methods can be avoided only if investigators carefully specify the methods used in their research.

The final consideration addressed in this paper is a mechanism that would facilitate more precise comparative and interpretive analysis dental pathology data.

ENHANCING COMPARABILITY: AN EXAMPLE FROM SOUTH ASIA

The Dental Pathology Profile (DPP) is introduced here as a useful conceptual and pragmatic approach to enhancing the comparability of dental pathology data sets. The DPP of a South Asian skeletal series from the Iron Age site of Sarai Khola is used to demonstrate the technique and illustrate the improved results that can be derived from its use.

The idea of a DPP is based on a recent survey of the prevalence of dental lesions associated with preagricultural and agricultural subsistence systems as presented in *Paleopathology at the Origins of Agriculture* (Cohen and Armelagos, 1984) and numerous other relevant sources. The DPP is proposed as an effective multipurpose research tool permitting 1) more precise reconstruction of dietary patterns for skeletal series whose diet and/or mode of subsistence is unknown from cultural, botanical, or zoological remains and 2) reduction of interobserver error by enhancing the precision with which comparative studies of dental disease are made. Shifts in the prevalence of dental diseases and changes in the robusticity of jaws and teeth accompany a dietary shift from hunting and gathering to intensive agriculture. The polarity for the range of variation in prevalence

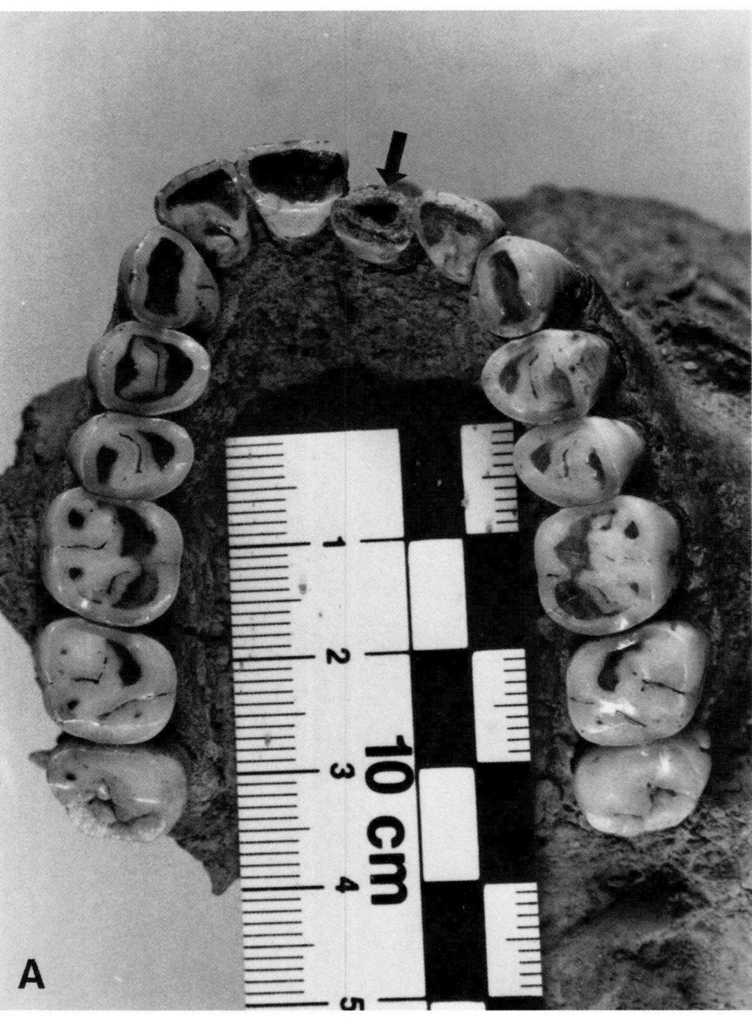
A
10 cm
1
2
3
4
5

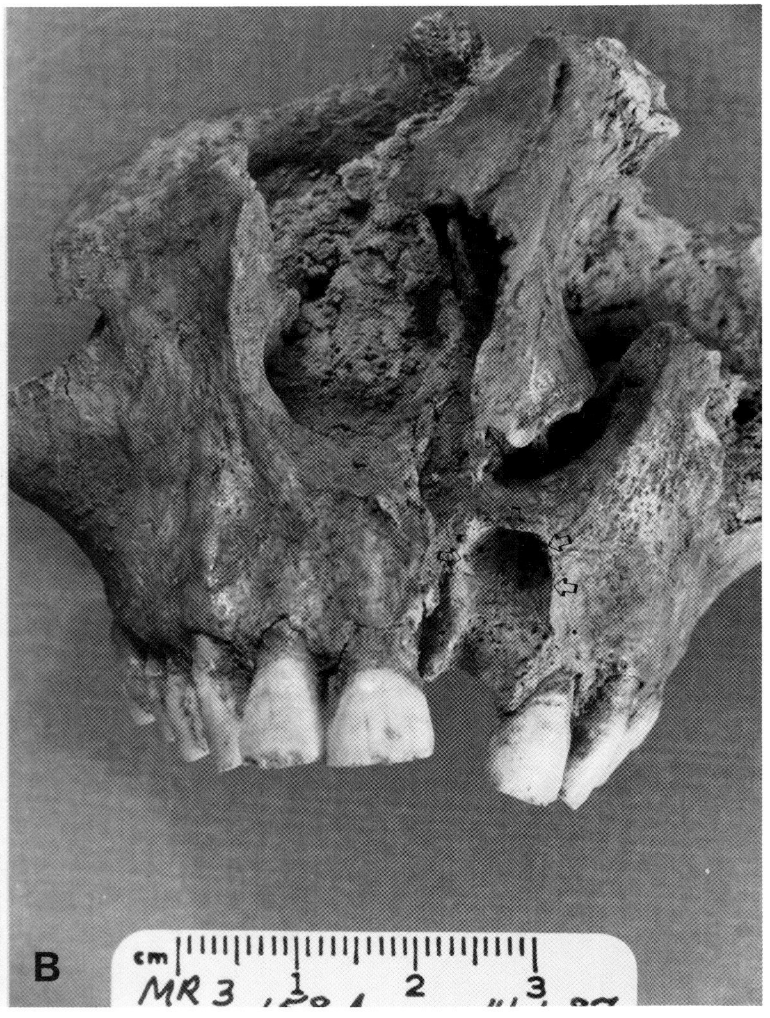
B
cm
1
2
3
MR 3

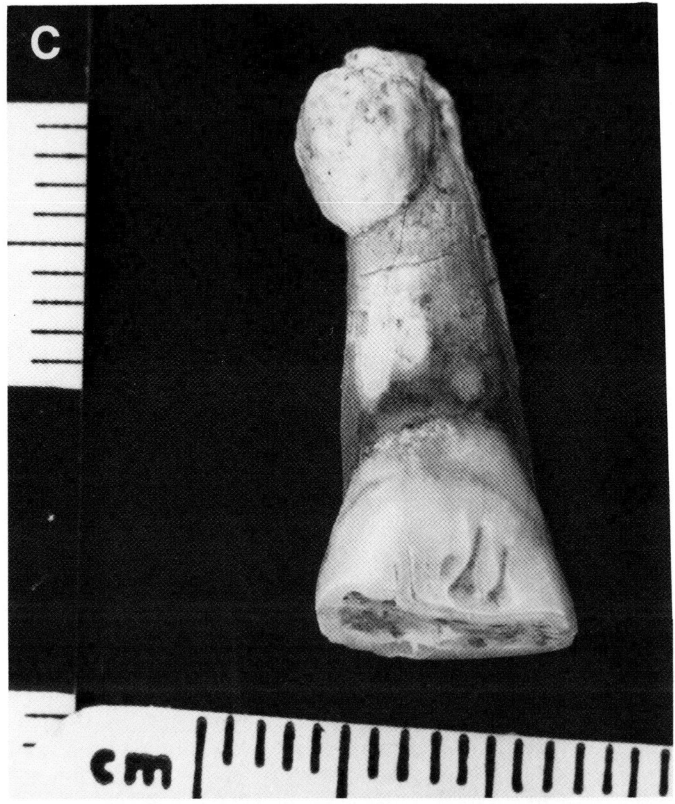

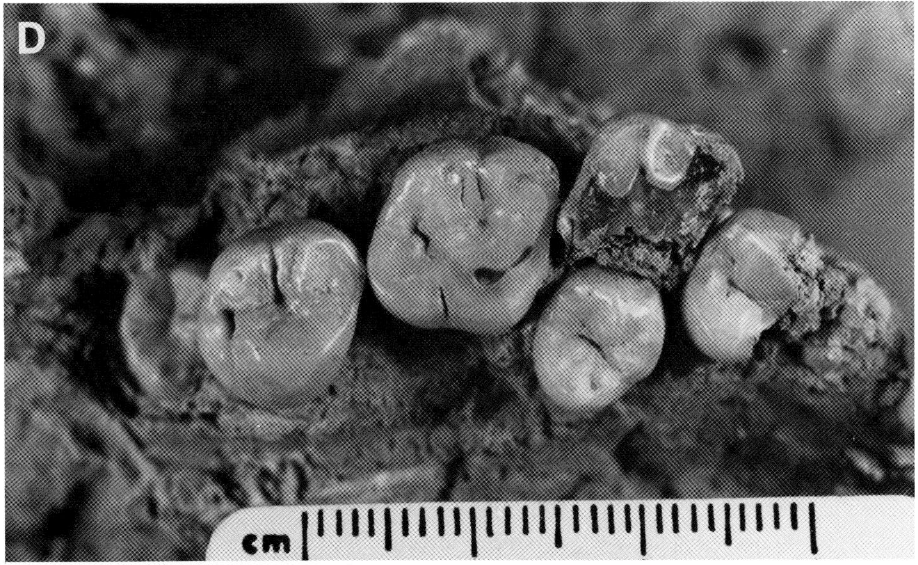

Fig. 6. Dental lesions. **a:** Traumatic fracture of LI^1 resulting in pulp exposure (arrows). **b:** Infection resulting in periapical abscess (arrow). **c:** Cemental dysplasia of LI^1. **d:** Prolonged retention of deciduous tooth (Rdm^2) with erupted RP^4.

TABLE 2. Dental Pathology Profiles for Different Subsistence Economies

Dental pathology	Hunter-gatherer	Transitional mixed	Agricultural
Dental caries	Low	Medium X[a]	High
Enamel hypoplasia	Low	Medium X	High
Dental calculus	Low	Medium	High X
Pulp exposure (caries)	Low	Medium X	High
Malocclusion	Low	Medium	High
Dental crowding	Low	Medium X	High
Alveolar resorption	Low	Medium X	High
Severity of attrition	High	Medium X	Low
Pulp exposure (attrition)	High	Medium	Low X
Robusticity of jaws	High	Medium	Low X
Relative jaw size	Large	Medium	Small
Antemortem tooth loss[b]			X
Periapical abscess[b]			X

[a] X, position of Sarai Khola skeletal series along the polarity gradient.
[b] Polarity uncertain; position of SKH based on the early age of onset of these diseases.

of each dental disease was established and is presented in Table 2.

Several diseases exhibit a positive polarity: the prevalence of a dental disease increases along the continuum from hunting and gathering to mixed economy to intensive agriculture. Dental diseases exhibiting positive polarity include caries, enamel hypoplasia, malocclusion, and dental crowding, among others. Negative polarity conditions are those whose prevalence decreases with the transition to agriculture; these include severe attrition, pulp exposure, and periapical osteitis due to attrition, size, and robusticity of the jaws. Polarity remains unestablished for certain conditions, including AMTL and periapical osteitis, because of their multiple etiological pathways and the absence of a clear-cut polarity profile in the dental paleopathology literature.

The DPP of a particular skeletal series is the prevalence with which each disease or condition occurs and, more importantly, the relative incidence of one disease to another. Once the DPP is established, through the application of methods outlined above for the description and reporting of dental lesions, it may then be employed in comparative investigations in two ways. First, the DPP can be evaluated against the standardized DPP (Table 2) and a probability statement generated regarding the dietary/subsistence pattern of the skeletal series. Second, the DPP of two or more skeletal series can be compared with one another as an indication of the degree of similarity or divergence in dietary or subsistence patterns. Caution must be exercised in using the second application; skeletal series to be compared must have a similar demographic structure for the results to be meaningful. The archaeological setting of Sarai Khola is reviewed below, followed by an interpretation of its dietary and subsistence patterns employing the DPP method.

Sarai Khola was discovered in 1967, and excavations were conducted by the Government of Pakistan Department of Archaeology under the direction of M.A. Halim. The site is located 33 km northwest of Islamabad (Fig. 7) and about 2 km southwest of Taxila (Bhir Mound). Reports on the excavations at Sarai Khola were published in *Pakistan Archaeology* by Halim (1968, 1970–71, 1972), who proposed the following chronology:

Period IV	
Medieval	A. D. 700–800
Period III	
Cemetery	B. C. 1000
Period II	
Kot Dijian	B. C. 2800–2400
Period I	
Late Neolithic	B. C. 3100–2800

However, the antiquity of Period III could be as young at 270 B.C. ± 60 years, based on a single radiometric date on bone (Bernhard, 1967, 1969).

Period I at Sarai Khola yielded handmade red burnished wares, ground stone tools, microliths, and bone points, artifacts that show similarities to the Neolithic of Burzahom in

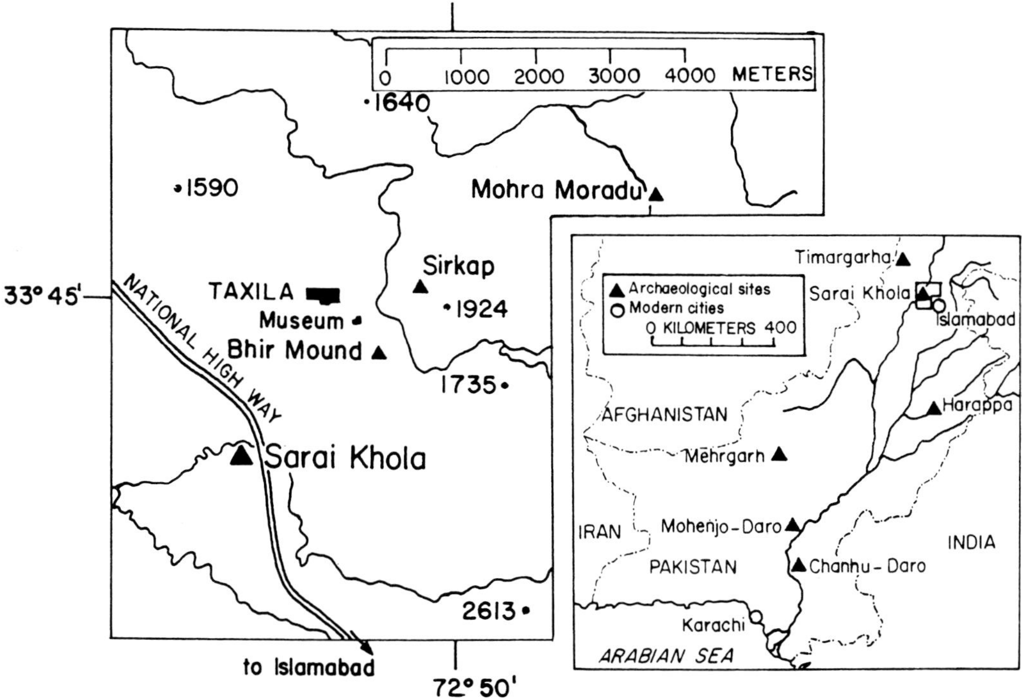

Fig. 7. Location map of Sarai Khola, Pakistan.

Kashmir and Yang-Shao in North China (Halim, 1972). Wheel-made pottery is found in Period II (Bronze Age) along with copper and stone objects, terra-cotta female figurines, bracelets, and beads. The great thickness of occupation layers in Period II suggests a settlement of long duration. Period III consisted of a cemetery with two phases, an early cemetery (SKH II) and a late cemetery (SKH I). After a long period of abandonment, Sarai Khola was reoccupied in the seventh and eighth centuries A.D.

Sarai Khola graves lack burial goods, but several iron artifacts (two rings, an iron rod, and bracelet clasps) were found in SKH I graves. The absence of cultural evidence from Period III graves severely limits our knowledge of the cultural affinities, food preparation methods, and dietary patterns at Sarai Khola. This situation is generally true of the Iron Age in South Asia which, with the exception of a few habitation sites in central India (Maski, Paiyampali, Takalghat), is known primarily through the excavation of megalithic mortuary sites (Deo, 1984, 1985a; Kennedy, 1975b). Because Iron Age graves in South Asia often lack cultural remains, the evidence of skeletal and dental pathology is the only direct method of assessing the diet and subsistence pattern. The degree of dependence on agriculture among megalith builders is controversial, but dental evidence from Mahurjhari suggests a mixed economy (Lukacs, 1981; Deo, 1985b).

The frequency of dental pathology at Sarai Khola is presented in Tables 3–5 and Figure 8; Sarai Khola data are compared with data from Mahurjhari (central India; Lukacs, 1981) and Timargarha (northern Pakistan; Dani, 1966, 1967, 1980) in Table 6 and Figure 9. Sarai Khola (SKH) and Mahurjhari (MHR) are similar in the percentage of individuals affected by dental caries and enamel hypoplasia, whereas SKH and Timargarha (TMG) are similar in the prevalence of AMTL and periapical abscess. SKH exhibits a high frequency of individuals with dental calculus.

The prevalence of dental caries (based on tooth count) in selected South Asian skeletal

TABLE 3. Prevalence of Dental Diseases at Sarai Khola: By Sex and Cemetery (Individual Count)

	Male		Female		Cemetery total		Site total	
Disease	Frequency	N	Frequency	N	Frequency	N	Frequency	N
Caries								
SKH I	0.67	3	0.14	7	0.30	10		
SKH II	0.56	18	0.15	8	0.62	26		
Total	0.57	21	0.47	15			0.53	36
Hypoplasia								
SKH I	0.66	3	0.00	7	0.20	10		
SKH II	0.28	18	0.25	8	0.27	26		
Total	0.33	21	0.13	15			0.25	36
Calculus								
SKH I	0.33	3	0.57	7	0.50	10		
SKH II	0.67	18	0.50	8	0.62	26		
Total	0.62	21	0.53	15			0.58	36
Crowding								
SKH I	0.50	2	0.67	3	0.60	5		
SKH II	0.50	16	0.50	8	0.50	24		
Total	0.52	18	0.55	11			0.52	29
Antemortem tooth loss								
SKH I	0.00	2	0.43	7	0.33	9		
SKH II	0.44	18	0.38	8	0.42	26		
Total	0.40	20	0.40	15			0.40	35
Alveolar resorption								
SKH I	0.50	2	0.57	7	0.56	9		
SKH II	0.44	18	0.38	8	0.42	26		
Total	0.45	20	0.47	15			0.46	35
Periapical abscess								
SKH I	0.50	2	0.00	7	0.11	9		
SKH II	0.17	18	0.13	8	0.15	26		
Total	0.20	20	0.07	15			0.14	35

samples is presented in Table 7. The figures reported by Pal (1981) are for culture groups consisting of from one to five skeletal series; consequently these caries rates are composite figures. The caries prevalence at SKH is 4.4%, the lowest caries rate reported by Lukacs (1976, 1981) for four Iron Age skeletal series. If caries rates for the four sites studied by Lukacs are averaged, a mean caries rate of about 6.0% (N = 1,705) is obtained for Iron Age

TABLE 4. Dental Caries Prevalence at Sarai Khola: By Cemetery and Tooth Class (Tooth Count)

Cemetery	Carious teeth (N)	Total teeth (N)	Unerupted teeth (N)	Possibly carious (N)	Caries rate (%)
SKH I	7	177	27	150	4.67
SKH II	29	671	6	665	4.36
Total	36	848	33	815	4.42

	Maxilla			Mandible		
		Carious			Carious	
Tooth class	Total N	N	%	Total N	N	%
Incisor	80	0	0.0	103	0	0.0
Canine	45	0	0.0	57	0	0.0
Premolar	92	6	6.52	125	1	0.80
Molar	131	5	3.82	182	24	13.19
Total	348	11	3.16	467	25	5.35

TABLE 5. Prevalence of Dental Diseases at Sarai Khola: By Tooth Class (Based on Tooth Count)

Tooth class	Enamel hypoplasia %	Enamel hypoplasia N	Caries (%)	Calculus (%)	AMTL (%)	Alveolar resorption (%)	Periapical abscess (%)	N
Incisor	10.6	199	0.0	19.7	5.5	0.0	0.5	183
Canine	18.7	107	0.0	11.8	1.0	1.0	0.0	102
Premolar	0.9	219	2.3	12.4	1.8	2.8	0.5	217
Molar	2.5	323	12.5	26.5	4.8	11.2	1.6	313
Total	6.0	848	4.4	19.4	3.6	5.2	0.9	815

South Asia. If Pal's figure of 2.5% is included, the Iron Age mean drops to 5.3% (N = 2,718). The SKH caries rate (4.4%) is almost 2% higher than that reported by Pal (1981) for megalithic populations (2.5%) in southern India; whereas the Iron Age mean value (6.0%) is about 3.5% higher.

The low caries rates (1.8%) reported for five Harappan sites (Pal, 1981) that are known to be agricultural from artifactual and botanical evidence is anomalous. The possibility exists that Harappan populations acquired immunity to dental caries due to naturally fluoridated drinking water known to be present in parts of the Punjab and Gujarat. This type of natural caries resistence was documented for early Neolithic Mehrgarh (Lukacs et al., 1985; Lukacs, 1985b), but further study of Harappan dental pathology and ecology are required to confirm this hypothesis for Indus Civilization sites.

The range of caries prevalence values reported here (2.5–7.7%) for Iron Age India are low compared with figures for prehistoric populations known archaeologically to be dependent on an agricultural base, such as American Indians from Georgia (11.6%, N = 4,189; Larsen, 1984), and the Ohio River Valley (24.8%, N = 953; Perzigian et al., 1984). The mean Iron Age caries prevalence

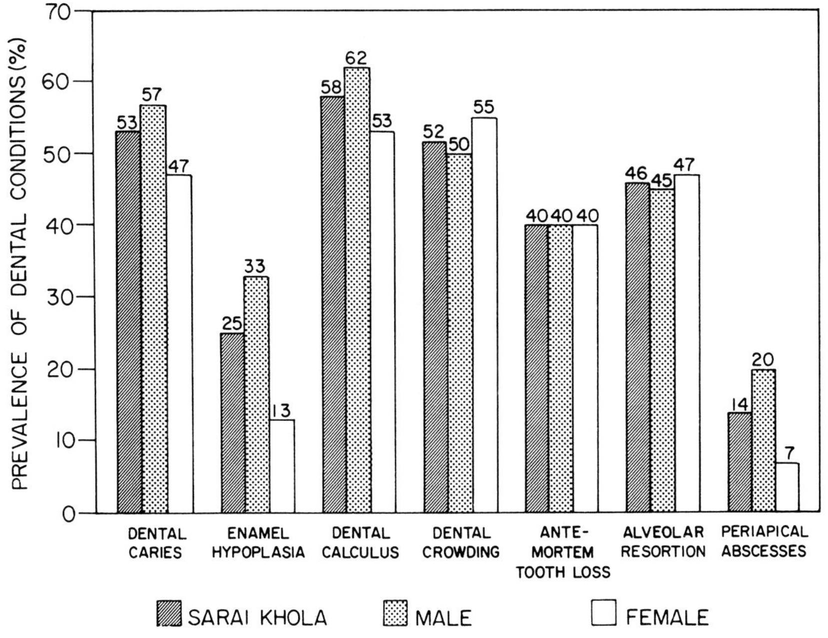

Fig. 8. Prevalence of dental lesions at Sarai Khola.

TABLE 6. Dental Pathology Profiles of Three Iron Age Sites in South Asia (Individual Count)[a]

	Tooth lesions			Jaw lesions		
Site[b]	Caries	Hypoplasia	Calculus	AMTL	Resorption	Abscess
SKH	52.8 (36)	25.0 (36)	58.3 (36)	40.0 (36)	47.2 (36)	14.3 (35)
TMG	34.9 (83)	12.7 (79)	5.1 (79)	32.0 (50)	— —	12.0 (50)
MRH	53.3 (15)	20.0 (15)	6.7 (15)	7.7 (13)	15.4 (13)	0.0 (13)

[a] Values are given as percentages; number of individuals is given in parentheses.
[b] SKH, Sarai Khola; TMG, Timargarha; MHR, Mahurjhari.

falls above the hunter-gatherer range (Table 7), but is within the caries rate ranges of agricultural and mixed economic systems (Turner, 1979).

The tooth count caries rate at SKH, while low, is not inconsistent with a mixed economy. However, when the percentage of individuals affected with caries is considered (52.8%), this value falls into the medium range, suggesting an economic base reliant to some extent on agriculture. MHR and SKH are similar in the percentage of specimens with caries to agricultural populations from Georgia (58.9%; N = 275; Larsen, 1984). The individual count method of computing caries rate suggests a medium caries prevalence and a subsistence economy that is mixed, but with an important agricultural component.

The discrepancy between caries rates determined by tooth count vs. individual count is related to the mean number of caries per person, which at Sarai Khola is low (1.0). Rose et al. (1984) consider a mean of 2.5 caries per person and higher to be indicative of maize agriculture in the Lower Mississippi River Valley; populations with a mean of less than 2.0 caries per person are considered nonagricultural. The generally higher caries rates quoted above, especially by tooth count and caries per person, may be due to the higher cariogenic properties

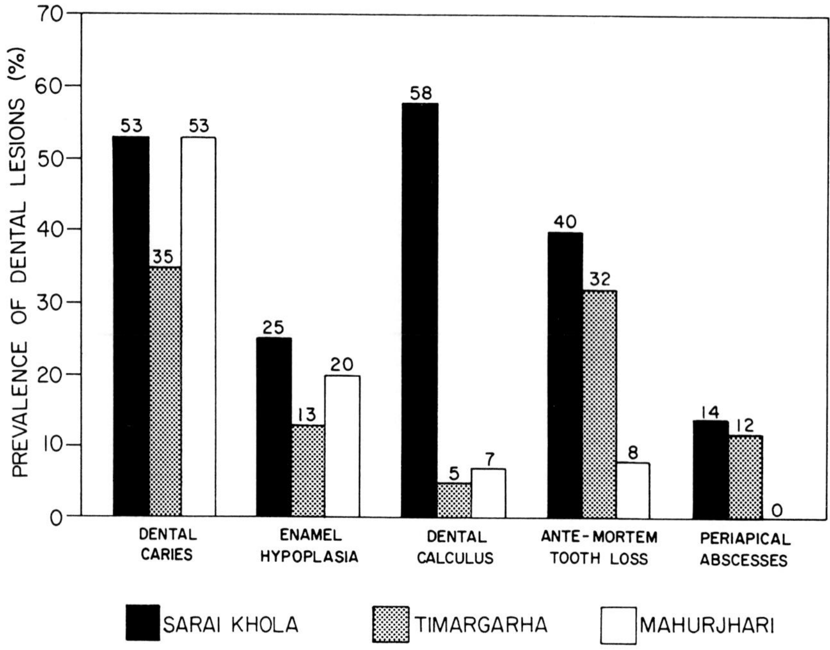

Fig. 9. Comparison of dental pathology prevalence for three South Asian Iron Age sites.

TABLE 7. **Dental Caries Prevalence in Prehistoric South Asia and in Different Subsistence Economies**

Study sample	Culture level	Caries rate %	Caries rate N	Source
Sarai Khola	Iron Age	4.4	815	This study
Timargarha	Iron Age	7.2	615	This study
Mahurjhari	Iron Age	7.7	196	Lukacs (1981)
Pomparippu	Iron Age	5.1	79	Lukacs (1976)
Megalithic (3)[a]	Iron Age	2.5	1,013	Pal (1981)
Kumhar Tekri (1)	Early Historic	2.1	431	Pal (1981)
Neo-Chalcolithic (4)	—	0.3	567	Pal (1981)
Harappan (5)	Bronze Age	1.8	1,501	Pal (1981)

Subsistence pattern	No. of groups	Mean percentage of carious teeth	Range: percentage of carious teeth
Hunting and gathering	17	1.30	0.0–5.3
Mixed economy	13	4.84	0.4–10.3
Agricultural	32	10.43	2.3–26.9

Prevalence data for subsistence groups was compiled by Lukacs (1981) from data presented in Turner (1979).

[a] Number in parentheses is the number of sites included in the study sample.

of maize vs. wheat, the latter cereal being the probable staple at Sarai Khola.

The caries rates at SKH and MHR are consistent with a subsistence pattern based on a mixed economic system in which agriculture and hunting and collecting formed important roles. The farming component of the SKH subsistence base, and possibly also the food preparation methods, produced a diet that, while not as highly cariogenic as maize, affected a large segment of the SKH population.

In *Paleopathology at the Origins of Agriculture* (Cohen and Armelagos, 1984), ten authors found that the frequency and/or severity of enamel hypoplasias increased in farming and later populations in comparison with hunters and gatherers, suggesting more frequent and/or more severe episodes of stress among farmers. Anywhere from 20 to 80% of individuals in farming series may exhibit enamel hypoplasia, and some sites (Dickson Mounds, Illinois) document its gradually increasing frequency from hunter-gatherer (45%) to transitional (60%) to intensively agricultural (80%) subsistence bases (Goodman et al., 1984). A very high rate of enamel hypoplasia was reported by Rathbun (1981) for the Iron Age site of Dinkha Tepe, Iran (77%). Against these comparative figures the prevalence of enamel hypoplasia at SKH (25%), MHR (20.0%), and TMG (12.5%) must be regarded as low, for intensively agricultural populations.

Enamel hypoplasia frequencies were not widely available for other prehistoric South Asian skeletal series (Kennedy, 1975a, 1984), but Lukacs et al. (1985) reported that 56% of the specimens from early Neolithic levels at Mehrgarh exhibit hypoplastic defects. This frequency is typical for a transitional economic system, but may reflect both natural fluorides interfering with calcium absorption and effects of the Mehrgarh diet. The higher frequency of enamel hypoplasias in SKH males than in females suggests that males were more susceptible to stresses causing growth disruption. This observation agrees with findings for Bronze Age Iran (Rathbun, 1981), Apache children (Infante and Gillespie, 1974), and medieval Swedish populations (Swarstedt, 1966), but not with American Indians from Dickson Mounds (Goodman et al., 1980).

The frequency of enamel hypoplasia at SKH indicates a population with a diverse nutritional base of good quality, characteristic of a transitional or mixed economic system. Agriculture at SKH was probably not intensive in nature and was regularly supplemented by food acquired by hunting and gathering. Much higher rates of enamel hypoplasia would be expected at all Iron Age sites in South Asia if intensive agriculture was practiced by the inhabitants of SKH, TMG, and MHR.

Prehistoric American Indians from various sites in North America (Leigh, 1925), the Central Ohio River Valley (Cassidy, 1984), and Mesoamerica (Evans, 1973) exhibited larger and/or more frequent deposits of calculus in association with sedentary farming economies. The percentage of individuals with calculus at SKH is high (58.3%, N = 36), suggesting an economy in which agriculture formed an important role and/or a diet conducive to the formation of alkaline plaque. Large differences in the prevalence of dental calculus among Iron Age skeletal samples from South Asia (TMG, 5.1%; MHR, 6.7%; SKH, 58.3%; individual count) may also suggest different levels of oral hygiene, different food preparation methods, and/or different dietary staples. Further documentation of dental calculus, including data on the size, distribution, and prevalence, are required for South Asian skeletal samples, especially those that bridge the development of agriculture.

Although dental crowding at SKH is common, the severity is mild in most cases. In the absence of corroborative evidence for chronic nutritional stress from enamel hypoplasia or stature, it is best to interpret dental crowding at SKH as part of the evolutionary reduction in jaw size. Crowding occurred in this interpretation because tooth size, which is evolutionarily more conservative than jaw size, produced relatively large teeth in small jaws (Lavelle, 1972).

Increased frequencies of periodontal disease, as indicated by the degree of alveolar resorption, were associated with the advent of intensive agriculture and/or lower quality food resources. Early documentation of this association among North American Indians by Leigh (1925) was more recently confirmed for Nubia by Martin et al. (1984) and for the Central Ohio River Valley by Cassidy (1984).

Variation in periodontal disease according to status group may reflect status-based differences in diet. Blakely (1980) showed that lower-status individuals had a higher frequency of periodontal disease than high-status individuals at Etowah, a Mississippian ceremonial site in northwestern Georgia. The status-based difference in frequency of periodontal disease reflects more maize in the diet of low-class individuals. The advent of agriculture, adoption of new foods of low nutritional value, and new food preparation methods may differentially stress age, sex, and status subgroups within a population. Much can be learned about the biological adaptation of prehistoric South Asians by applying these methods to appropriate skeletal series in the subcontinent.

At SKH the frequency of alveolar resorption is moderate, and in most instances the severity is mild. The relatively young mean age at death (36 years) in conjunction with a mixed economy could account for the moderate level of alveolar resorption at SKH.

Interpreting the moderate prevalence of AMTL at SKH (40%, N = 35) is difficult because of conflicting reports on the changing frequency of this dental pathology with the onset of agriculture. An increase in AMTL with increased dependence on farming is reported for the Levant (Smith et al., 1984) and for the Lower Illinois Valley (Cook, 1984). High frequencies of AMTL are also found among Mesolithic Europeans (Meikeljohn et al., 1984) and in Paleolithic southwest Asia (Rathbun, 1981). Anderson (1965), on the other hand, found a dramatic decrease in AMTL from preagricultural (41.6%) to agricultural (6.2%) periods at Tehuacan. In the Central Ohio River Valley, changes in AMTL were small and of less importance than the shift in causal agent from heavy attrition in preagricultural to caries in postagricultural skeletal series (Cassidy, 1984).

The conflicting evidence makes it difficult to establish the polarity of the pathology profile for AMTL. Part of the problem may be lack of control for age structure in comparing populations; therefore, a comparison of the age at which AMTL first occurs in a population may be a more reliable and more meaningful index of stress than AMTL prevalence. Cassidy (1984) noted that in Archaic hunter-gatherers, pulp exposure, apical abscessing, and AMTL primarily affected older individuals, whereas these afflictions have an earlier onset (childhood or adolescence) in farming groups.

The mean age of specimens with AMTL at SKH is 39.4 years (S.D. 10.8), but the earliest occurrence is between 16 and 20 years (SKH, 16), and 28% of individuals with AMTL are under 30 years of age. The occurrence of AMTL among adolescents and young adults is more suggestive of an agricultural component at SKH than the prevalence of AMTL among individuals.

Recent descriptions of dental pathology omit or give little attention to the incidence of periapical osteitic foci, perhaps for reasons outlined in the methodology section. Consequently, like AMTL, the polarity of the pathology profile for periapical osteitis (abscess) does not show a definite association with the transition from hunting and collecting to farming. However, a shift in the ultimate cause of periapical abscesses from heavy attrition to dental caries was reported by several investigators (Alexandersen, 1967; Cassidy, 1984).

Periapical abscesses are infrequent at SKH (0.9%, N = 815, tooth count; 14%, N = 35, individual count) and are more often due to attrition than to caries. This suggests heavy, but not severe, masticatory stress of the type associated with a mixed economy. There is no attrition-induced pulp exposure at Sarai Khola, and the youngest individual exhibiting a periapical abscess at SKH is 16–20 years, coincident with the earlier age of onset expected in societies with some degree of dependence on agriculture (Cassidy, 1984).

CONCLUSIONS

1. Variations in the perception of what constitutes dental disease and lack of standardized methods for data collection and analysis are factors that have limited the insights derived from research in comparative dental pathology.

2. The dental pathology profile of earlier human populations yields valuable clues regarding diet, food preparation, nutrition, and subsistence. The distribution of dental diseases by age, sex, and status group can aid in identifying the differential effects of nutritional stress within a population.

3. The overall dental pathology profile for Sarai Khola suggests a subsistence system that was based on a mixed economy, implying a moderate degree of dependence on farming with regular supplementation through hunting and collecting. The inhabitants of Sarai Khola and Mahurjhari had similar subsistence systems, though differences in diet and food preparation must have been present.

4. The possibility that the Sarai Khola diet was diversified and included foods with higher nutrient values than the intensive maize agriculture of North America may account for the low rate of enamel hypoplasia and moderate caries rate. Males clearly suffered childhood growth disruptions to a greater extent than females.

5. The Sarai Khola diet did not emphasize a single, soft, high-carbohydrate staple, but had a diversity of medium course foods. Moderate to heavy levels of masticatory stress were indicated by attrition-induced periapical osteitis, AMTL, and hypercementosis. An alkaline oral environment and poor dental hygiene were responsible for the high prevalence of dental calculus and contributed to the medium caries rate.

6. Changes in oral health that accompany subsistence and dietary shifts in prehistory need to be documented in greater detail for the South Asian subcontinent, especially for sites that bridge the origins of agriculture.

7. A quantitative expression of the dental pathology profile needs to be developed in order to further aid in paleodietary reconstruction and comparative studies of dental pathology.

ACKNOWLEDGMENTS

This research was completed with the helpful cooperation of Dr. Wolfram Bernhard (Anthropologisches Institut, Universitat Mainz, FRG), Mr. M.A. Halim (Department of Archaeology, National Museum, Karachi), and with the permission of the Department of Archaeology of the Government of Pakistan.

Research grants from the Alexander von Humboldt Foundation, Fulbright Commission, National Geographic Society, and National Science Foundation made this project possible. Mr. P.C. Jenkins and Mr. S. Radosevich assisted with research on the SKH I skeletons in Karachi. Mr. A. Bertinoudis and Mr. Brian E. Hemphill statistically summarized the raw dental data. Graphics were designed by Mr. Charley Kiefer.

The author is indebted to Drs. M. Y. İşcan and K. A. R. Kennedy for their cooperation in providing comments and criticism of the manuscript.

REFERENCES

Alexandersen V (1967) The pathology of the jaws and the temporomandibular joint. In D Brothwell and AT Sandison (eds): Diseases in Antiquity. Springfield, IL: Charles C Thomas, pp 551–595.

Anderson JE (1965) Human skeletons of Tehuacan. Science 148:496–497.

Anderson JE (1969) The Human Skeleton: A Manual for Archaeologists. Ottawa: National Museum of Man.

Baker J, and Brothwell D (1980) Animal Diseases in Archaeology. London: Academic Press.

Bass WM (1971) Human Osteology: A Laboratory and Field Manual of the Human Skeleton, 2nd Ed. Columbia: Missouri Archaeological Society.

Bernhard W (1967) Human skeletal remains from the cemetery of Timargarha. Ancient Pakistan 3:291–407.

Bernhard W (1969) Human skeletal remains from the prehistoric cemetery of Sarai Khola. Pakistan Archaeol 6: 100–116.

Bernhard W (1981) Ethnic and morphological affinities of the Iron Age cemetery of Sarai Khola near Taxila (Pakistan). J Mediter Anthropol Archaeol 1:180–210.

Blakely RL (1980) Sociocultural implications of pathology between the village area and Mound C skeletal material from Etowah, Georgia. In P Willey and FH Smith (eds): The Skeletal Biology of Aboriginal Populations in the Southeastern United States. Tennessee Anthropological Association Miscellaneous Paper No. 5, pp 28–38.

Brabant H (1967) Palaeostomatology. In D Brothwell and AT Sandison (eds): Diseases in Antiquity. Springfield, IL: Charles C Thomas, pp 538–550.

Brothwell DR (1963) The macroscopic dental pathology of some earlier human populations. In DR Brothwell (ed): Dental Anthropology. London: Pergamon Press, pp 271–288.

Brothwell DR (1965) Digging up Bones. London: British Museum (Natural History).

Brothwell DR (1972) Digging up Bones, 2nd Ed. London: British Museum (Natural History).

Brothwell DR (1981) Digging up Bones, 3rd Ed. Ithaca: Cornell University Press.

Cassidy CM (1984) Skeletal evidence for prehistoric subsistence adaptation in the Central Ohio River Valley. In MN Cohen and GJ Armelagos (eds): Paleopathology at the Origins of Agriculture. New York: Academic Press, pp 307–345.

Clement AJ (1963) Variations in the microstructure and biochemistry of human teeth. In DR Brothwell (ed): Dental Anthropology. Oxford: Pergamon Press, pp 245–269.

Cohen MN, and Armelagos GJ (eds) (1984) Paleopathology at the Origins of Agriculture. New York: Academic Press.

Cook DC (1984) Subsistence and health in the Lower Illinois Valley: Osteological evidence. In MN Cohen and GJ Armelagos (eds): Paleopathology at the Origins of Agriculture. New York: Academic Press, pp 235–269.

Corruccini RS, and Whitely LD (1981) Occlusal variation in a rural Kentucky community. Am J Orthod 79:250–262.

Dani AH (1966) Gandhara grave complex in West Pakistan. Asian Perspect 11:99–110.

Dani AH (1967) Timargarha and the Gandhara grave culture. Ancient Pakistan 3:1–407.

Dani AH (1980) Northwest frontier burial rites and their wider archaeological setting. In HHE Loofs-Wissowa (ed): The Diffusion of Material Culture. Asian and Pacific Archaeology Series No. 9. Manoa: University of Hawaii, pp 121–137.

DeNiro MJ (1987) Stable isotopy and archaeology. Am Sci 75(2):182–191.

Deo SB (1984) Megalithic problems of the Deccan. In B Allchin (ed): South Asian Archaeology 1981. Cambridge: Cambridge University Press, pp 221–224.

Deo SB (1985a) The Megalithic problem: A review. In VN Misra and P Bellwood (eds): Recent Advances in Indo-Pacific Prehistory. New Delhi: Oxford and IBH Publishing Co., pp 447–453.

Deo SB (1985b) The Megaliths: Their culture, ecology, economy and technology. In Recent Advances in Indian Archaeology. Proceedings of a symposium held at Deccan College, Pune, December 10–12, 1983, pp 89–99.

Enoki K, and Dahlberg AA (1958) Rotated maxillary central incisors. Orthod J Jpn 17:157–169.

Evans DT (1973) A preliminary evaluation of the Tayasal area, El Peten, Guatemala. Am Antiq 38(4):489–493.

Gilbert RI, and Mielke JH (1985) The Analysis of Prehistoric Diets. Orlando, FL: Academic Press.

Goodman AH, and Armelagos GJ (1985) Factors affecting the distribution of enamel hypoplasias within the human permanent dentition. Am J Phys Anthropol 68(4):479–493.

Goodman AH, Armelagos GJ, and Rose JC (1980) Enamel hypoplasias as indicators of stress in three prehistoric populations from Illinois. Hum Biol 52:515–528.

Goodman AH, Lallo J, Armelagos GJ, and Rose JC (1984) Health changes at Dickson Mounds, IL (A.D. 950–1300). In MN Cohen and GJ Armelagos (eds): Paleopathology at the Origins of Agriculture. New York: Academic Press, pp 271–305.

Grine FE (1981) Trophic differences between "gracile" and "robust" Australopithecines: A scanning electron microscope analysis of occlusal events. S Afr J Sci 77:203–230.

Hadjimarkos DM, and Bornhorst CW (1962) Fluoride- and selenium-levels in contemporary and ancient Greek teeth in relation to dental caries. Nature 193:177–178.

Halim MA (1968) Preliminary report on the excavations at Sarai Khola. Pakistan Archaeol 5:28–40.

Halim MA (1970–71) Excavations at Sarai Khola, Part I. Pakistan Archaeol 7:23–89.

Halim MA (1972) Excavations at Sarai Khola, Part II. Pakistan Archaeol 8:3–112.

Hart GD (1983) Disease in Ancient Man. Toronto: Clarke Irwin.

Haviland WA (1967) Stature at Tikal, Guatemala: Implications for ancient Maya demography and social organization. Am Antiq 32(5):316–325.

Hillson SW (1979) Diet and dental disease. World Archaeol 11(2):147–162.

Hillson SW (1986) Teeth. Cambridge: Cambridge University Press.

Huss-Ashmore R, Goodman AH, and Armelagos GJ (1982) Nutritional inference from paleopathology. In MB Schiffer (ed): Advances in Archaeological Method and Theory, Vol. 5. New York: Academic Press, pp 395–474.

Infante P, and Gillespie GM (1974) Enamel hypoplasia in Apache Indian children. Ecol Food Nutr 2:155–156.

Janssens PA (1970) Paleopathology. London: John Baker.

Kaul SS, and Corruccini RS (1984) The epidemiological transition in dental occlusion in a North Indian population. In JR Lukacs (ed): People of South Asia. New York: Plenum Press, pp 201–216.

Kennedy KAR (1975a) Biological adaptations of prehistoric South Asian populations to different and changing ecological settings. In E Watts, FE Johnston, and GW Lasker (eds): Biosocial Interrelations in Population Adaptation. The Hague: Mouton, pp 65–90.

Kennedy KAR (1975b) The Physical Anthropology of the Megalith-builders of South India and Sri Lanka. Canberra: Australian National Museum.

Kennedy KAR (1984) Growth, nutrition and pathology in changing paleodemographic settings in South Asia. In MN Cohen and GJ Armelagos (eds): Paleopathology at the Origins of Agriculture. New York: Academic Press, pp 169–192.

King DL (1983) The etiology of malocclusion. In RJ Jorgenson (ed): Dentition: Genetic Effects. New York: Alan R. Liss, pp 83–94.

Krogman WM, and İşcan MY (1986) The Human Skeleton in Forensic Medicine. Springfield, IL: Charles C Thomas.

Larsen CS (1983) Behavioural implications of temporal change in cariogenesis. J Archaeol Sci 10:1–8.

Larsen CS (1984) Health and disease in prehistoric Georgia: The transition to agriculture. In MN Cohen and GJ Armelagos (eds): Paleopathology at the Origins of Agriculture. New York: Academic Press, pp 367–392.

Lavelle CLB (1972) A comparison between the mandibles of Romano-British and nineteenth century periods. Am J Phys Anthropol 36(2):213–220.

Leigh RW (1925) Dental pathology of Indian tribes of varied environments and food conditions. Am J Phys Anthropol 8(2):179–199.

Leverett DH (1982) Fluorides and the changing prevalence of dental caries. Science 217:26–30.

Lukacs JR (1976) Dental anthropology and the biological affinities of an Iron Age population from Pomparippu, Sri Lanka. In KAR Kennedy and GL Possehl (eds): Ecological Backgrounds of South Asian Prehistory. Occasional Paper No. 4. Ithaca: Cornell University, South Asia Program, pp 197–215.

Lukacs JR (1981) Dental pathology and nutritional patterns of South Asian megalith-builders: The evidence from Iron Age Mahurjhari. Proc Am Philos Soc 125:220–237.

Lukacs JR (1983) Dental anthropology and the origins of two Iron Age populations from northern Pakistan. Homo 34:1–15.

Lukacs JR (1985a) Dental anthropology of human skeletal remains from Iron Age Mahurjhari. In SB Deo (ed): Excavations at Mahurjhari. Pune: Deccan College Press (in press).

Lukacs JR (1985b) Dental pathology and tooth size at early Neolithic Mehrgarh: An anthropological perspective. In M Taddei (ed): South Asian Archaeology 1983. Naples: Instituto Universitario Orientale, pp 121–150.

Lukacs JR, Retief DH, and Jarrige JF (1985) Dental disease in prehistoric Baluchistan. Natl Geogr Res 1(2):184–197.

Mandel ID (1979) Dental caries. Am Sci 67:680–688.

Martin DL, Armelagos GJ, Goodman AH, and Van Gerven DP (1984) The effects of socioeconomic change in prehistoric Africa: Sudanese Nubia as a case study. In MN Cohen and GJ Armelagos (eds): Paleopathology at the Origins of Agriculture. New York: Academic Press, pp 193–214.

Meikeljohn C, Schentag C, Venema A, and Key P (1984) Socioeconomic change and patterns of pathology and variation in the Mesolithic and Neolithic of western Europe: Some suggestions. In MN Cohen and GJ Armelagos (eds): Paleopathology at the Origins of Agriculture. New York: Academic Press, pp 75–100.

Metress JF, and Conway T (1975) Standardized system for recording dental caries in prehistoric skeletons. J Dent Res 54(4):908.

Molnar S, and Molnar I (1985) Observations of dental diseases among the prehistoric populations of Hungary. Am J Phys Anthropol 67(1):51–63.

Molnar S, and Ward SC (1975) Mineral metabolism and microstructural defects in primate teeth. Am J Phys Anthropol 43(1):3–18.

Moore WJ, and Corbett ME (1983) Dental and alveolar infection. In GD Hart (ed): Disease in Ancient Man. Toronto: Clarke Irwin, pp 139–155.

National Research Council Subcommittee on Selenium, Committee on Animal Nutrition, Board on Agriculture (1983) Selenium in Nutrition, Rev. Ed. Washington, DC: National Academy Press.

Oppenheimer A (1964) Tool use and crowded teeth in Australopithecines. Curr Anthropol 5(5):419–421.

Ortner DJ, and Putschar WGJ (1981) Identification of pathological conditions in human skeletal remains. Smithsonian Contrib Anthropol 28.

Pal A (1981) Dental health in ancient India. J Indian Anthropol Soc 16:171–177.

Pedersen PO (1949) The East Greenland Eskimo dentition, numerical variations and anatomy. Med Gronland 142:1–244.

Perzigian AJ, Tench PA, and Braun DJ (1984) Prehistoric health in the Ohio River Valley. In MN Cohen and GJ Armelagos (eds): Paleopathology at the Origins of Agriculture. New York: Academic Press, pp 347–366.

Pindborg JJ (1970) Pathology of the Dental Hard Tissues. Copenhagen: Munksgaard.

Powell ML (1985) The analysis of dental wear and caries for dietary reconstruction. In RI Gilbert and JH Mielke (eds): The Analysis of Prehistoric Diets. Orlando, FL: Academic Press, pp 307–338.

Rathbun TA (1981) Harris lines and dentition as indirect evidence of nutritional states in early Iron Age Iran. Am J Phys Anthropol 54(3):266.

Rose JC (1977) Defective enamel histology of prehistoric teeth from Illinois. Am J Phys Anthropol 46:439–446.

Rose JC, Burnett BA, Nassaney MS, and Blaeuer NW (1984) Paleopathology and the origins of maize agriculture in the Lower Mississippi Valley and Caddoan culture areas. In MN Cohen and GJ Armelagos (eds): Paleopathology at the Origins of Agriculture. New York: Academic Press, pp 393–424.

Rose JC, Condon KW, and Goodman AH (1985) Diet and dentition: Developmental disturbances. In RI Gilbert and JH Mielke (eds): Analysis and Prehistoric Diets. Orlando, FL: Academic Press, pp 281–305.

St. Hoyme LE, and Koritzer RT (1976) Ecology of dental disease. Am J Phys Anthropol 45:673–686.

Schoeninger M (1979) Diet and status of Chalcatzingo: Some empirical and technical aspects of strontium analysis. Am J Phys Anthropol 51:295–310.

Scott JH, and Symons NBB (1982) Introduction to Dental Anatomy, 9th Ed. Baltimore: Williams and Wilkins.

Shapiro SD, and Farrington FH (1983) A potpourri of syndromes with anomalies of the dentition. In RJ Jorgensen (ed): Dentition: Genetic Effects. New York: Alan R. Liss, pp 129–140.

Shipman P, Walker A, and Bichell D (1985) The Human Skeleton. Cambridge, MA: Harvard University Press.

Sillen A, and Kavanagh M (1982) Strontium and paleodietary research: A review. Yrbk Phys Anthropol 25:67–90.

Smith BH (1984) Patterns of molar wear in hunter-gatherers and agriculturalists. Am J Phys Anthropol 63(1):39–56.

Smith P, Bar-Yosef O, and Sillen A (1984) Archaeological and skeletal evidence for dietary change during the late Pleistocene/early Holocene in the Levant. In MN Cohen and GJ Armelagos (eds): Paleopathology at the Origins of Agriculture. New York: Academic Press, pp 101–136.

Sognnaes RF (1956) Histologic evidence of developmental lesions in teeth originating from Paleolithic, prehistoric and ancient man. Am J Pathol 32:547–577.

Steadman LT, Brudevold F, Smith FA, Gardiner DE, and Little MF (1959) Trace elements in ancient Indian teeth. J Dent Res 38:285–292.

Steinbock RT (1976) Paleopathological Diagnosis and Interpretation: Bone Diseases in Ancient Human Populations. Springfield, IL: Charles C Thomas.

Swarstedt T (1966) Odontological Aspects of a Medieval Population in the Province of Jamtland/MidSweden. Stockholm: Tiden-Barnagen Tryckerien.

Thoma KH, and Goldman HM (1960) Oral Pathology. St. Louis: C.V. Mosby.

Turner CG II (1978) Dental caries and early Ecuadorian agriculture. Am Antiq 43:694–697.

Turner CG II (1979) Dental anthropological indications of agriculture among the Jomon people of central Japan. Am J Phys Anthropol 51:619–636.

Ubelaker DH (1978) Human Skeletal Remains: Excavation, Analysis, Interpretation. Chicago: Aldine.

Walker AC (1981) Dietary hypotheses and human evolution. Philos Trans R Soc Lond [Biol] 292(1057):57–63.

Wells C (1964) Bones, Bodies and Disease. New York: Praeger.

Wells C (1967) Pseudopathology. In D Brothwell and AT Sandison (eds): Diseases in Antiquity. Springfield, IL: Charles C Thomas, pp 5–19.

Wing ES, and Brown AB (1979) Paleonutrition: Method and Theory in Prehistoric Foodways. New York: Academic Press.

Zimmerman MR, and Kelley MA (1982) Atlas of Paleopathology. New York: Praeger.

Zivanovic S (1982) Ancient Diseases. New York: Pica Press.

Reconstruction of Life From the Skeleton
 pages 287–302

Chapter 15

Osteobiography: A Maya Example

Frank P. Saul and Julie Mather Saul
Department of Anatomy, Medical College of Ohio, Toledo, Ohio 43699

THE "OSTEOBIOGRAPHIC" APPROACH TO STUDYING SKELETAL REMAINS

For us, reconstruction of life from the skeleton has its roots in the late Larry Angel's intensive studies of often fragmentary ancient Greek skeletons. Angel, in turn, had been inspired by his (and F.P.S.'s) teacher E.A. Hooton's monumental study of better-preserved material from the Pecos Pueblo (Hooton, 1930).

Based on our own experiences with the usually fragmentary remains of the Maya (sometimes referred to as the "Greeks of the New World"), we suspect that it is highly likely that poor preservation played an important role in Angel's choosing to emphasize a functional interpretation (both individual and populational). This was a welcome departure from merely publishing lists of measurements as appendices to archaeological reports, measurements that are virtually meaningless if uninterpreted and often unobtainable from fragmented and incomplete remains ("I have examined the skeletal remains of about eighty males and fifty females, represented by at least one bone, from all periods from Neolithic through Byzantine . . . only fifteen skeletons are fully measurable" [Angel, 1946:69]).

Fortunately (serendipitously?), the mind that confronted these scraps was not only well trained in physical anthropology but had also absorbed classical culture in his youth and had then taught gross anatomy to medical students (there were only a few full-time jobs in physical anthropology in those days), as is apparent in his analysis of Greek "posture" (Angel, 1946: 77–78).

> Greek countryside is not only steeply mountainous with almost no gently sloping roads, but slippery talus covers most of the slopes traversed on a foot journey. This demands a springy and flexible gait with knees bent like those of a skier especially in descending slopes. The three indispensable elements in this gait are flexible balance with sidesway at waist and hips, well-bent knees to lower and easily shift the centre of gravity, and easily flexed, strong feet to adapt to sliding irregularities of surface. This is an efficient rather than slouching posture, is normal among modern Greek shepherds and farmers, and of course is never used on level ground.

Each of the "three indispensable elements" is then analyzed in terms of specific muscles and associated attachments and columns as found in Greek skeletons and then related briefly to late sixth or early fifth century vase paintings and sculpture (Angel adding with his typical honesty that he cannot be certain that his interpretation of skeletal detail may have been subconsciously influenced by his cultural knowledge). Diet, disease, and seemingly anything else that can be discovered in the bones or the cultural record are factored in as Angel seeks to understand the interaction of heredity and environment in Greek history.

It is this truly ecologic or total interaction approach that we have sought to follow in our work with ancient Maya remains.

We have been further influenced by the late Calvin Wells, the English physician who so effectively applied his broad clinical experience to the study of ancient British skeletons as in this selection from his analysis of the Iona remains:

> Two general comments may be made about these Iona fractures. Firstly, they are all ones which normally occur after accidental injuries, not deliberate aggression. Fractures of truculence are wholly absent here. There are no cracked skulls from brandished clubs, no broken noses or jaws from a vicious fist and no parry fractures of the forearm from warding off the blow of a cudgel. There is not even a snapped rib which might have resulted from an aggressive elbow. Secondly, it is worth noting that, although almost all these breaks have healed well with much less deformity than is often found, in no case does it appear possible to give any credit to surgeon or leech. Unaided nature has healed these fractures—despite any palliatives, splinting or other attention they may have received. (Wells, 1981:90)

It will always be difficult to match the knowledge (and also writing skills) of these men, but we have attempted to follow both Larry Angel's broad approach with regard to relating skeletal change to ecology and culture history and Calvin Wells's more specific emphasis on relating observed bone pathology to how the individual and group actually functioned in life.

In 1961, F.P.S. coined the terms "osteobiography" (life history as recorded in bone, from the Greek *osteon* = bone, Greek *bios* = life, mode of life, Greek *graphia* from *graphein* = to write), and "osteobiographic analysis" to further emphasize that skeletons record the life history of their occupants in various ways and that we should be extracting these life histories from their bones instead of making lists of often uninterpreted measurements.

What follows is a specific example of how we applied the work of Angel, Wells, and others within an osteobiographic context to reconstruct the way of life of the ancient Maya of Mexico and Central America. The chapter is organized in terms of "Who was there?," "Where did they come from?" (originally and over time), "What happened to them?," and "What can be said about their way of life?" (see Table 1).

INTRODUCTION TO THE MAYA

The Maya Empire of Mexico and Central America was one of the major civilizations of the Western Hemisphere (see Adams, 1977; Stuart and Stuart, 1977; Willey, 1966). While building great ceremonial centers with temple pyramids, they also produced exquisite works of art and developed a very accurate calendar with the aid of their independent invention of the mathematical concept of zero.

The decline of their civilization occurred by about A.D. 900–1000, well before the arrival of the Europeans who were responsible for the destruction of the Aztec and Inca civilizations in Mexico and Peru, respectively. Many explanations have been offered for this pre-Columbian collapse, ranging from disease and crop failure on through revolt and invasion (Culbert, 1973; Sabloff and Willey, 1967). Primarily cultural or ecological data have been used to support these explanations inasmuch as pertinent data from Maya skeletons were mostly unavailable because of the poor preservation and extremely fragmentary nature of the remains. In addition, the lack of information on ancient skeletal remains has resulted in the poor health of the modern-day Maya being contrasted with the presumed good health of the ancient Maya (PAHO 1968:166).

Since 1962 we have attempted to compensate for this gap in our knowledge of the ancient Maya by studying the skeletal remains recovered from archaeological sites in Guatemala (Altar de Sacrificios, Rio Azul, Seibal), Mexico (Tancah, Cozumel, Chichen Itza), and Belize (Cuello, Lubaantun, Nohmul). In addition, we have surveyed the remains recovered from many other sites in the Maya area (see Hammond et al., 1975, 1979; Saul, 1972a,b, 1973, 1975a,b, 1977, 1982; and Hammond, 1974; and Saul and Saul, 1984a,b, 1985).

The Maya people themselves did not disappear, but rather abandoned their ceremonial centers and dispersed to villages. Thus they were still available for exposure to European diseases as part of the "Columbian Exchange," (Crosby, 1972). Much cultural continuity, as well as an apparent genetic continuity, can be seen to this day in the Maya area, making the Maya ideal subjects for our studies of the history and ecology of certain diseases.

WHO WAS THERE?

Infectious Disease or Sacrifice?

In its most basic sense, "who was there?" can be answered in terms of sex and age. Sometimes this information, along with "how many?" and combined with historical and cultural information, is all that is needed to support (or negate) a hypothesis. For example, such demographic data proved useful in interpreting a mass burial, potentially associated with a smallpox epidemic known to have occurred in 1524 on the island of Cozumel (Sabloff, 1980; Sabloff and Rathje, 1975). This stone-lined pit proved to contain the commingled skeletal remains of at least 67 individuals (based on nonduplication of left femora or thigh bones). The suspected postcontact time frame was confirmed by the presence of Spanish beads. Size and degree of robusticity of the mature remains indicate that 24 were probably male and 11 were probably female, while three were of uncertain sex. The immature remains include only one infant (differential preservation?), nine young children, 18 older children or early adolescents, and one late adolescent (Saul and Saul, 1985).

Aside from the apparent lack of infant remains, this distribution is consistent with what is known of the effects of infectious disease on a "virgin soil population" that has not had an opportunity to develop immunity through prior exposure. Not only do the young and the old succumb, but also those in the prime of life—and all in great numbers (Cockburn, 1963).

Although most infectious diseases usually kill before leaving a record in the skeleton, their tracks can sometimes be seen in the sex and age distribution of their victims, as well as total numbers.

It is known that the Spanish brought smallpox, measles, and typhus to the New World, thus conquering native Amerindians through disease as well as warfare (Stewart, 1973). This mass burial would appear to be further evidence of the power of this "secret weapon."

"Inhabitants" of the Sacred Well

The importance of basic age and sex determination is demonstrated again in a study of the "inhabitants" of the Sacred Well of Sacrifice at Chichen Itza. For years, tour guides have been regaling visitors with lurid tales of "virgin maidens" having been hurled into the Sacred Well as offerings to the gods. Who was (actually) there?

In 1940 the late Earnest Hooton, professor of anthropology at Harvard, examined the Peabody Museum's collection of skeletal material from the legendary well and found that at least one-half of the remains were those of young children, mostly between 4 and 12 years of age. The degree of formation and eruption of deciduous and permanent dentition of the cranial remains, plus the diaphyseal length of long bones and epiphyseal union or lack thereof, are indicators of the age of immature remains. (See Johnston and Zimmer, Chapter 2, this volume, for more information on growth and age changes.)

Of the adult "inhabitants" of the well, more than half were found to be male. The pelvis is the ideal structure to examine for sex information, as the configuration of the female pelvis has evolved through generation after generation of selection for success in childbearing. In order to get that large-headed infant through the bony birth canal quickly and safely, the "horizontal" dimensions of the pelvic inlet and outlet need to be as large and open as possible, and the "vertical" dimensions between inlet and outlet as short as possible. From there, common sense dictates, for instance, that the female sacrum will be short and wide, whereas the male sacrum will be longer and more narrow, and outlet-related female subpubic arches and sciatic notches will be more open. In addition, since males are larger than females on the average (within a population), the size and robusticity-related contours of the skull and mandible, size and ruggedness of long bones (especially joints), and all

TABLE 1. Some Potential Applications of Osteobiographic Analysis

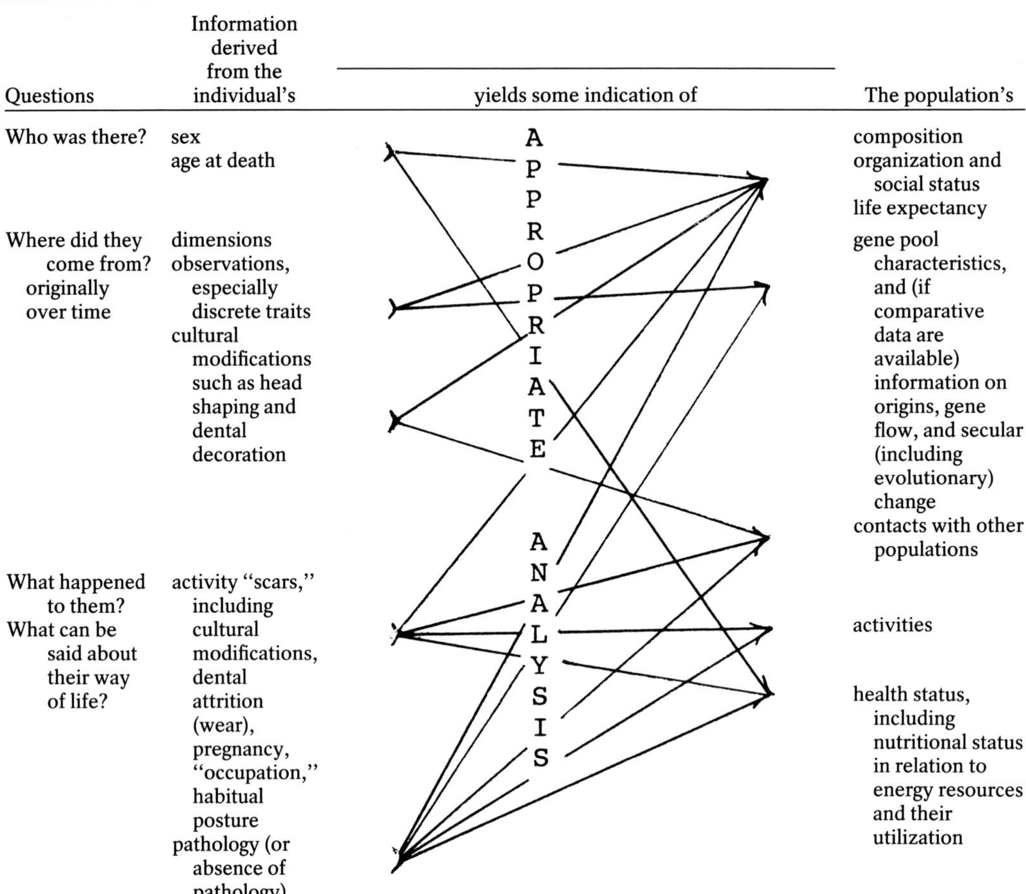

Questions	Information derived from the individual's	yields some indication of	The population's
Who was there?	sex age at death	APPROPRIATE ANALYSIS	composition organization and social status life expectancy
Where did they come from? originally over time	dimensions observations, especially discrete traits cultural modifications such as head shaping and dental decoration		gene pool characteristics, and (if comparative data are available) information on origins, gene flow, and secular (including evolutionary) change contacts with other populations
What happened to them? What can be said about their way of life?	activity "scars," including cultural modifications, dental attrition (wear), pregnancy, "occupation," habitual posture pathology (or absence of pathology)		activities health status, including nutritional status in relation to energy resources and their utilization

available indicators of sex must be evaluated before coming to a conclusion. (See St. Hoyme and İşcan, Chapter 5, this volume, for more information on sex assessment.)

Hooton further stated that "all of the individuals involved (or rather immersed) may have been virgins, but the osteologic evidence does not permit a determination of this nice point" (Hooton, 1940:273). Our examination of a later collection located in Mexico City confirms the earlier age and sex ratios. However, osteological science has advanced, allowing us to "read" the "scars" of pregnancy and parturition on the left hip bone of one of the females from the well; at least one of the females had probably borne a child. The scar of pregnancy, or preauricular sulcus, is a gouged-out area just anterior to the auricular area of the hip bone. This is formed during the later stages of pregnancy when the hormone relaxin is released to "relax" or loosen the ligaments tying the bony birth canal together in anticipation of the demands of childbirth. A combination of chemical and mechanical factors work to produce this chisled-out groove. When the head of the child is large in relation to the size of the bony birth canal, there may be a tearing of attachments at the pubic symphysis; in modern times this tearing is sometimes severe enough to require pinning. The bleeding caused by this trauma leads to dissolution of bone and the formation of pits of varying size on the dorsal surface of the pubic bones adjacent to the pubic symphysis. The above-described hip bone from the Sacred Well shows both of these scars, leaving the question of this individual's virginity in grave doubt.

So the legend of "virgin maidens" being hurled into the waters as a sacrifice to the gods has been challenged by a "reading" of the bones. About one-half of the real "occupants" of the Sacred Well were young children, more than one-quarter were adult males, and less than one-quarter were adult females (at least one of them a mother). How they got into the well and the actual cause of death are questions not yet answered.

A Maya Ball Team?

Information on age and physical condition as well as sex draws a more complete picture of a Maya ball team at Seibal, and in so doing provides some insight into the game itself.

The ancient Maya played a very rugged ball game. In Maya art one can see players in "uniform"—heavily padded and shielded from injury. We know from glyphs, art, and legends that this ritualized game often ended in the sacrifice of players. A very tough game indeed. A mass burial was found under a ball court at Seibal. Who was there? A group of young athletes in their prime?

Eleven individuals were found, and as expected from figurines, etc., all were male. Based on known age changes in the pubic symphysis, their ages were determined to range from the late teens through the later forties or early fifties (see chapters by Johnston and Zimmer and Işcan and Loth, this volume, on skeletal age markers). Scarcely "healthy" specimens of athletic young manhood, these team members suffered from the same disorders as the rest of the Maya population, manifesting skeletal lesions indicative of nutritional disorders (vitamin C deficiency, iron-deficiency anemia, "weanling disease"), treponema, arthritis, and dental problems as discussed below.

The actual composition of the group points toward a ritualistic, rather than an athletic, interpretation of the ball game.

The Ladies and the Vase

Interpretation of the Altar Vase combined with interpretation of the skeletal remains from the same tomb result in a fascinating story and also provide information on the status of women and clues to the ritual life of the Maya ruling class.

A Late Classic tomb at Altar de Sacrificios yielded a particularly fine polychrome vase. With this vase were found the skeletal remains of a young (25–29) female. Her skull showed the very pronounced tabular oblique cranial shaping typical of Late Classic males and females, as well as osteitic lesions on the frontal bone indicative of probable treponema. She was relatively short, with gracile although fairly well-muscled bones, and had borne at least one child.

She, however, was not the main occupant of the tomb. The remains in the position of honor were also those of a female. She appears to have been between the ages of 40 and 44, and her skull also was shaped in the typical tabular oblique style, although not as extreme as the younger woman. This high-status female was more robust than the younger and was taller than average (perhaps rank has its privileges where the food supply is concerned). She, too, had borne at least one child. The jaws and teeth of both women showed that they suffered from the same dental problems found in other ancient Maya: caries, periodontal degeneration, dental abscess, calculus, linear enamel hypoplasia (see below; also see Stuart-Macadam, Chapter 11, and Lukacs, Chapter 14, this volume).

The glyphs on the vase give the names of Maya rulers, and there are scenes believed to show ceremonies involving the gathering together of prominent Maya in honor of the older woman's death. Included is a scene that apparently depicts the autosacrifice by the younger woman upon this important occasion. The face of this cross-legged seated figure is painted dead white, with bulging black-rimmed eye and the sign of death painted upon her cheek. She holds a laurel-leaf flint blade in her right hand and her left is raised to her neck, from which red (blood) spurts. She wears a belt of "death eyes." The dominant symbolic references indicate death. Furthermore, a laurel-leaf blade, similar to that shown in the hand of the seated figure, was found in the tomb. All of this took place on A.D. 21 April 754, as determined from glyphs on the vase and translated from the Maya calendar to ours (Adams, 1971).

At this time, therefore, we presume that at least one Maya female held a fairly high status, and her death was an event of such magnitude that rulers from other parts of the Maya world gathered in her honor for ceremonies that included the autosacrifice of another, younger female.[1]

WHERE DID THEY COME FROM?

The dramatic nature of Maya architecture and art and other accomplishments during the Classic period, together with an apparent lack of archaeological antecedents, has led some scholars to postulate that Maya high culture was derived from the Olmecs of the Mexican Gulf Coast. A more extreme "theory" by one pseudoscholar suggests that Maya culture was brought from outer space.

Physical characteristics such as cranial shape and size and the presence or absence of variable bones and foramina have been used (in conjunction with appropriate mathematical formulas and computers) in attempts to determine genetic relationships among populations. Unfortunately, artificial shaping of Maya skulls and the fragmentary nature of Maya remains has limited the application of these techniques in the Maya area.

Fortunately, however, dental remains have sometimes survived where other portions of the skeleton have not, and teeth are considered to be ideal for genetic analyses because certain dental traits (cusp numbers and patterns) are inherited.

Our former colleague, Dr. Donald Austin, has used the frequencies of 11 of these dental traits to determine the genetic distance coefficients (DK^2) between early and late population subsamples from the nearby sites of Altar de Sacrificios and Seibal in Guatemala. The results of his analysis (Austin, personal communication) suggest that while the population of Altar may have been fairly homogeneous over time ($DK^2 = 1.47$), the later Seibal population appears to have changed more through time ($DK^2 = 3.38$). Early Altar and early Seibal show some differences ($DK^2 = 4.28$), but seem to become more similar over time (late Altar vs. late Seibal $DK^2 = 2.53$).

A Mexican colleague, J.A. Pompa y Padilla (1984) has compared the Altar dental data with similar information from the Yucatecan sites of Jaina and Chichen Itza and believes that the three populations share certain characteristics that define them as Maya and distinguish them from the people of Tlatilolco in central Mexico. Chichen Itza shows a tendency to separate itself a little from Jaina and Altar perhaps because of contact with non-Maya groups from the Caribbean and possible European influence, as it was used as a sacrificial site until the middle of the sixteenth century.

An as yet unfinished study that includes the Altar and Seibal dental remains but will emphasize the similarly early remains from Cuello, Belize, is being carried out by our associate, Richard Harrington.

Thus far, therefore, the very limited dental genetics data indicate a basic genetic continuity over time and between past Maya communities, with the possible exceptions of some late mixture at Chichen Itza and Seibal. This is in essential agreement with the cultural record as interpreted by archaeologists.

Dental data aside, the less quantifiable Maya profile (sloping forehead, high and convex bridged nose with protruding dentition and receding chin) is found again and again in ancient skulls (when those parts are present) and ancient art (paintings and sculptures) and persists in the faces of the modern Maya. The slope of the forehead may in some instances have been accentuated by intentional shaping (in ancient times) and unintentionally by use of the "tump line" or sling across the forehead for carrying burdens on the back (in both ancient and modern times).

A post-European contact burial from Tancah, Mexico, is especially interesting, because the traits that indicate and support his Maya affinity (shovel-shaped incisors, short stature, a dental enameloma, linear dental enamel hypoplasia, and moderate to marked dental attrition) are accompanied by a cranium that is not only not shaped but has a cranial index (79.0) that is low for Maya (ancient Altar range, 82.2–91.5 [Saul, 1972a: 112]; modern mean, 85.2 [Williams, 1931:105]) but similar to the ce-

[1] We have recently determined that the very fragmentary remains found in an Early Classic Maya tomb at Rio Azul, Guatemala, are those of another high-status female.

phalic index means for three modern Spanish series (77.7–79.1 [Williams, 1931:105]). In addition, he lacks the alveolar prognathism and receding chin that we have come to associate with so many ancient and modern Maya profiles. He is apparently a composite or hybrid of Maya and European physical characteristics, thus lending special significance to his burial within a Christian context.

WHAT HAPPENED TO THEM? WHAT CAN BE SAID ABOUT THEIR WAY OF LIFE?

Activities That May "Scar" or Mark the Skeleton

Activities that may "scar" or mark the skeleton range from both unintentional and intentional head shaping on through habitual working postures and even include the act of giving birth (see earlier, "Inhabitants" of the Sacred Well).

Head shaping. Head shaping among the Maya may have begun by accident as the soft, thin occipital bones of an infant were unintentionally molded by being pressed for long periods of time against the hard surface of a cradleboard or similar child carrier. The resulting head shape (lambdoid flattening?) may have seemed pleasing to the eyes of adults and attempts made to improve upon the accident through the use of shaping boards and/or bandages. Carrying burdens on the back with the aid of a sling or "tump line" across the frontal bone (forehead) may also unintentionally shape growing (and perhaps even mature) bones.

At any rate, the Maya and other populations in various parts of the Old and New Worlds have unintentionally and intentionally shaped their heads in distinctive fashion. Several head shaping (we prefer the neutral term "shaping" rather than the often-used but pejorative term "deformation") classifications have been established based on shapes and/or presumed shaping devices. We have followed Imbelloni's and Dembo's 1938 classification as presented in Comas (1960:391–395), because it seemed to be the most frequently used classification in Latin America. It consists of a "Tabular" category produced by fronto-occipital compression

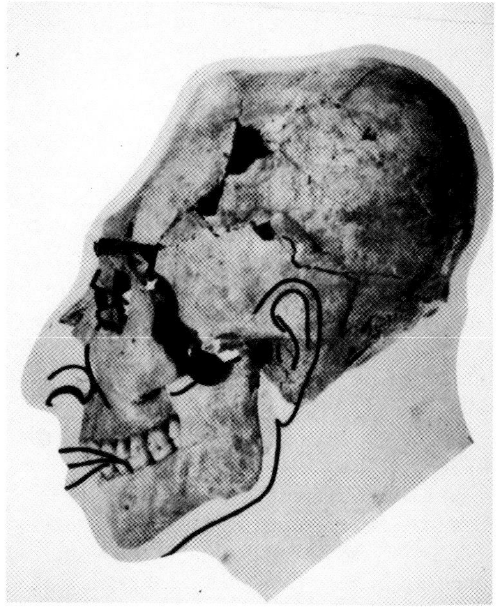

Fig. 1. Flesh reconstruction, male, mid-adult. Pronounced tabular oblique deformation. Reconstruction by F.P.S. using soft tissue thicknesses and alignments based on Krogman and İşcan (1986). Altar, ca. A.D. 775–900.

between thin boards and an "Orbicular" (sometimes called "Annular") category produced by compressing the head circumferentially with the aid of bandages or elastic bands.

Each category was further subdivided into Erect and Oblique varieties according to the inclination of the occipital area upon the Frankfort plane. In the Erect variety, pressure was confined to the upper portion of the occipital and adjacent portions of the parietalia (the lambdoid area) resulting in an essentially vertical orientation or occasionally an anterior inclination of the occipital bone. The Oblique variety was subjected to overall pressure on the occipital bone to such an extent that the entire occipital was flattened and tilted posteriorly (see Fig. 1).

Normal skulls with or without varying degrees of lambdoid flattening seemed to have been the rule during pre- and Early Classic times at Altar de Sacrificios, whereas intentional shaping was likely during later periods (although normal skulls do occur). Tabular Oblique shaping is frequently found among both males and females in Late Classic skulls that could be evaluated at Altar, whereas the Tabular Erect category seems to have been later (post-Classic) and is seen in both sexes.

Dental decoration. The Maya were not content to just shape their children's heads. They also occasionally decorated (we avoid the more often used but value-loaded term "mutilated") their teeth by filing the incisive edges of incisors (and sometimes canines) and/or drilling shallow holes for jadite or hematite inserts in the labial (lip) surfaces of maxillary teeth. Again, like head shaping, dental decoration is found in both the Old and New Worlds, but the types found in Mexico and Central America have been classified by Romero (in Stewart, 1970:50–67). In addition to those listed by Romero, we have encountered previously unreported oversize (mushroom-shaped) jadite and hematite inserts in an individual from Copan and incised decorations upon the labial surfaces of two teeth of an individual from Nohmul (Saul and Saul, 1984a,b).

Dental attrition (tooth wear). Moderate to extreme dental attrition (tooth wear) is of course not limited to the Maya. In traditional societies, fibrous foods and adhering "grit" may hasten dental attrition. (In our roles as forensic anthropologists we often use degree of tooth wear to help us distinguish between recent and ancient remains.) Grinding maize or other foods between two stones was (and is) still common among the Maya (and some other Amerindians); this process introduces additional "grit" into the diet because the stones grind each other as well as the foodstuff between them. In fact, the British physician-archaeologist Gann (1918:71) quotes the modern Maya as saying that "an old man eats two rubbing stones and six rubbers during his life."

The above somewhat self-explanatory horizontal attrition has recently been found accompanied by an unusual oblique attrition of the lingual (tongue) surface of the maxillary anterior teeth. This unique type of wear (LSAMAT or lingual surface attrition of the maxillary anterior teeth with no corresponding diagonal wear of the mandibular teeth) was first defined and described by Turner and Machado (1983) in an Archaic Brazilian site, and Irish and Turner (1987) in prehistoric Panamanians. LSAMAT was found in combination with a high incidence of caries. Turner, Irish and Machado theorize that the use of the maxillary incisors and tongue to manipulate and consume (much as we eat artichokes) a gritty, high carbohydrate cariogenic food such as manioc root might account for this unusual wear coupled with caries. We have found LSAMAT (plus caries) in 8 out of 10 of the earliest evaluable Preclassic dentitions and 18 out of 35 of the later (Cocos Chicanel) evaluable Preclassic individuals at Cuello. Found in both males and females, this wear persisted over a long period of time and does not appear to be related to a sexually limited activity—further support that a similar basic local food item may have been involved. The particular foodstuff responsible for LSAMAT was perhaps relied upon to a lesser degree by some during the Late Formative period. As many climates are not conducive to the survival of organic material in an archaeologic context, tooth wear patterns may provide the only clues.

Other activities. We have not noted articular surface extensions of the sort that indicate habitual postures (in squatting) or other joint changes that may indicate habitual usage ("atlatl" or spear thrower elbow, etc.) because of the uneven condition of the Maya remains. We were, however, startled to note that left humerus least circumference was greater in five of seven paired male humeri (+8, +5, +4, +2, and +1 mm, respectively) at Seibal as compared with only two of 14 paired male humeri (+5 and +2 mm) at Altar, leading us to *speculate* that most of these Seibal males may have used their left arms vigorously (perhaps to habitually support a substantial weight like a ceremonial ball player's shield or a ruler's chair, etc.?).

Diagnostic Problems in Paleopathology

Arriving at a diagnosis in a living patient is often difficult, even though the patient can provide the physician with clues such as symptoms as well as fluids and tissues for study and testing.

Obviously, dry bone determinations are more difficult in the absence of the additional information available from living patients. The problem is further compounded by the fact that

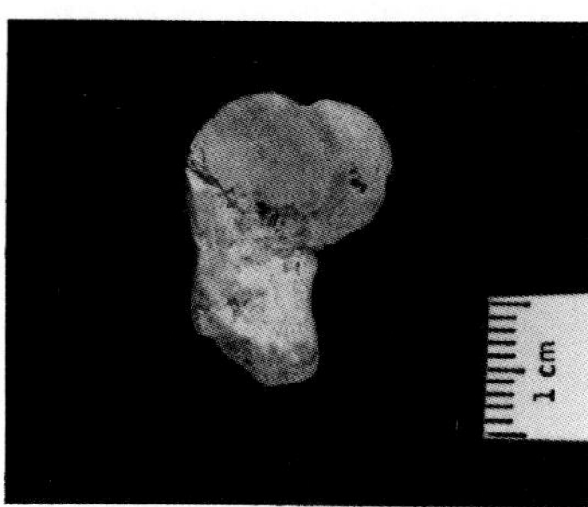

Fig. 2. Fragmentary right superior articular process of a lower lumbar vertebra. Although fragmentary, the distinctive surface that indicates a defect (spondylolysis) at the pars interarticularis has survived. Further changes suggest slippage (spondylolisthesis) has also occurred probably due to the accumulation of stress microfractures over time. Cuello, ca. 400 B.C.

not all diseases leave their mark on the skeleton, and when they do, the "mark" may be ambiguous (found in more than one disease) rather than pathognomonic or specific.

For those of us working in the Maya area (and some other areas as well), postmortem forces of nature sometimes intervene to create pseudopathology that resembles the real thing. Rodent gnawing on bone produces bone damage that is usually easily distinguished because of the distinctive patterns left by the teeth of various rodents. Insect activity and vegetation can, however, produce bone destruction that can mimic the destructive lesions of cancer and the caries sicca associated with syphilis. The thirsty vegetation of the savannas of Belize is especially noteworthy because we have found living vegetation reaching 4.7 meters below the surface to fragment bone with penetrating roots while also scouring or destroying dental enamel with the aid of the acid secreted by tiny rootlets.

On the positive side, occasionally one may encounter a disorder so distinctive that even a small fragment may yield the diagnosis. For instance, a bit of bone smaller than a small fingertip (see Fig. 2) from a mass burial at Cuello (400 B.C.) was identified as the right superior articular process of a lower lumbar vertebra from a mature individual (sex could not be determined, but all "sexable" bones in this burial appear to be male). Although fragmentary, enough bone was present to indicate that the bony bridge between the superior and inferior articular processes had "dissolved" in life (spondylolysis), resulting in the anterior slippage of the vertebral body and the upper articular processes known as spondylolisthesis. Fortunately, the low level of the slippage does not ordinarily cause nerve damage, but can be painful in some individuals. This condition was fairly common in certain groups of ancient Eskimos and is also well known among professional football players and other athletes. Although once suspected of having genetic overtones because of its preponderance in Eskimos, it is now believed to be due to accumulated stress fractures at the pars interarticularis (the place between the superior and inferior articular process) that result from frequent flexion and especially extension of the lower back of the sort involved in athletics, heavy lifting, and also in sitting in kayaks (Merbs, 1983). As no other bone fragments can be definitely linked to this individual, the lack of other "activity" markers leaves us "clueless" as to the activity responsible in this case. (See chapters by Kennedy and Merbs, this volume, for more on occupational stress and trauma.) Rare successes and frequent difficulties aside, the following examples should help demonstrate that paleopathology can provide useful information for historians of medicine and archaeologists alike.

Trauma and Invasions

Trauma is a category of potentially great interest to the Maya specialist in relation to postulations of invasions and/or civil warfare that might have contributed to the decline of the Maya. Some authorities (especially Sabloff and Willey, 1967) have noted cultural discontinuities, possibly due to invasions and/or internal unrest, that might have brought about the collapse of the classic Maya. Furthermore, stature estimates based on long bone lengths have shown that the earliest Maya males were taller than later ancient Maya males, who in turn were taller than modern Maya males (the situation is similar but more complicated for females). This is again suggestive of population intrusions.

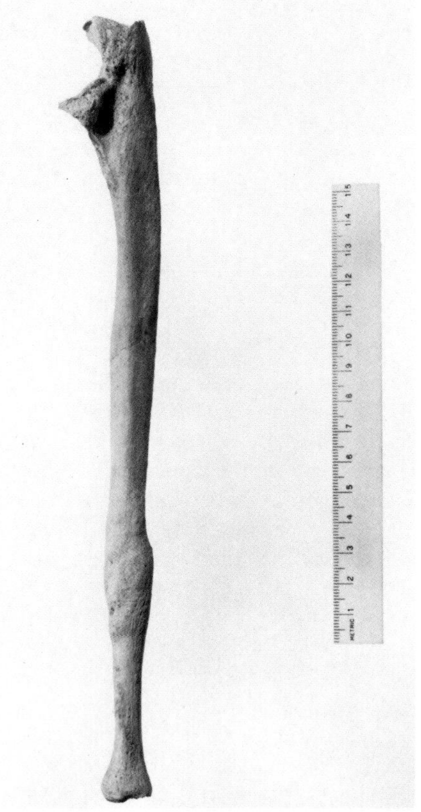

Fig. 3. Right ulna, male, old adult, showing a healed, well-aligned fracture. The associated right radius shows no sign of fracture. This type of injury is often referred to as a "parry" (or "night-stick") fracture in accordance with the idea that the forearm was injured while attempting to shield its owner from a blow. The extent of the callus surrounding the break zone indicates that the injury occurred a few months prior to his death. Additional pathologic lesions found in this individual include a fused sacroiliac joint and a vermiform ossified subperiosteal hemorrhage. Altar, ca. A.D. 450–575.

We have, therefore, searched for traces of warlike injuries in Maya bones. We have found only a few healed fractures (Fig. 3) and one well-healed hacking wound on a skull (Fig. 4) in the Mexican (Museo Nacional de Antropologia) collection from Chichen Itza (while also downgrading a previously noted "old, healed and depressed circular fracture" from the Harvard collection from Chichen Itza to a congenital dysraphism-encephalocele; Fig. 5).

However, we have found a great variety of disorders ranging from the prosaic (dental decay) on through lesions of interest to historians of medicine (possible pre-Columbian syphilis or yaws, tuberculosis, Paget's disease) as well as a series of lesions relating to malnutrition that may help explain the decline of the Maya while also providing new time depth for present-day health problems in the area.

Treponemal Disease? Osteitis or Bone Inflammation and the Questions of pre-Columbian Syphilis and/or Yaws

Inflammation is a general category involving enlargement and deformation of bone in response to various external stimuli, including both infectious disease and trauma or injury (sometimes in conjunction), as well as various internal disorders. Most authorities distinguish between periostitis, or inflammation of the periosteum or outer bone, and osteomyelitis, or involvement of the marrow and other deeper tissues. The majority of the Maya specimens seem to emphasize periostitis, and these and other osteitic lesions, both cranial and postcranial (especially those of the tibia), are very similar to those associated with present-day treponemal infections such as syphilis or yaws (see Fig. 6).

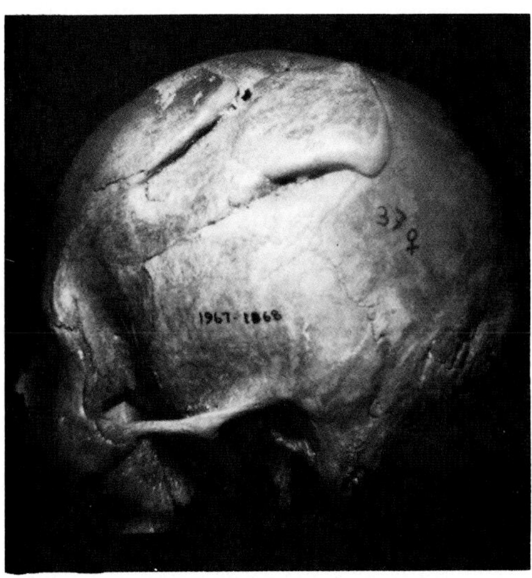

Fig. 4. Skull, left side, male (disregard female symbol in picture), mid-adult, showing a well-healed massive hacking injury that might have been produced by an obsidian-edged club. Chichen Itza, ca. A.D. 900–1200.

The pre-Columbian history of syphilis remains uncertain and controversial after centuries of discussion. Among the items of controversy is the question of the pre-Columbian presence of syphilis in the Americas, since this obviously bears on the possibility of transmitting the disease to Europe by way of Columbus' returned crews, as has been suggested by several authorities.

Various reviews touch upon the difficulties of diagnosis in old and dry bone. Hudson (1965) and Brothwell (1970) further emphasize the continuities between syphilis and yaws and other treponemal infections, together with the possibility of change over time.

Therefore, at this time it can only be said that at least several Maya who are definitely pre-Columbian in date present osteitic lesions on their crania and long bones that are very reminiscent of syphilis or yaws as seen today.

Anemia? Spongy or Porotic Hyperostosis Cranii (Alias Osteoporosis Symmetrica) and the Possibility of Anemia

The dominant characteristic involved is the hypertrophy of marrow tissue within the diploe

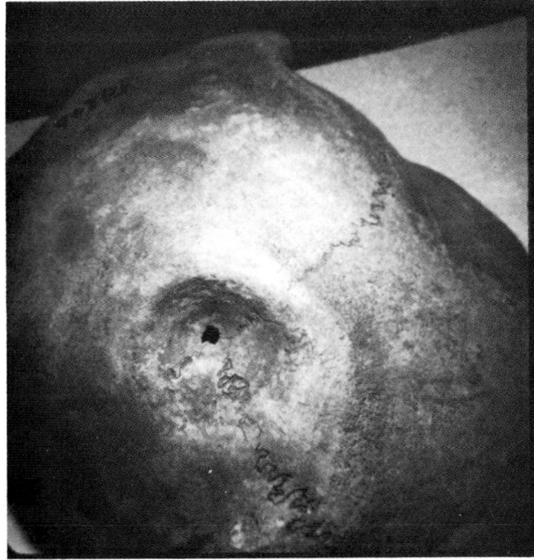

Fig. 5. Skull, bregma area, male, young adult, showing congenital dysraphism-encephalocele caused by herniation of brain tissue through what was then the anterior fontanelle. This was originally classified as an "old, healed and depressed circular lesion," caused by a "good bang . . . on . . . the head." Chichen Itza, ca. A.D. 900–1200.

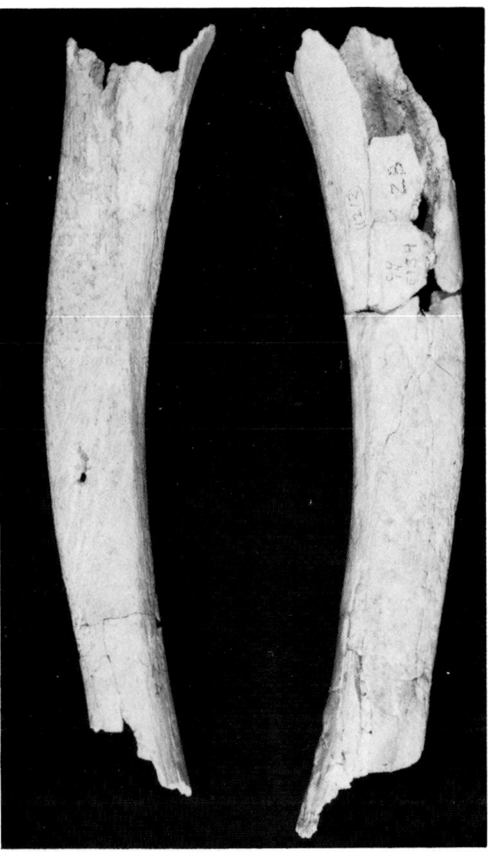

Fig. 6. Left and right tibiae of a young to mid-adult female showing osteitic swelling and curvature ("saber shin") that, together with anterior "build up" revealed by radiology, is suggestive of syphilis or yaws. This female was buried with another young to mid-adult female whose tibiae show similar swelling and curvature. Cuello, A.D. 200.

between the inner and outer tables, with a consequent thickening of the bone itself. It is in fact the reorientation of the diploe that helps produce a pressure atrophy or erosion of the outer table, thus giving the bones their characteristic coral or sieve-like appearance in advanced "active" cases.

Recently, many studies have amplified and "seconded" the relationship between hereditary anemias and spongy hyperostosis to such an extent that other possible bases for the condition tend to have been obscured or ignored. Moseley (1965) not only commented on this unfortunate attitude but provided, in addition to a long list of congenital hemolytic anemias, a brief list of disorders such as iron-deficiency anemia, cyanotic congenital heart disease, and polycythemia vera (in childhood) that can produce similar bone symptoms. The form and location of the lesions as seen among the ancient Maya are consistent with an association with anemia.

Although there is no generally accepted evidence for the presence of hereditary anemias among the ancient Maya or unmixed modern Maya, iron-deficiency and similar anemias are common in the Maya area at the present time, and their underlying causes are likely to have been present in ancient times. According to Davidson and Passmore (1969:41), "iron deficiency is by far the most common cause of anemia in every part of the world." Both males and females have increasing iron requirements during childhood, and females have increased requirements during pregnancy and lactation as well as increased loss during menses. These normal requirements and losses are further heightened in the tropics by iron absorption problems associated with chronic diarrhea (often involving parasitic infestation) and high-carbohydrate, low-protein diets, as well as increased iron loss associated with intestinal bleeding due to parasitic infestation and increased sweating. Lawson and Stewart (1967: 22) state that "the daily iron requirement for the pregnant or lactating woman in the tropics should reasonably be twice that of her temperate zone counterpart."

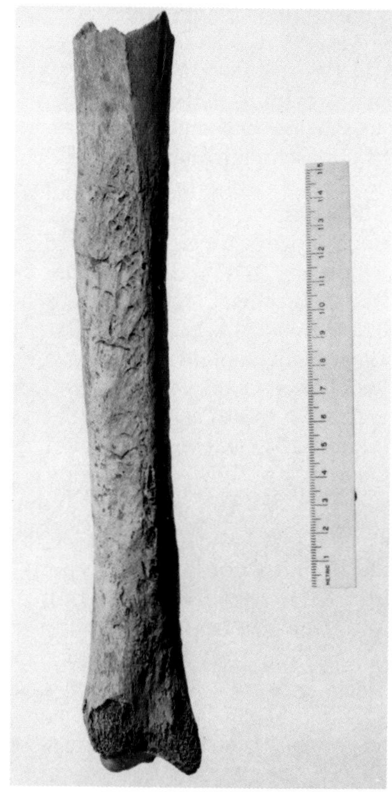

Fig. 7. Left tibia, male, age 60+ years, showing ossified remains of a massive subperiosteal hemorrhage that, together with the severe peridontal degeneration shown in his mandible, is suggestive of vitamin C deficiency or scurvy. Altar, ca. A.D. 900–950.

An anemic mother is highly likely to produce an infant with low iron stores, and the prolonged (three to four years) breast-feeding common to the Maya area not only cannot reverse the situation, but makes it worse. Upon weaning, the anemic child is put on the high-carbohydrate, low-protein, maize-dependent Maya diet. The low iron content of this diet is further diminished by the presence of stone grit—stones used to grind the maize are gradually incorporated into the ground maize until too thin to use. This stone dust acts as a chelating agent, bonding to what little iron is present and making it inaccessible to the body.

Furthermore, the soils of the Peten are iron deficient, and the ancient Maya were apparently enthusiastic ceremonial bleeders. Ascorbic acid, or vitamin C, deficiency may also be involved in terms of both retardation of iron reduction and the anemia of extreme ascorbic acid deficiency or scurvy. Protein deficiency may also be associated with anemia (see Stuart-Macadam, Chapter 11, this volume).

Scurvy? Ossified Subperiosteal Hemorrhages Together With Periodontoclasia and the Possibility of Vitamin C Deficiency

Ossified subperiosteal hemorrhages are blood flows outside of the normal channels, in this case just below the fibrous membrane surrounding bone in life, that become calcified or eventually ossified and are thus preserved after death (see Fig. 7). The initial impetus for such a flow would probably be trauma or injury of some sort (such as a blow), but the possibility of hemorrhaging is enhanced by previous soft tissue (especially capillary wall) structural weakness due, for instance, to inadequate vitamin C in the diet.

Periodontoclasia is a form of soft tissue and bone degeneration of the alveoli (tooth socket ridges) and may involve a number of factors, including mechanical irritation, infection, and tissue breakdown due to vitamin C deficiency. When periodontoclasia occurs in conjunction with ossified subperiosteal hemorrhages, then vitamin C deficiency should be suspected.

In seeking an explanation for the high frequency of periodontoclasia and the sometimes associated ossified subperiosteal hemorrhages seen in Maya skeletons, it has become apparent that a good circumstantial case can be made for vitamin C insufficiency resulting in various degrees of deficiency through to scorbutus or "scurvy." Trauma or injury leading to hemorrhaging and calculus irritation and dental decay leading to periodontal degeneration are all probably implicated, but vitamin C insufficiency resulting in blood vessel and tissue weakness is likely to have set the scene for them.

The possibility of vitamin C insufficiency, in what is often thought of as a lush tropical paradise filled with fruit, peppers, and other sources of vitamin C, seems unlikely at first, but further thought and investigation suggest otherwise; for example, the following are comments on diet in recent Yucatan and the Peten:

> After five seasons in Yucatan, Morris Steggerda is confident that the Maya Indians eat little fruit as compared with white people in the northern United States. Fresh fruits are available throughout the year, and in most yards belonging to the Indians some fruit is grown; yet they eat fruit sparingly. (Benedict and Steggerda, 1936:165)

> Years ago a high percentage of *chicleros* (= gum gatherers) used to have scurvy and many died from it. Since 1931, antiscorbutic remedies have been sent to the camps and, consequently, the disease has become rare. (Shattuck, 1938:70)

In addition, it must be remembered that food preparation and storage such as boiling and drying, respectively, can diminish or destroy the fragile vitamin C content of foods. The traditional drying of peppers for use as condiments in this area drastically reduces their vitamin C content.

Weanling Disease? Enamel Hypoplasia and Childhood Illness

Tooth crown formation proceeds gradually from what will eventually be the occlusal or chewing surface on through to the crown–root junction (the roots will form gradually in similar fashion). Enamel hypoplasia represents a developmental arrest of enamel or underlying tissue formation during the process of crown formation. Such arrests have been related to a wide range of systemic disturbances, including malnutrition and various other disease processes that occur during childhood. The location of the arrest line serves as a clue to the timing of the disturbance, since the timing of enamel formation has been studied in modern populations.

The location of most of the lesions seen in the Maya indicate that they occurred at about 3 to 4 years of age. This is the age of weaning among the Maya as recorded by Landa at the time of European contact (Tozzer, 1941). Weaning has long been considered to be a critical period from many points of view; the following is from an investigation among modern highland Maya:

> Weanling diarrhea was established by these studies as a classical example of synergistic interaction of malnutrition and infectious disease and, in developing countries, as probably the most important single factor in growth and development of children in their most formative years. (Scrimshaw et al., 1969:55)

The negative consequences of weaning might be reduced in 3- to 4-year-old ancient Maya as compared with the 25-month-old (median age of completed weaning) modern Maya cited above, but the possibility remains that there is a relationship between at least some of the ancient Maya lesions and the rigors of weaning.

Collapse of the Ancient Maya and the Roots of Modern Health Problems

Although trauma and osteitis may have been involved in the decline of the Maya, the skeletal lesions indicating an apparently high and continuing incidence of malnutrition and/or parasitic disorders and perhaps childhood infection are probably the most significant in relation to the functional ability of the ancient Maya. This group of lesions involves disorders that, while not always leading to death in childhood or, occasionally, in adulthood, do at least debilitate and impair normal function, often on a long-term basis.

Some potential implications of debilitating and chronic disease among the recent Maya were dramatically expressed by the physician-archaeologist Gann, who in speaking of the recent Maya of southern Yucatan and northern British Honduras stated:

> Indian men and women of all ages and classes, when attacked by any serious malady, are found to be lacking in vitality and stamina; they relinquish hope, and relax their grip on life very easily, seeming to hold it lightly and as not worth a fight to retain. An elderly man or woman will sometimes take to the hammock without apparent physical symptoms of disease beyond the anemia and splenitis from which nearly all suffer, and merely announce *Ile in ci mli,* "I am going to die." They refuse to eat, drink, or talk, wrap them selves in a sheet from head to foot, and finally do succumb in a very short time apparently from sheer lack of vitality and absence of desire to continue living. (Gann, 1918:36)

The present meaning of our findings, in relation to the decline of the Maya, is that skeletal lesions indicate the presence of important health problems throughout the known past as well as in modern times, and a chronic precarious health status would be likely to magnify the impact of invasions or crop failures or any similar sudden negative occurrences and thus could set the scene for the "collapse" of the Classic Maya.

In addition, this disease burden would help to explain the decrease in size of these people from ancient to modern times. A precarious health status, compounded by poor nutrition during growth and maturation, may prevent an individual from attaining maximum stature. Only those who can live and reproduce themselves can pass their genetic characteristics on to the next generations. We assume that since individuals with the genetic potential for short (small) bodies would require less food for survival than tall (big) ones, it was the shorter Maya, for the most part, whose characteristics were passed on. The more recent (and modern) Maya represent the survivors—their small size being the result of a process of successful adaptation through microevolution.

Our skeletal evidence of debilitating disease provides a new time depth for present-day health problems in Mexico and Central America. It would seem that many modern-day health problems have their roots in "ancient" civilization, not "modern" civilization as has been assumed.

CONCLUSIONS

During the preceding pages our focus has been on using information derived from the life histories of individuals to make projections onto the life history of the population (as in attempting to explain the pre-Columbian "collapse" of the Maya). We use much the same approach in our efforts to reconstruct the lives of individuals whose remains are brought to us by the police. Dealing with ancient remains prepares us for these occasional high-pressure identifications. Our Maya studies have trained us to carefully examine the smallest bit of bone, searching for clues that might help to "put the people back on their bones." (A rural friend once insightfully defined skeletons as "bones with the people scraped off of them.")

Forensic cases test us. Rarely are we questioned on our ancient Maya evaluations, but every time we make a determination of sex, age, ancestry, etc. (draw up a "life history") in a police case, we are putting our reputations on the line. Fortunately, our reputations seem to be intact (so far).

In addition, our interpretations of activity "scars" and pathology and their effects on an individual's life-style can also be confirmed or questioned. For instance, the dentition of an unidentified elderly male whose skeletonized remains were found in a cave was in such dreadful shape that we postulated that this person probably had great difficulty chewing and quite possibly was on a soft diet. Quite the contrary. Upon identification (based on the other information we supplied), we learned that his last meals had been normal, hearty ones, eaten with no signs of discomfort. From this and other forensic work we have learned to be very cautious about interpreting the functional impact that various disease processes and trauma might have on the life of an individual or population, be it ancient or modern.

On the other hand, it is sometimes appropriate to speculate on the *possible* consequences in life of conditions determined from bony remains. For example, hyperostosis frontalis interna (HFI) is frequently seen in our dissecting rooms in otherwise normal, elderly (60+) females. We were intrigued to find this internal thickening of the frontal bone in a dismembered female whose other characteristics indicated an age in the late forties to early fifties. After reviewing the literature, we postulated that she may have had either an early menopause and/or mental problems, headaches, etc. (We knew from soft tissue remains that she was also obese, which is part of an HFI syndrome). This is still too recent a case for all information to be checked, but we have learned (upon her positive identification) that she was 50, postmenopausal, and being treated for mental and physical problems.

Therefore, based on our personal experience, we strongly encourage that this sort of interaction between forensic and archaeologic work take place. One sphere of activity enhances and can learn from the other.

ACKNOWLEDGMENTS

Many people and institutions have helped us with the research reviewed in this chapter, but in particular we are grateful to A. Romano, M.T. Jaen, R.T. Steinbock, R.A. Burns, D.M. Austin, L. Vargas, L. Marquez de Gonzales, M.E. Salas Cuesta, J.A. Pompa y Padilla, and R. Harrington for biomedical guidance; G.R. Willey, R.E.W. Adams, N. Hammond, A. Miller, J.A. Sabloff, R.M. Leventhal, and W.L. Rathje for archaeological guidance; and W.G. Mather III and D. Dobson for photographic assistance. For financial support we thank the National Science Foundation, National Institutes of Health, and the National Geographic Society. Finally, we thank B.A. Carlson for preparing this manuscript.

REFERENCES

Adams REW (1971) The ceramics of Altar de Sacrificios. Papers Peabody Museum 63:1.

Adams REW (1977) Prehistoric Mesoamerica. Boston: Little, Brown.

Angel JL (1946) Skeletal change in ancient Greece. Am J Phys Anthropol 4:1:69–97.

Benedict FG, and Steggerda M (1936) The food of the present-day Maya Indians of the Yucatan. Contrib Am Archaeol 18.

Brothwell DR (1970) The real history of syphilis. Science Journal 6:27–32.

Cockburn TA (1963) The Evolution and Eradication of Infectious Diseases. Baltimore: Johns Hopkins University Press.

Comas J (1960) Manual of Physical Anthropology. Springfield, IL: Charles C Thomas.

Crosby Jr AW (1972) The Columbian Exchange: Biological and Cultural Consequences of 1492. Westport: Greenwood Press.

Culbert TP (ed) (1973) The Classic Maya Collapse. Albuquerque: University of New Mexico Press.

Davidson S, and Passmore R (1969) Human Nutrition and Dietetics. Baltimore: Williams and Wilkins.

Gann TWF (1918) The Maya Indians of southern Yucatan and northern British Honduras. Bureau Am Ethnol Bull 64.

Hammond N, Pretty K, and Saul FP (1975) A classic Maya family tomb. World Archaeol 7:1:57–78.

Hammond N, Pring D, Wilk R, Donaghey S, Saul FP, Wing ES, Miller AV, and Feldman LH (1979) The earliest lowland Maya: Definition of the Swasey Phase. Am Antiq 44: 1:92–110.

Hooton EA (1930) The Indians of Pecos Pueblo. New Haven: Yale University Press.

Hooton EA (1940) Skeletons from the Cenote of sacrifice at Chichen Itza. In C. L. Hay et al. (eds): The Maya and Their Neighbors. New York: Appleton-Century, pp 272–280.

Hudson EH (1965) Treponematosis and man's social evolution. Am Anthropol 67:885–901.

Irish JD, and Turner II CG (1987) More lingual surface attrition of the maxillary anterior teeth in American Indians: Prehistoric Panamanians. Am J Phys Anthropol 73:209–213.

Krogman WM, İşcan MY (1986) The Human Skeleton in Forensic Medicine. Springfield, IL: Charles C Thomas.

Lawson JB, and Stewart DB (1967) Obstetrics and Gynaecology in the Tropics (and Developing Countries). London: Arnold.

Merbs CF (1983) Patterns of activity-induced pathology in a Canadian Inuit population. National Museum of Man Mercury Series, Archaeological Survey of Canada Paper No. 119.

Moseley JE (1965) The paleopathological riddle of symmetrical osteoporosis. Am J Roentgenol Radium Ther 95: 135–142.

PAHO (1968) Food and nutrition of the Maya before the conquest and at the present time. In: Biomedical Challenges Presented by the American Indian. Washington DC: Pan American Health Organization, pp 114–119.

Pompa y Padilla JA (1984) Jaina y Chichen-Itza: Morfologia Dentaria Normal de Dos Muestras de la Poblacion Maya Prehispanica. Investigaciones Recientes en el Area Maya: XVII Mesa Redonda. Sociedad Mexicana de Antropologia, Sn. Cristobal de las Casas, Chiapas, Mexico, Tomo II: 481–489.

Sabloff JA, and Willey GR (1967) The collapse of Maya civilization in the southern lowlands: A consideration of history and process. Southwest J Anthropol 23:311–336.

Sabloff JA, and Rathje WL (1975) Changing pre-Columbian commercial systems. Monogr Peabody Museum 3.

Sabloff JA (1980) Archeological research on the island of Cozumel, Mexico. Natl Geogr Soc Res Rep 12:595–599.

Saul FP (1972a) The human skeletal remains from Altar de Sacrificios, Guatemala: An osteobiographic analysis. Papers Peabody Museum 63:2:1–123.

Saul FP (1972b) The Physical Anthropology of the Ancient Maya: An Appraisal. Verhandlungen des XXXVIII. Internationales Amerikanistenkongresses Stuttgart-München, 1968, Vol. 4, pp 383–394.

Saul FP (1973) Disease in the Maya area: The pre-Columbian evidence. In TP Culbert (ed): The Classic Maya Collapse. Albuquerque: University of New Mexico Press, pp 301–324.

Saul FP, and Hammond N (1974) A classic Maya tooth cache from Lubaantun, Belize. Man 9:123–127.

Saul FP (1975a) As recorded in their skeletons. In GR Willey, JA Sabloff, EZ Vogt, and FP Saul (eds): The Maya and Their Neighbors, 1974: A Symposium. Cambridge, MA: Peabody Museum of Harvard Press, pp 45–50.

Saul FP (1975b) The human remains from Lubaantun. In N Hammond (ed): Lubaantun. Cambridge, MA: Peabody Museum Monographs No. 2, Appendix 8, pp 389–410.

Saul FP (1977) The paleopathology of anemia in Mexico and Guatemala. In E. Cockburn (ed): Porotic Hyperostosis: An Enquiry. Detroit: Paleopathology Association Monograph, No. 2, pp 10–15, 18.

Saul FP (1982) The human skeletal remains from Tancah, Mexico. In AG Miller (ed): On the Edge of the Sea: Mural Painting at Tancah-Tulum. Washington, DC: Dumbarton Oaks Trustees for Harvard University, Appendix II, pp 115–128.

Saul FP, and Saul JM (1984a) Paleobiologia en la Zona Maya. Investigaciones Recientes en el Area Maya, XVII Mesa Redonda, Sociedad Mexicana de Antropologia, Tomo 1:23–42.

Saul FP, and Saul JM (1984b) La osteopatologia de los Mayas de las Tierras Bajas del Sur. In A. Lopez Austin and C. Viesca Trevino (eds): Mexico Antiguo, Tomo I of Historia General de la Medicina en Mexico. Mexico, D. F: Universidad Nacional Autonoma de Mexico, Facultad de Medicina, and the Academia Nacional de Medicina, pp 313–321.

Saul FP, and Saul JM (1985) Life history as recorded in Maya skeletons from Cozumel, Mexico. In W Swanson (ed): National Geographic Society Research Reports for 1979. Washington, DC: National Geographic Society Press, pp 583–587.

Scrimshaw NS, Behar M, Guzman MA, and Gordon JE (1969) Nutrition and infection field study in Guatemalan villages, 1959–1964. IX: An evaluation of medical, social, and public health benefits, with suggestions for future field study. Arch Environ Health 18:51–62.

Shattuck GC (1938) A medical survey of the republic of Guatemala. Carnegie Institution of Washington Publication 499.

Stewart TD (ed) (1970) Handbook of Middle American Indians, Vol. 9. Physical Anthropology. Austin: University of Texas Press, Austin.

Stewart TD (1973) The People of America. London: Weidenfeld and Nicolson.

Stuart GE, and Stuart GS (1977) The Mysterious Maya. Washington, DC: National Geographic Society.

Tozzer AM (ed) (1941) Landa's relacion de las cosas de Yucatan. Papers Peabody Museum Archaeol Ethnol 18.

Turner II CG, and Machado LMC (1983) A new dental wear pattern and evidence for high carbohydrate consumption in a Brazilian archaic skeletal population. Am J Phys Anthropol 61:125–130.

Wells C (1981) Excavations in Iona 1964–1974: Discussion of the skeletal material. Institute of Archaeology Occasional Publications No. 5, pp 85–101.

Willey GR (1966) An Introduction to American Archaeology, Vol. 1. North and Middle America. Englewood Cliffs, NJ: Prentice-Hall.

Williams GD (1931) Maya—Spanish crosses in Yucatan. Papers Peabody Museum Archaeol Ethnol 13:1.

Index